Y0-AFZ-450

# Female Infertility Therapy

# Female Infertility Therapy
# Current Practice

*Edited by*

**ZEEV SHOHAM, MD**
Professor of Obstetrics, Gynaecology and
Infertility
Department of Obstetrics and Gynaecology
Kaplan Medical Centre
affiliated to the Medical School of the Hebrew
University and Hadassah
Jerusalem, Israel

**COLIN M HOWLES, PhD, FRSM**
Ares-Serono International SA
Geneva, Switzerland

**HOWARD S JACOBS, MD, FRCP, FRCOG**
Professor of Reproductive Endocrinology
The Endocrine Unit
University College London Medical School
The Middlesex Hospital
London, UK

MARTIN DUNITZ

© Martin Dunitz Ltd 1999

First published in the United Kingdom in 1999
by Martin Dunitz Ltd, The Livery House, 7–9 Pratt Street, London
NW1 0AE

Telephone    (44)(0)171 482 2202
Fascimile     (44)(0)171 267 0159
http://www.dunitz.co.uk

A CIP record for this book is available from the British Library.

ISBN 1 85317 593 5

Distributed in the United States by:
Blackwell Science Inc.
Commerce Place, 350 Main Street
Malden, MA 02148, USA
Tel: 1–800–215–1000

Distributed in Canada by:
Login Brothers Book Company
324 Salteaux Crescent
Winnipeg, Manitoba, R3J 3T2
Canada
Tel: 204–224–4068

Distributed in Brazil by:
Ernesto Reichmann Distribuidora de Livros, Ltda
Rua Coronel Marques 335, Tatuape 03440–000
Sao Paulo,
Brazil

Composition by Wearset, Boldon, Tyne and Wear

Printed and bound in Great Britain by
Biddles Limited, Guildford and King's Lynn

# Contents

# List of Contributors

**Eli Y Adashi**
Division of Reproductive Sciences
Department of Obstetrics and Gynecology
University of Utah Health Sciences Center
546 Chipeta Way, Mailbox #20
Salt Lake City, Utah 84108, USA

**Rina Agrawal**
Cobbold Laboratories
University College London School of Medicine
The Middlesex Hospital
Mortimer Street
London W1N 8AA, UK

**Juan Balasch**
Department of Obstetrics and Gynecology
Faculty of Medicine
University of Barcelona
Casanova 143
08036 Barcelona, Spain

**Adam Balen**
Department of Obstetrics and Gynaecology
Clarendon Wing
The General Infirmary
Leeds LS2 9NS, UK

**Ami Barash**
Department of Obststrics and Gynecology
Kaplan Medical Center
Rehovot 76100, Israel

**David Barlow**
Nuffield Department of Obstetrics and
Gynaecology
University of Oxford
John Radcliffe Hospital
Oxford OX3 9DU, UK

**Marinko M Biljan**
McGill Reproductive Center
Department of Obstetrics and Gynecology
Women's Pavilion
Royal Victoria Hospital
687 Pine Avenue West
Montreal H3A 1A1, Quebec, Canada

**Maryse Bonduelle**
Centre for Medical Genetics
Dutch-Speaking Brussels Free University
Laarbeeklaan 101
1090 Brussels, Belgium

**Frank Broekmans**
Subdivision of Reproductive Medicine
Department of Obstetrics and Gynaecology
Academic Hospital Utrecht
Heidelberglaan 100
3584 CX Utrecht
The Netherlands

**Ivo Brosens**
Leuven Institute for Fertility and Embryology
Tiensevest 168
3000 Leuven, Belgium

**Barbara Cantelli**
Reproductive Endocrinology Center
Clinica Ostetrica e Ginecologica
Via Massarenti 13
40138 Bologna, Italy

**Benjamin Caspi**
Department of Obststrics and Gynecology
Kaplan Medical Center
Rehovot 76100, Israel

**Scott Chappel**
Science and Technology
Ares Advanced Technology Inc
280 Pond Street
Randolph, MA 02368, USA

**Graciela Estela Cognigni**
Reproductive Endocrinology Center
Clinica Ostetrica e Ginecologica
Via Massarenti 13
40138 Bologna, Italy

**Salim Daya**
Departments of Obstetrics and Gynaecology
*and* Clinical Epidemiology and Biostatistics
McMaster University
1200 Main Street West
Hamilton, Ontario, Canada L8N 3Z5

**Guy Delacrétaz**
Institut d'Optique Appliquée
École Polytechnique Fédérale de Lausanne
CH-1015 Lausanne, Switzerland

**Anick De Vos**
Centre for Reproductive Medicine
Dutch-Speaking Brussels Free University
Laarbeeklaan 101
1090 Brussels, Belgium

**Paul Devroey**
Centre for Reproductive Medicine
Dutch-Speaking Brussels Free University
Laarbeeklaan 101
1090 Brussels, Belgium

**Klaus Diedrich**
Department of Obstetrics and Gynecology
Medical University of Lübeck
Ratzeburger Allee 160
23538 Lübeck, Germany

**Eduardo Díez**
Servicio de Ginecología (Reproducción
Humana)
Hospital Universario La Fe
Avenida de Campanar, 21
46009 Valencia, Spain

**Patrick Engrand**
Corporate Medical Affairs Department
Ares-Serono International SA
CH-1211 Geneva, Switzerland

**Raffaella Fabbri**
Infertility and IVF Center
Reproductive Medicine Unit
Department of Obstetrics and Gynecology
Università degli Studi di Bologna
Via G Massarenti 13
I-40138 Bologna, Italy

**Bart CJM Fauser**
Department of Obstetrics and Gynecology
Division of Reproductive Medicine
Dijkzigt University Hospital
Dr Molewaterplein 40
3015 GD Rotterdam, The Netherlands

**Ricardo Felberbaum**
Department of Obstetrics and Gynecology
Medical University of Lübeck
Ratzeburger Allee 160
23538 Lübeck, Germany

**Marco Filicori**
Reproductive Endocrinology Center
Clinica Ostetrica e Ginecologica
Via Massarenti 13
40138 Bologna, Italy

**Carlo Flamigni**
Infertility and IVF Center
Reproductive Medicine Unit
Department of Obstetrics and Gynecology
Università degli Studi di Bologna
Via G Massarenti 13
I-40138 Bologna, Italy

**Stephen Franks**
Reproductive Endocrinology Group
Department of Obstetrics and Gynaecology
Imperial College School of Medicine
St Mary's Hospital
London W2 1PG, UK

**David K Gardner**
Colorado Center for Reproductive Medicine
799 East Hampden Avenue, Suite 300
Englewood, Colorado 80110, USA

**Marc Germond**
Unite de Médecine de la Reproduction
Maternité du CHUV
1011 Lausanne, Switzerland

**Giuseppe Gessa**
Reproductive Endocrinology Center
Clinica Ostetrica e Ginecologica
Via Massarenti 13
40138 Bologna, Italy

**Roger G Gosden**
Centre for Reproduction Growth and
Development
Research School of Medicine
University of Leeds
Clarendon Wing (D103)
Leeds General Infirmary
Leeds LS2 9NS, UK

**Asnat Groutz**
Department of Obststrics and Gynecology
Kaplan Medical Center
Rehovot 76100, Israel

**Lars Hamberger**
Department of Obstetrics and Gynecology
Sahlgrenska Hospital
Göteborg University
S-413 45 Göteborg, Sweden

**David L Healy**
Monash University Department of Obstetrics
and Gynaecology
Level 5, Monash Medical Centre
246 Clayton Road
Clayton
3168 Melbourne, Australia

**Roy Homburg**
Fertility Unit
Department of Obstetrics and Gynaecology
Rabin Medical Centre
Hasharon Hospital
Golda Campus
Petah Tikva 49372, Israel

**Colin M Howles**
Ares-Serono International SA
15 bis, chemin des Mines
Case Postale 54
1211 Geneva 20, Switzerland

**Jean Noel Hugues**
Service de Médecine de la Reproduction
Hôpital Jean Verdier
Avenue du 14 Juillet
93143 Bondy Cedex, France

**Babek Imani**
Department of Obstetrics and Gynecology
Division of Reproductive Medicine
Dijkzigt University Hospital
Dr Molewaterplein 40
3015 GD Rotterdam, The Netherlands

**Howard S Jacobs**
Cobbold Laboratories
University College London School of Medicine
The Middlesex Hospital
Mortimer Street
London W1N 8AA, UK

**Per Olof Janson**
Department of Obstetrics and Gynecology
Sahlgrenska Hospital
Göteborg University
S-413 45 Göteborg, Sweden

**Ruth Janssens**
Department of Obstetrics and Gynaecology
Free University Hospital
Postbus 7057
1007 MB Amsterdam, The Netherlands

**Christine Kelton**
Science and Technology
Ares Advanced Technology Inc
280 Pond Street
Randolph, MA 02368, USA

**Stephen Kennedy**
Nuffield Department of Obstetrics and
Gynaecology
University of Oxford
John Radcliffe Hospital
Oxford OX3 9DU, UK

**Philippe R Koninckx**
Department of Obstetrics and Gynaecology
University Hospital Gasthuisberg
*and* Center for Surgical Technologies
Catholic University of Leuven
B-3000 Leuven, Belgium

**Liat Lerner-Geva**
Department of Clinical Epidemiology
Chaim Sheba Medical Center
Tel-Hashomer 52621, Israel

**Ernest Loumaye**
Corporate Medical Affairs Department
Ares-Serono International SA
CH-1211 Geneva, Switzerland

**Bruno Lunenfeld**
Department of Life Sciences
Bar-Ilan University
Ramat Gan 52900, Israel

**Nicholas S Macklon**
Department of Obstetrics and Gynecology
Division of Reproductive Medicine
Dijkzigt University Hospital
Dr Molewaterplein 40
3015 GD Rotterdam, The Netherlands

**Ana Monzó**
Servicio de Ginecología (Reproducción
Humana)
Hospital Universario La Fe
Avenida de Campanar, 21
46009 Valencia, Spain

**Carlos Moreno**
Instituto Valenciano de Infertilidad
Guardia Civil 23
46020 Valencia, Spain

**Noreen Nugent**
Science and Technology
Ares Advanced Technology Inc
280 Pond Street
Randolph, MA 02368, USA

**Antonio Pellicer**
Instituto Valenciano de Infertilidad
Guardia Civil 23
46020 Valencia, Spain

**Angela Piazzi**
Corporate Medical Affairs Department
Ares-Serono International SA
CH-1211 Geneva, Switzerland

**Helen M Picton**
Centre for Reproduction Growth and
Development
Research School of Medicine
University of Leeds
Clarendon Wing (D103)
Leeds General Infirmary
Leeds LS2 9NS, UK

**Tomás Pieró**
Servicio de Ginecología (Reproducción
Humana)
Hospital Universario La Fe
Avenida de Campanar, 21
46009 Valencia, Spain

**Eleonora Porcu**
Infertility and IVF Center
Reproductive Medicine Unit
Department of Obstetrics and Gynecology
Università degli Studi di Bologna
Via G Massarenti 13
I-40138 Bologna, Italy

**Marie-Pierre Primi**
Unite de Médecine de la Reproduction
Maternité du CHUV
1011 Lausanne, Switzerland

**Luis Alberto Quintero**
Servicio de Ginecología (Reproducción
Humana)
Hospital Universario La Fe
Avenida de Campanar, 21
46009 Valencia, Spain

**Klaus Rink**
Medical Technologies Montreux
Parc scientifique
CH-1015 Lausanne, Switzerland

**Alberto Romeu**
Servicio de Ginecología (Reproducción Humana)
Hospital Universario La Fe
Avenida de Campanar, 21
46009 Valencia, Spain

**Anthony J Rutherford**
Obstetrics and Gynaecology
Leeds General Infirmary
Leeds LS2 9NS, UK

**Fedde Scheele**
Department of Obstetrics and Gynaecology
St Lucas/Andreas Hospital
Postbus 9243
1006 AE Amsterdam
The Netherlands

**Joop Schoemaker**
Department of Obstetrics and Gynaecology
Free University Hospital
Postbus 7057
1007 MB Amsterdam, The Netherlands

**William B Schoolcraft**
Colorado Center for Reproductive Medicine
799 East Hampden Avenue, Suite 300
Englewood, Colorado 80110, USA

**Alfred Senn**
Unite de Médecine de la Reproduction
Maternité du CHUV
1011 Lausanne, Switzerland

**Zeev Shoham**
Department of Obstetrics and Gynecology
Kaplan Medical Center
Rehovot 76100, Israel

**Carlos Simón**
Instituto Valenciano de Infertilidad
Guardia Civil 23
46020 Valencia, Spain

**Stephen K Smith**
Department of Obstetrics and Gynaecology
University of Cambridge
The Rosie Hospital
Robinson Way
Cambridge CB2 2SW, UK

**Catherine Staessen**
Centre for Reproductive Medicine
Dutch-Speaking Brussels Free University
Laarbeeklaan 101
1090 Brussels, Belgium

**Cristina Tabarelli**
Reproductive Endocrinology Center
Clinica Ostetrica e Ginecologica
Via Massarenti 13
40138 Bologna, Italy

**Seang Lin Tan**
Department of Obstetrics and Gynecology
McGill University
Women's Pavilion
Royal Victoria Hospital
687 Pine Avenue West
Montreal H3A 1A1, Quebec, Canada

**Karel Van Loon**
Ares-Serono International SA
15 bis, chemin des Mines
Case Postale 54
1211 Geneva 20, Switzerland

**André Van Steirteghem**
Centre for Reproductive Medicine
Dutch-Speaking Brussels Free University
Laarbeeklaan 101
1090 Brussels, Belgium

**Stefano Venturoli**
Infertility and IVF Center
Reproductive Medicine Unit
Department of Obstetrics and Gynecology
Università degli Studi di Bologna
Via G Massarenti 13
I-40138 Bologna, Italy

**Greta Verheyen**
Centre for Reproductive Medicine
Dutch-Speaking Brussels Free University
Laarbeeklaan 101
1090 Brussels, Belgium

**Ariel Weissman**
Division of Reproductive Sciences
Department of Obstetrics and Gynaecology
University of Toronto
The Toronto Hospital
6-246 Eaton Wing North
200 Elizabeth Street
Toronto, Ontario M5G 2C4, Canada

**Matts Wikland**
Fertilitetscentrum
Carlanderska sjukhemmet
Carlandersplatsen 1
S–41255 Göteborg, Sweden

**Patrick Wynn**
Centre for Reproduction Growth and
Development
Research School of Medicine
University of Leeds
Clarendon Wing (D103)
Leeds General Infirmary
Leeds LS2 9NS, UK

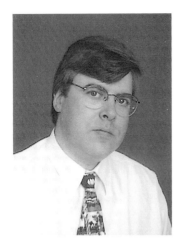

Zeev Shoham was born in Israel in 1951. He graduated at the Hadassah Medical School in Jerusalem and currently is an Associate Professor at the Department of Obstetrics and Gynecology at the Kaplan Medical Center, Rehovot, Israel. Professor Shoham teaches at the Faculty of Medicine at the Hebrew University, Jerusalem, Israel, and is well known for his academic work in the field of Reproductive Medicine.

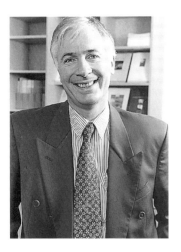

Colin Howles started working in the field of human assisted reproduction in 1984, when he joined the in vitro fertilization pioneers Professor Robert Edwards and the late Mr Patrick Steptoe at Bourn Hall Clinic, Cambridge, UK. Since leaving Bourn Hall, Dr Howles worked as Scientific Director for Serono Laboratories in the UK and then moved to the Ares-Serono Corporate Headquarters in Geneva, Switzerland, where he now has worldwide responsibilities for the group in the field of Reproductive Endocrinology.

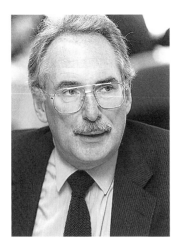

Howard Jacobs is Professor of Reproductive Endocrinology at University College London Medical School, Past Chairman and Current President of the British Fertility Society, and has been active in research, teaching and practice in the areas of Reproductive Medicine and Fertility for many years.

# Preface

The collection of papers contained in the volume cover a wide range of reproductive medicine and science. They represent the cutting-edges of our discipline and are written by acknowledged experts in the field. They complement a Serono Symposium held at the Royal College of Physicians in London on 16–17 September 1998, whose purpose was to mark the retirement of Professor Howard S Jacobs.

Professor Jacobs's career has spanned a golden age of pathophysiological research, that is, of the study of systems rather than of cells, or indeed of subcellular processes. His first experience of endocrine research began very shortly after the invention of radioimmuno-assay and he was fortunate to receive laboratory training in the department of Professor Roger Elkins, which no doubt accounts for his longstanding interest in problems of hormone measurement and their interpretation. For many years he provided clinical liaison to the UK National Quality Assessment Scheme and more recently has been involved with the National Institute of Biological Standards and Control, serving both on its Scientific Advisory Committee and its Board of Management.

After his initial research fellowship with the late Sir John Nabarro, Howard Jacobs spent two years at Harbor General Hospital, the southern campus of UCLA, learning reproductive endocrinology from Professors Bill Odell and Ron Swerdloff. Using rat models, his research at that time focused on the control of the onset of puberty, determinants of the midcycle surge of luteinizing hormone and factors that control the secretion of follicle-stimulating hormone. On his return to England, he completed his endocrine training at The Middlesex Hospital and then joined Professors Richard Beard (Obstetrics and Gynaecology) and Vivian James (Chemical Pathology) as Senior Lecturer at St Mary's Hospital Medical School.

Over the next eight years studies of the menopause, hyperprolactinaemia and hyperandrogenism were initiated. He subsequently returned to The Middlesex Hospital and, together with a number of collaborators, developed an innovative ovulation induction clinic which, for instance, saw the introduction of pulsatile gonadotrophin-releasing hormone and growth hormone treatment, the use of superactive analogues for ovulation induction and in vitro fertilization and, of course, the exploitation of ultrasound for the diagnosis of polycystic ovary syndrome and for monitoring the outcome of ovarian stimulation.

Serono Symposia, the educational division of the Ares-Serono Group, is committed to furthering the advancement of medicine within the medical, scientific, allied health professional and consumer communities. Exchange and dissemination of information relating to important clinical research are accomplished through a range of educational programs and materials, including international scientific symposia, and the publication of research results and proceedings of scientific meetings, primarily in the fields of endocrinology and reproduction, immunology, neurology and oncology. It is an honor for Serono Symposia to be involved in the publication of this volume and to coordinate the organization of the prestigious meeting to mark the retirement of Professor Howard S Jacobs.

*ZS*
*CMH*

# Part I
# Drug Regulation and Effects

# 1

# In utero exposure to gonadotrophins

Karel Van Loon

**Preclinical safety data** • **Pharmacology** • **Accidental exposure to fertility drugs during early pregnancy** • **Epidemiological data** • **Conclusion**

In general, medical treatment aims to reverse a particular disease process or relieve an incapacitating sign or symptom, whereas fertility treatment is targeted at the birth of a healthy baby. During pregnancy, there is always concern over the use of drugs. With fertility drugs, however, the situation is different in several respects. First, the drugs used are often exact copies of human hormones, which are usually produced by and circulating in the human body. Second, treatment aims to influence the process of human germ cell development itself. Third, to a large extent the safety of fertility treatment is expressed in terms of mutagenicity, teratogenicity, and the possibly deleterious effects on pregnancy and pregnancy outcome. The effects of fertility treatment on the fetus, pregnancy and pregnancy outcome may be viewed from various angles, and each approach requires a specific field of research.

One may consider the effects of ovulation induction or superovulation drug regimens on the ovum itself, as well as on the earliest development of the embryo in successful cycles. This approach requires pharmacology research to determine the drug levels present during the early embryonic stages. The effects of remaining levels of ovulation-inducing drugs on the uterine function during early pregnancy would also be studied. Toxicology studies will identify whether the drug or its metabolites have deleterious effects, looking particularly at the risk of chromosomal aberrations – including the pathology of spontaneous abortion products – and congenital malformations.

Alternatively, it is possible to look at the effects of exogenous gonadotrophins on an existing viable gestation, as in the case of accidental gonadotrophin treatment during early pregnancy. This approach aims to answer the straightforward question of the clinical reproductive safety of fertility drugs. Series of case reports of accidental exposure to gonadotrophin-releasing hormone (GnRH) agonists and exogenous gonadotrophins during early pregnancy provide the main body of evidence, through assessment of pregnancy outcomes.

Last, one may simply compare the risk of unfavourable pregnancy outcomes or birth defects after fertility treatment or assisted reproduction techniques (ART) with outcomes after natural conception. This research comprises maternal parameters as well as fertility drugs and ART procedures. The approach requires large datasets or applied observational studies, and the methods of data collection and analysis are epidemiological.

In a classic down-regulation in vitro fertilization (IVF) schedule, the patient receives a GnRH agonist, a follicle-stimulating hormone (FSH) preparation and an injection of human chorionic gonadotrophin (hCG). Several GnRH agonist molecules are on the market: most are synthetic human luteinizing hormone-releasing hormone (LHRH) analogues, such as goserelin acetate, triptorelin and leuprolide acetate. FSH and hCG are pharmacological formulations of recombinant hormone or hormone extracted from human urine. The data presented in this chapter are based on published results on GnRH agonists and Profasi (urine (u)-derived hCG, Ares-Serono, Geneva), and from the research programmes of Gonal-F (recombinant human (r-h) FSH, Ares-Serono, Geneva) and Ovidrel (r-hCG, Ares-Serono, Geneva).

## PRECLINICAL SAFETY DATA

LHRH (either human synthetic or porcine) was not found to have teratogenic effects in animals. The same was true for goserelin acetate.[1] Studies with triptorelin in rats, rabbits and monkeys did not show any mutagenic potential, but a number of preimplantation losses were observed in rats and rabbits.[2] Leuprolide acetate was found to cause fetal malformations in rabbits, but not in rats, whereas mutagenicity studies in bacterial and mammalian systems did not demonstrate evidence of mutagenic potential.[3] Further animal data suggested that leuprolide may have detrimental effects on corpus luteum function by a direct action on the ovary.[4]

The reproductive toxicology programme for Gonal-F included fertility studies in rats, teratology studies in rats and rabbits, and peri- and postnatal studies in rats. In the fertility studies the drug was administered before and during the mating period, in the teratology studies the drug was administered during gestation, and in the peri- and postnatal studies the drug was administered during late gestation and lactation. The doses by body mass used in the animal toxicology studies were far greater than those used in clinical practice: 5–320 IU/kg per day. No congenital abnormalities were observed in any of the studies. The toxicology programme concluded that Gonal-F was not found to be a teratogen, even at the highest doses (toxicology carried out by RBM Spa, Ivrea, Italy).

The mutagenic and clastogenic potentials of Gonal-F were assessed in a series of tests in vitro and in vivo. The tests basically focused on mechanisms involving induction of point mutation and chromosomal damage. No mutagenic effects were found in the Ames test and in the gene mutation test in V79 Chinese hamster lung cells. Gonal-F was also not found to have clastogenic effects either in cultured human lymphocytes or in the micronucleus test.

Ovidrel was found to be devoid of any intrinsic toxicity. Mutagenicity and clastogenicity of the drug were tested in the same way for Gonal-F, with the same conclusions (toxicology carried out by RBM Spa, Ivrea, Italy).

## PHARMACOLOGY

Pharmacodynamic studies have clearly demonstrated that r-hFSH is functionally similar to human pituitary FSH. When injected subcutaneously, the product is absorbed quickly. After repeated administration, it accumulates threefold at the steady state, which is reached after 3–4 days. Gonal-F is eliminated from the body, with a terminal half-life of less than 24 hours. During fertility treatment with r-hFSH, and particularly during superovulation, blood levels of FSH at the time of ovulation are higher than during natural cycles. By the time of early embryo development, however, particularly with IVF, exogenous FSH used for the induction of superovulation is all but eliminated from the body.

Pharmacological research with Profasi and Ovidrel led to a comparable dataset for hCG. The products were shown to be functionally similar to natural hCG, and both have a terminal half-life of about 30 hours. From a pharmacokinetic viewpoint, hCG levels all but return to pre-treatment levels within 2 weeks of the last injection.[5] This does not, of course, take into account the endogenous hCG produced by a developing fetoplacental unit. Indeed, it should be borne in mind that the levels of endogenous hCG during pregnancy are far greater than the hCG levels observed after a single injection of 5000–10 000 IU.

GnRH agonists are classically used for down-regulation of the pituitary before ovulation induction with gonadotrophins, particularly for IVF. The use of long-acting (more than 1 month) products has added to concerns over the possible deleterious effects on fetal development, because GnRH agonists are present in the blood at the time of embryo transfer.[6] As GnRH agonists comprise various molecules and formulations, both short and long acting, it is not possible to present a single set of pharmacometric figures that would apply to all.

## ACCIDENTAL EXPOSURE TO FERTILITY DRUGS DURING EARLY PREGNANCY

As well as being used for down-regulation of the pituitary before superovulation with gonadotrophins, GnRH agonists are also licensed for indications such as fibroma and endometriosis. With these two groups of indications, accidental exposure to GnRH agonists during pregnancy has become less uncommon, and the published case series have been growing over the years.[1,2,7,8] Large series of cases were presented by both Chang and Soong[7] and Elefant et al[8] Chang and Soong[7] reviewed the literature and found 69 cases of inadvertent use of GnRH agonists during early pregnancy, to which they added six from their own experience. In their series, a total of 49 babies were born. Two of these 49 babies presented congenital malformations: one had a minor degree of cleft palate and another presented bilateral talipes. Two cases of malformation out of 49 live births represents a proportion that is comparable with rates seen after spontaneous pregnancies. Elefant et al[8] presented a series of 28

pregnancies with exposure to triptorelin. Injections were given up to week 21 of amenorrhoea. Twenty-four of the 28 patients successfully delivered a baby. Of three early abortions (less than 12 weeks of amenorrhoea), no fetal pathology could be obtained. The fetal pathology of the fourth abortion was normal. In the 24 live births, one case of trisomy 13 was reported. In this case, the GnRH agonist had been administered 15 days after fertilization, and therefore the defect was unlikely to have been caused by the drug. The other 23 pregnancies were uneventful and the babies were in good health.

It is clear that the above data are not sufficient to draw a conclusion about the safe use of GnRH agonists during pregnancy. At this point in time, however, the available evidence of accidental administration of GnRH agonists during early pregnancy does not indicate any major hazards to the fetus.

Product information for all gonadotrophin preparations available on the market, whether they are urine-derived or recombinant products, clearly states that pregnancy is a contraindication for their use. Consequently, pregnancy should be excluded immediately before starting treatment. Nevertheless, infertile patients may feel that their chances of conceiving without treatment are remote, and it is possible to imagine a number of scenarios in which, regardless of warnings, a patient starts a new cycle without realizing that she is already pregnant. Once it becomes clear that there was a viable pregnancy at the time of treatment, the physician may have concerns over the possible untoward effects on the fetus and may consider therapeutic abortion. In these situations, Ares-Serono's medical information services (Geneva) may be addressed for information and guidance. Several such cases have come to our attention in this way. Follow-up information with respect to pregnancy and pregnancy outcome is, however, rare. So far, only two of these cases have been reported in the medical literature.

As early as 1985, the first case of inadvertent use of gonadotrophins for ovulation induction in a pregnant woman was reported.[9] The observation of successful ovulation induction during pregnancy confirmed previous animal experiments with regard to the absence of ovarian refractoriness to gonadotrophins during pregnancy.[10] As the ongoing pregnancy was ectopic in this case, no relevant information could be gained about pregnancy outcome. Shortly thereafter, Diamond et al[11] published a second case of successful stimulation of multiple follicular development during pregnancy. The patient had become spontaneously pregnant (unnoticed) between two ART attempts and the pregnancy was intrauterine. During the second assisted cycle, the patient received human menopausal gonadotrophin (hMG) 225 IU/day from day 12 to day 21 after fertilization, and hCG 10 000 IU on about day 22. There did not seem to be any untoward effect on the fetus or pregnancy – the pregnancy developed uneventfully and the infant was delivered healthy, at term, with a birth weight of 3021 grams.

Four years later, Lessing et al[12] reported a second case of ovarian superovulation in a patient with an undiagnosed intrauterine pregnancy. The patient in this case report had a history of two induced first-trimester abortions, complicated by severe pelvic inflammatory disease. This patient also conceived between two IVF attempts, in spite of a diagnosis of mechanical infertility. The stimulation protocol was the same as described by Diamond et al[11] – hMG 225 IU/day for 8–9 days and hCG 10 000 IU on the following day. Lessing et al[12] estimated that this treatment schedule must have corresponded to days 3–13 after fertilization of the existing pregnancy. The course of pregnancy was uneventful until week 23 of gestation, at which time the patient had severe uterine contractions and vaginal bleeding. Shortly thereafter, the patient delivered an immature fetus of 425 grams. The placenta showed clear signs of premature separation. The fetus underwent a postmortem examination, but did not reveal any pathology.

Among other indications, Profasi is licensed for threatened and habitual abortion.[13] The usual treatment schedule for this indication is 10 000 IU once, followed by 5000 IU twice weekly until week 14 of gestation. This schedule was not found to be associated with an increased risk of congenital malformations or adverse pregnancy outcomes.

## EPIDEMIOLOGICAL DATA

The early publications on untoward effects of fertility drugs on the fetus were inspired by the idea that inducing pregnancy after a long period of infertility carried a risk.[14,15] With the increasing use of ovulation-inducing treatment, doubts about the safety of fertility drugs were fuelled by case reports and short series of unfavourable outcomes, first with clomiphene citrate[16] and later with gonadotrophins and IVF,[17,18] as well as with ART in general. Concerns over the safety of the fetus in ART are basically of three different kinds. One concern has to do with early fetal development. This is expressed by case reports of all kinds on developmental congenital malformations.[19] Another concern is the possible induction of chromosomal abnormalities, because it has been suggested that factors associated with ART, such as gamete manipulation or sperm ageing, may increase the risk of chromosomal damage.[20] A third concern pertains to the fetoplacental function and the pregnancy after ovulation induction and superovulation. The latter concerns are reflected in publications regarding the risk of abortion associated with IVF and the birthweight of ART babies.

With the increasing use of ART over the last decade, the body of experience has been growing steadily, and a number of large series have been published on pregnancies and pregnancy outcomes after ART. More and more countries have set up national registries and publish data at regular intervals. With the increasing amount of evidence grew the conviction that IVF is not associated with an increased risk of birth defects.[21,22] Certain issues, such as neural tube defects, kept on surfacing in the medical literature and it took powerful datasets to settle the issue adequately. Large case–control studies[23,24] concluded that there was no increase in the risk of neural tube defects with the use of fertility drugs, and pooled analysis of large datasets[25,26] confirmed the findings of the case–control studies. Although it is important to remain vigilant, the data available to date do not indicate any increased risk of developmental defects in relation to the use of fertility drugs or the practice of IVF.

To a large extent, concern over chromosomal abnormalities followed the 'congenital malformations' discussion. Indeed, as with developmental defects, some early published data indicated an increased risk of chromosomal aberrations related to ovulation-inducing drugs.[27] These findings were not, however, reproduced by others, who found no increased risk of chromosomal defects after IVF drug regimens.[28] The total prevalence of birth defects after ART does not seem to be increased when compared with birth defects after spontaneous conception. Where data are provided separately, the same conclusions may be drawn for chromosomal anomalies.

More recently, new concern has arisen after the observation of high numbers of sex chromosomal abnormalities after intracytoplasmic sperm injection (ICSI).[29] ICSI is used predominantly for the treatment of male subfertility, and was introduced relatively recently. Therefore, the number of outcomes are still limited and do not allow powerful analysis. The concerns with ICSI are of two kinds: one is that spermatozoa, which would otherwise fail to fertilize because they are genetically deficient, are 'forced' into the ovum, and may lead to embryo defects;[30] the other is that, by micromanipulation (mechanical aspects, exposure to media, etc), the zygote or embryo is somehow damaged, which may lead to malformation.[31] A closer look at the original data series showed that the unfavourable findings in ICSI offspring may be explained by observation bias,[32] and a further series did not indicate an increased risk.[33] The public debate has widened and includes delicate aspects, such as systematic genetic testing and other ethical questions,[34] genetic counselling of couples[35] and preimplantation screening.[36] The European Society of Human Reproduction and Embryology has set up a worldwide database of ICSI procedures and outcomes, and publishes regular reports.

So far, although the numbers are still relatively small, the findings are reassuring.[37]

Since the use of ovulation inducing drugs became widespread, and later with IVF, treatment outcomes have been scrutinized, and the early reports showed an increased spontaneous abortion rate. Published figures range from 15% to 30% of pregnancies, which is clearly higher than the generally accepted range of 10–15% in pregnancies after spontaneous conception. Several explanations have been suggested for these apparent differences, but none seems to be adequate.[38] Observation bias certainly accounts for a fraction (if not all) of the observed difference. Indeed, IVF pregnancies are usually confirmed very early, and fetal wastage at the very early stages will be recognized promptly, whereas in natural cycles a pregnancy may have gone unnoticed and early loss may be passed off as a late menstrual period.[39] The risk of fetal wastage was found to be influenced by hormonal profiles during the conceptual cycles[40] as well as by high levels of LH on the day of hCG administration,[41] the prevalence of chromosomal abnormalities[27] and the number of siblings.[42] Babies born after IVF were found to have a lower birthweight, shorter gestation and longer hospitalization. Multiple gestations accounted for most of the neonatal morbidity.[43] However, when considering only singletons, the birthweight of babies born after assisted conception was still lower when compared with that of natural conceptions.[44] The observed difference decreases, but does not disappear, after correcting for gestational age.[45] Several authors suggested that the remaining difference should be attributed to the maternal infertility status itself.[46,47]

**CONCLUSION**

GnRH agonists and gonadotrophins for the stimulation of multiple follicular development in infertile women seem to have little or no untoward effect on the resulting pregnancy and pregnancy outcome. Toxicology data on GnRH agonists, r-hFSH and r-hCG give little cause for concern. Pharmacology data show that most of the exogenous gonadotrophins have been eliminated by the time of early embryo development. Human chorionic gonadotrophin is used in the case of threatened abortion in the first trimester. Observations of accidental exposure of viable pregnancies to either GnRH agonists or exogenous gonadotrophins do not indicate particular hazards for the fetus, although the data are largely insufficient for conclusions of any kind. With the growing volume of data on pregnancy outcomes after ART, it becomes clear that gonadotrophins do not increase the risk of congenital malformations or chromosomal aberrations. The risk of abortion after IVF may be somewhat higher, although this could be the result of observational bias. Birthweights of singleton babies born after IVF are lower than those of babies from spontaneous conceptions, but this is probably the result of the infertility status of the mother.

## REFERENCES

1. *ABPI Compendium of Data Sheets and Summaries of Product Characteristics 1998–1999.* London: Datapharm Publications Limited, 1998: 1372, 1549.
2. Drieu K, Osterburg I. Etude de Décapeptyl sur les fonctions de reproduction. *Contracept Fertil Sex* 1989;**17**:1105–8.
3. *Physicians' Desk Reference*, 52nd edition. Montvale: Medical Economics Company, 1998: 2905.
4. Wishire GB, Emmi AM, Gagliardi CC, et al. Gonadotropin-releasing hormone agonist administration in early human pregnancy is associated with normal outcomes. *Fertil Steril* 1993;**60**:980–3.
5. Damewood MD, Shen W, Zacur HA, Schlaff WD, Rock JA, Wallach EE. Disappearance of exogenously administered human chorionic gonadotropin. *Fertil Steril* 1989;**52**:398–400.
6. Golan A, Ron-El R, Herman A, Weinraub Z, Soffer Y, Caspi E. Fetal outcome following inadvertent administration of long-acting DTRP⁶ microcapsules during pregnancy: a case report. *Hum Reprod* 1990;**5**:123–4.
7. Chang SY, Soong YK. Unexpected pregnancies exposed to leuprolide acetate administered after mid-luteal phase for ovarian stimulation. *Hum Reprod* 1995;**10**:204–6.
8. Elefant E, Biour B, Blumberg-Tick J, Roux C, Thomas F. Administration of a gonadotropin-releasing hormone agonist during pregnancy: follow-up of 28 pregnancies exposed to triptoreline. *Fertil Steril* 1995;**63**:1111–13.
9. Serafini P, Yee B, Vargyas J, Marrs RP. Development of multiple ovarian follicles for in vitro fertilization in a patient with an undiagnosed ectopic pregnancy. *Fertil Steril* 1985; **43**:656–8.
10. diZerega G, Hodgen GP. Pregnancy-associated ovarian refractoriness to gonadotropin: a myth. *Am J Obstet Gynecol* 1979;**134**:819–22.
11. Diamond MP, Tarlatzi BC, DeCherney AH. Recruitment of multiple follicular development for in vitro fertilization in the presence of a viable intrauterine pregnancy. *Obstet Gynecol* 1987;**70**:498–9.
12. Lessing JB, Kogosowski A, Amit A, et al. Successful ovarian superovulation in a patient with an undiagnosed intrauterine pregnancy. *J in vitro Fertil Embryo Transf* 1991;**8**:237–40.
13. Blumenfeld Z, Ruach M. Early pregnancy wastage: the role of repetitive human chorionic gonadotropin supplementation during the first 8 weeks of gestation. *Fertil Steril* 1992;**58**:19–23.
14. Sandler B. Anencephaly and ovulation stimulation (letter) *Lancet* 1973;**ii**:379.
15. James WH. Anencephaly and ovulation stimulation (letter) *Lancet* 1974;**i**:1353.
16. Biale Y, Leventhal M, Altaras M, Ben-Aderet N. Anencephaly and clomiphene-induced pregnancy. *Acta Obstet Gynaecol Scand* 1978;**57**:483–4.
17. Lancaster PAL. Congenital malformations after in vitro fertilisation (letter). *Lancet* 1987;**ii**:1392–3.
18. Cornel MC, Ten Kate LP, Dukes MNG, et al. Ovulation induction and neural tube defects (letter). *Lancet* 1989;**i**:1386.
19. Rejjal ARA, Abu-Osba YK. Discordant anencephaly with cleft lip and palate in a Pergonal-induced triplet pregnancy. *J Perinat Med* 1992;**20**:241–4.
20. Bernabeu R, Bonada M, Cremades N, Galan F. Deletion of chromosome 13:46,XY,del(13)(q14→qter) after in vitro fertilization and tubal embryo transfer. *J Assist Reprod Genet* 1996;**13**:519–22.

21. American Fertility Society, Society for Assisted Reproductive Technology. Assisted reproductive technology in the United States and Canada: 1992 results generated from the AFS/SART registry. *Fertil Steril* 1994;**62:**1121–8.

22. FIVNAT. Pregnancies and births resulting from in vitro fertilization. French national registry, analysis of data 1986–1990. *Fertil Steril* 1995;**64:**746–56.

23. Mills LJ, Simpson JL, Rhoads GG, et al. Risk of neural tube defects in relation to maternal fertility and fertility drug use. *Lancet* 1990;**335:**103–4.

24. Werler M, Louik C, Shapiro S, Mitchell A. Ovulation induction and risk of neural tube defects. *Lancet* 1994;**334:**445–6.

25. Van Loon K, Besseghir K, Eshkol A. Neural tube defects after infertility treatment: a review. *Fertil Steril* 1992;**58:**875–84.

26. Greenland S, Ackerman DL. Clomiphene citrate and neural tube defects: a pooled analysis of controlled epidemiologic studies and recommendations for the future. *Fertil Steril* 1995;**64:**936–41.

27. Boué JG, Boué A. Increased frequency of chromosomal anomalies in abortions after induced ovulation. *Lancet* 1973;**i:**679.

28. Tejada MI, Mendoza R, Corcostegui B, Benito JA. Chromosome studies in human unfertilized oocytes and uncleaved zygotes after treatment with gonadotropin-releasing hormone analogs. *Fertil Steril* 1991;**56:**874–80.

29. In'tVeld P, Brandenburg H, Verhoeff A, et al. Sex chromosomal abnormalities and intracytoplasmic sperm injection (letter). *Lancet* 1995;**346:**773.

30. Foresta C, Garolla A, Ferlin A, Galeazzi C, Rossato M. Use of intracytoplasmic sperm injection in severe male factor infertility. *Lancet* 1996;**348:**59.

31. Meschede D, De Geyter C, Nieschlag E, Horst J. Genetic risk in manipulative assisted reproduction. *Hum Reprod* 1995;**10:**2880–6.

32. Bonduelle M, Devroey P, Liebaers I, Van Steirteghem A. Commentary: major defects are overestimated. *BMJ* 1997;**315:**1265–6.

33. Bonduelle M, Wilikens Y, Buysse A, et al. Prospective follow-up study of 877 children born after intracytoplasmic sperm injection (ICSI), with ejaculated epididymal and testicular spermatozoa and after replacement of cryopreserved embryos obtained after ICI. *Hum Reprod* 1997;**11**(suppl 4):131–55.

34. Persson JW, Peters GB, Saunders DM. Genetic consequences of ICSI. Is ICSI associated with risks of genetic disease? Implications for counselling, practice and research. *Hum Reprod* 1996;**11:**921–32.

35. Meschede D, Horst J. Sex chromosomal anomalies in pregnancies conceived through intracytoplasmic sperm injection: a case for genetic counselling. *Hum Reprod* 1997;**12:**1125–7.

36. Pellestor F, Girardet A, Andreo B, Lefort G, Charlieu JP. The PRINS technique: potential use for rapid preimplantation embryo chromosome screening. *Mol Hum Reprod* 1996;**2:**135–8.

37. Tarlatzis BS. Report on the activities of the ESHRE Task Force on intracytoplasmic sperm injection. *Hum Reprod* 1996;**11**(suppl 4):160–85; discussion 186.

38. Ron-El R. Complications of ovulation induction. *Baillière's Clin Obstet Gynaecol* 1993;**7:**435–53.

39. Scialli AR. The reproductive toxicity of ovulation induction. *Fertil Steril* 1986;**45:**315–23.

40. Suk-Yee L, Baker HW, Evans JH, Pepperell RJ. Factors affecting fetal loss in induction of ovulation with gonadotropins: increased abortion rates related to hormonal profiles in conceptual cycles. *Am J Obstet Gynecol* 1989;**160:**621–8.

41. Howles CM, Macnamee MC, Edwards RG, et al. Effects of high tonic levels of luteinizing hormone on outcome of in vitro fertilization. *Lancet* 1986;**ii:**521–2.

42. Kurachi K, Aono T, Suzuki M, et al. Results of hMG (Humegon)-hCG therapy in 6096 treatment cycles of 2166 Japanese women with anovulatory infertility. *Eur J Obstet Gynecol Reprod Biol* 1985;**19:**43–51.

43. Tallo CP, Vohr B, Oh W, et al. Maternal and neonatal morbidity associated with in vitro fertilization. *J Pediatr* 1995;**127:**794–800.

44. MRC Working Party on Children Conceived by IVF. Births in Great Britain resulting from assisted conception, 1978–87. *BMJ* 1990;**300:**1229–33.

45. Petersen K, Hornnes PJ, Ellingsen S, et al. Perinatal outcome after in vitro fertilisation. *Acta Obstet Gynecol Scand* 1995;**74:**129–31.

46. Ghazi HA, Spielberger C, Källén B. Delivery outcome after infertility – a registry study. *Fertil Steril* 1991;**55:**726–32.

47. Williams M, Goldman M, Mittendorf R, et al. Subfertility and the risk of low birth weight. *Fertil Steril* 1991;**56:**913–17.

# 2

# Risk and the use of drugs in infertility treatment

David L Healy

**Can consent ever be completely informed?** • **What is a material risk?** • **What is the risk of the ovarian hyperstimulation syndrome?** • **What is the risk of cancer?** • **Conclusions and future directions** • **Acknowledgements**

No drug is safe when used for infertility treatment. No operation is safe when used for infertility treatment. Media allegations that drugs used in infertility treatment caused cancer in women has probably been the greatest threat to the trust between infertile couples and their doctors in the past 10 years. This crisis in infertility therapy introduced very clearly to all patients and their doctors the concept of risk and, in particular, the concept of epidemiological risk. It reinforced for many of us that no medical treatment is completely safe. Quantitative assessment of health risks for informed consent with any medical or surgical treatment is still in its infancy. The aim of this chapter is to give our current approach to providing this information to the infertile woman. We also review current knowledge of cancer risk with drugs in infertility treatment.

## CAN CONSENT EVER BE COMPLETELY INFORMED?

Informed consent in the USA evolved from medicolegal practice which established that the medical practitioner breaches the duty owed to a patient if he or she withholds any facts that are necessary to form the basis of an intelligent consent by the patient to the proposed treatment (*Salgo v Leiland Stanform Junior* 1957).

This doctrine of informed consent was based on the notion that patients have a right to body integrity and self-determination which should not be interfered with. The focus is upon the patient's decision to accept or refuse medical treatment. This cannot be made without full information about the risks, complications and side effects of a procedure. In, for example, an in vitro fertilization (IVF) cycle, this would include the risks associated with drug administration to induce multiple folliculogenesis as well as the risks of oocyte retrieval by vaginal ultrasonography or laparoscopy, and those associated with subsequent embryo transfer.

In several parts of the USA, a duty to take reasonable care in relation to the provision of information has evolved as a separate duty from the ordinary duty related to diagnosis and treatment. It is considered that the latter duty focuses on the medical practitioner's obligation rather than on the patient's rights.

In the UK, prevailing medical opinion has historically been the standard of care expected of medical practitioners. In the medicolegal case of *Bolam v Friern Hospital Management Committee* 1957, the appropriate standard of care was to be determined by the practices adopted by the relevant sectors of the medical profession at that time. This test was applied not only to situations involving negligent performance of treatment, but also to situations involving negligent failure to disclose.

Since 1979, Australian courts have rejected the view that the standard of care is to be determined by reference to the standard practices of the medical profession. Rather, several court decisions have stated that the standard of medical care is to be determined by reference to what the law courts consider appropriate. Many doctors find this bewildering to say the least!

For the typical clinician providing infertility therapy, these issues can be a nightmare. In one sense, totally informed consent is impossible. A patient cannot be given all information about all possible complications of her medical and surgical treatments, even if the patient's doctor was able to make such a list.

## WHAT IS A MATERIAL RISK?

These obligations have been focused by the High Court of Australia which determined that a doctor has a duty to warn a patient of a material risk inherent in any proposed treatment. A material risk is, in the circumstances of the particular case, a risk that a reasonable person in the patient's position, if warned of the risk, would be likely to attach significance to (*Rogers v Whitaker* 1992). A risk is also material if the medical practitioner is, or should reasonably be, aware that the particular patient, if warned of the risk, would be likely to attach significance to it.

At least the High Court of Australia has determined that there was no need for a patient herself to express a desire for information about a particular risk in a precise manner. The High Court expressed the view that, even if the patient had not expressed a desire for information, the medical practitioner would have been negligent in not providing the information. In the particular case involved in *Rogers v Whitaker*, the risk of blindness to the remaining good eye of the patient in an ophthalmological case was one in 14 000 in the circumstances of the case.

In dealing with these issues of informed consent and material risk, we have found it useful to attempt to provide infertile patients with information about their proposed medical and surgical treatments which are related to the general risks of death in community activities.[1] For example, all infertile couples are interested in having a pregnancy and a baby. Even in Western democracies, there is nevertheless a risk of dying from pregnancy. In most developed countries this risk is about one in 14 000 in urban communities as indicated in Table 1. We found that a risk of one in 14 000 of a woman dying in pregnancy is still difficult for many infertile couples to put into context of other life risks.

The Perinatal Society of Australia identified in 1995 (Table 1) that even normal couples have a risk of miscarriage of about one in seven in the general community. Quite clearly, some infertile couples will have a significantly higher risk than this. Nevertheless, a risk of one in

| Table 1 Information sheet of risks for pregnancy for an infertile couple | |
|---|---|
| **Event** | **Material risk** |
| Miscarriage | 1 in 7 |
| Premature birth | 1 in 15 |
| Birth defect in the baby | 1 in 20 |
| Death of the baby | 1 in 100 |
| Cerebral palsy in the baby | 1 in 400 |
| Death of the mother | 1 in 14 000 |

Adapted from ref. 2.

seven is understandable by most infertile patients. The risk of pre-term birth, again in the general community, is about one in 15. It surprises many patients in Australia to know that the rate of notifiable birth defect in the Australian community is one in 20, as indicated by the Royal Australian College of Paediatricians. Although the risk of any couple having a baby with cerebral palsy is one in 400, most infertile couples are relieved to know that their risks are so low and that, conversely, they have 399 chances out of 400 of having a baby without cerebral palsy.

A similar approach can be taken to a woman's lifetime risk of development of cancer. In industrialized societies, the lifetime risk of the development of breast cancer is about one in 14. In a woman aged 50 years, with no known family history, the chance of the development of breast carcinoma over the next 12 months is about one in 500. Ovarian carcinoma will occur in about one woman in 90 in our general community. Once again, it is possible to put such risks into some sort of general community reference as indicated in Table 2. The Australian Bureau of Statistics data indicate that a fit and healthy 40-year-old woman has a one in 1000 chance of dying within the next year. At 50 years of age, this risk is one in 500 in one year and at 60 years of age the risk is one in 170.

Risks associated with ovulation induction treatment, laparoscopy and various IVF-related procedures can also be addressed in this general matter. Table 3 indicates some of those risks; we incorporated these into the general risks of death from a range of community and personal activities which most of us have undertaken at some time or another. We provide such a Material Risk Information Sheet to our infertile patients. Many are greatly relieved to know that risk of death from laparoscopy or related procedures is so low! Most are amazed to learn that sexual intercourse can actually kill a woman from subsequent acute pelvic inflammatory disease!

## WHAT IS THE RISK OF THE OVARIAN HYPERSTIMULATION SYNDROME?

Jacobs and colleagues[5] reported on the risk of the ovarian hyperstimulation syndrome after IVF. These authors studied 1302 patients undergoing ovarian stimulation for IVF. They reported eight women who developed a severe hyperstimulation syndrome. Seven additional patients developed a moderate ovarian hyperstimulation syndrome. In the context of material risk, this means that a previously fit but infertile woman had one chance in 160 of being seriously ill from the ovarian hyperstimulation syndrome after one IVF cycle.

Patients who develop the severe ovarian

| Table 2  Material risks related to a woman's age | |
| --- | --- |
| **Activity** | **Chance of death in one year** |
| Fit and healthy at 40 years | 1 in 1000 |
| Fit and healthy at 50 years | 1 in 500 |
| Fit and healthy at 60 years | 1 in 170 |

Adapted from ref. 3

**Table 3 Material risks with various events and community activities**

| Activity | Chance of death in one year |
| --- | --- |
| Motor cycling | 1 in 1000 |
| Hysterectomy | 1 in 1600 |
| Driving a car | 1 in 6000 |
| Power boating | 1 in 6000 |
| Rock climbing | 1 in 7500 |
| Continuing pregnancy | 1 in 14 000 |
| Playing football | 1 in 25 000 |
| Laparoscopy | 1 in 67 000 |
| Canoeing | 1 in 100 000 |
| Having sexual intercourse (PID) | 1 in 100 000 |
| RU486 use | 1 in 200 000 |
| Using tampons | 1 in 300 000 |
| Legal termination of pregnancy: <9 weeks | 1 in 500 000 |
| Jumbo jet flight | 1 in 2 000 000 |

Adapted from refs 3, 4.

hyperstimulation syndrome are at significant risk for stroke, renal failure and death. In the above study, five of the eight women had polycystic ovaries diagnosed on ultrasonography. Six of the eight patients were undergoing their first attempt at IVF. The mean serum oestradiol concentration on the day of human chorionic gonadotrophin (hCG) administration was 8200 pmol/l. A mean number of 13 oocytes were recovered at transvaginal ultrasonographically directed oocyte recovery.

In patients with the severe ovarian hyperstimulation syndrome, there were five multiple pregnancies and two singleton pregnancies. The five multiple pregnancies comprised one set of twins, three sets of triplets and one set of quadruplets. The risk of most obstetric complications is increased in multiple pregnancy. Multiple pregnancy increases the risks of death to the babies and to the mother, but it also increases risks of mental or physical disability to the babies (see Table 1).

Ovarian hyperstimulation is an iatrogenic condition. Its cause is not known, although vascular endothelial growth factor is thought to be a major capillary permeability agent in the pathogenesis of the ovarian hyperstimulation syndrome.[6] Patients with the polycystic ovary syndrome should be started on a lower dosage of gonadotrophin to minimize the risk of the ovarian hyperstimulation syndrome. As gonadotrophin-releasing hormone (GnRH) agonists appear to increase the risk of the ovarian hyperstimulation syndrome, close monitoring of follicle numbers in such IVF patients is necessary. Patients with serum oestradiol concentrations above 15 000 pmol/l on the day of hCG administration should have their embryos cryopreserved for elective transfer in a subsequent cycle. The use of hCG for luteal support in all patients at risk of the ovarian hyperstimulation syndrome should be avoided obstetrically; it could be argued that no more than two embryos should ever be transferred.

## WHAT IS THE RISK OF CANCER?

The use of fertility drugs in women with ovulation disorders has held an important place in infertility treatment for 30 years.[7] The aim is to stimulate the production of a limited number of oocytes, preferably one per cycle. However, the use of fertility drugs with assisted conception such as IVF and gamete intrafallopian transfer (GIFT) is different. In IVF, combinations and different dosages of fertility drugs are given to stimulate production of multiple oocytes to improve the chances of fertilization in any given treatment cycle.[8]

Two important studies suggested an association between exposure to fertility drugs and an increased risk of ovarian cancer. A pooled analysis of three case-controlled studies showed an odds ratio (OR) of 2.8 (95% Confidence Interval or 95%CI = 1.3–6.1) for ovarian cancer in infertile women treated with fertility drugs compared with women with no diagnosis of infertility or fertility drug treatment.[9] In 1994, Rossing and colleagues,[10] using record linkage with a population-based cancer registry, identified an increased incidence of ovarian cancer (invasive or borderline malignant tumours) with a standardized incidence rate (SIR) of 2.5 (95%CI = 1.3–4.5) in a cohort of infertile women compared with age-standardized general population rates. An increased relative risk (RR = 11.1; 95%CI = 1.5–82.3) was also found in women, with or without ovarian abnormalities, who had been treated with the fertility drug clomiphene citrate for more than one year, compared with infertile women who had not taken the drug.

Studies of cancer after infertility and infertility treatment are different to undertake. A common problem is the limitations placed upon the conclusions of the study by low statistical power. Other problems are the difficulties in distinguishing possible effects of fertility drug exposure from the underlying ovulation disorder that they were used to treat. Important contributions in this area were the publications of Ron and colleagues, Brinton and associates and Gammon and Thompson.[11–13]

More recently, Shushan and associates[14] undertook a case-controlled study of ovarian cancer by examining self-reported fertility drug use in 200 women with epithelial ovarian tumours. One hundred and sixty-four patients had invasive ovarian malignancy and 36 had borderline ovarian cancers; there were 408 controls. They found no significant association between fertility drug use and epithelial ovarian tumours (OR = 1.31; 95%CI = 0.63–2.74). Fertility drug use was significantly associated with borderline tumours in this study (OR = 3.52; 95%CI = 1.23–10.29). The strongest association was seen in women who had used human menopausal gonadotrophins (OR = 9.38; 95%CI = 1.66–52.08). This study shows the difficulties, strengths and weaknesses of these methods in trying to provide the best data about risks from the use of drugs in infertility treatment. For example, women who had died of ovarian cancer were not included in this study. Their families were not approached. Such studies were further limited by the lack of verification of medical records of fertility drug use.

At Monash, we have taken a different approach with a cohort study.[15] As ovulation disorders are not in themselves an indication for IVF, and because most patients exposed to ovarian stimulation for IVF have normal ovulatory cycles, studies of cancer incidence after IVF enable any effect of fertility drug exposure to be distinguished from underlying ovulation disorders. We studied a cohort of women who were referred for IVF to examine whether exposure to fertility drugs to induce multiple folliculogenesis was associated with an increased cancer rate.

Our cohort was 10 358 women registered with the Monash IVF programme in Melbourne, Australia. To be eligible for the study, patients were known to have been treated or referred for IVF treatment. They were normally resident in Australia at the time of registration with a known date of birth or age and a known time of entry into the cohort between 1 June 1978 and 31 December 1992. Women resident outside the State of Victoria (11.9% of the cohort) were included if their date of entry was up to 31 December one year before the end of complete data collection for their state's cancer registry. From 11 129 women identified as being treated or referred for IVF in the time period, 771 were excluded because of overseas residence, unknown date of birth, unknown age or unknown date of entry into the cohort.

## Data collection

Data were retrieved from computerized records kept by Monash IVF from August 1990, onwards. Data for patients who registered or were treated before that time were retrieved manually from medical histories or registration forms kept by the clinic. Data items collected included: name and date of birth, husband's name, address, type of infertility, date of registration (unexposed), date of first stimulated treatment cycle (exposed) and total number of stimulated treatment cycles (exposed). Infertility was classified as tubal, male factor, endometriosis, ovarian disorders (ovulation disorders, polycystic ovary syndrome, donor egg recipients for premature menopause and oophorectomy), unexplained or other (cervical factors, other uterine abnormalities, donor egg recipients for genetic disease and altruistic egg donors). Women could be included in more than one cause-of-infertility group; unexplained infertility was however, a unique classification.

## Exposure ascertainment

Women who had had one or more IVF treatment cycles with ovarian stimulation to induce multiple folliculogenesis were allocated to the exposed group ($n = 5564$), including women who had started but not completed a stimulated IVF cycle. The drug regimens used for ovarian stimulation were similar to those used in other IVF programmes around the world. Until 1987 most stimulated IVF cycles used clomiphene citrate in combination with human menopausal gonadotrophins (hMG) to induce multiple folliculogenesis, followed by hCG for oocyte maturation before retrieval. From 1987

the GnRH agonists leuprolide and buserelin were introduced to replace clomiphene and to prevent untimely surges of leutinizing hormone (LH). From 1990 to 1992 the main drug regimen was an GnRH agonist in combination with hMG or follicle-stimulating hormone (FSH) followed by hCG. With this regimen oocytes retrieved per stimulated cycle averaged nine; with clomiphene–hMG–hCG the average had been six.

Information about fertility drug exposures outside the Monash IVF programme was not available, except for those women who had also attended the other major IVF programme in Victoria at the Royal Women's Hospital and Melbourne IVF clinic (RWH/Melbourne IVF). The two Victorian programmes were the first to be established in Australia and have provided most IVF services to women in the state. Record linkage showed that 414 women had registered with both programmes, and data were adjusted to include exposure to stimulated cycles on the RWH/Melbourne IVF programme. The number of women who attended Monash IVF and other Australian IVF programmes was not known but was expected to be small. Exposure to fertility drugs outside IVF programmes was also not known but was expected to have occurred for only those women in the cohort who had ovulation disorders and who might have had prior exposure to conventional ovulation induction.

Women in the unexposed group (4794) were those who had registered for IVF but had not received treatment (93.4%) or who had 'natural cycle' treatment only, without ovarian stimulation (6.6%). Women who did not receive treatment withdrew of their own accord. Their reasons were not usually recorded but included pregnancy while on the waiting list, other treatment options pursued (for example, tubal surgery), financial or relationship difficulties, and change of mind as a result of perceived discomforts and risks or other personal reasons.

## Follow-up and case ascertainment

Ascertainment of cancer cases was by record linkage with the population-based Victorian

Cancer Registry (VCR) for Victorian residents (88.1% of the cohort) and the National Cancer Statistics Clearing House (NCSCH), which compiles data from all Australian state cancer registries, for residents of other states. Data collection at the VCR was complete from 1982 to the end of 1993, with over 90% notification between 1978 and 1982 from the major Victorian hospitals. The NCSCH had complete data from 1982 to the end of 1988–93, depending on the state. Follow-up was from the time each woman entered the cohort until 31 December for the year to complete cancer data for her state of residence. All women had at least one year of follow-up. Cancers of all types were identified from the VCR for Victorian residents, and invasive breast cancers (International Classification of Disease, after revision or ICD-9 code 1740–1749) and ovarian cancers (ICD-9 code 1830) from the NCSCH for residents of other states.

Attempts were made to locate women to do a sensitivity analysis of the possible effect of loss to follow-up. Loss to follow-up was expected to occur mainly as a result of name change and migration. There was no contact with women in the study. Location searches, based on woman's name, husband's name and last known address, used 1993 Australian electoral roll listings on microfiche and electronic telephone listings. The electoral roll has compulsory enrolment for Australian citizens aged 18 or over.

## Statistical methods

Expected numbers of cancers were calculated from the person-years in exposed and unexposed groups, assuming the age-specific rates for the Victorian female population in 1982–91. From these it was estimated that the study had 80% power at the 5% level, to detect SIRs of 1.7 for breast cancer in both exposed and unexposed groups and an SIR of 4.0 for ovarian cancer in both groups. The study had also had 80% power at the 5% level for detecting an RR of 2.15 for breast cancer in the exposed group and an RR of 5.05 for ovarian cancer.

All women registered in the cohort were included for the SIR estimation of breast and ovarian cancer risk. For analysis of other cancers, only those women whose original address was Victoria were included because linkage was not made with other than Victorian registries for those cancers. Sensitivity analyses for the SIRs estimated were performed for breast and ovarian cancers. Using only those women who were located in a 1993 address or who had died from cancer (and an adjustment to the denominator to account for the number of women expected to have died from all causes), an upper limit of association was estimated. To allow for a possible latency period, further SIR estimates were made using only those women with at least 5 years of follow-up.

The proportional hazards models, including age at diagnosis or (censored) time to end of follow-up and type of infertility as co-variates, were fitted to estimate the relative risk for the exposed group for various cancers. Relative risks were also estimated for each type of infertility, with absence of that type of infertility as the reference group.

The DATAB and PEANUTS modules of the EPICURE software package were used for the SIR and RR calculations.

## Results

The median age at entry into the cohort was 32 for the exposed group (range 18–49) and 31 for the unexposed group (19–51). At the end of follow-up, the median age was 38 (21–57) in the exposed group and 38 (22–59) in the unexposed group. The median length of follow-up for the exposed group (5.2; range = 1–15.1) was less than that in the unexposed group (7.6; 1–15.5). More women in the unexposed group entered the cohort in the earlier years when waiting times for IVF treatment were as long as 3 years. The figure shows the person-years distribution by age group for women in the exposed and unexposed groups. The total person-years contributed was 31 272 for the exposed group and 33 655 for the unexposed group.

*Standardized incidence rate*

In Table 4 are shown the observed number of cases identified, the expected number and the SIR estimates for the exposed group, the unexposed group and both groups combined. There was no evidence of an increase in breast cancer incidence in the exposed or unexposed groups compared with the female population of Victoria. The median time to diagnosis from time of registration (unexposed) or first stimulated treatment cycle (exposed) was 3.5 years (range 0.7–6.7) for the exposed group and 4.7 years (0.8–11.0) for the unexposed group. The median time between the last stimulated cycle and diagnosis for the exposed group was 3.1 years (0.1–5.3). The median age at diagnosis was 39.7 years (33–49) for the unexposed group. Seven women were known to have died.

Invasive ovarian cancer occurred in six women (three exposed, three unexposed). The SIR estimates suggested an increased incidence of ovarian cancer in the cohort, irrespective of exposure status, which was not significant. The ovarian tumours were serous and mucinous adenocarcinomas. Women were aged 28–42 at diagnosis and three were known to have died. The times to diagnosis were 3.4, 6.6 and 7.5 years in the exposed group and 1.9, 6.5 and 7.6 years in the unexposed group. Three additional ovarian tumours (ICD-9 code 2362) were identified (two exposed, one unexposed) and all were mature cystic teratomas, which were benign. The times to diagnosis were 0.7 and 2.4 years in the exposed group and 0.2 year in the unexposed group. Combining invasive ovarian cancers and mature cystic teratomas gave SIR estimates of 2.17 (0.90–5.20) for the exposed group, 1.65 (0.62–4.39) for the unexposed group and 1.90 (0.99–3.65) for the groups combined. No borderline ovarian tumours were identified.

The incidence of other cancers identified in the VCR (see Table 4) showed an increased incidence of cancer of the body of the uterus (ICD-9 code 182), irrespective of exposure status, with an SIR for the groups combined of 2.84 (1.18–6.81). Of the five tumours four were endometrial adenocarcinomas and one (unexposed to IVF treatment) was a leiomyosarcoma. It was not possible to obtain morphology-specific population cancer rates for these two types of uterine cancer. Removal of the leiomyosarcoma gave an SIR of 2.27 (0.85–6.04) which was not significant. The times to diagnosis were 0.7 and 3.4 years in the exposed group and 0.1, 2.1 and 9.2 years in the unexposed group. Women were aged 35–48 at diagnosis. Melanomas and colorectal cancer (the most common cancers in Victorian women after breast cancer) showed a similar incidence to that of the general population. The incidence of invasive cervical cancer and that of all cancers (excluding in situ cancers) in the exposed and unexposed groups was found to be not significantly different from age-standardized general population rates. However, the incidence of carcinoma in situ (CIS) of the cervix was significantly less in both the exposed and unexposed groups than in the general population (SIR for groups combined 0.53; 0.38–0.74).

*Exposure dosage: number of stimulated IVF treatment cycles*

For the exposed group, the distribution of the number of stimulated cycles and the cancer incidence is shown in Table 5. The median number of cycles with ovarian stimulation was 2 (range 1–22). Of the women 77% had three or fewer stimulated cycles; 1.9% (104 women) had 10 or more cycles. Of incident cancers 74% occurred in women having only one or two stimulated cycles. There was no apparent increase in risk associated with level of exposure to stimulated treatment cycles. For breast cancer the SIR was 1.02 (0.46–2.27) for women exposed to one stimulated cycle and 0.83 (0.45–1.55) for women exposed to more than one. For all cancers these SIRs were 1.13 (0.69–1.84) and 0.86 (0.58–1.26), respectively. There was no evidence for a trend effect with dose ($\chi^2 = 0.5$ for breast cancer and 0.8 for all cancers). Other cancers had too few numbers for a dose effect to be studied.

*Type of infertility*

Infertility for both groups was classified as tubal 43.4%, male factor 23.2%, endometriosis 13.2%, ovarian disorders 6.2%, unexplained

**Table 4 Observed and expected cases, SIRs and confidence intervals by cancer and exposure to IVF treatment**

| | ICD-9 Code | Exposed | | | | Unexposed | | | | Combined | | | |
|---|---|---|---|---|---|---|---|---|---|---|---|---|---|
| | | Observed | Expected | SIR | 95%CI | Observed | Expected | SIR | 95%CI | Observed | Expected | SIR | 95%CI |
| *Cancer* | | | | | | | | | | | | | |
| Breast | 1740–1749 | 16 | 17.90 | 0.89 | 0.55–1.46 | 18* | 18.29 | 0.98 | 0.62–1.56 | 34 | 36.19 | 0.94 | 0.67–1.31 |
| Ovarian | 1830 | 3 | 1.77 | 1.70 | 0.55–5.27 | 3 | 1.85 | 1.62 | 0.52–5.02 | 6 | 3.62 | 1.66 | 0.75–3.69 |
| Body of uterus | 1820–1828 | 2 | 0.90 | 2.22 | 0.55–8.87 | 3 | 0.86 | 3.48 | 1.12–10.8 | 5 | 1.76 | 2.84 | 1.18–1.75 |
| Melanoma | 1720–1729 | 7 | 7.36 | 0.95 | 0.45–1.99 | 9 | 7.55 | 1.19 | 0.62–2.29 | 16 | 14.92 | 1.07 | 0.66–1.75 |
| Colorectal | 1530–1549 | 1 | 2.75 | 0.36 | 0.05–2.58 | 3 | 2.66 | 1.13 | 0.36–3.50 | 4 | 5.41 | 0.74 | 0.28–1.97 |
| Cervix | 1800–1809 | 5 | 5.03 | 0.99 | 0.41–2.39 | 1 | 5.16 | 0.19 | 0.03–1.38 | 6 | 10.19 | 0.59 | 0.26–1.31 |
| Other† | | 8 | 8.79 | 0.91 | 0.45–1.82 | 12 | 7.87 | 1.53 | 0.87–2.69 | 20 | 16.66 | 1.20 | 0.77–1.86 |
| All cancers‡ | 1400–2089 | 42 | 44.51 | 0.94 | 0.70–1.28 | 48 | 44.24 | 1.08 | 0.82–1.44 | 90 | 88.75 | 1.01 | 0.82–1.25 |
| CIS cervix | 2331 | 18 | 30.52 | 0.59 | 0.37–0.94 | 16 | 33.99 | 0.47 | 0.29–0.77 | 34 | 64.51 | 0.53 | 0.38–0.74 |
| *Sensitivity analysis* | | | | | | | | | | | | | |
| Including only women located in electoral roll, electronic telephone directory, or who had died | | | | | | | | | | | | | |
| Breast | 1740–1749 | 13 | 13.53 | 0.96 | 0.56–1.65 | 13 | 11.51 | 1.13 | 0.66–1.95 | 26 | 25.04 | 1.04 | 0.71–1.53 |
| Ovarian | 1830 | 3 | 1.34 | 2.25 | 0.72–6.97 | 2 | 1.17 | 1.72 | 0.43–6.86 | 5 | 2.50 | 2.00 | 0.83–4.80 |
| Including only women with at least 5 years of follow-up | | | | | | | | | | | | | |
| Breast | 1740–1749 | 12 | 14.46 | 0.83 | 0.47–1.46 | 15 | 16.99 | 0.88 | 0.53–1.46 | 27 | 31.45 | 0.86 | 0.59–1.25 |
| Ovarian | 1830 | 3 | 1.40 | 2.14 | 0.69–6.63 | 3 | 1.71 | 1.75 | 0.57–5.44 | 6 | 3.11 | 1.93 | 0.87–4.29 |

*One breast cancer case not resident in Victoria therefore not included in 'All' cancer category; see methods, follow-up and case ascertainment. †Other cancers not including those above or CIS. ‡Sum of above.

**Table 5 Distribution of exposed group and incident cancers in that number of IVF cycles**

| | Number of IVF cycles | | | | | | | |
|---|---|---|---|---|---|---|---|---|
| | 1 | 2 | 3 | 4 | 5 | 6 | 7 | 8+ |
| **Cancer** | 2052 | 1362 | 869 | 469 | 299 | 191 | 122 | 200 |
| | (37%)* | (24%) | (16%) | (8%) | (5%) | (3%) | (2%) | (4%) |
| Breast | 6† | 5 | 2 | 2 | | 1 | | |
| Ovarian | 1 | 1 | | | 1 | | | |
| Other | 10 | 10 | 1 | 1 | | 1 | | |
| | | | | | | | | 1 |
| All cancers | 17 | 16 | 3 | 3 | 1 | 2 | 0 | 1 |

*Number exposed (% of total exposed). †Number of cancers, excluding CIS.

infertility 18.7% and other causes 3.5%. Information on type of infertility was missing for 8.4% of the women in the cohort. Some women had more than one type of infertility recorded, but unexplained and missing were unique classifications. Table 6 shows the distribution of type of infertility by breast cancer incidence and exposure status, and the SIR and 95%CI for the groups combined. There was no association between infertility type and breast cancer or exposure to IVF. None of the women with ovarian cancer was recorded as having ovarian disorders as their cause of infertility. For cancers of both the ovaries and the body of the uterus an unexpectedly high number of women had unexplained infertility recorded. For those with unexplained infertility, the SIR for ovarian cancer was 6.98 (2.90–16.7) and for cancer of the body of the uterus 8.30 (2.77–25.7).

*Adjusted RR assessment*
Cancers of the breast, ovary, body of the uterus and all cancers combined were not associated with exposure to stimulated IVF cycles. The rel-ative risks of these four cancer groups, estimated by proportional hazards modelling and adjusting for age at diagnosis or end of follow-up (depending on disease status) and infertility type, were 1.11 (0.56–2.20), 1.45 (0.26–7.55), 0.65 (0.11–3.94) and 0.96 (0.62–1.47), respectively (Table 7). Also shown are relative risks, adjusted for exposure of unexplained infertility (with all other types of infertility as the reference group). For cancers of the ovaries and the body of the uterus, the effect of unexplained infertility was independent of exposure status and gave significant adjusted relative risks of 19.19 (2.23–165; $p = 0.0007$) and 6.34 (1.06–38; $p = 0.04$), respectively.

*Cancers diagnosed before cohort entry*
Ninety-eight tumours (invasive cancers, mature cystic teratomas and CIS of the cervix), identified by record linkage with the VCR, had been diagnosed before the women registered or received IVF treatment (58 exposed, 40 unexposed). These included two breast cancers, four mature cystic teratomas and four invasive cer-

**Table 6 Observed and expected and SIRs for combined groups by certain cancers by type of infertility**

| Site and type of infertility | Observed | | | Expected | SIR | CI 95% |
|---|---|---|---|---|---|---|
| | Exposed | Unexpected | Combined | | | |
| *Breast cancer* | | | | | | |
| Tubal | 6 | 7 | 13 | 19.28 | 0.67 | 0.39–1.16 |
| Male factor | 3 | 8 | 7 | 6.57 | 1.06 | 0.51–2.23 |
| Endometriosis | 2 | 0 | 2 | 3.99 | 0.50 | 0.13–2.00 |
| Ovarian disorders | 1 | 2 | 3 | 1.66 | 1.81 | 0.58–5.60 |
| Unexplained | 2 | 4 | 6 | 7.16 | 0.84 | 0.38–1.87 |
| Other | 0 | 0 | 0 | 0.48 | 0.00 | – |
| Missing | 1 | 2 | 3 | 1.86 | 1.62 | 0.52–5.01 |
| *Ovarian cancer* | | | | | | |
| Ovarian disorders | 0 | 0 | 0 | 0.17 | 0.00 | – |
| Unexplained | 3 | 2 | 5 | 0.72 | 6.98 | 2.90–16.8 |
| *Cancer of body of uterus* | | | | | | |
| Ovarian disorders | 0 | 0 | 0 | 0.08 | 0.00 | – |
| Unexplained | 1 | 2 | 3 | 0.36 | 8.30 | 2.68–25.7 |
| *All cancers* | | | | | | |
| Ovarian disorders | 1 | 4 | 5 | 4.19 | 1.19 | 0.50–2.86 |
| Unexplained | 12 | 12 | 24 | 18.10 | 1.33 | 0.89–1.98 |

vical cancers, with equal numbers of each cancer in the exposed and unexposed groups. There were no prior cancers of the body of the uterus. There were 64 prior diagnoses of CIS of the cervix (42 exposed, 22 unexposed, compared with the expected 41 and 23, respectively).

There was one case of Hodgkin's lymphoma in the exposed group and four in the unexposed group, and there were two cases of chronic myeloid leukaemia in the unexposed group. For five of these six women in the unexposed group, treatment had caused ovarian failure and infertility, as noted in their clinic records.

*Sensitivity analyses*
Analysis based on only those women who were located in 1993 (79% of the exposed and 66% of the unexposed group) gave estimates of SIRs for breast cancer of 0.96 (0.56–1.65) for the exposed and 1.13 (0.66–1.95) for the unexposed group. For invasive ovarian cancer, SIRs were 2.25 (0.72–6.97) for exposed and 1.72 (0.43–6.86) for unexposed. The adjusted relative risks calculated from the located cohort were 1.06 (0.48–2.31) for breast cancer in the exposed group relative to the unexposed group, and 2.09 (0.33–13.2) for ovarian cancer. A further sensitivity analysis, which included only women with at least 5 years of follow-up (51%

**Table 7** For various cancers, relative risk estimates for IVF exposure adjusted for age and infertility type, and relative risk estimates for unexplained infertility versus known causes of infertility, adjusted for age and IVF exposure

| Cancer | RR adjusted | 95%CI | p |
|---|---|---|---|
| *Breast cancer* | | | |
| IVF exposure | 1.11 | 0.56–2.20 | 0.8 |
| Unexplained infertility | 0.77 | 0.19–3.10 | 0.07 |
| *Ovarian cancer* | | | |
| IVF exposure | 1.45 | 0.28–7.55 | 0.7 |
| Unexplained infertility | 19.19 | 2.23–165 | 0.007 |
| *Cancer of body of uterus* | | | |
| IVF exposure | 0.65 | 0.11–3.94 | 0.6 |
| Unexplained infertility | 6.34 | 1.06–38.0 | 0.04 |
| *All cancers* | | | |
| IVF exposure | 0.96 | 0.62–1.47 | 0.8 |
| Unexplained infertility | 2.01 | 0.84–4.78 | 0.11 |

of the exposed and 78% of the unexposed group) gave SIRs for breast cancer in the exposed group of 0.83 (0.47–1.46) and in the unexposed group of 0.88 (0.53–1.48). For ovarian cancer the SIRs were 2.14 (0.69–6.63) and 1.75 (0.57–5.44), respectively (see Table 4). The adjusted relative risk for breast cancer was 1.27 (0.58–2.77) and for ovarian cancer it was 1.81 (0.35–9.70).

## CONCLUSIONS AND FUTURE DIRECTIONS

Our results showed that the incidence of breast cancer in women who have had IVF treatment with ovarian stimulation was no different from the incidence in women referred for IVF but not treated. The incidence in breast cancer in women who have been infertile was also no different than the incidence of this malignancy in the general population.

This cohort study showed the limitations of this type of epidemiological approach. Our study had limited power to detect differences in the incidence of gynaecological cancers. It did suggest that the incidence of cancer of the body of the uterus appeared significantly higher, irrespective of whether IVF treatment was undertaken or not. An increased risk of endometrial adenocarcinoma has been associated with the unopposed action of oestrogens, postmenopausal status, obesity, the polycystic ovary syndrome and nulliparity.

We found that the incidence of ovarian cancer in the cohort was higher than that in the general population. However, this increase was not significant. Once again, the findings were limited by the low power of the study and the rarity of ovarian cancer in this age group. In contrast to Rossing and colleagues,[15] we found no evidence to suggest an increased risk of borderline ovarian tumours associated with exposure to fertility drugs.

An unexpected finding from our study was the significant association between unexplained infertility and both invasive ovarian cancer as well as invasive cancer of the body of the uterus. This was independent of exposure status (see Tables 6 and 7). It is unlikely that early cancer was a cause of infertility for women in our exposed group with unexplained infertility, because endometrial sampling was common practice in the diagnostic work-up and all cancers were diagnosed at least 3 years after the first IVF treatment.

Our study also showed a reduced incidence of in situ and invasive carcinoma of the cervix. This finding has subsequently been confirmed by Rossing and colleagues.[16] These authors studied the incidence of cancer in a cohort of 3837 women evaluated for infertility between 1974 and 1985 in Seattle, USA. The incidence of cancer was determined by record linkage with a population-based cancer registry. The incidence of in situ and invasive carcinoma of the cervix was less than expected (36 cases observed, 67 expected) giving an SIR of 0.5

(95%CI = 0.4–0.7). Women with tubal causes of infertility had relatively more incidences of cervical carcinoma than women with other causes. By contrast, we did not observe a relatively increased incidence in women with tubal infertility. We suggested that the higher levels of screening for cervical abnormalities in the infertile women may account for the lower incidence of cervical carcinoma observed.

An Australian multicentre study of cancer after infertility and IVF is currently being undertaken. Our study will allow for larger numbers of patients (about 30 000), as well as a longer latency effect between exposure to fertility drugs and the possible later development of cancer. This study will also include a nested case–control study. We hope to contact patients who may have developed cancer, or their relatives, after infertility or IVF treatment.

## ACKNOWLEDGEMENTS

The author thanks all his colleagues at Monash and Melbourne for advice and assistance in this work. The professional example of Professor Howard Jacobs has been an inspiration for many in Australia.

## REFERENCES

1. Healy DL, Petrucco O. *Effective Gynaecological Day Surgery*. London: Thompson Scientific, 1998.
2. Consensus statement: cerebral palsy. *Med J Austr* 1995;**162**:86–91.
3. Australian Bureau of Statistics (personal communication).
4. Hatcher RD, Stewart F, Trusell J, et al. *Contraceptive Technology*. New York: Irvington, 1990–2.
5. McDougall MJ, Tan SL, Jacobs HS. In vitro fertilisation and the ovarian hyperstimulation syndrome. *Hum Reprod* 1992;**7**:597–600.
6. McClure N, Healy DL, Rogers PAW, et al. Vascular endothelian growth factor as capillary permeability agent in ovarian hyperstimulation syndrome. *Lancet* 1994;**344**:235–6.
7. Healy DL, Trounson AO, Andersen AN. Female Infertility: pathogenesis and management. *Lancet* 1994;**343**:1539–44.
8. Trounson AO, Leeton JF, Wood EC, Webb J, Wood J. Pregnancies in humans by fertilisation in vitro and embryo transfer in the controlled ovulatory cycle. *Science* 1981;**212**:616–19.
9. Whittemore A, Harris R, Itnyre J and the Collaborative Ovarian Cancer Group. Characteristics related to ovarian cancer risk; collaborative analysis of 12 US case–control studies. II: invasive epithelial cancer in white women. *Am J Epidemiol* 1992;**136**:1184–203.
10. Rossing MA, Daling JR, Weiss NS, Moore DE, Self SG. Ovarian tumours in a cohort of infertile women. *N Engl J Med* 1994;**331**:771–6.

11. Ron E, Lunenfeld B, Menczer J. Cancer incidence in a cohort of infertile women. *Am J Epidemiol* 1987;**125:**780–90.

12. Brinton LA, Melton J, Malkasian GD, Bond A, Hoover R. Cancer risk after evaluation for infertility. *Am J Epidemiol* 1989;**129:**712–22.

13. Gammon MD, Thompson WD. Infertility and breast cancer; a population-based case-controlled study. *Am J Epidemiol* 1990;**132:**708–16.

14. Shushan A, Paltiel O, Oiscovich J, Elchalal U, Peretz T, Schenker JG. Human menopausal gonadotrophin and the risk of epithelial ovarian cancer. *Fertil Steril* 1996;**65:**13–18.

15. Venn A, Watson L, Lumley J, Giles G, King C, Healy DL. Breast and ovarian cancer incidence after infertility and in vitro fertilization. *The Lancet* 1995;**346:**995–1000.

16. Rossing MA, Daling JR, Weiss NS, Moore DE, Self SG. In situ and invasive cervical carcinoma in a cohort of infertile women. *Fertil Steril* 1996;**65:**19–22.

## TABLE OF CASES

Bolam v Friern Hospital Management Committee [1957] 1 WLR 582.
Rogers v Whitaker [1992] High Court of Australia.
Salgo v Leiland Stanform Jnr [1957] University Board of Trustees.

# Part II
# Reproductive Dysfunction

# 3

# Genetically determined reproductive dysfunction in women

Eli Y Adashi

**Gonadotropin-releasing hormone resistance • Isolated follicle-stimulating hormone deficiency • Hypergonadotropic hypogonadal ovarian failure • LH resistance**

## GONADOTROPIN-RELEASING HORMONE RESISTANCE

Although the gonadotropin-releasing hormone (GnRH) gene is potentially subject to mutations, as evident from the existence of a murine paradigm,[1] several studies failed to document any such abnormality in either men or women with idiopathic hypogonadotropic hypogonadism. However, mutations of the G protein-coupled/membrane-spanning GnRH receptor were recently documented by de Roux and associates in a kindred who had the condition.[2] The female proband aged 37 years, presented with the chief complaint of amenorrhea after a single episode of spontaneous uterine bleeding (at the age of 18) and infertility. Spontaneous thelarche had occurred at the age of 14. Upon presentation, the circulating levels of estradiol and pituitary gonadotropins were in the low–normal range for the early follicular phase of the menstrual cycle.

Using leukocytic DNA from the subject being studied, intronic primers for the three exons comprising the GnRH receptor gene, polymerase chain reaction (PCR) amplification, and direct sequencing of the resultant PCR prod-

ucts, Roux et al were able to document a compound heterozygotic mutation in the GnRH receptor (Arg for Gln-106 and Gln for Arg-262 substitutions).[2] A similarly affected brother was also reported. The phenotypically normal parents and a normal sister proved to be heterozygous, suggesting that the partial hypogonadotropic hypogonadism is transmitted as an autosomal recessive trait.

Expression vectors encoding the wild-type and mutant receptors were used to transfect COS-7 cells in order to study binding of GnRH to its receptor and the stimulation of cellular phospholipase C activity. The Gln 106 Arg substitution, localized to the first extracellular loop, markedly impaired binding of GnRH to its receptor and its ability to stimulate the activity of cellular phospholipase C. The Arg 262 Gln mutation, localized to the third intracellular loop, did not affect the binding of GnRH to its receptor but impaired GnRH-induced activation of cellular phospholipase C.

The partial phenotype encountered (resulting from the mutation of the GnRH receptor causing partial loss of function) raises the possibility that genetically determined cycling disorders may well be underestimated when the presentation is clinically subtle. Indeed, many of the entities discussed in this chapter represent extreme examples of reproductive dysfunction. It would therefore appear desirable for renewed attention to be paid to subtle forms of reproductive dysfunction and the possibility of an underlying genetic cause. Further studies will be necessary to establish the prevalence of mutations in the GnRH receptor and to devise appropriate tests to improve the detection of such patients. Clearly, mutations of the GnRH receptor gene should be considered in the differential diagnosis of hypogonadotropic hypogonadism.

## ISOLATED FOLLICLE-STIMULATING HORMONE DEFICIENCY

The first proband described presented with primary amenorrhea, sexual infantilism, and a sex steroid-responsive endometrium.[3–5] Physical findings revealed a eunochoid habitus (height > arm span) and limited secondary sexual characteristics. Dynamic pituitary testing revealed normal release of growth hormone, adrenocorticotropic hormone (ACTH), and thyroid-stimulating hormone (TSH). Evaluation of basal hormones disclosed high circulating levels of luteinizing hormone (LH), undetectable circulating levels of follicle stimulating hormone (FSH), and circulating levels of estradiol in the castrate range. Several years earlier, a cortical ovarian biopsy was performed disclosing an apparently normal complement of primordial follicles, thereby ruling out premature ovarian failure. Reasoning that replacement therapy was called for, Rabin et al[3] proceeded to provide the proband with a 14-day course of human menopausal gonadotropins, a bioactive LH- and FSH-containing preparation derived from the urine of postmenopausal subjects. Follow-up disclosed progressive increments in the circulating levels of estradiol coupled with enhanced production of cervical mucus, which indicates an estrogenic endpoint. After the provision of an ovulatory trigger (10 000 units of human chorionic gonadotropin or hCG) on day 14 of the simulated cycle, Rabin et al were able to document progressive increments in the circulating levels of progesterone as well as a basal body temperature shift, both compatible with presumptive ovulation. Conception was documented in due course.

It took over 20 more years before the molecular basis of isolated FSH deficiency was elucidated by Matthews and associates.[6] The clinical presentation and laboratory assessment of the proband reported by Matthews et al proved to be identical to those reported by Rabin and associates. Using the reasoning that the common α subunit (of pituitary glycoproteins) is unlikely to be the culprit, because LH proved to be both biologically and immunologically intact, Matthews et al focused on the FSH β subunit. Using leukocytic DNA, intronic primers for exons 2 and 3 (coding region of the FSH β subunit gene), PCR (polymerase chain reaction) amplification, and direct sequencing of the resultant PCR products, Matthews et al were able to demonstrate a two-nucleotide (T and G) frameshift deletion in codon 61, a finding predicted to produce a truncated version of the protein. Autosomal recessive transmission was ascertained, as the mother and a brother proved to be obligatory heterozygotes. Paternal DNA was not available for analysis. More importantly, based on established structure–function correlations,[6] the resultant protein product was predicted to lack key 'cassettes' that had previously been determined as essential to the promotion of steroidogenesis, the binding to specific cognate cell surface receptors, and the association with the common α subunit. In all probability, little if any functional heterodimeric FSH would be formed, thereby explaining the absence of FSH immuno- and bioactivity. A 14-day course of treatment with purified bioactive human FSH (Metrodin) yielded ovulation and conception in keeping with the observations of Rabin et al.

There was recently an additional report of isolated FSH deficiency resulting from mutations in the FSH β gene from Layman et al. The proband presented with clinical manifestations similar to those described by Mathews et al.[6] Molecular analysis of both FSH β alleles demonstrated the presence of a compound heterozygote mutation. One allele possessed the same premature stop mutation at codon 61 described by Mathews et al,[6] whereas the other allele possessed a T to G conversion in codon 51 of exon 3. This leads to the substitution of cysteine for glycine within the FSH β subunit. Both mutations are projected to have profound functional consequences on the FSH β subunit protein as described above.

As such, these observations documented that FSH is indispensible only during the last 14 days of the follicular life cycle, during which a secondary early antral follicle is recruited into the exponential growth phase leading to pre-ovulatory/graafian status. Qualitatively comparable phenotypic features were noted for the recently recorded murine knock-out paradigm.[8]

## HYPERGONADOTROPIC HYPOGONADAL OVARIAN FAILURE

In 1995, Aittomaki and associates described a cycling disorder attributable to mutations at the level of the FSH receptor.[9] This discovery was part of a larger concerted effort to delineate the genetic determinants of hypergonadotropic hypogonadal ovarian failure. To this end, Aittomaki et al embarked on a state-wide search for potential eligible subjects using karyotype and outpatient registries from a network of university hospitals in Finland. The study inclusion criteria consisted of primary or secondary amenorrhea before the age of 20, a 46XX karyotype, circulating FSH levels in excess of 40 mIU/ml (indicative of ovarian failure), a date of birth between 1950 and 1976, and no other known etiology of ovarian failure such as surgery, chemotherapy, or radiotherapy. At the conclusion of the survey, a total of 3856 subjects were found of whom only 75 proved to be eligible in terms of meeting the relevant inclusion criteria; 57 were labeled as sporadic in that they represented the sole affected individual in their family and the remaining 18 were labeled familial because they had similarly affected sibs. In all, one in 8300 newborn girls (46XX) in Finland was destined to develop hypergonadotropic

hypogonadism as a result of causes other than surgery, chemotherapy, or radiotherapy.

Armed with this information, Aittomake and associates undertook a conventional linkage approach using 37 subjects from six multiplex families. That effort localized the trait in question to the short arm of chromosome 2 (2p), the marker in question (D2S391) yielding a log of the odds (LOD) score of 4.71. As both the LH and FSH receptors were previously localized to the short arm of chromosome 2, Aittomake and associates undertook to sequence the FSH receptor gene in the subjects identified. Each exon was amplified by PCR and then analyzed for mutations by multiple approaches, including denaturing gradient gel electrophoresis and direct sequencing. PCR amplification of exon 7, using intronic primers and direct sequencing of the product, ultimately led to the discovery of the disease that caused mutation. The analysis revealed that 29% of the subjects studied displayed a single nucleotide missense mutation (a C to T conversion) at position 566 in exon 7 of the FSH receptor. This observation places the deranged protein sequence in the extracellular domain of the receptor, so suggesting a possible disruption of ligand binding. To establish the significance of this mutation. Aittomake et al undertook to transfect MSC-1 cells with mutant or wild-type cDNA constructs of the FSH receptor. The results indicated that cells transfected with mutant FSH receptor constructs displayed limited FSH receptor binding as well as limited FSH-induced generation of cAMP compared with wild-type-transfected (FSH receptor-expressing) counterparts. These findings suggested that the mutation in question is functionally significant and associated with reduced FSH receptor binding and activation of adenylate cyclase present. Interestingly, several of the subjects studied in this way underwent cortical ovarian biopsy, which revealed an apparently normal complement of primordial follicles, so ruling out premature ovarian failure.[10] Thus these findings reaffirm the notion that congenital FSH and/or FSH receptor deficiency is compatible with the formation of a morphologically intact follicular apparatus.

It may be of interest to note that a somatic

mutation at the level of the FSH receptor has recently been reported for nine of thirteen sex cord ovarian tumors and for two of three ovarian small cell carcinomas.[11] The mutation in question, a heterozygous T to C conversion at nucleotide 1777, changed the phenylalanine, normally at codon 591, to a serine. This sixth transmembrane domain mutation was not present in normal ovaries, non-sex-cord ovarian tumors, thyroid tumors, or leukocytic DNA, suggesting that the mutation in question is not a polymorphism. Assessment of the functional significance of the above mutation in COS-7 cells revealed all but absent FSH-stimulated cAMP production. These observations suggest that a somatic mutation at the level of the FSH receptor may play a role in the development of certain ovarian tumors.

## LH RESISTANCE

A cycling disorder attributable to mutations at the level of the LH receptor was first reported in 1996. The proband reported by Toledo et al[12] presented with prolonged periods of amenorrhea, punctuated by irregular episodes of apparently anovulatory uterine bleeding. Two brothers of the above proband have previously been reported to have Leydig cell hypoplasia attributable to a single missense mutation within the transmembranous region of the LH receptor.[13] Basal laboratory assessment of the female proband revealed a modest elevation of the circulating levels of gonadotropins. However, the circulating levels of estradiol, progesterone, 17α-hydroxyprogesterone, dehydroepiandrosterone, dehydroepiandrosterone sulfate, androstenedione, and cortisol all proved to be within normal limits. Leukocytic DNA and appropriate primers were used to amplify the region encoding the sixth transmembrane region of the LH receptor gene. The resultant PCR products were sequenced directly. The proband displayed a single nucleotide missense mutation (G to C) at position 1787, leading to an Ala 593 Pro substitution, a mutation identical to that observed in the two brothers.[13] Sequence analysis of the

paternal LH receptor revealed a heterozygous condition, suggesting autosomal recessive transmission. To establish the significance of the above mutation, Toledo et al designed mutant and wild-type cDNA constructs of the LH receptor in order to assess their function after transfection into human embryonic kidney 293 cells. The overall binding of hCG proved markedly reduced in mutant-transfected cells compared with wild-type-transfected counterparts. In addition, the ability of hCG to stimulate the generation of cAMP was practically negated in mutant-transfected cells compared with wild-type controls. These findings suggest that the single missense mutation at the transmembranous domain of the LH receptor was associated with a marked reduction in LH/hCG binding, as well as secondary reduction in the activation of the attendant adenylate cyclase. It is assumed that the mutation-induced perturbation of the transmembranous region may have affected the intracellular processing of the LH receptor, resulting in limited translocation of the mature protein to the plasma membrane.

In the same year, an additional proband was reported by Latronico et al;[14] the chief complaint of this woman was prolonged amenorrhea after a single episode of vaginal bleeding.[14] Sequencing of PCR-amplified exon 11 of the LH receptor gene revealed a nonsense mutation which produced a stop codon at position 1660. Inevitably, the resultant protein was truncated at a point beyond the fifth transmembranous loop. COS-7 cells transfected with a vector containing the mutant receptor exhibited no LH binding or LH-induced cAMP production, although COS-7 cells expressing the wild-type LH receptor were normal with regard to ligand binding and LH-induced cAMP generation. These results demonstrate that the truncated protein is biologically inactive because of the deletion of the region that encompasses not only the remaining two adjacent transmembranous loops but also the cytosolic component of the receptor.

Taken together, these observations document the existence of cycling disorders attributable to mutations at the level of the LH receptor.[15] Subject to the severity of the condition, LH resistance is not only associated with ovulatory failure but may also contribute to severe steroidogenic dysfunction because the folliculogenic process itself may also be deranged. Consequently, this clinical entity must be taken into account in the differential diagnosis of either primary or secondary amenorrhea. Although the full-blown variant of LH resistance may well constitute a rare phenomenon, the possibility cannot be ruled out that incomplete forms of LH resistance may be more common than previously thought. This testable hypothesis would require examples of subtle reproductive dysfunction to be screened for the possibility of loss of function mutations at the level of the LH receptor.

## REFERENCES

1. Mason AJ, Hayflick JS, Zoeller RT, et al. A deletion truncating the gonadotropin-releasing hormone gene is responsible for hypogonadism in the hpg mouse. *Science* 1986;**234:**1366–71.
2. de Roux ND, Young J, Mishrahi M, et al. Mutations in the GnRH receptor: A novel cause of hypogonadotropic hypogonadism. *N Engl J Med* 1997;**337:**1597–602.
3. Rabin D, Spitz I, Bercovici B, et al. Isolated deficiency of follicle-stimulating hormone. Clinical and laboratory features. *N Engl J Med* 1972;**287:**1313–17.
4. Rabinowitz D, Benveniste R, Linder J, et al. Isolated follicle-stimulating hormone deficiency revisited. Ovulation and conception in presence of circulating antibody to follicle-stimulating hormone. *N Engl J Med* 1979;**300:**126–8.
5. Spitz IM, Diamant Y, Rosen E, et al. Isolated gonadotropin deficiency. A heterogenous syndrome. *N Engl J Med* 1974;**290:**10–15.
6. Matthews CH, Borgato S, Beck-Peccoz P, et al. Primary amenorrhoea and infertility due to a mutation in the B-subunit of follicle-stimulating hormone. *Nature Genet* 1993;**5:**83–6.
7. Layman LC, Lee EJ, Peak DB, et al. Delayed puberty and hypogonadism caused by mutations in the follicle-stimulating hormone beta-subunit gene. *N Engl J Med* 1997;**337:**607–11.
8. Kumar TR, Wang Y, Lu N, Matzuk MM. Follicle stimulating hormone is required for ovarian follicle maturation but not male fertility. *Nature Genet* 1997;**15:**201–4.
9. Aittomaki K, Lucena JLD, Pakarinen P, et al. Mutation in the follicle-stimulating hormone receptor gene causes hereditary hypergonadotropic ovarian failure. *Cell* 1995;**82:**959–68.
10. Aittomaki K, Herva R, Stenman UH, et al. Clinical features of primary ovarian failure caused by a point mutation in the follicle-stimulating hormone receptor gene. *J Clin Endocrinol Metab* 1996;**81:**3722–6.
11. Kotlar TJ, Young RH, Albanese C, et al. A mutation in the follicle-stimulating hormone receptor occurs frequently in human ovarian sex cord tumors. *J Clin Endocrinol Metab* 1997;**82:**1020–6.
12. Toledo SPA, Brunner HG, Kraaij R, et al. An inactivating mutation of the luteinizing hormone receptor causes amenorrhea in a 46,XX female. *J Clin Endocrinol Metab* 1996;**81:**3850–4.
13. Kremer H, Kraaij R, Toledo SPA, et al. Male pseudohermaphroditism due to a homozygous missense mutation of the luteinizing hormone receptor gene. *Nature Genet* 1995;**9:**160–4.
14. Latronico AC, Anasti J, Arnhold IJ, et al. Brief report: testicular and ovarian resistance to luteinizing hormone caused by inactivating mutations of the luteinizing hormone-receptor gene. *N Engl J Med* 1996;**334:**507–12.
15. Themmen A, Brunner H. Luteinizing hormone receptor mutations and sex differentiation. *Eur J Endocrinol* 1996;**134:**533–40.

# Part III
# Polycystic Ovaries

# 4

# Molecular genetics of the polycystic ovary syndrome

Stephen Franks

**Physiological basis for the candidate gene approach • Investigation of candidate genes in the aetiology of the PCOS • Conclusion**

The polycystic ovary syndrome (PCOS) is the most common endocrine disorder in women of reproductive age. It is estimated to be the major cause of anovulatory infertility (accounting for 73% of cases) and of hirsutism.[1] In recent years, it has become clear that the PCOS is also associated with characteristic metabolic abnormalities which include hyperinsulinaemia, insulin resistance and dyslipidaemia.[1,2] These findings, in young women with the syndrome, have been linked to a significantly increased risk (six- to sevenfold) of type 2 or non-insulin-dependent diabetes mellitus (NIDDM) in later life.[3] In other words, diagnosis of the PCOS in young women may have major implications for long-term health.

The aetiology of the PCOS remains unclear. It is heterogeneous in its clinical and biochemical presentation and several possible causes have been suggested. The typical ovarian morphology – multiple follicles and increased stroma – and hypersecretion of androgens are almost invariable features and suggest that abnormalities of folliculogenesis and steroidogenesis are central to the disorder. Hyperinsulinaemia and insulin resistance are prominent features of patients with the 'classic'

syndrome (that is, anovulation and hyperandrogenism,[1,4] thus raising the question of aetiological role for insulin. Work in our laboratory, indicating that insulin has profound effects on steroidogenesis and ovarian stromal cell growth in both normal and polycystic ovaries, supports this concept.

There is strong evidence that genetic factors play a major part in the aetiology of the PCOS.[1,5] There is familial aggregation of cases but the mode of inheritance is far from clear. Clinical genetic data from this centre point to an autosomal dominant trait,[6] but results of our more recent studies suggest that more than one gene is likely to be involved in the aetiology of the PCOS, indicating that it is likely to represent a complex trait.[7] Taking a candidate gene approach, we have focused, primarily, on genes involved in androgen production and in insulin secretion or action.

## PHYSIOLOGICAL BASIS FOR THE CANDIDATE GENE APPROACH

### Ovarian androgens and the PCOS

*Clinical evidence for ovarian hyperandrogenism*
The ovary appears to be the main source of hyperandrogenaemia in the PCOS.[1] Selective suppression of the pituitary–ovarian axis by the chronic administration of agonist analogues of gonadotrophin-releasing hormone (GnRH) results in a fall in circulating androstenedione and testosterone, to levels that are similar to those in ovariectomized or menopausal women, whereas the slightly raised serum concentrations of the weak adrenal androgen, dehydroepiandrosterone sulphate (DHAS), remain unchanged by this treatment.[8]

A series of clinical studies by Rosenfield and colleagues have pointed to dysregulation of cytochrome P450c17α as a central abnormality in the genesis of excessive ovarian androgen production.[9,10] These workers assessed the response of the pituitary and ovary to a single dose of the GnRH agonist, nafarelin, in hyperandrogenaemic women with the PCOS, after suppression of adrenal androgen production by the administration of dexamethasone. They observed that serum concentrations of both androstenedione and 17-hydroxyprogesterone were significantly higher than normal both before and for 24 hours after nafarelin. Luteinizing hormone (LH) levels were also higher than normal but the difference in ovarian steroid response to GnRH agonist could not be explained on the basis of hyperresponsiveness of LH to GnRH agonist. These findings have since been confirmed in studies of both anovulatory women with the PCOS and hyperandrogenaemic women with polycystic ovaries who have regular, ovulatory cycles.[11]

These data support the concept of abnormal regulation of 17-hydroxylase/17,20-lyase activity in the ovary.[10] The finding of an equal degree of hyperandrogenaemia in ovulatory and anovulatory groups with polycystic ovaries,[11] even though LH levels were much higher in the latter, suggests that hypersecretion of LH is not the primary cause of ovarian hyperandrogenism. Hyperandrogenism in the PCOS may therefore represent an intrinsic abnormality of ovarian theca–interstitial cell function.

*In vitro evidence for ovarian hyperandrogenism in the PCOS*
Our hypothesis was that hypersecretion of androgens is an intrinsic function of the polycystic ovary. Production of androstenedione and its precursors by monolayer cultures of theca cells, obtained from nine women with polycystic ovaries, was studied and the results compared with those observed in theca cell cultures from five subjects with normal ovaries.[12] Accumulation of androstenedione (both basal and LH stimulated) in theca cell-conditioned medium was much greater (median 20-fold) in cultures from polycystic ovaries compared with normal ovaries. Production of 17-hydroxyprogesterone was also significantly (median sevenfold) higher than normal in polycystic ovarian theca cell cultures, suggesting increased activity of both 17-hydroxylase and 17,20-lyase. In addition, enhancement of steroidogenesis was also observed with respect to progesterone accumulation in culture medium (Figure 1). There was more overlap in progesterone production between normal and polycystic ovarian theca, but cells from polycystic ovaries nevertheless produced four to five times more progesterone than cells from normal ovaries.

The finding of greatly increased levels of androstenedione and 17-hydroxyprogesterone is consistent with the view that increased activity of 17-hydroxylase/17,20-lyase is an intrinsic feature of polycystic ovarian theca cells, but these data suggest the possibility that abnormal steroidogenesis by polycystic ovarian theca includes upregulation of the activity of cytochrome P450 cholesterol side chain cleavage (P450$_{scc}$). The magnitude of response of steroids to LH was similar in polycystic ovaries to that in normal ovaries which, taken together with the results of in vivo studies, implies that neither elevated serum concentrations of LH nor increased sensitivity of the ovary to LH can explain the profound differences in androgen

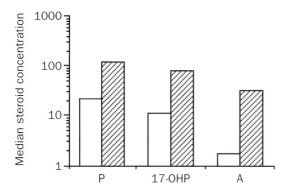

**Figure 1** Steroid concentrations (pmol/1000 cells/48 h) in theca cell cultures from normal and polycystic ovaries. Data bars shown are median values of progesterone (P), 17-hydroxyprogesterone (17-OHP) and androstenedione (A) in cultures of theca from 9 pairs of polycystic (shaded column) and 5 pairs of normal (blank column) ovaries (see Gilling Smith et al[12] and Franks et al[26]).

production between normal and polycystic ovaries.

## Abnormalities of insulin secretion and action in the PCOS

Women with the PCOS are both hyperinsulin-aemic and insulin resistant in relation to weight-matched control groups.[13,14] There is a close correlation between body fat topography and both hyperinsulinaemia and insulin resistance, so that, if polycystic ovary and non-polycystic ovary groups are matched for waist:hip ratio rather than body mass index, the difference in insulin concentrations and sensitivity between women with the PCOS and controls is no longer significant.[14] There is a complex interrelationship of hyperandrogenism, central adiposity and insulin resistance. Suppression of ovarian androgen production does not change the pattern of insulin secretion but, conversely, insulin stimulates androgen secretion.[1,13,14] Addition of insulin augments the androgen response to LH in human ovarian interstitial tissue in vitro and positive correlations have been observed between circulating concentrations of androgens and insulin.[1,13,14]

Insulin resistance in women with the PCOS can be distinguished, clinically and biochemically, from the rarer, genetically determined syndromes of severe insulin resistance (such as type A and leprechaunism) and can justly be regarded as a distinct aetiological entity.[13] Decreased sensitivity to insulin is found in peripheral tissues, notably muscle and adipose, but not in the liver.[13,14] The mechanism of insulin resistance in the PCOS remains the subject of much interest and speculation but the weight of evidence supports the view that there is a postreceptor defect which is characterized by an abnormality of serine–threonine phosphorylation in response to insulin.[15] Interestingly, serine phosphorylation appears to be an important step in post-translational regulation of 17,20-lyase activity in steroidogenic tissue.[16] These findings have lead Miller and colleagues[16] to put forward the hypothesis that a common, perhaps genetically determined, biochemical abnormality could result in both insulin resistance and hyperandrogenism in patients with the PCOS.

Hyperinsulinemia and insulin resistance are not universal features of women with hyperandrogenism. Hyperandrogenaemic women with polycystic ovaries who have regular menstrual cycles have fasting and glucose-stimulated serum insulin concentrations that are similar to those in weight-matched normal subjects.[4,17] Likewise, reduced insulin sensitivity is characteristic of women with the PCOS who have oligomenorrhoea or amenorrhoea, but equally hyperandrogenaemic, weight- and age-matched patients with polycystic ovaries who have regular cycles have normal insulin-mediated glucose disposal.[4] The probable explanation of this phenomenon is that hyperinsulinaemia/insulin resistance contributes to the mechanism of anovulation, for example, changes in insulin concentrations during energy intake restriction precede resumption of ovulatory cycles in obese women with the PCOS.[18]

The distinction in insulin dynamics between anovulatory and ovulatory women with equal degrees of hyperandrogenaemia is of some importance, both in assessing the role of insulin resistance in the aetiology of the PCOS and in determining which hyperandrogenic women may be at long-term risk of the metabolic and cardiovascular sequelae of insulin resistance. Thus, it seems unlikely that insulin resistance has an *obligatory* role in development of ovarian hyperandrogenism, although its presence may determine whether a woman with this condition becomes anovulatory.[19]

## INVESTIGATION OF CANDIDATE GENES IN THE AETIOLOGY OF THE PCOS

### Genes involved in androgen biosynthesis

*The 17-hydroxylase/17,20-lyase gene (CYP17)*
The physiological data regarding ovarian hyperandrogenism inevitably pointed to the 17-hydroxylase/17,20-lyase gene as a candidate in the genetic aetiology of the PCOS. Cytochrome P450c17α is the product of a single gene, *CYP17*, which has been localized to the long arm of chromosome 10 (10q24.3).[20] We investigated the possibility that polycystic ovaries are caused by an abnormality in the expression of *CYP17* in the ovary, leading to increased activity of cytochrome P450c17α. We performed a case–control study to investigate whether variation in the promoter region of *CYP17* was associated with polycystic ovaries.[21] Using linkage analysis, we also examined whether polymorphic, microsatellite markers close to the gene segregated with polycystic ovaries (or with the putative male phenotype – premature balding)[6] within the families, to determine whether this was likely to be the major causative gene.

A 459 base-pair (bp) fragment from the 5' promoter region of *CYP17* was generated by a polymerase chain reaction (PCR), using primers designed by reference to the published sequence of this area of the gene.[20] Heteroduplex analysis – a sensitive technique which allows the detection of a single base-pair mismatch[22] – was applied to the PCR product and revealed a single base change (substitution of a T by a C) 34 base-pairs upstream from the proposed site of the initiation of translation. This base change conveniently results in a recognition site for the restriction enzyme *MspA*1, leading to the generation of fragments of 124 and 335 bps in size (restriction fragment length polymorphisms or RFLPs), which can be identified after polyacrylamide gel electrophoresis of the DNA. Thus, the presence of the variant A2 allele can be detected by simple screening using RFLPs.

In our preliminary study, the prevalence of the variant, A2 allele was found to be as high as 69% in 71 consecutive patients with the PCOS whose DNA was examined. It was also found in 69% of affected family members (including 68% of men with premature balding). Examination of the appropriate control populations showed the prevalence of this allele to be around 40%.[21] The difference between affected and non-affected subjects was statistically significant and estimation of the odds ratios indicated that the presence of the variant allele conferred an increased 'risk' of polycystic ovaries of threefold in the general population and twofold within the families.

We were, however, surprised to observe that there was no correlation of genotype with serum testosterone concentrations. This prompted us to extend our study to include a larger population of both affected and control subjects and, on subsequent analysis, we found no significant difference in the prevalence of the A2 allele between the two groups.[23] This finding is in keeping with results of other studies which have since been published.[24,25]

From linkage analysis, using microsatellite markers close to *CYP17*, we were able to demonstrate that, despite the association of the variant A2 allele with affected status, *CYP17* could be excluded as the major gene causing polycystic ovaries or premature balding in the 14 families studied.[21]

In summary, a single base change has been found in the promoter region of *CYP17*, the gene encoding cytochrome P450c17α, which appears to a common, non-functional polymorphism and can be excluded as the primary genetic defect.

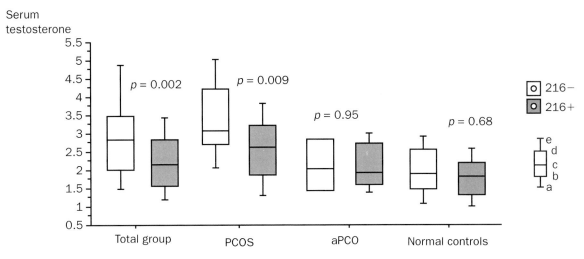

**Figure 2** Association of *CYP11a* with total serum testosterone levels (nmol/L) in a case control data-set. Values shown are 10th, 25th, 50th, 75th and 90th centiles (a, b, c, d, e respectively) of testosterone concentrations, grouped according to genotype (216− or 216+) in all subjects (total group), subjects with PCO *syndrome* (PCOS), asymptomatic PCO (aPCO) and normal controls (see Gharani et al[27]).

### The cholesterol side chain cleavage gene (CYP11a)

The results of studies of ovarian theca cells in culture, mentioned above, demonstrated that polycystic ovarian theca cells produce an excess of progesterone as well as 17-hydroxyprogesterone and androstenedione, suggesting that there is upregulation of P450$_{scc}$ as well as P450c.17.[12,26] We therefore turned our attention to the examination of *CYP11a* as a possible candidate gene for abnormal steroidogenesis.[27] Association (case–control) studies were performed in 148 consecutively recruited, premenopausal women with polycystic ovaries on ultrasonography and in 59 matched control women (with normal ovaries) from a similar ethnic background (all were white European). An informative, microsatellite marker in the promoter region of *CYP11a* was identified – a pentanucleotide repeat (tttta)$_n$, −528 bp from the AGT start of translation site. In the case–control study, subjects were allocated to

one of two groups according to the presence or absence of the most common polymorphism (216−). Our results showed that variation at the *CYP11a* gene was associated with both the PCOS and serum testosterone concentrations[27] (Figure 2).

We examined the segregation of *CYP11a* in 20 families: using a number of polymorphic markers in the region of *CYP11a*, we carried out non-parametric linkage analysis using the GENEHUNTER (multipoint linkage) program.[28] We found evidence for excess allele sharing (that is, linkage) at the *CYP11a* locus, giving a maximum non-parametric linkage (NPL) score of 3.03 ($p = 0.003$). The data from both association and linkage studies suggest that *CYP11a* is a major genetic susceptibility locus for the PCOS.

## Genes affecting the secretion or action of insulin

### The insulin receptor gene

The occurrence of peripheral insulin resistance in women with the PCOS (see above) raises the possibility that genetic abnormalities of the insulin receptor and/or postreceptor signalling are involved in the aetiology of the PCOS. There have been occasional reports of a PCOS-like phenotype occurring in patients with severe insulin resistance associated with defects of the insulin receptor gene.[29] Molecular screening of the insulin receptor gene in populations of well-characterized, hyperinsulinaemic women with the PCOS has, however, revealed no significant abnormalities.[30,31]

It remains conceivable that there is a genetic cause for the reported abnormality of serine–threonine phosphorylation in insulin signalling which was found in a significant proportion of women with typical PCOS studied by Dunaif and colleagues.[15] As mentioned previously, serine–threonine phosphorylation has recently been shown also to be involved in the post-translational regulation of 17,20-lyase activity (and therefore androgen secretion) in steroidogenic tissue.[16] It is possible, therefore, that there is a common aetiology for both insulin resistance and hyperandrogenism in the PCOS, although this seems, at present, somewhat speculative.

### The insulin gene variable number tandem repeat (INS-VNTR)

The results of recent studies have pointed to abnormalities of first phase insulin secretion in hyperinsulinaemic women with the PCOS.[32–35] Importantly, Holte and colleagues[35] have demonstrated that these abnormalities persist after weight reduction, despite improved insulin sensitivity, thus raising the question of a primary disorder in pancreatic β-cell function. We have therefore investigated the role of the insulin gene in the aetiology of the PCOS and, in particular, we examined the variable number tandem repeat (VNTR) minisatellite 5' to the insulin gene on chromosome 11p15.5, a locus that has been implicated in regulation of insulin

secretion and in susceptibility to NIDDM.[36]

We examined linkage of the PCOS to the 11p15.5 locus in 17 families with multiple cases of the PCOS. We also looked for an association between the insulin gene VNTR (particularly class I and class III alleles) and polycystic ovaries in two additional populations of women (all white European) presenting with symptoms of the PCOS at two different endocrine centres.[37] We looked for association of insulin VNTR genotypes with the PCOS using either a conventional case–control approach or (in a separate, independent population) by the use of affected family-based controls (AFBAC) and the related transmission disequilibrium test (TDT).[38]

We found that class III alleles were associated with the PCOS in each of the three populations and were most strongly associated with *anovulatory* PCOS. This is in keeping with the

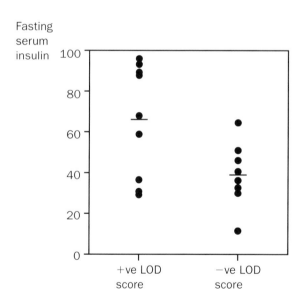

**Figure 3** Geometric mean (●) of fasting specific serum insulin (pmol/L) in each family, grouped according to whether polycystic ovaries in families are linked to *INS*-VNTR gene locus. (___ = mean value in each LOD [log of the odds] score group.) (From Waterworth et al.[37])

observation that hyperinsulinaemia is more prominent in women with polycystic ovaries who are anovulatory than in hyperandrogenaemic subjects with regular menses.[4,17]

We performed non-parametric linkage analysis (GENEHUNTER program) in those families with the PCOS using polymorphic markers in the region of 11p15 and found evidence for excess allele sharing at the *INS*-VNTR locus, giving a maximum NPL score of 3.250 ($p = 0.002$). Furthermore, we found that there was a relationship between fasting specific insulin levels and genotype[37] (Figure 3).

## CONCLUSION

The polycystic ovary syndrome is a familial condition. Clinical genetic studies have pointed to an autosomal dominant mode of inheritance but a complex trait with an oligogenic basis seems more likely. We have found evidence, so far, for the involvement of two key genes in the aetiology of the PCOS. The results of both linkage and association studies suggest that the steroid synthesis gene *CYP11a* and the insulin VNTR regulatory polymorphism are important factors in the genetic basis of the PCOS and may explain, in part, the heterogeneity of the syndrome. Thus, differences in expression of *CYP11a* could account for variation in androgen production in women who have polycystic ovaries. We postulate that those subjects carrying class III alleles at the insulin gene VNTR locus are more likely to be hyperinsulinaemic and to suffer from menstrual disturbances, and may be at higher than normal risk of NIDDM.

## REFERENCES

1. Franks S. Medical progress article: polycystic ovary syndrome. *N Engl J Med* 1995;**333**:853–61.
2. Dahlgren E, Johansson S, Lindstedt G, et al. Women with polycystic ovary syndrome wedge resected in 1956 to 1965: a long-term follow-up focusing on natural history and circulating hormones. *Fertil Steril* 1992;**57**:505–13.
3. Conway GS, Agarwal R, Betteridge DJ, Jacobs HS. Risk factors for coronary artery disease in lean and obese women with the polycystic ovary syndrome. *Clin Endocrinol (Oxf)* 1992;**37**:119–25.
4. Robinson S, Kiddy D, Gelding SV, et al. The relationship of insulin sensitivity to menstrual pattern in women with hyperandrogenism and polycystic ovaries. *Clin Endocrinol (Oxf)* 1993;**39**:351–5.
5. Simpson JL. Elucidating the genetics of polycystic ovary syndrome. In: *Polycystic Ovary Syndrome* (Dunaif A, Givens JR, Haseltine FP, Merriam GR, eds). Oxford: Blackwell Scientific, 1992: 59–77.
6. Carey AH, Chan KL, Short F, White DM, Williamson R, Franks S. Evidence for a single gene effect in polycystic ovaries and male pattern baldness. *Clin Endocrinol (Oxf)* 1993;**38**:653–8.
7. Franks S, Gharani N, Waterworth D, et al. The genetic basis of polycystic ovary syndrome. *Hum Reprod* 1997;**12**:2641–8.
8. Steingold K, De Ziegler D, Cedars M, et al. Clinical and hormonal effects of chronic gonadotropin-releasing hormone agonist treatment in polycystic ovarian disease. *J Clin Endocrinol Metab* 1987;**65**:773–8.
9. Barnes RB, Rosenfield RL, Burstein S, Ehrmann DA. Pituitary–ovarian responses to nafarelin testing in the polycystic ovary syndrome. *N Engl J Med* 1989;**320**:559–65.
10. Rosenfield RL, Barnes RB, Cara JF, Lucky AW. Dysregulation of cytochrome P450c 17 alpha as the cause of polycystic ovarian syndrome. *Fertil Steril* 1990;**53**:785–91.
11. White DW, Leigh A, Wilson C, Donaldson A, Franks S. Gonadotrophin and gonadal steroid response to a single dose of a long-acting agonist of gonadotrophin-releasing hormone in ovulatory and anovulatory women with polycystic ovary syndrome. *Clin Endocrinol (Oxf)* 1995;**42**:475–81.
12. Gilling-Smith C, Willis DS, Beard RW, Franks S. Hypersecretion of androstenedione by isolated theca cells from polycystic ovaries. *J Clin Endocrinol Metab* 1994;**79**:1158–65.
13. Dunaif A. Hyperandrogenic anovulation

(PCOS): a unique disorder of insulin action associated with an increased risk of non-insulin-dependent diabetes mellitus. *Am J Med* 1995;**98**:33S–9S.

14. Holte J. Disturbances in insulin secretion and sensitivity in women with the polycystic ovary syndrome. *Baillière's Clin Endocrinol Metab* 1996;**10**:221–47.

15. Dunaif A, Xia J, Book C-B, Schenker E, Tang Z. Excessive insulin receptor phosphorylation in cultured fibroblasts and in skeletal muscle. *J Clin Invest* 1995;**96**:801–10.

16. Zhang LH, Rodriguez H, Ohno S, Miller WL. Serine phosphorylation of human P450c17 increases 17,20-lyase activity: implications for adrenarche and the polycystic ovary syndrome. *Proc Natl Acad Sci USA* 1995;**92**:10619–23.

17. Dunaif A, Graf M, Mandeli J, Laumas V, Dobrjansky A. Characterization of groups of hyperandrogenic women with acanthosis nigricans, impaired glucose tolerance, and/or hyperinsulinemia. *J Clin Endocrinol Metab* 1987;**65**:499–507.

18. Kiddy DS, Hamilton-Fairley D, Bush A, et al. Improvement in endocrine and ovarian function during dietary treatment of obese women with polycystic ovary syndrome. *Clin Endocrinol (Oxf)* 1992;**36**:105–11.

19. Franks S, Robinson S, Willis D. Nutrition, insulin and polycystic ovary syndrome. *Rev Reprod* 1996;**1**:47–53.

20. Picado-Lenard J, Miller WL. Cloning and sequencing of the human gene for P450c17. *DNA* 1987;**6**:439–88.

21. Carey AH, Waterworth D, Patel K, et al. Polycystic ovaries and premature male pattern baldness are associated with one allele of the steroid metabolism gene *CYP17. Hum Mol Genet* 1994;**3**:1873–6.

22. Keen J, Lester D, Inglehearn C, Curtis A, Battacharya S. Rapid detection of a single base mismatch as heteroduplexes on HydroLinkgels. *Trends Genet* 1991;**7**:5–10.

23. Gharani N, Waterworth DM, Williamson R, Franks S. 5' polymorphism of the *CYP17* gene is not associated with serum testosterone levels in women with polycystic ovaries (letter). *J Clin Endocrinol Metab* 1996;**81**:4174.

24. Tetchatraisak K, Conway GS, Rumsby G. Frequency of a polymorphism in the regulatory region of the 17α-hydroxylase–17,20 lyase (*CYP17*) gene in hyperandrogenic states. *Clin Endocrinol (Oxf)* 1997;**46**:131–4.

25. Franks S. The 17α-hydroxylase–17,20-lyase gene (*CYP17*) and polycystic ovary syndrome (commentary). *Clin Endocrinol* 1997;**46**:135–6.

26. Franks S, Willis D, Mason H, Gilling-Smith C. Comparative androgen production from theca cells of normal women and women with polycystic ovaries. In: *Polycystic Ovary Syndrome* (Chang RJ, ed.). New York: Springer, 1996: 154–64.

27. Gharani N, Waterworth DM, Batty S, et al. Association of the steroid synthesis gene *CYP11a* with polycystic ovary syndrome and hyperandrogenism. *Hum Mol Genet* 1997;**6**:397–402.

28. Kruglyak L, Daly MJ, Reeve-Daly MP, et al. Parametric and non-parametric linkage analysis: a unified multipoint approach. *Am J Hum Genet* 1996;**58**:1347–63.

29. Moller DE, Flier JS. Detection of an alteration in the insulin receptor gene in a patient with insulin resistance, acanthosis nigricans and the polycystic ovary syndrome. *N Engl J Med* 1988;**319**:1526–9.

30. Conway GS, Avey C, Rumsby G. The tyrosine kinase domain of the insulin receptor gene is normal in women with hyperinsulinaemia and polycystic ovary syndrome. *Hum Reprod* 1994;**9**:1681–3.

31. Talbot JA, Bicknell EJ, Rajkhowa M, Krook A, O'Rahilly S, Clayton RN. Molecular scanning of the insulin receptor gene in women with polycystic ovary syndrome. *J Clin Endocrinol Metab* 1996;**81**:1979–83.

32. O'Meara N, Blackman JD, Ehrmann DA, et al. Defects in B-cell function in functional ovarian hyperandrogenism. *J Clin Endocrinol Metab* 1993;**76**:1241–7.

33. Ehrmann D, Sturis J, Byrne M, Karrison T, Rosenfield R, Polonsky K. Insulin secretory defects in polycystic ovary syndrome: relationship to insulin sensitivity and family history of non-insulin-dependent diabetes mellitus. *J Clin Invest* 1995;**96**:520–7.

34. Holte J, Bergh T, Berne C, Berglund L, Lithell H. Enhanced early insulin response to glucose in relation to insulin resistance in women with polycystic ovary syndrome and normal glucose tolerance. *J Clin Endocrinol Metab* 1994;**78**: 1052–8.

35. Holte J, Bergh T, Berne C, et al. Restored insulin sensitivity but persistently increased early insulin secretion after weight loss in obese women with polycystic ovary syndrome. *J Clin Endocrinol Metab* 1995;**80**:2586–93.

36. Bennett ST, Todd JA. Human type 1 diabetes and the insulin gene: Principles of mapping polygenes. *Annu Rev Genet* 1996;**30:**343–70.

37. Waterworth DM, Bennett ST, Gharani N, et al. Linkage and association of insulin gene VNTR regulatory polymorphism with polycystic ovary syndrome. *Lancet* 1997;**349:**986–9.

38. Spielman RS, Ewens WJ. The TDT and other family-based tests for linkage disequilibrium and association. *Am J Hum Genet* 1996;**59:**983–9.

# 5

# Polycystic ovary syndrome: mode of treatment

Adam Balen

**Definition of the PCOS/anovulatory infertility** • **Pre-treatment considerations** • **Ovulation-induction strategies** • **Medical therapies for inducing ovulation** • **Adjuncts to gonadotrophin therapy** • **Surgical ovulation induction** • **Medical or surgical ovulation induction? Arguments for and against**

The principles of the management of anovulatory infertility in women with the polycystic ovary syndrome (PCOS) are first to optimize health before starting therapy (for example, weight loss for those who are overweight) and then to induce regular unifollicular ovulation, while minimizing the risks of the ovarian hyperstimulation syndrome (OHSS) and multiple pregnancy. This chapter deals with the induction of ovulation and does not discuss broader issues, for example, whether women with regular ovulatory cycles and polycystic ovaries are less fertile than those with ovulatory cycles and normal ovaries. The issue of miscarriage is, however, discussed because it has a bearing on the successful outcome of treatment.

## DEFINITION OF THE PCOS/ANOVULATORY INFERTILITY

The polycystic ovary syndrome is one of the most common endocrine disorders, although its aetiology remains unknown. This heterogeneous disorder may present, at one end of the spectrum, with the single finding of polycystic ovarian morphology as detected by pelvic ultrasonography. At the other end of the spectrum, symptoms such as obesity, hyperandrogenism, menstrual cycle disturbance and infertility may occur either singly or in combination. Endocrine and metabolic disturbances (elevated serum concentrations of luteinizing hormone (LH), testosterone, insulin and prolactin) are common and may have profound implications for the long-term health of women with the PCOS.

In this chapter, the polycystic ovary syndrome is defined as the detection of polycystic ovaries by ultrasonography (enlarged ovaries with more than 10 cysts 2–8 mm in diameter, scattered either around or through an echodense, thickened central stroma)[1] plus symptoms of oligo-/amenorrhoea, obesity and hyperandrogenism (acne, hirsutism).[2] We studied over 1800 women with polycystic ovaries at the Middlesex Hospital, London, and found that the original descriptive triad of amenorrhoea, obesity and hirsutism (the Stein–Leventhal syndrome) appears to be at the extreme end of the disorder's spectrum.[2] Indeed, many women with polycystic ovaries detected by ultrasonography do not have symptoms of the PCOS, although symptoms may develop later in life, for example, after weight gain. Ovarian morphology appears to be the most sensitive marker for the PCOS compared with the classic endocrine features of a raised serum LH and/or testosterone concentration, which were found in only 39.8% and 47.8% of our patients, respectively, whereas the symptoms of obesity, hyperandrogenism (acne, hirsutism and alopecia) and menstrual cycle disturbances occurred in 38.4%, 70.3% and 66.2% of patients, respectively.[2] We therefore found it preferable to make the diagnosis of the polycystic ovary *syndrome* when, in addition to the ultrasound finding of polycystic ovaries, there are associated symptoms (menstrual irregularity, hyperandrogenization, obesity) or endocrine abnormalities (raised serum LH and testosterone concentrations).

It should be said from the outset that a universally agreed definition of either the polycystic ovary or the polycystic ovary *syndrome* is not available. The polycystic ovary is usually detected by ultrasonography, which correlates well with histopathological studies.[3,4] The original definition was provided by transabdominal ultrasonography,[1,5] which was used in recent publications.[2,6] Although Swanson et al[5] described a characteristic appearance without the need for a particular number of cysts, Adams et al[1] proposed a quantifiable definition, with a prerequisite number of at least 10 cysts in a single plane. It is now accepted that transvaginal ultrasonography provides greater resolution and the need to rethink the ultrasound criteria for the polycystic ovary.[7] Indeed, Fox et al[7] suggested the requirement of at least 15 cysts per ovary in their study. Apart from the number of cysts, it is necessary to consider the stromal thickness or density – the latter being a subjective assessment – and the ovarian volume, none of which is clearly defined.[8–10] Van Santbrink et al[11] have recently characterized the PCOS by taking values for the diagnostic criteria of the syndrome (increased follicle number and ovarian volume, elevated serum concentrations of testosterone, androstenedione and LH) as the 95th percentile of a control population. They found considerable overlap between the ultrasonographic and endocrine criteria for the

diagnosis of the PCOS in women with normogonadotrophic oligomenorrhoea or infertile women with amenorrhoea. The predictive value of polycystic ovaries detected by ultrasonography for endocrine parameters was, however, limited[11] – a finding supported by others.[12]

There have been many reviews over the years which have attempted to piece together the complexities of the syndrome;[13–22] these are beyond the scope of this chapter. It is fascinating to follow the evolving ideas on the spectrum and pathogenesis of the PCOS, but at the same time frustrating that a definition cannot be accepted. When we turn to the literature on the treatment of the condition, it is impossible to compare studies from different centres that use different starting points.

Hypersecretion of LH is associated particularly with menstrual disturbances and infertility. Indeed, it is this endocrine feature that appears to result in reduced conception rates and increased rates of miscarriage in both natural and assisted conception.[23] The finding of a persistently elevated early to mid-follicular phase LH concentration (> 10 IU/l with our assay) in a woman who is trying to conceive suggests the need to suppress LH levels by either pituitary desensitization, using a gonadotrophin-releasing hormone (GnRH) agonist, or laparoscopic ovarian diathermy. There are, however, no large, prospectively randomized trials that demonstrate a therapeutic benefit from a reduction in serum LH concentrations during ovulation induction protocols.

We and others have found that the patient's body mass index (BMI) correlated with both an increased rate of hirsutism, cycle disturbance and infertility.[2,24] Obese women with the PCOS hypersecrete insulin, which stimulates ovarian secretion of androgens and is associated with hirsutism, menstrual disturbance and infertility. It is seldom necessary to measure the serum insulin concentration, because this will not affect the management of the patient, but the prevalence of diabetes in obese women with the PCOS is 11%,[25] so a measurement of glucose tolerance is important in these women. Obese women (BMI > 30 kg/m$^2$) should therefore be encouraged to lose weight, because this improves the symptoms of the PCOS and improves the patient's endocrine profile.[24,26]

## PRE-TREATMENT CONSIDERATIONS

Although there is no doubt that a semen analysis should be performed before ovulation induction therapy is commenced, there is debate about the appropriate time for testing tubal patency. Until recently, if there had been no clear indication of the possibility of tubal damage (for example, past history of pelvic infection, pelvic pain), a reasonable policy was to delay a test of tubal patency until there had been up to three or even six ovulatory cycles. In the light of recent evidence suggesting a possible link between ovulation-induction therapy and a long-term risk of ovarian cancer (reviewed by Nugent et al[27]), we should perhaps now be thinking about performing a complete assessment of every woman before choosing her appropriate therapy. Tubal patency should therefore be assessed by either hysterosalpingography or laparoscopy before embarking on any form of ovulation-induction therapy.

## OVULATION-INDUCTION STRATEGIES

Once the diagnosis of anovulatory infertility has been made it is necessary to direct the patient to the appropriate therapy. It should be remembered, however, that the diagnosis is not absolute: amenorrhoeic women *are* anovulatory (although they may ovulate sporadically), whereas oligomenorrhoeic women may well ovulate erratically, albeit infrequently. Women with regular 4-weekly cycles have the opportunity to conceive 13 times a year, and with less frequent ovulations the chances of conception over a given period of time obviously decline. It is therefore appropriate to treat oligo-ovulatory women, but it is sometimes difficult to provide a unifying diagnosis for use when comparing the results of different treatments.

## Weight loss

An increasing BMI has been found to be correlated with an increased rate of hirsutism, cycle disturbance and infertility.[2,28] Even moderate obesity (BMI > 27 kg/m$^2$) is associated with a reduced chance of ovulation[29] and a body fat distribution leading to an increased waist:hip ratio appears to have a more important effect than body weight alone.[30] Obese women (BMI > 30 kg/m$^2$) should therefore be encouraged to lose weight. Weight loss improves the endocrine profile,[24,31] and the likelihood of ovulation and a healthy pregnancy. Achieving weight reduction is, however, extremely difficult, particularly as the metabolic status of a patient with the PCOS conspires against weight loss.[32,33]

A recent study by Clark et al[26] looked at the effect of a weight loss and exercise programme on women with at least a 2-year history of anovulatory infertility, clomiphene resistance and a BMI > 30 kg/m$^2$. The emphasis of the study was a realistic exercise schedule combined with positive reinforcement of a suitable eating programme over a 6-month period of time; 13 of the 18 women who enrolled completed the study. Weight loss had a significant effect on endocrine function, ovulation and subsequent pregnancy. Fasting insulin and serum testosterone concentrations fell and 12 of the 13 women resumed ovulation, 11 becoming pregnant (five spontaneously). Thus, with appropriate support, patients may ovulate spontaneously without medical therapy.

Weight loss should also be encouraged before ovulation-induction treatments are started, since they appear to be less effective when the BMI is greater than 28–30 kg/m$^2$.[34,35] Monitoring treatment is harder when the patient is obese and it may be difficult to see the ovaries clearly, thus risking multiple ovulation and multiple pregnancy. Furthermore, pregnancy carries greater risks in the obese (miscarriage, gestational diabetes, hypertension, problems with delivery),[34,36] which is a further incentive to lose weight.

## Weight reduction therapies

A number of agents have been used to aid weight loss, although there is really no substitute for a continued programme of exercise and diet. Appetite suppressants should be reserved for the extremely obese (BMI > 35 kg/m$^2$) because of the potential for serious adverse effects (for example, pulmonary hypertension) and close medical supervision is essential. Over the past 20 years or so it has increasingly become recognized that the PCOS and hyperinsulinaemia are intimately related[37–39] with respect to pathogenesis, endocrine disturbances and molecular genetics (see the literature[25,40–42]). Metformin inhibits the production of hepatic glucose and enhances the sensitivity of peripheral tissue to insulin, thereby decreasing insulin secretion.[43] It has been shown that metformin ameliorates hyperandrogenism and abnormalities of gonadotrophin secretion in women with the PCOS,[44–46] and can restore menstrual cyclicity and fertility.[47] Not all authors agree with these findings,[48] particularly if there is no weight loss with metformin therapy.[49] The insulin-sensitizing agent troglitazone also appears to cause a significant improvement in the metabolic and reproductive abnormalities in women with the PCOS,[50,51] although this product has unfortunately been withdrawn recently because of reports of deaths from hepatotoxicity. Newer insulin-sensitizing agents are currently being evaluated in phase III studies.

## MEDICAL THERAPIES FOR INDUCING OVULATION

### Clomiphene citrate/tamoxifen

Women with the PCOS who are anovulatory have traditionally been treated with antioestrogens (clomiphene citrate or tamoxifen) as first-line therapy. Clomiphene citrate has been available for many years, is administered orally for 5 days (usually starting on day 2 of a spontaneous or progestogen-induced bleed) and has on the whole not been closely monitored. It is now time to rethink this approach because there have been inadequate, prospective, randomized studies comparing the efficacy of clomiphene citrate with other therapies.

Clomiphene citrate induces ovulation in about 70–85% of patients, although only 40–50% conceive.[52] It has been suggested that the most important reason for reduced overall pregnancy rates with clomiphene citrate therapy is discontinuation of the therapy; cumulative conception rates approach 100% after 10 cycles, when corrected for those who discontinue therapy (which is possibly a rather biased approach to analysing data).[53] Nevertheless, there is no doubt that most cycles of clomiphene citrate treatment go unmonitored and it is recommended that at least the first cycle of treatment, if not all cycles, should be monitored with a combination of serial ultrasound scans and serum endocrinology.[54,55] Kousta et al[56] have recently reported their experiences in the treatment of 167 patients and also found good cumulative conception rates (67.3% over 6 months in those who had no other subfertility factors), which continued to rise up to 12 cycles of therapy. They reported a multiple pregnancy rate of 11%, similar to that described in other series, and a miscarriage rate of 23.6%, with those who miscarried tending to have a higher serum LH concentration immediately after clomiphene administration. Recent reviews about the safety of clomiphene citrate with respect to congenital anomalies indicate that there is no increased risk.[57,58]

Shoham et al[59] studied the hormonal profiles in a series of 41 women treated with clomiphene citrate, of whom 28 ovulated. In those who ovulated, 17 exhibited normal patterns of hormone secretion and 5 conceived, whereas 11 exhibited an abnormal response, characterized by significantly elevated serum concentrations of LH from day 9 until the LH surge, together with premature luteinization and higher serum levels of oestradiol throughout the cycle; none of the patients with this abnormal response conceived. This strengthens the argument for careful monitoring of therapy and discontinuation if the response is abnormal.

It is therefore useful to measure serum LH

levels in the mid-follicular phase (we aim for day 8 ± 1 day), and if they are abnormally high (> 10 IU/l) the chance of success is reduced and the rate of miscarriage raised. If there is an exuberant response to 50 mg, as in some women with the PCOS, the dose can be decreased to 25 mg. Antioestrogen therapy should be discontinued if the patient is anovulatory after the dose has been increased in consecutive cycles (up to 100 mg for clomiphene citrate or 40 mg for tamoxifen). A daily dose of more than 100 mg rarely confers any benefit. If the patient is ovulating, it is not necessary to increase the dose because conception is expected to occur at a rate determined by factors such as the patient's age etc. Clomiphene, via its antioestrogenic action, can cause thickening of the cervical mucus (although this is a matter of some debate) which may impede passage of sperm through the cervix. A postcoital test should be considered when treatment is started.

It is thought by some that doses of 150 mg or more confer no benefit;[56,60] they only worsen the side effects, particularly of a thickened cervical mucus, and might also have an antioestrogenic effect on the endometrium.[61] In the USA, the maximum dose of clomiphene citrate approved for use by the Food and Drug Administration (FDA) is 100 mg/day for 5 days. Some authors, however, have found that higher doses are required, particularly in women who are overweight.[62–64] Dickey et al[64] reported a series of 1681 pregnancies that occurred with a combination of clomiphene citrate and intrauterine insemination (in patients who did not necessarily have the PCOS and may have had other subfertility factors). They used doses of up to 250 mg for 5 days and found that overweight women required higher doses to achieve a pregnancy, with no apparent increase in the rate of miscarriage or multiple pregnancy.

Another approach for women who are unresponsive to 5 days of clomiphene citrate (≥150 mg) is to increase the duration of therapy to 10 days, which in one study enabled 14 previously unresponsive women to ovulate in 65% of 48 cycles, during which 5 conceived.[65] Alternatively, adjunctive therapy with naltrexone, which by its action as an opioid receptor blocker can normalize gonadotrophin secretion in women with the PCOS, has been found to increase the efficacy of clomiphene citrate in previously unresponsive patients.[66]

Another attractive approach in clomiphene-resistant patients is the administration of progesterone before clomiphene citrate treatment,[67] which at an intramuscular dose of 50 mg over 5 days caused a suppression of follicle-stimulating hormone (FSH) and LH secretion. LH levels fell in seven of ten women treated with progesterone, all became responsive to clomiphene (those whose LH levels were not suppressed remained unresponsive) and three conceived in the first cycle of treatment.

An ovulatory trigger in the form of human chorionic gonadotrophin (hCG) is very rarely required and should only be given if there has been repeated evidence of an unruptured follicle by ultrasound monitoring, as the majority (80%) of treatment cycles in which ovulation does not occur are characterized by failure of development of a dominant follicle.[68]

Clomiphene is currently licensed for only 6 months use in the UK because of the putative increased risk of ovarian cancer (there are no data on this association and tamoxifen). The paper on which this ruling was based found an association between clomiphene and ovarian cancer with more than 12 months of therapy and in most cases of prolonged use the indication was unexplained infertility rather than anovulation.[69] It would seem reasonable that patients should be counselled about the possible risks if treatment is to continue beyond 6 months; for example, some patients might not respond to a dose of 50 mg that has been prescribed for 3 months and then ovulate in response to 100 mg. They can expect an increasing cumulative chance of conception over at least the next 9 months and so it is reasonable to suggest that they take clomiphene for a total of 12 months, provided that a full explanation is given.[54,56] If pregnancy has not occurred after 10–12 normal ovulatory cycles, it is then appropriate to offer the couple assisted conception.

The therapeutic options for patients with anovulatory infertility who are resistant to antioestrogens are either parenteral gonadotrophin therapy or laparoscopic ovarian diathermy. Here lies another problem with definition, because some, including ourselves, consider clomiphene resistance to mean failure to ovulate (that is, no response), while others take it to mean failure to conceive despite ovulation (which we would call clomiphene failure). Here too is a cause of considerable confusion when it comes to comparing pregnancy rates with either gonadotrophin therapy or laparoscopic ovarian diathermy.

## Gonadotrophin therapy

Gonadotrophin therapy is indicated for women with anovulatory polycystic ovary syndrome who have been treated with antioestrogens if either they have failed to ovulate or they have a response to clomiphene that is likely to reduce their chance of conception (for example, persistent hypersecretion of LH, or negative postcoital tests resulting from the antioestrogenic effect on cervical mucus). Whether gonadotrophin therapy should be offered to women who have responded normally to clomiphene citrate but failed to conceive is another issue of some debate, with some (in particular manufacturers of gonadotrophin preparations) suggesting transfer to gonadotrophin therapy after six, or sometimes fewer, clomiphene-stimulated ovulatory cycles. In our experience there is a greater consensus for the view, argued above, in which there is provision of careful monitoring of clomiphene therapy and the assumption that, if conception has not occurred after 9–12 cycles of treatment, the next step is assisted conception and not alternative methods of ovulation induction.

It is essential to scrutinize carefully the criteria used to define patients who are selected for gonadotrophin therapy in published studies. It should be remembered that, using the criteria suggested above, that is, the 20% or so who are resistant to clomiphene therapy, it will be the most 'resistant' of patients who require gonadotrophin therapy. We have recently published the cumulative conception and livebirth rates in 103 women with the PCOS who did not

ovulate with antioestrogen therapy.[70] Although the cumulative conception and livebirth rates after 6 months were 62% and 54%, respectively, and after 12 months 73% and 62%, respectively, the rate of multiple pregnancy was 19% and there were three cases of moderate-to-severe ovarian hyperstimulation syndrome. We found that the rate of multiple pregnancy fell to 4% after the introduction of real-time transvaginal ultrasonographic monitoring of follicular development. This emphasizes the central role of effective surveillance in programmes of ovulation induction. If conception has failed to occur after six ovulatory cycles in a woman younger than 25 years, or after 12 ovulatory cycles in women aged over 25, then it can be assumed that anovulation is unlikely to be the cause of the couple's infertility and assisted conception (usually in vitro fertilization) is now indicated.

Gonadotrophins are available in the form of human menopausal gonadotrophins derived from urine (hMG) or FSH. The gonadotrophins are glycoprotein hormones, with the degree of glycosylation affecting the biological activity (half-life) (see Rose et al[71] for a recent review). This can only be measured by bioassay and not by immunoassay. Pharmacopoeial monographs taking account of the inherent precision of the methods in bioassays allow 95% confidence limits of 80–125% of the stated dose on estimates of activity, that is, between 60 and 94 units of activity in a 75 unit ampoule (a potential variation of up to 57% between ampoules from different batches). The same pharmacopoeial requirements apply to the recombinantly derived FSH preparations. There is also evidence that there is heterogeneity between the different recombinantly derived preparations. The preparations of hMG are administered intramuscularly, although more highly purified preparations can now be given by subcutaneous injection, which can be self-administered and appear to be tolerated better by the patient.

Our current protocol is that treatment with gonadotrophins should be commenced within the first 5 days of a natural or induced menstrual bleed, when pelvic ultrasonography indicates that the endometrium is thin (< 6 mm in depth) and that there are no ovarian cysts. The initial dose, until recently one ampoule per day of either hMG (75 IU FSH + 75 IU LH) or FSH (75 IU), is increased by one ampoule per day after 14 days in the first cycle of treatment (and 7 days in subsequent cycles) if there is an inadequate response, as assessed by ultrasonography. There is no value in increasing the initial dose before the fifth day (at the earliest) because recruitment of follicles takes between 5 and 15 days. Further increases are made at 4- to 7-day intervals. In subsequent cycles the starting dose is determined by the patient's previous response and can be reduced in some cases to half an ampoule and increased in others to two ampoules per day.[54]

To prevent the risks of overstimulation and multiple pregnancy, the traditional standard step-up regimens (when 75–150 IU are increased by 75 IU every 3–5 days)[72–74] have been replaced by either low-dose step-up regimens[70,75–78] or step-down regimens.[79] The low-dose step-up regimen employs a starting dose usually of 1 ampoule (or as low as 37.5 IU), which is only increased after 14 days if there is no response and then by only half an ampoule every 7 days.[76] Treatment cycles using this approach can be quite long – up to 28–35 days – but the risk of multiple follicular growth appears to be small compared with conventional step-up regimens. With the 'step-down' protocol, follicular recruitment is achieved using two or three ampoules daily for 3–4 days before decreasing the dose to one ampoule to maintain follicular development.[79,80] Experimental studies have indicated that initiation of follicular growth requires a 10–30% increment in the dose of exogenous FSH and the threshold changes with follicular growth, caused by an increased number of FSH receptors, so that the concentration of FSH required to maintain growth is less than that required to initiate it.[81] More recently, a 'sequential', step-up, step-down protocol has been employed, in which the FSH threshold dose is reduced by half when the leading follicle has reached 14 mm.[82] This approach also appears to reduce the number of lead follicles when compared with a classic step-up protocol.[82]

The rationale behind the development of low-dose stimulation regimens is to reduce the risks of both multiple pregnancy and the ovarian hyperstimulation syndrome (OHSS), both of which are increased in women with polycystic ovaries compared with those with normal ovaries. The reduction in these harmful side effects has been further aided by the use of transvaginal ultrasonographic monitoring; in the early days of the development of gonadotrophin therapy the only means of monitoring treatment was the measurement of urinary oestrogen metabolites – at best a semiquantitative system.

Ovulation is triggered with a single intramuscular injection of hCG 10 000 units (occasionally 5000 units are given). The inclusion criterion for hCG administration should be the development of at least one follicle that is at least 17 mm in its largest diameter, and there may be some benefit to waiting until the largest follicle is over 20 mm.[83] To reduce the risks of multiple pregnancy and the OHSS, the exclusion criteria for hCG administration are the development of two or more follicles larger than 16 mm in diameter and/or more than four follicles larger than 14 mm in diameter. In overstimulated cycles hCG is withheld, and the patient counselled about the risks and advised to refrain from sexual intercourse.

Multiple pregnancy and OHSS are avoidable and this should be a matter, not of controversy, but of responsible clinical practice. Multiple pregnancy is an undesirable side effect of fertility therapy because of the increased rates of perinatal morbidity and mortality. In the UK it is the unmonitored use of oral antioestrogens that accounts for more cases of triplets than gonadotrophin therapy or assisted conception.[84] High-order multiple pregnancies (quadruplets or more) result almost exclusively from ovulation-induction therapies.[86] Gonadotrophins should be given in low doses to women with anovulatory infertility and strict criteria employed before the administration of the ovulatory trigger. Hull[86] reviewed the results of six studies of conventional dose gonadotrophin therapy (111 patients) and compared them with six studies of low-dose therapy (243 patients). The pregnancy rates per cycle (23%) and per ovulatory cycle (30%) were higher in the standard dose cycles than during low-dose therapy (11% and 15%, respectively). The miscarriage rate was also lower in the standard dose cycles (17% versus 37%), resulting in an ongoing pregnancy rate per cycle of 20% compared with 7% in the low-dose cycles. The multiple pregnancy rate was, however, 23% in the standard dose cycles compared with 9% in the low-dose cycles. Homburg et al[87] compared 25 women treated with a conventional protocol with 25 treated with a low-dose protocol, and found a slightly higher pregnancy rate with the latter (40% vs 24% – not significant) and no multiple pregnancies or cases of OHSS, compared with 33% and 11%, respectively, in the conventional group.

It can be extremely difficult to predict the response to stimulation of a woman with polycystic ovaries – indeed this is the greatest therapeutic challenge in all ovulation-induction therapies. The polycystic ovary is characteristically quiescent – at least when viewed by ultrasonography – before exhibiting an exuberant and explosive response to stimulation. It can be very challenging to stimulate the development of a single dominant follicle and, although attempts have been made to predict a multifollicular response[88] by looking at midfollicular endocrine profiles and numbers of small follicles, it is harder to do so before starting ovarian stimulation and hence to determine the required starting dose of gonadotrophin. To prevent OHSS and multiple pregnancy, however, the strategy of cancelling cycles on day 8 of stimulation, if there are more than seven follicles ($\geq$8 mm) and an FSH:LH ratio of $\geq$1.6[88] would seem to be reasonable.

White and colleagues[89] have recently reported their extensive experience of the low-dose regimen in 225 women, over 934 cycles of treatment, resulting in 109 pregnancies in 102 women (45%). Seventy-two per cent of the cycles were ovulatory (fewer than 5% of patients failed to ovulate) and 77% of these were uniovulatory. The multiple pregnancy rate was 6%. Despite the low-dose protocol 18% of cycles were abandoned because more than three large follicles developed – a further reminder of the sensitivity of the polycystic ovary even when attempts are made to reduce the response. At the start of their series the initial starting dose was 75 IU but this was reduced to 0.7 of an ampoule (that is, 52.5 IU) for the last 429 cycles of treatment in order to try to reduce further the rate of multiple follicle development (84% of ovulatory cycles with the lower starting dose were uniovulatory). The incidence of cancelled cycles due to more than three follicles developing was 13.5% (58/429) and the multiple pregnancy rate was still 6%. Starting with 52.5 IU unfortunately did not result in a reduction in complications. However, compared to their previously reported series a relatively high miscarriage rate of 35% was associated with the higher starting dose and this fell to 20% with the 52.5 IU starting dose.[89] Once again it was noted that the only factor that influenced the outcome significantly was the patient's BMI. Those with a BMI of over 25 kg/m$^2$ had a higher rate of abandoned cycles (31% vs 15% in those of normal weight), a lower cumulative conception rate over six cycles (46.8% vs 57% for the whole group) and a miscarriage rate of 31%. This confirms earlier findings of the adverse effects of obesity on outcome.[34]

We have recently reported the first observational study of the use of recombinantly derived FSH (Follitropin beta, Puregon) in the induction of ovulation in 11 patients with clomiphene-resistant PCOS using a starting dose of 50 IU FSH and increasing by 50 IU after 7 days.[90] All of the patients exhibited a follicular response: six ovulated of whom two conceived. Four (36%) were cancelled because of overstimulation and one was anovulatory despite the development of a follicle. We have therefore demonstrated that like urinary FSH[89] recombinant FSH (rFSH) can be used to stimulate follicular growth at a starting dose of 50 IU; however a reduction in complications was not demonstrated.

There are many published series in the literature which support the notion that carefully conducted ovulation-induction therapy results in good cumulative conception rates in women with the PCOS. It is beyond the scope of this chapter to provide details of each publication and interested readers are referred to some relevant references: Schoot et al;[91] Fauser;[92] Schoot;[93] van Santbrink et al;[94] Tadokoro et al.[95]

## Different gonadotrophin preparations

The 'purified' FSH preparations, or those with a reduced LH content, seem to confer no therapeutic advantage over hMG, as described in small comparative studies, since the LH content in hMG is low in comparison with the endogenous secretion of LH.[96–99] Some pharmacokinetic studies indicate a significant difference when hMG and FSH are administered. LH levels decrease significantly more after FSH vs HMG administration.[100,101] It is our experience that serum LH concentrations usually fall in response to normal ovarian–pituitary feedback as the dominant follicle grows, although some women with the PCOS continue to oversecrete LH in the presence of follicular growth – a phenomenon that may result from disordered production of non-steroidal ovarian factors in these patients.[102]

There have been two meta-analyses carried out on FSH vs HMG treatment. In one, of eight randomized studies of patients undergoing in vitro fertilization (IVF), treatment with FSH resulted in 50% higher pregnancy rates[103] with an overall odds ratio of 1.71 (95% CI = 1.12–2.62). In a second study in OI, there was no difference in terms of pregnancy rates, but FSH appeared to be associated with a reduction in moderate to severe OHSS (odds ratio 0.2, 95% CI = 0.009–0.46).[104] Arguably, the papers that made up the meta-analysis had small numbers and the result was skewed by small studies that needed to be combined in order to achieve significance – a possible drawback of such reviews.[105]

## ADJUNCTS TO GONADOTROPHIN THERAPY

A number of pre-stimulation protocols have been used in order to suppress endogenous pituitary gonadotrophin secretion and ovarian activity before commencing gonadotrophin therapy. These include 2–3 months of the combined oral contraceptive pill or a GnRH agonist for 6–8 weeks. It is our view that this approach simply prolongs the treatment cycle, resulting in fewer ovulations and hence fewer chances of conception in a given period of time without conferring a significant benefit on the pregnancy rates.

### GnRH agonists

Hypersecretion of LH has a profound effect on conception and miscarriage.[23,106] Initial, non-randomized reports of GnRH agonist therapy in the PCOS described encouraging rates of pregnancy,[107] but prospective randomized studies have indicated that GnRH agonists provide no benefit over hMG therapy alone and, in particular, do not reduce the tendency of the polycystic ovary to multifollicular development, cyst formation or the OHSS.[97,108,109] Miscarriage related to LH hypersecretion is one condition that might benefit from pituitary desensitization, as suggested by preliminary studies of women with polycystic ovaries undergoing ovulation induction for in vivo and in vitro fertilization.[110–112]

One potential advantage of the use of GnRH agonists is to enable accurate timing of ovulation and hence either intercourse or intrauterine insemination (the latter being used by some to enhance the efficacy of treatment further). Luteal support is, of course, required after a GnRH agonist is used either throughout the follicular phase[113] or simply instead of hCG to trigger ovulation.[114] The latter is an approach for preventing the development of the OHSS.[115]

Pulsatile GnRH has been used in an attempt to stimulate unifollicular growth in women with the PCOS and thereby avoid the risks of exogenous gonadotrophins. Rates of ovulation are, however, disappointing[35,116] and miscarriage rates are as high as 45%.[35,117] Pulsatile GnRH therapy is ideally suited to women with hypogonadotrophic hypogonadism and it is interesting that some women with this condition also have polycystic ovaries, responding in a typically 'polycystic' fashion to stimulation with respect to both ultrasonographic and endocrine findings.[118,119] The effect of pulsatile GnRH may be improved when given together with gonadotrophins[120] or clomiphene citrate,[121] or after pre-treatment with an GnRH agonist.[35] Alternatively GnRH antagonists have been proposed as a possible therapy to permit normalization of LH secretion when exogenous pulsatile GnRH is superimposed.[122] Although there was certainly an improvement in the endocrinopathy, an ovarian response was not obtained and so the theoretical promise of this approach has not been pursued.[122] Thus pulsatile GnRH therapy is rarely used nowadays for women with the PCOS.[123]

*Growth hormone and somatostatin*
The co-administration of growth hormone with gonadotrophins showed initial promise, particularly in women with pituitary insufficiency (and hence growth hormone deficiency) or those with elevated serum FSH concentrations.[124] Growth hormone is not, however, now thought to have a significant role as a cogonadotrophin in the treatment of anovulatory PCOS.[124] The long-acting somatostatin analogue octreotide suppresses the hyperinsulinaemia, hyperandrogenaemia and LH concentrations in women with the PCOS, and improves the endocrine milieu and ovulatory performance when given with hMG,[125] but, perhaps because of cost or complexity of therapy, has yet to be widely adopted.

## SURGICAL OVULATION INDUCTION

### Laparoscopic ovarian surgery

Laparoscopic ovarian surgery has replaced ovarian wedge resection as the surgical treatment for clomiphene resistance in women with the PCOS. It is free of the risks of multiple pregnancy and ovarian hyperstimulation and does not require intensive ultrasound monitoring. Furthermore, ovarian diathermy appears to be as effective as routine gonadotrophin therapy in the treatment of clomiphene-insensitive PCOS.[126–128] In addition, laparoscopic ovarian surgery is a useful therapy for anovulatory women with the PCOS who fail to respond to clomiphene and who either persistently hypersecrete LH, need a laparoscopic assessment of their pelvis or who live too far away from the hospital to be able to attend for the intensive monitoring required of gonadotrophin therapy.

Surgery does of course carry its own risks and should be performed only by properly trained laparoscopic surgeons.

### Wedge resection

Resection of the ovaries was initially described by Stein and Leventhal[129] at the time that polycystic ovaries were diagnosed during a laparotomy. It was found that ovarian biopsies taken to make the diagnosis led to subsequent ovulation. The rationale was to 'normalize' ovarian size and hence the endocrinopathy by removing between 50% and 75% of each ovary. Until the introduction of clomiphene citrate therapy in 1961, wedge resection was the only treatment for anovulatory PCOS, and it is interesting to note that, despite this, over a 30-year period such great care was taken in the selection of patients for treatment that Stein reported a personal experience of only 108 cases.[130] Stein found that 95% of patients resumed normal menstrual cycles and 87% of those wishing to conceive did so on at least one occasion. Furthermore he stated that surgery cured the condition such that the ovarian pathology did not recur.[131,132]

A large review of 187 reports summarized data on 1079 ovarian wedge resections, with an overall rate of ovulation of 80% and pregnancy of 62.5% (range: 13.5–89.5%).[13] Another 30 or so years later Donesky and Adashi[25] were able to increase the summated experience in the literature to 1766 treatments, with an average pregnancy rate of 58.8%. Wedge resection went out of favour in the 1970s because of the realization that there was significant postoperative adhesion formation and that initial favourable reports of pregnancy rates were not sustained.[133–135] In one series of seven patients, all were found to have extensive pelvic adhesions after wedge resection.[136] A microsurgical approach has been recommended,[137] but this did not become popular. The operation is therefore rarely performed these days. Donesky and Adashi[127] provide an excellent history of the surgical management of the PCOS, which is recommended for a more comprehensive overview.

## Mechanism of action of wedge resection/laparoscopic ovarian surgery and endocrine changes

An unfortunate feature of most of the papers that describe wedge resection is the poor characterization of the patients, so that many appear to have been ovulating before treatment. This problem is also a feature in many of the papers that describe laparoscopic treatment, so that it is unclear whether patients are anovulatory before treatment, let alone whether they have polycystic ovaries in all cases. Herein lie further problems, as already described for medical ovulation induction therapies, in comparing the results from different published series.

Another issue that is difficult to qualify is the aim of the surgery, that is, whether the surgery is directed at reducing ovarian volume, destroying the cysts or stroma or causing non-specific local tissue injury. The uncertainties concerning the aim of the surgery stem in part from incomplete understanding about its mechanism of action. Is the restoration of cyclical ovarian activity a result of (1) reducing the size of enlarged ovaries, (2) reducing abnormal hormone secretion (for example, testosterone), (3) reducing secretion of inhibitory factors (for example, inhibin), (4) sensitizing the (smaller) ovary to circulating gonadotrophins, (5) the release of growth factors in response to injury which augment the effect of FSH on folliculogenesis, or (6) complete destruction of the cysts allowing the development of new follicles?

Whatever the mechanism of action of laparoscopic ovarian surgery, there is no doubt that with restoration of ovarian activity serum concentrations of LH and testosterone fall. The endocrine changes after ovarian diathermy have been explored in detail by a number of groups. Greenblatt and Casper[138] studied six patients and found that serum androgen concentrations fell to a nadir by the third postoperative day and that this preceded a fall in serum oestradiol and LH concentrations, which then coincided with a rise in serum FSH concentration by days 2–3. It was postulated that ovarian trauma impaired local production of androgens and hence a reduction in extraovarian production of oestrone, which in turn would decrease positive feedback on LH secretion. Negative feedback on FSH secretion would diminish concurrently, caused by both a decrease in peripheral oestrogens and also, possibly, ovarian inhibin.[138] Abdel Gadir et al[139] found a significant fall in serum LH and testosterone concentrations and examined LH pulse frequency, which was unaltered following laparoscopic ovarian diathermy (LOD). In a study of 11 patients treated by laser to the ovary, Rossmanith et al[140] also noted no change in pulse frequency of LH secretion and observed an attenuation in GnRH-stimulated LH after treatment, suggesting an alteration of ovarian–pituitary feedback which affects the sensitivity of the pituitary to GnRH.

In two small series ovulation was induced in about 70% of patients and the serum testosterone concentrations fell significantly, although there was no change in the mean serum LH concentrations.[141,142] Naether et al[143] observed a decline in serum androgen concentrations and a slight increase in serum gonadotrophin levels. Most series, however, report a fall in both androgen and LH concentrations and an increase in FSH concentrations.[140,144–146] A fall in serum LH concentrations both increases the chance of conception and reduces the risk of miscarriage, as demonstrated by Armar and Lachelin,[147] who observed a miscarriage rate of 14% in 58 pregnancies compared with the expected miscarriage rate of 30–40% seen in reports of hormonal induction of ovulation in women with the PCOS.[104]

Whether patients respond to LOD appears to depend on their pre-treatment characteristics, with patients with high basal LH concentrations having a better clinical and endocrine response.[148] In Abdel Gadir's study[148] it was found that the pre-treatment testosterone level, BMI or ovarian volume could not be used to predict outcome. We performed a small prospective study in which women were randomized to receive either unilateral or bilateral LOD.[149] We found that unilateral diathermy restored bilateral ovarian activity, with the contralateral, untreated ovary often being the first to ovulate after the diathermy treatment. We also found that the only significant difference between the responders and non-responders was a fall in serum LH concentration after diathermy.

Although the mechanism of ovulation induction by LOD is uncertain, it appears that minimal damage to an unresponsive ovary either restores an ovulatory cycle or increases the sensitivity of the ovary to exogenous stimulation. Furthermore, the finding of an attenuated response of LH secretion to stimulation with GnRH[140] suggests an effect on ovarian–pituitary feedback and hence pituitary sensitivity to GnRH. Our study goes one step further by demonstrating that unilateral diathermy leads to bilateral ovarian activity, suggesting that ovarian diathermy achieves its effect by correcting a perturbation of ovarian–pituitary feedback.[149] Our own hypothesis is that the response of the ovary to injury leads to a local cascade of growth factors and those such as insulin-like growth factor I (IGF-I), which interact with FSH, result in stimulation of follicular growth and the production of the hormone gonadotrophin surge attenuating/inhibitory factor (GnSAF/GnSIF), which in turn leads to a fall in serum LH concentrations.[149]

## Methods of laparoscopic ovarian surgery and results

Laparoscopic surgery has several obvious advantages over laparotomy and was first reported by Palmer and de Brux[150] some years after the invention of their ovarian biopsy forceps. The initial reports were of multiple biopsies with additional cautery only to stop bleeding. Commonly employed methods for laparoscopic surgery include monopolar electrocautery (diathermy)[36] and laser[151] whereas multiple biopsy alone is less commonly used. In the first reported series, ovarian diathermy resulted in ovulation in 90% and conception in 70% of the 62 women treated.[36] The outcome of 62 pregnancies was no different from the normal population[152] and the miscarriage rate was 15%.

A number of subsequent studies have produced similarly encouraging results, although the techniques used and degree of ovarian damage vary considerably. Gjoannaess[36] cauterized each ovary at five to eight points, for 5–6 seconds at each point with 300–400 watts (W). Using the same technique as Gjoannaess, Dabirashrafi et al[153] reported mild-to-moderate adhesion formation in 20% of patients. Naether et al[143] treated 5–20 points per ovary, with 400 W for approximately 1 second. They found that the rate of adhesions was 19.3% and that this was reduced to 16.6% by peritoneal lavage with saline.[154] In an earlier study, Naether et al[155] found that the fall in serum testosterone concentration after diathermy was proportional to the degree of ovarian damage, with up to 40 cauterization sites being used in some patients. The greater the amount of damage to the surface of the ovary the greater the risk of periovarian adhesion formation. This lead Armar et al[144] to develop a strategy of minimizing the number of diathermy points. We have employed Armar's technique, in which the ovary is simply cauterized at four points. We have not performed routine follow-up laparoscopy on our patients, but the high pregnancy rate (86% of those with no other pelvic abnormality) reported by Armar and Lachelin[147] indicates that the small number of diathermy points used in our method leads to a low rate of significant adhesion formation.

The risk of periovarian adhesion formation may be reduced by abdominal lavage and early second-look laparoscopy, with adhesiolysis if necessary.[156] Others have also used liberal peritoneal lavage to good effect.[54,145] Greenblatt and Casper[157] found no correlation between the degree of ovarian damage and subsequent adhesion formation, nor did they find benefit from the adhesion barrier Interceed (Ethicon Ltd), as assessed by second-look laparoscopy. In another interesting study 40 women undergoing laser photocoagulation of the ovaries using a neodymium:yttrium–aluminium–garnet–(Nd:YAG) laser set at 50 W at 20–25 points per ovary were randomized to a second-look laparoscopy and adhesiolysis.[158] Of those who underwent a second-look laparoscopy adhesions that were described as minimal or mild were found in 68%, yet adhesiolysis did not appear to be necessary, because the cumulative conception rate after 6 months was 47% compared with 55% in the expectantly managed group (not significant).

The difficulty when deciding how to perform LOD is not knowing the 'dose–response' for a particular patient. Although we have shown that LOD using 40 W for 4 seconds in four places on one ovary can lead to bilateral ovarian activity and ovulation (our usual protocol involves the same on each ovary),[149] our ovulation rate was 50% and conception rate 40% (some patients were sensitized to exogenous stimulation). It has been proposed that the degree of ovarian destruction should be determined by the size of the ovary.[159] Naether has reported their method of laparoscopic electrocautery of the ovarian surface (LEOS) which causes greater destruction of the ovary than the method used by us, because they apply 400 W at 5–20 sites on each ovary.[159] Despite such a large amount of ovarian destruction, in Naether's series of 206 patients 45.2% of those who conceived required additional ovarian stimulation (with an 8% multiple pregnancy rate) and the overall miscarriage rate was 20%.[157] We also believe that we are dealing with different patient populations, because we only recommend operation for women with irregular, anovulatory cycles who have not responded to antioestrogen therapy, whereas in Naether's series about 24% of the women operated on had regular cycles and 15% were ovulating before their operation.

Although unilateral ovarian diathermy might be insufficient to induce spontaneous ovulations and pregnancies in all patients, we would like to quantify better the 'dose' of diathermy that is required and evaluate how it should be adjusted for individual patients. We therefore urge caution to those who practise any form of ovarian destruction because we believe that we should be striving to cause only the necessary damage in order to induce ovulation. In general, the correct dose of any therapy is the lowest one that works. Furthermore, a combined approach may be suitable for some women whereby low-dose diathermy is followed by low-dose ovarian stimulation. Ostrzenski,[160] for example, started all his

patients on either clomiphene or FSH therapy immediately after laser wedge resection and Farhi et al[161] also demonstrated an increased ovarian sensitivity to gonadotrophin therapy after LOD.

An additional concern is the possibility of ovarian destruction leading to ovarian failure – an obvious disaster in women wishing to conceive. Cases of ovarian failure have been reported after both wedge resection and laparoscopic surgery.[128,136] An unfortunate vogue has developed whereby women with polycystic ovaries who have over-responded to superovulation for IVF are subjected to ovarian diathermy as a way of reducing the likelihood of subsequent OHSS.[162] If one accepts that appropriately performed ovarian diathermy works by sensitizing the ovary to FSH (and ovarian diathermy certainly makes the clomiphene-resistant polycystic ovary sensitive to clomiphene)[127,144,149] then one could extrapolate that ovarian diathermy before superovulation for IVF should make the ovary more and not less likely to overstimulate. The amount of ovarian destruction that is required to reduce the chance of overstimulation is therefore likely to be considerable (as is indeed the case: MR Rimington, personal communication). We would therefore urge great caution before proceeding with such an approach because of concerns about permanent ovarian atrophy.

LOD appears to be as effective as routine gonadotrophin therapy in the treatment of clomiphene-insensitive PCOS.[126] Abdel Gadir et al[126] prospectively randomized 88 patients, who had failed to conceive after six cycles of clomiphene citrate, to receiving LOD, hMG or FSH. There were no differences in the rates of ovulation or pregnancy between the two groups, although those treated with LOD had fewer cycles with multiple follicular growth and a lower rate of miscarriage.[126] This is the only prospective randomized study to have attempted to compare the two therapies and it really should be repeated with larger numbers.

Laser treatment seems to be as efficacious as diathermy and it has been suggested that it may result in less adhesion formation,[151,163,164] although the only study to compare the two techniques was non-randomized, reported similar ovulation and pregnancy rates, and did not examine adhesion formation.[165] Various types of laser have been used from the $CO_2$ laser, to the Nd:YAG and KTP (potassium–titanyl–phosphate) lasers. As with the use of lasers in other spheres of laparoscopic surgery, whether laser or diathermy is employed appears to depend upon the preference of the surgeon and the availability of the equipment.

### Transvaginal approach

As early as 1938 Zondek attempted multiple follicular ovarian puncture through the cul de sac, with 'good success',[166] yet the transvaginal approach to the ovary, now so familiar to practitioners of IVF with transvaginal ultrasonography, has never really been developed. Paldi et al[167] performed culdoscopy and delivered the ovary into the vagina to do a classic wedge resection. More recently, Mio et al[168] performed transvaginal ultrasound-guided follicular aspiration in the midluteal phase of a cycle stimulated by a variety of ovulation induction agents. This strategy was chosen because these patients had failed to ovulate previously using their standard ovulation induction protocol. In Mio's study, hCG was administered when a follicle exceeded 18 mm in diameter and the patient was monitored daily for evidence of ovulation. If ovulation did not occur after 3 days, follicular aspiration of all persistent cysts (even < 10 mm) was undertaken. In subsequent cycles patients were stimulated with the same regimen (all received clomiphene with or without step-up hMG and prednisolone or bromocriptine). Two groups were established: eight patients had the PCOS and ten had ultrasonographic evidence of PCO without other manifestations of the syndrome. None conceived with the aspiration cycle. In the first group, seven of eight had at least one ovulatory cycle in the following 8 months. The overall rate of ovulation was 52.6% per cycle for this group. Three conceptions occurred in the second, fourth and fifth cycles after aspiration. In the second group all patients ovulated at least once, with an ovulation rate

per cycle of 63.3%. Five conceptions occurred in cycles 2, 4, 5, 7 and 10. We have been examining the response of unstimulated women with anovulatory PCOS who have undergone transvaginal, ultrasound-guided cyst aspiration for research into in vitro maturation of oocytes (K Hayden, P Wynn, A Rutherford and A Balen, unpublished observations) and have found so far that ovulatory cycles are restored without the aid of adjunctive ovulation induction therapy.

## MEDICAL OR SURGICAL OVULATION INDUCTION? ARGUMENTS FOR AND AGAINST

Compared with medical ovulation induction, the additional advantage of laparoscopic diathermy is that it need only be performed once and intensive monitoring is not required because there is no danger of multiple ovulation or ovarian hyperstimulation. Furthermore, only minimal ovarian damage is required to achieve this effect. We are, however, still unsure of the right dose of diathermy to stimulate the resumption of ovulatory cycles reliably. Nor are we certain about the degree of permanent damage done to the ovary by different amounts (duration, power, number of sites) of treatment. We are therefore currently performing studies to quantify the effects of different amounts of diathermy on cell death in the ovarian stroma and the oocyte pool.

One of the most cogent arguments for the use of LOD as a therapy is its avoidance of multiple pregnancy. The risks of multiple pregnancy are significant[169] with greater monitoring of the pregnancy being required, problems with prenatal screening (particularly if there is discordancy for abnormality), increased incidence of pregnancy-induced hypertension, antepartum haemorrhage, pre-term labour and surgical delivery. Neonatal mortality is seven times higher in twins than in singletons and 20 times higher in triplets and higher-order births, whereas survivors have an increased risk of cerebral palsy and other neurological impairments. Furthermore, multiple pregnancies that occur in subfertile women appear to fare worse than those in otherwise normal women.[169] Even if all children are born healthy, the parenting problems and stresses to the family unit are immense.

The possible association between epithelial ovarian cancer and ovulation-induction therapies has been widely discussed after a retrospective case-controlled study from the USA,[170] which did not provide adequate information about the drugs used and concerned a small number of cases of different histological types. Infertility is associated with an increased risk of ovarian cancer and suppression of ovarian activity (oral contraceptive use, pregnancy, etc.) reduces the risk. There might, therefore, be an association between induced multiple ovulations or superovulation therapies (for assisted conception procedures such as IVF) and ovarian cancer. Do the resultant pregnancies counterbalance this risk? The recent debate has alerted clinicians to study these associations further by careful follow-up of our patients, although there are, as yet, no reliable screening techniques for ovarian cancer. We have recently reviewed the literature on the association between ovulation induction and ovarian cancer and conclude, along with others, that more prospective data collection is required.[27] It is not known whether laparoscopic ovarian surgery causes sufficient epithelial damage to increase the long-term risk of ovarian cancer.

Unifollicular ovulation induction requires a subtle approach, particularly in women with the PCOS. Superovulation induction is, on the other hand, one of the least subtle of therapeutic procedures because the ovaries are farmed in the quest for eggs.[171] Although many eggs lead to the chance of many embryos, with the possibility of freezing some for later use, we have seen tremendous advances in assisted reproductive techniques. The ever-continuing improvements in the embryology laboratory might one day lead to improved chances of conception after the transfer of a single pre-embryo and so avoid the need for superovulation for IVF as well. Equally feasible is the prospect of in vitro culture of follicles or oocytes, and the avoidance of gonadotrophin therapy altogether, which has particular attractions for women with sensitive polycystic ovaries.

Gonadotrophin therapy adds appreciably to the cost of the treatment of assisted reproduction therapies (although it is hoped that the recombinant preparations will be produced in sufficient quantities to enable the prices to be reduced dramatically). It is, unfortunately, always necessary to discuss the financial costs of a treatment. These days with the high costs of gonadotrophins, even for unifollicular ovulation induction, there is little to choose between ovulation induction and laparoscopic ovarian diathermy. The potential financial costs of a multiple pregnancy, particularly if neonatal intensive care facilities are required, are of course immense. Other costs have to be counted in terms of the successful outcome of treatment with a low rate of miscarriage and the birth of healthy, preferably singleton, babies, with no health risks to their mothers. It is here that laparoscopic ovarian surgery appears to provide a significant advantage: it is a single treatment that results in unifollicular ovulation, with correction of the endocrinopathy and an apparent low rate of miscarriage. Although there are risks associated with surgery and an anaesthetic, women require a test of tubal patency before gonadotrophin therapy and so many would be subjected to a laparoscopy in any case. The main concern is the formation of adhesions and the potential for significant reduction in viable ovarian tissue, with the possibility of inducing premature ovarian failure. The evidence to date, however, is reassuring. The underlying principle of all methods of ovulation induction for women with the PCOS must always be to use the lowest possible dose (of drug or surgery) to achieve unifollicular ovulation.

## REFERENCES

1. Adams J, Franks S, Polson DW, et al. Multifollicular ovaries: clinical and endocrine features and response to pulsatile gonadotrophin-releasing hormone. *Lancet* 1985; **ii:**1375–8.
2. Balen AH, Conway GS, Kaltsas G, et al. Polycystic ovary syndrome: The spectrum of the disorder in 1741 patients. *Hum Reprod* 1995;**8:**2107–11.
3. Saxton DW, Farquhar CM, Rae T, Beard RW, Anderson MC, Wadsworth J. Accuracy of ultrasound measurements of female pelvic organs. *Br J Obstet Gynaecol* 1990;**97:**695–9.
4. Takahashi K, Eda Y, Okada S, Abu-Musa A, Yoshino K, Kitao M. Morphological assessment of polycystic ovaries using transvaginal ultrasound. *Hum Reprod* 1993;**6:**844–9.
5. Swanson M, Sauerbrei EE, Cooperberg PL. Medical implications of ultrasonically detected polycystic ovaries. *J Clin Ultrasound* 1981; **9:**219–22.
6. Robinson S, Rodin DA, Deacon A, Wheeler MJ, Clayton RN. Which hormone tests for the diagnosis of polycystic ovary disease? *Br J Obstet Gynaecol* 1992;**99:**232–8.
7. Fox R, Corrigan E, Thomas PA, Hull MGR. The diagnosis of polycystic ovaries in women with oligo-amenorrhoea: predictive power of endocrine tests. *Clin Endocrinol* 1991;**34:**127–31.
8. Puzigaca Z, Prelevic GM, Stretenovic Z, Balint-Peric L. Ovarian enlargement as a possible marker of androgen activity in polycystic ovary syndrome. *Gynecol Endocrinol* 1991;**5:** 167–74.
9. Pache TD, de Jong FH, Hop WC, Fauser BCJM. Association between ovarian changes assessed by transvaginal sonography and clinical and endocrin signs of the polycystic ovary syndrome. *Fertil Steril* 1993;**59:**544–9.
10. Dewailly D, Robert Y, Helin I, et al. Ovarian stromal hypertrophy in hyperandrogenic women. *Clin Endocrinol* 1994;**41:**557–62.
11. van Santbrink EJP, Hop WC, Fauser BCJM. Classification of normogonadotrophic infertility: polycystic ovaries diagnosed by ultrasound versus endocrine characteristics of polycystic ovary syndrome. *Fertil Steril* 1997;**67:**452–8.
12. Abdel Gadir A, Khatim MS, Mowafi RS, Alnaser HMI, Muharib NS, Shaw RW. Implications of ultrasonically diagnosed poly-cystic ovaries. I. Correlations which basal hormonal profiles. *Hum Reprod* 1992;**4:**453–7.
13. Goldzieher JW, Axelrod LR. Clinical and bio-chemical features of polycystic ovarian disease. *Fertil Steril* 1963;**14:**631–53.
14. Leventhal ML. The Stein–Leventhal syndrome. *Am J Obstet Gynecol* 1958;**76:**825–38.
15. Yen SSC. The polycystic ovary syndrome. *Clin Endocrinol* 1980;**12:**177–208.
16. Vaitukaitis JL. Polycystic ovary syndrome – What is it? *N Engl J Med* 1983;**309:**1245–6.
17. Hull MGR. Epidemiology of infertility and polycystic ovarian disease: endocrinological and demographic studies. *Gynaecol Edinocrinol* 1987;**1:**235–45.
18. Jacobs HS. Polycystic ovaries and polycystic ovary syndrome. *Gynecol Endocrinol* 1987; **1:**113–31.
19. Barnes R, Rosenfield RL. The polycystic ovary syndrome: Pathogenesis and treatment. *Ann Intern Med* 1989;**110:**386–99.
20. Franks S. Polycystic ovary syndrome: a changing perspective. *Clin Endocrinol* 1989;**31:**87–120.
21. Insler V, Lunenfeld B. Pathophysiology of poly-cystic ovarian disease: new insights. *Hum Reprod* 1991;**6:**1025–9.
22. Homburg R. Polycystic ovary syndrome – from gynaecological curiosity to multisystem endocrinopathy. *Hum Reprod* 1996;**11:**29–39.
23. Balen AH, Tan SL, Jacobs HS. Hypersecretion of luteinising hormone – a significant cause of subfertility and miscarriage. *Br J Obstet Gynaecol* 1993;**100:**1082–9.
24. Kiddy DS, Hamilton-Fairley D, Bush A, Anyaoku V, Reed MJ, Franks S. Improvement in endocrine and ovarian function during dietary treatment of obese women with polycystic ovary syndrome. *Clin Endocrinol* 1992; **36:**105–11.
25. Conway GS. Insulin resistance and the polycystic ovary syndrome. *Contemp Rev Obstet Gynaecol* 1990;**2:**34–9.
26. Clark AM, Ledger W, Galletly C, et al. Weight loss results in significant improvement in pregnancy and ovulation rates in anovulatory obese women. *Hum Reprod* 1995;**10:**2705–12.
27. Nugent D, Salha O, Balen AH, Rutherford AJ. Ovarian neoplasia and subfertility treatments. *Br J Obstet Gynaecol* 1998; (in press).
28. Kiddy DS, Sharp PS, White DM, et al. Differences in clinical and endocrine features

between obese and non-obese subjects with polycystic ovary syndrome: an analysis of 263 consecutive cases. *Clin Endocrinol* 1990;**32:** 213–20.

29. Grodstein F, Goldman MB, Cramer DW. Body mass index and ovulatory infertility. *Epidemiology* 1994;**5:**247–50.

30. Zaazdstra BM, Seidell JC, Van Noord PA, et al. Fat and female fecundity: prospective study of effect of body fat distribution on conception rates. *BMJ* 1993;**306:**484–7.

31. Kiddy DS, Hamilton Fairley D, Seppala M, et al. Diet-induced changes in sex hormone binding globulin and free testosterone in women with normal or polycystic ovaries: correlation with serum insulin and insulin-like growth factor-I. *Clin Endocrinol* 1989;**31:**757–63.

32. Nestler JE, Clore JN, Blackard WG. The central role of obesity (hyperinsulinemia in the pathogenesis of polycystic ovary syndrome. *Am J Obstet Gynecol* 1989;**5:**1095–7.

33. Michelmore K, Balen AH, Dunger D, Vessey M. Polycystic ovary syndrome: is the diagnosis important? *Br J Obstet Gynaecol* 1998; in press.

34. Hamilton-Fairley D, Kiddy D, Watson H, Paterson C, Franks S. Association of moderate obesity with poor pregnancy outcome in women with polycystic ovary syndrome treated with low dose gonadotrophins. *Br J Obstet Gynaecol* 1992;**99:**128–31.

35. Filicori M, Flamigni C, Dellai P, Cognigni G, et al. Treatment of anovulation with pulsatile GnRH: prognostic factors and clinical results in 600 cycles. *J Clin Endocrinol Metab* 1994; **79:**1215–20.

36. Gjoannaess H. Polycystic ovarian syndrome treated by ovarian electrocautery through the laparoscope. *Fertil Steril* 1984;**41:**20–5.

37. Burghen GA, Givens JR, Kitabchi AE. Correlation of hyperandrogenism with hyperinsulinism in polycystic ovarian disease. *J Clin Endocrinol Metab* 1980;**50:**113–16.

38. Dunaif A, Segal KR, Futterweit W, Dobrjansky A. Profound peripheral insulin resistance, independent of obesity in polycystic ovary syndrome. *Diabetes* 1989;**38:**1165–73.

39. Rajkhowa M, Bicknell J, Jones M, Clayton RN. Insulin sensitivity in women with polycystic ovary syndrome: relationship to hyperandrogenaemia. *Fertil Steril* 1994;**61:**605–12.

40. Rajkhowa M, Clayton RN. Polycystic ovary syndrome. *Curr Obstet Gynaecol* 1995;**5:**191–200.

41. Prelevic GM. Insulin resistance and polycystic ovary syndrome. *Curr Opin Obstet Gynecol* 1997;**9:**193–201.

42. Franks S, Gharani N, Waterworth D, et al. The genetic basis of polycystic ovary syndrome. *Hum Reprod* 1997;**12:**2641–8.

43. DeFronzo RA, Barzilai N, Simonson DC. Mechanism of action of metformin in obese and lean noninsulin-dependent diabetic subjects. *J Clin Endocrinol Metab* 1991;**73:**1294–301.

44. Nestler JE, Jakubowicz DJ. Decreases in ovarian cytochrome P450c17alpha activity and serum free testosterone after reduction of insulin secretion in polycystic ovary syndrome. *N Engl J Med* 1996;**335:**617–23.

45. Velazquez EM, Mendoza S, Hamer T, Sosa F, Glueck CJ. Metformin therapy in polycystic ovary syndrome reduces hyperinsulinaemia, insulin resistance, hyperandrogenaemia and systolic blood pressure, while facilitating normal menses and pregnancy. *Metabolism* 1994;**43:**647–54.

46. Velazquez EM, Mendoza SG, Wang P, Glueck CJ. Metformin therapy is associated with a decrease in plasminogen activator inhibitor-1, lipoprotein(a) and immunoreactive insulin levels in patients with PCOS. *J Clin Endocrinol Metab* 1997;**82:**524–30.

47. Velazquez EM, Acosta A, Mendoza SG. Menstrual cyclicity after metformin therapy in PCOS. *Obstet Gynecol* 1997;**90:**392–5.

48. Acbay O, Gundogdu S. Can metformin reduce insulin resistance in polycystic ovary syndrome? *Fertil Steril* 1996;**65:**946–9.

49. Ehrmann DA, Cavaghan MK, Imperial J, Sturis J, Rosenfield RL, Polonsky KS. Effects of metformin on insulin secretion, insulin action and ovarian steroidogenesis in women with polycystic ovary syndrome. *J Clin Endocrinol Metab* 1997;**82:**1241–7.

50. Dunaif A, Scott D, Finegood D, Quintana B, Whitcomb R. The insulin-sensitizing agent troglitazone improves metabolic and reproductive abnormalities in polycystic ovary syndrome. *J Clin Endocrinol Metab* 1996; **81:**3299–306.

51. Ehrmann DA, Schneider DJ, Sobel BE, et al. Troglitazone improves defects in insulin action, insulin secretion ovarian steroidogenesis and fibrinolysis in women with polycystic ovary syndrome. *J Clin Endocrinol Metab* 1997; **82:**2108–116.

52. ESHRE. Female infertility: treatment options for complicated cases. The ESHRE Capri

Workshop. *Hum Reprod* 1997;**12:**1191–6.

53. Hammond MG, Halme JK, Talbert LM. Factors affecting the pregnancy rate in clomiphene citrate induction of ovulation. *Obstet Gynecol* 1983;**62:**196–202.

54. Balen AH, Jacobs HS. Ovulation induction. In: *Infertility in Practice* (Balen AH, Jacobs HS, eds). Edinburgh: Churchill Livingstone, 1997: 131–80.

55. Balen AH. Anovulatory infertility and ovulation induction – Recommendations for good clinical practice. *J Br Fertil Soc*, 1997;**2:**83–7.

56. Kousta E, White DM, Franks S. Modern use of clomiphene citrate in induction of ovulation. *Hum Reprod Update* 1997;**3:**359–65.

57. Shoham Z, Zosmer A, Insler V. Early miscarriage and fetal malformations after induction of ovulation (by clomiphene citrate and/or human menopausal gonadotrophins), *in vitro* fertilisation and gamete intrafallopian transfer. *Fertil Steril* 1991;**55:**1–11.

58. Venn A, Lumley J. Clomiphene citrate and pregnancy outcome. *Aust NZ J Obstet Gynaecol* 1994;**34:**56–66.

59. Shoham Z, Borenstein R, Lunenfeld B, Pariente C. Hormonal profiles following clomiphene citrate therapy in conception and nonconception cycles. *Clin Endocrinol* 1990;**33:**271–8.

60. Franks S. Induction of ovulation. In: *Infertility* (Templeton AA, Drife JO, eds). London: Springer Verlag, 1992: 237–52.

61. Dickey RP, Olar TT, Taylor SN, et al. Relationship of biochemical pregnancy to preovulatory endometrial thickness and pattern in ovulation induction patients. *Hum Reprod* 1993;**8:**327–90.

62. Shepard MK, Balmaceda JP, Leija CG. Relationship of weight to successful induction of ovulation with clomiphene citrate. *Fertil Steril* 1979;**32:**641–5.

63. Lobo RA, Gysler M, March CM, et al. Clinical and laboratory predictors of clomiphene response. *Fertil Steril* 1982;**37:**168–74.

64. Dickey RP, Taylor SN, Curole DN, Rye P, Lu PY, Pyrzak R. Relationship of clomiphene dose and patient weight to successful treatment. *Hum Reprod* 1997;**12:**449–53.

65. Fluker MR, Wang I, Rowe TC. An extended 10-day course of clomiphene citrate in women with CC-resistant ovulatory disorders. *Fertil Steril* 1996;**66:**761–4.

66. Roozenberg BJ, van Dessel HJHM, Evers JLH, Bots RSGM. Successful induction of ovulation in normogonadotrophic clomiphene resistant anovulatory women by combined naltrexone and clomiphene citrate treatment. *Human Reprod* 1997;**12:**1720–2.

67. Homburg R, Weissglass L, Goldman J. Improved treatment for anovulation in polycystic ovarian disease utilizing the effect of progesterone on the inappropriate gonadotrophin release and clomiphene citrate response. *Hum Reprod* 1988;**3:**285–8.

68. Polson DW, Kiddy DS, Mason HD, Franks S. Induction of ovulation with clomiphene citrate in women with polycystic ovary syndrome: the difference between responders and non-responders. *Fertil Steril* 1989;**51:**30–4.

69. Rossing MA, Dalling JR, Weiss NS et al. Ovarian tumours in a cohort of infertile women. *N Engl J Med* 1994;**331:**335–9.

70. Balen AH, Braat DDM, West C, Patel A, Jacobs HS. Cumulative conception and live birth rates after the treatment of anovulatory infertility. An analysis of the safety and efficacy of ovulation induction in 200 patients. *Hum Reprod* 1994;**9:**1563–70.

71. Rose MP, Gaines Das RE, Balen AH. Definition and measurement of FSH. *Endocrine Rev* 1998; in press.

72. Thompson CR, Hansen LM. Pergonal (menotropins): a summary of clinical experience in the induction of ovulation and pregnancy. *Fertil Steril* 1970;**21:**844–53.

73. Lunenfeld B, Insler V. Classification of amenorrhoeic states and their treatment by ovulation induction. *Clin Endocrinol* 1974;**3:**223–37.

74. Wang CF, Gemzell C. The use of human gonadotrophins for induction of ovulation in women with polycystic ovarian disease. *Fertil Steril* 1980;**33:**479–86.

75. Brown JB, Evans JH, Adey FD, Taft HP, Townsend L. Factors involved in the induction of fertile ovulation with human gonadotrophins. *J Obstet Gynaecol Br Commun* 1969;**76:**289–307.

76. Hamilton-Fairley D, Kiddy DS, Watson H, Sagle M, Franks S. Low-dose gonadotrophin therapy for induction of ovulation in 100 women with polycystic ovary syndrome. *Hum Reprod* 1991;**6:**1095–9.

77. Shoham Z, Patel A, Jacobs HS. Polycystic ovary syndrome: safety and effectiveness of stepwise and low-dose administration of purified follicle stimulating hormone. *Fertil Steril* 1991; **55:**1051–6.

78. Schoemaker J, van Weissenbruch MM, Scheele F, van der Meer M. The FSH threshold concept

79. Fauser BC, Donderwinkel PFJ, Schoot DC. The step-down principle in gonadotrophin treatment and the role of GnRH analogues. *Baillière's Clin Obstet Gynaecol* 1993;**7**:309–30.

80. van Santbrink EJP, Donderwinkel PFJ, van Dessel TJHM, Fauser BCJM. Gonadotrophin induction of ovulation using a step-down dose regimen: single centre clinical experience in 82 patients. *Hum Reprod* 1995;**10**:1048–53.

81. Ben Rafael Z, Levy T and Schoemaker J. Pharmacokinetics of follicle-stimulating hormone: clinical significance. *Fertil Steril* 1995;**63**:689–700.

82. Hugues J-N, Cedrin-Dumerin I, Avril C, Bulwa S, Herve F, Uzan M. Sequential step-up and step-down dose regimen: an alternative method for ovulation induction with FSH in polycystic ovary syndrome. *Hum Reprod* 1996;**11**:2581–4.

83. Silverberg KM, Olive DL, Burns WN, Johnson JV, Groff TR, Schenken RS. Follicular size at the time of human chorionic gonadotrophin administration predicts ovulation outcome in human menopausal gonadotrophin-stimulated cycles. *Fertil Steril* 1991;**56**:296–300.

84. Levene MI, Wild J, Steer P. Higher multiple births and the modern management of infertility in Britain. *Br J Obstet Gynaecol* 1992;**99**:607–13.

85. Botting BJ, Macfarlane AJ, Price FV (eds). *Three, Four and More. A study of triplet and higher order births.* London: HMSO, 1990.

86. Hull MGR. Gonadotrophin therapy in anovulatory infertility. In: *Gonadotrophins, Gonadotrophin Hormone Releasing Analogues and Growth Factors in Infertility: Future Perspectives* (Howles CM, ed). Sussex: Medifax International, 1992: 56–70.

87. Homburg R, Levy T, Ben-Rafael Z. A comparative prospective study of conventional regimen with chronic low-dose administration of FSH for anovulation associated with polycystic ovary syndrome. *Fertil Steril* 1995;**59**:729–33.

88. Farhi J, Jacobs HS. Early prediction of ovarian multifollicular response during ovulation induction in patients with polycystic ovary syndrome. *Fertil Steril* 1997;**67**:459–62.

89. White DM, Polson DW, Kiddy D, et al. Induction of ovulation with low-dose gonadotrophins in polycystic ovary syndrome: An analysis of 109 pregnancies in 225 women. *J Clin Endocrinol Metab* 1996;**81**:3821–4.

90. Hayden C, Rutherford AJ, Balen AH. Induction of ovulation using a starting dose of 50 units of recombinant human follicle stimulating hormone (Puregon). British Fertility Society Meeting 1998; abstr.

91. Schoot DC, Pache TD, Hop WC, de Jong FH, Fauser BCJM. Growth patterns of ovarian follicles during induction of ovulation with decreasing doses of human menopausal gonadotrophin following presumed selection in polycystic ovary syndrome. *Fertil Steril* 1992;**57**:1117–20.

92. Fauser BCJM. Observations in favor of normal early follicle development and disturbed dominant follicle selection in polycystic ovary syndrome. *Gynecol Endocrinol* 1994;**8**:75–82.

93. Schoot DC. *Exogenous Follicle Stimulating Hormone and Development of Human Ovarian Follicles.* Carnforth: Parthenon Publishing group, 1995.

94. van Santbrink EJP, Hop WC, van Dessel TJHM, de Jong FH, Fauser BCJM. Decremental FSH and dominant follicle development during the normal menstrual cycle. *Fertil Steril* 1995;**64**:37–43.

95. Tadokoro N, Vollenhoven B, Clark S, et al. Cumulative pregnancy rates in couples with anovulatory infertility compared with unexplained infertility in an ovulation induction programme. *Hum Reprod* 1997;**12**:1939–44.

96. Jacobs HS, Porter R, Eshel A, Craft I. Profertility uses of luteinising hormone releasing hormone agonist analogues. In: *LHRH and its Analogs* (Vickery BH, Nestor JJ, eds). Lancaster: MTP Press, 1987: 303–22.

97. Homburg R, Eshel A, Kilborn J, Adams J, Jacobs HS. Combined luteinising hormone releasing hormone analogue and exogenous gonadotrophins for the treatment of infertility associated with polycystic ovaries. *Hum Reprod* 1990;**5**:32–5.

98. Sagle MA, Hamilton-Fairley D, Kiddy D, Franks S. A comparative, randomised study of low-dose human menopausal gonadotrophin and FSH in women with polycystic ovary syndrome. *Fertil Steril* 1991;**55**:56–60.

99. Fulghesu AM, Lanzone A, Gida C, et al. Ovulation induction with human menopausal gonadotrophin versus follicle stimulating hormone after pituitary suppression by gonadotrophin-releasing hormone agonist in polycystic ovary disease: A cross over study. *J Reprod Med* 1992;**37**:834–40.

100. Venturoli S, Paradisi R, Fubbri R, et al. Comparison between human urinary follicle-

stimulating hormone and human menopausal gonadotropin treatment in polycystic ovary. *Obst Gyn* 1984;**63**:6–11.

101. Anderson RE, Cragun JM, Chary RJ, et al. A pharmacodynamic comparison of human urinary follicle-stimulating hormone and human menopausal gonadotropin in normal women and polycystic ovary syndrome. *Fertil Steril* 1989;**52**:216–20.

102. Balen AH, Rose M. The control of luteinising hormone secretion in the polycystic ovary syndrome. *Contemp Rev Obstet Gynaecol* 1994;**6**:201–7.

103. Daya S. Follicle stimulating hormone versus human menopausal gonadotropin for in vitro fertilisation: results of a meta-analysis. *Horm Res* 1995;**43**:224–9.

104. Hughes E, Collins J, Vandekerckhove P. Ovulation induction with urinary follicle stimulating hormone vs human menopausal gonadotropin for clomiphene-resistant polycystic ovary syndrome. In: Subfertility Module of the *Cochrane database of systematic reviews* (Lilford R, Hughes E, Vanderkerckhove P, eds). Oxford: The Cochrane Collaboration, 1997: issue 3.

105. Gardosi J. Systematic reviews: insufficient evidence on which to base medicine. *Br J Obstet Gynaecol* 1998;**105**:1–4.

106. Homburg R, Armar NA, Eshel A, Adams J, Jacobs HS. Influence of serum luteinising hormone concentrations on ovulation, conception and early pregnancy loss in polycystic ovary syndrome. *BMJ* 1998;**297**:1024–6.

107. Fleming R, Haxton MJ, Hamilton MPR, et al. Successful treatment of infertile women with oligomenorrhoea using a combination of an LHRH agonist and exogenous gonadotrophins. *Br J Obstet Gynaecol* 1985;**92**:369–73.

108. Buckler HM, Critchley HO, Cantrill JA, Shalet SM, Anderson DC, Robertson WR. Efficacy of low dose purified FSH in ovulation induction following pituitary desensitisation in polycystic ovary syndrome. *Clin Endocrinol* 1993; **38b**:209–17.

109. Scheele F, Hompes PGA, van der Meer M, Schoute E, Schoemaker J. The effects of a gonadotrophin-releasing hormone agonist on treatment with low dose FSH in polycystic ovary syndrome. *Hum Reprod* 1993;**8**:699–704.

110. Balen AH, Tan SL, MacDougall J, Jacobs HS. Miscarriage rates following in vitro fertilisation are increased in women with polycystic ovaries

and reduced by pituitary desensitisation with buserelin. *Hum Reprod* 1993;**8**:959–64.

111. Farhi J, Homburg R, Lerner A, Ben-Rafael Z. The choice of treatment for anovulation associated with polycystic ovary syndrome following failure to conceive with clomiphene. *Hum Reprod* 1993;**8**:1367–71.

112. Homburg R, Levy T, Berkovitz D, et al. Gonadotropin-releasing hormone agonist reduces the miscarriage rate for pregnancies achieved in women with polycystic ovary syndrome. *Fertil Steril* 1993;**59**:527–31.

113. Donderwinkel PFJ, Schoot DC, Pache TD, de Jong FH, Fauser BCJM. Luteal function following ovulation induction in polycystic ovary syndrome patients using exogenous gonadotrophins in combination with a gonadotrophin-releasing hormone agonist. *Hum Reprod* 1993;**8**:2027–32.

114. Fraser HM. Risk of luteal phase inadequacy after GnRH agonist-induced ovulation. In: *The Triggering of Ovulation in Stimulated Cycles: hCG or LH?* (Emperaire JC, ed.). Carnforth: Parthenon Publishing Group, 1994: 229–38.

115. Emperaire JC, Ruffie A. Triggering of ovulation with endogenous LH may prevent ovarian hyperstimulation syndrome. *Hum Reprod* 1991;**6**:506–10.

116. Eshel A, Abdulwahid NA, Armar NA, Jacobs HS. Pulsatile LHRH therapy in women with polycystic ovary syndrome. *Fertil Steril* 1988;**49**:956–60.

117. Shoham Z, Homburg R, Jacobs HS. Induction of ovulation with pulsatile GnRH. *Baillière's Clin Obstet Gynaecol* 1990;**4**:589–608.

118. Shoham Z, Conway GS, Patel A, Jacobs HS. Polycystic ovaries in patients with hypogonadotrophic hypogonadism: similarity of ovarian response to gonadotrophin stimulation in patients with polycystic ovary syndrome. *Fertil Steril* 1992;**58**:37–45.

119. Schachter M, Balen AH, Patel A, Jacobs HS. Hypogonadotrophic patients with ultrasonographically diagnosed polycystic ovaries have aberrant gonadotropin secretion when treated with pulsatile gonadotrophin releasing hormone – a new insight into the pathophysiology of polycystic ovary syndrome. *Gynecol Endocrinol* 1996;**10**:327–35.

120. Homburg R, Kilborn J, West C, Jacobs HS. Treatment with pulsatile luteinising hormone-releasing hormone modulates folliculogenesis

in response to ovarian stimulation with exogenous gonadotrophins in patients with polycystic ovaries. *Fertil Steril* 1990;**54**:737–40.

121. Tan SL, Farhi J, Homburg R, Jacobs HS. Induction of ovulation in clomiphene-resistant polycystic ovary syndrome with pulsatile GnRH. *Obstet Gynecol* 1996;**88**:221–6.

122. Dubourdieu S, Nestour EL, Spitz IM, Charbonnel B, Bouchard P. The combination of gonadotrophin-releasing hormone antagonist and pulsatile GnRH normalises LH secretion in polycystic ovarian disease but fails to induce follicular maturation. *Hum Reprod* 1993; **8**:2056–60.

123. Homburg R. Polycystic ovary syndrome – induction of ovulation. *Hum Reprod* 1996; **11**:29–39.

124. Homburg R. Ovulation induction in gonadotrophin-resistant women. *Baillière's Clin Obstet Gynaecol* 1993;**7**:349–61.

125. Prelevic GM, Ginsburg J, Maletic D, et al. The effects of the somatostatin analogue octreotide on ovulatory performance in women with polycystic ovaries. *Hum Reprod* 1995;**10**:28–32.

126. Abdel Gadir A, Mowafi RS, Alnaser HMI, Alrashid AH, Alonezi OM, Shaw RW. Ovarian electrocautery versus human menopausal gonadotrophins and pure follicle stimulating hormone therapy in the treatment of patients with polycystic ovarian disease. *Clin Endocrinol* 1990;**33**:585–92.

127. Donesky BW, Adashi EY. Surgically induced ovulation in the polycystic ovary syndrome: wedge resection revisited in the age of laparoscopy. *Fertil Steril* 1995;**63**:439–63.

128. Cohen BM. Laser laparoscopy for polycystic ovaries. *Fertil Steril* 1989;**52**:167–8.

129. Stein IF, Leventhal ML. Amenorrhoea associated with bilateral polycystic ovaries. *Am J Obstet Gynecol* 1935;**29**:181–91.

130. Stein IF. Wedge resection of the ovaries: The Stein–Leventhal Syndrome. In: *Ovulation: Stimulation, suppression, detection* (Greenblatt RB, ed.). Philadelphia: JB Lippincott, 1966: 150–7.

131. Stein IF. Ultimate results of bilateral ovarian wedge resection: twenty five years follow-up. *Int J Fertil* 1956;**1**:333–44.

132. Stein IF. Duration of fertility following ovarian wedge resection – Stein–Leventhal syndrome. *West J Surg* 1964;**78**:124–7.

133. Weinstein D, Polishuk W. The role of wedge resection of the ovary as a cause of mechanical sterility. *Surg Obstet Gynecol* 1975;**141**:417–18.

134. Buttram VC, Vaquero C. Post-ovarian wedge resection adhesive disease. *Fertil Steril* 1975;**26**:874–6.

135. Adashi EY, Rock JA, Guzick D, Wenz AC, Jones GS, Jones HW. Fertility following bilateral ovarian wedge resection; a critical analysis of 90 consecutive cases of the polycystic ovary syndrome. *Fertil Steril* 1981;**36**:320–5.

136. Toaff R, Toaff ME, Peyser MR. Infertility following wedge resection of the ovaries. *Am J Obstet Gynecol* 1976;**124**:92–6.

137. Eddy CA, Asch RH and Balmaceda JP. Pelvic adhesions following microsurgical and macrosurgical wedge resection of the ovaries. *Fertil Steril* 1980;**33**:557–61.

138. Greenblatt E, Casper RF. Endocrine changes after laparoscopic ovarian cautery in polycystic ovarian syndrome. *Am J Obstet Gynaecol* 1987;**42**:517–18.

139. Abdel Gadir A, Khatim MS, Mowafi RS, Alnaser HMI, Alzaid HGN, Shaw RW. Hormonal changes in patients with polycystic ovarian disease after ovarian electrocautery or pituitary desensitization. *Clin Endocrinol* 1990;**32**:749–54.

140. Rossmanith WG, Keckstein J, Spatzier K, Lauritzen C. The impact of ovarian laser surgery on the gonadotrophin secretion in women with polycystic ovarian disease. *Clin Endcrinol* 1991;**34**:223–30.

141. Van der Weiden RMF, Alberda AT, de Jong FH, Brandenburg H. Endocrine effects of laparoscopic ovarian electrocautery in patients with polycystic ovarian disease, resistant to clomiphene citrate. *Eur J Obstet Gynecol Reprod Biol* 1989;**32**:157–62.

142. Kovacs G, Buckler H, Bangah M, Outch K, Burger H, Healy D, Baker G, Phillips S. Treatment of anovulation due to PCOS by laparoscopic ovarian electrocautery. *Br J Obstet Gynecol* 1991;**98**:30–5.

143. Naether OGJ, Fischer R, Weise HC, Geiger-Kotzler L, Delfs T, Rudolf K. Laparoscopic electrocoagulation of the ovarian surface in infertile patients with polycystic ovarian disease. *Fertil Steril* 1993;**60**:88–94.

144. Armar NA, McGarrigie HHG, Honour JW, Holownia P, Jacobs HS, Lachelin GCL. Laparoscopic ovarian diathermy in the management of anovulatory infertility in women with polycystic ovaries: endocrine changes and clinical outcome. *Fertil Steril* 1990;**53**:45–9.

145. Sakata M, Tasaka K, Kurachi H, Terakawa N,

Miayake A, Tanizawa O. Changes of bio-active LH after laser laparoscopic ovarian cautery in patients with PCOS. *Fertil Steril* 1990;**53**:610–13.

146. Tasaka K, Sakata M, Kurachi H, Miayake A, Tanizawa O. Electrocautery in PCOS. *Horm Res* 1990;**33**:40–2.

147. Armar NA, Lachelin GCL. Laparoscopic ovarian diathermy: an effective treatment for antioestrogen resistant anovulatory infertility in women with polycystic ovaries. *Br J Obstet Gynaecol* 1993;**100**:161–4.

148. Abdel Gadir A, Alnaser HMI, Mowafi RS, Shaw RW. The response of patients with polycystic ovarian disease to human menopausal gonadotrophin therapy after ovarian electrocautery or a luteinizing hormone-releasing hormone agonist. *Fertil Steril* 1992;**57**:309–13.

149. Balen AH, Jacobs HS. A prospective study comparing unilateral and bilateral laparoscopic ovarian diathermy in women with the polycystic ovary syndrome. *Fertil Steril* 1994;**62**:921–5.

150. Palmer R, de Brux J. Resultants histologiques, biochemiques et therapeutiques obtenus chez les femmes dont les ovaires avaient été diagnostiques Stein–Leventhal à la coelioscopie. *Bull Fed Soc Gynaecol Obstet Lang Fr* 1967;**19**:405–12.

151. Daniell JF, Miller N. Polycystic ovaries treated by laparoscopic laser vaporization. *Fertil Steril* 1989;**51**:232–6.

152. Gjoannaess H. The course and outcome of pregnancy after ovarian electrocautery with PCOS: the influence of body weight. *Br J Obstet Gynaecol* 1989;**96**:714–19.

153. Dabirashrafi H, Mohamad K, Behjatnia Y, et al. Adhesion formation after ovarian electrocauterization on patients with PCO syndrome. *Fertil Steril* 1991;**55**:1200–1.

154. Naether OGJ, Fischer R. Adhesion formation after laparoscopic electrocoagulation of the ovarian surface in polycystic ovary patients. *Fertil Steril* 1993;**60**:95–9.

155. Naether O, Weise HC, Fischer R. Treatment with electrocautery in sterility patients with polycystic ovarian disease. *Geburtsh Frauenheilk* 1991;**51**:920–4.

156. Naether OGJ. Significant reduction in numbers of adnexal adhesions following laparoscopic electrocautery of the ovarian surface by lavage and artificial ascites. *Gynaecol Endosc* 1995;**4**:17–19.

157. Greenblatt E, Casper RF. Adhesion formation after laparoscopic ovarian cautery for POCS: lack of correlation with pregnancy rate. *Fertil Steril* 1993;**60**:766–9.

158. Gurgan T, Urman B, Aksu T, Develioghu O, Zeyneloghu H, Kisnisci HA. The effect of short internal laparoscopic lysis of adhesions in pregnancy rates following ND:YAG laser photocoagulation of PCO. *Obstet Gynecol* 1992;**80**:45–7.

159. Naether IGJ, Baukloh V, Fischer R, Kowalczyk T. Long-term follow-up in 206 infertility patients with polycystic ovarian syndrome after laparoscopic electrocautery of the ovarian surface. *Hum Reprod* 1994;**9**:2342–9.

160. Ostrzenski A. Endoscopic carbon dioxide laser ovarian wedge resection in resistant polycystic ovarian disease. *Int J Fertil* 1992;**37**:295–9.

161. Farhi J, Soule S, Jacobs H. Effect of laparoscopic ovarian electrocautery on ovarian response and outcome of treatment with gonadotrophins in clomiphene citrate resistant patients with PCOS. *Fertil Steril* 1995;**64**:930–5.

162. Rimmington MR, Walker SM, Shaw RW. The use of laparoscopic ovarian electrocautery in preventing cancellation of in-vitro fertilization treatment cycles due to risk of ovarian hyperstimulation syndrome in women with polycystic ovaries. *Hum Reprod* 1997;**7**:1443–7.

163. Huber J, Hosmann J, Spona J. Polycystic ovarian syndrome treated by laser through the laparoscope. *Lancet* 1988;**ii**:215.

164. Keckstein G, Rossmanith W, Spatzier K, Schneider V, Borchers K, Steiner R. The effect of laparoscopic treatment of polycystic ovarian disease by $CO_2$ laser or Nd:YAG laser. *Surg Endosc* 1990;**4**:103–7.

165. Heylen SM, Puttemans PJ, Brosens LH. Polycystic ovarian disease treated by laparoscopic argon laser capsule drilling: comparison of vaporization versus perforation technique. *Hum Reprod* 1994;**9**:1038–42.

166. Zondek B. Polyhormonal amenorrhoea and polyhormonal haemorrhage. *Harefuah* 1938;**14**:12–13.

167. Paldi F, Timor-Tritsch I, Brandes JM, Peretz A, Abramovici H, Fushs K. Operative culdoscopy as treatment for the polycystic ovary. *Int J Fertil* 1992;**17**:109–10.

168. Mio Y, Toda T, Tanikawa M, Terado H, Harada T, Terakawa N. Transvaginal ultrasound guided follicular aspiration in the management of anovulatory infertility associated with polycystic ovaries. *Fertil Steril* 1991;**56**:1060–5.

169. Doyle P. The outcome of multiple pregnancy. *Hum Reprod* 1996;**11**(suppl 4):110–20.

170. Whittemore AS, Harris R, Itnyre J and the Collaborative Ovarian Cancer Group. Char-

acteristics relating to ovarian cancer risk: collaborative analysis of 12 US case-control studies. II Invasive epithelial ovarian cancers in white women. *Am J Epidemiol* 1992;**136:**1184–203.

171. Balen AH. Effects of ovulation induction with gonadotrophins on the ovary and uterus and implications for assisted reproduction. *Hum Reprod* 1995;**10:**2233–7.

# 6

# Novel approaches to the management of the polycystic ovary syndrome with GnRH agonists

Marco Filicori, Graciela Estela Cognigni, Giuseppe Gessa, Cristina Tabarelli, Barbara Cantelli

**Diagnostic use of GnRH agonists** • **Management of hirsutism with GnRH agonists and oestroprogestins** • **Ovulation induction regimens**

In the last 15 years gonadotrophin-releasing hormone (GnRH) agonists have become an invaluable tool for the management and treatment of various reproductive and neoplastic disorders, ranging from precious puberty to prostate cancer.[1] Numerous GnRH agonists are currently available world wide and are listed in Table 1. All GnRH agonists share the replacement of amino acid number 6 with a D-amino acid which ensures enhanced potency and a more prolonged plasma half-life; most GnRH agonists are also characterized by the replacement of amino acid number 10 with an ethylamide residue that further increases their hydrophobicity and thus their potency (Table 1).

**Table 1 GnRH agonists amino acid replacements, names and manufacturers**

| Position 6 | Position 7 | Position 10 | Name | Company |
|---|---|---|---|---|
| D-Leu | – | NEt | Leuprorelin | Takeda, TAP |
| D-Trp | – | – | Triptorelin | Ferring, Ipsen |
| D-Trp | – | NEt | Deslorelin | Salk Institute |
| D-Trp | N-Me-Leu | NEt | Lutrelin | Wyeth |
| D-Ser(tBU) | – | NEt | Buserelin | Hoechst |
| D-Ser(tBU) | – | aza-Gly | Goserelin | Zeneca |
| D-His(Bzl) | – | NEt | Histrelin | Ortho, Roberts |
| D-Ala(2-Naph) | – | – | Nafarelin | Syntex |

GnRH agonists have a biphasic mode of action. In the first few days of administration these compounds stimulate gonadotrophin secretion and increase luteinizing hormone (LH) and follicle-stimulating hormone (FSH) plasma levels; thereafter, if an GnRH agonist administration is continued, pituitary desensitization ensues and LH levels are profoundly suppressed. Reduction of FSH plasma levels during chronic GnRH agonist administration is less marked and FSH levels tend to increase progressively if treatment is continued for several months.[2]

As a result of these characteristics, GnRH agonists have been employed with different goals in the diagnosis and management of patients with the polycystic ovary syndrome (PCOS). Short-term gonadotrophin and ovarian androgen stimulation has been used to give better definition of the endocrine derangements of this condition and to trigger ovulation after induction of ovulation by gonadotrophins. Conversely, administration of longer-term GnRH agonists has been used to supplement oestroprogestin and ovulation induction regimens for the improvement of clinical results in PCOS. This chapter summarizes these clinical applications of GnRH agonists in PCOS.

## DIAGNOSTIC USE OF GnRH AGONISTS

GnRH agonists can be used to assess 17-hydroxyprogesterone (170HP) responses in PCOS. The levels of 170HP were found to be raised more in PCOS than in controls after buserelin administration, and to be directly correlated with ovarian volume.[3] The stimulation of the increase in 170HP levels induced by GnRH agonists is comparable to that obtained with human chorionic gonadotrophin (hCG), thus suggesting that the deranged secretion of this ovarian hormone is not exclusively related to the well-known hypersecretion of LH.[4] Although androstenedione levels were found to be similarly elevated in ovulatory and anovulatory women with PCOS, LH response to a GnRH agonist was greater in anovulatory patients, suggesting that hyperandrogenism in

this condition is not directly proportional to LH hypersecretion but related to an intrinsic enzyme abnormality involving 17-hydroxylase and 17,20-lyase activity.[5]

The response of 170HP to GnRH agonists was also employed to assess cytochrome P450c17α activity after reduction in endogenous insulin induced by weight loss[6] or metformin.[7] Both approaches resulted in a reduction in GnRH agonist-stimulated 170HP and androgen levels, thus confirming that insulin plays a key role in the development of hyperandrogenism in this disorder. Finally, GnRH agonist suppression can be used to differentiate adrenal from ovarian causes of hyperandrogenemia.[8]

In summary, GnRH agonists can be used effectively to test for steroid hypersecretion and ovarian enzyme defects, as well as to give better characterization of the source of excess androgen production in PCOS.

## MANAGEMENT OF HIRSUTISM WITH GnRH AGONISTS AND OESTROPROGESTINS

Most of the excessive androgen secretion in the PCOS is from the ovary and is LH dependent. As GnRH agonists provide long-term suppression of LH and ovarian steroid secretion, there is no question that these drugs are able to reduce hyperandrogenism and hirsutism in PCOS.[9,10] However, management of these conditions requires that treatment be continued for many months or years, thus making administration of a GnRH agonist alone unfeasible because of the well-known side effects (for example, bone mass reduction). Thus, administration of a GnRH agonist has been supplemented with various types of oestroprogestin formulations.

Cyproterone acetate is an antiandrogenic progestin electively used with oestrogens for the management of hirsutism. This drug is widely available in Europe and other countries, but not in the USA. Combined regimens consisting of cyproterone acetate, ethinyloestradiol and GnRH agonists have been employed in several studies. Falsetti et al[11] found that this regimen effectively reduced moderate and severe hirsutism. Ciotta et al[12] found that a similar regimen reduced gonadotrophin and gonadal steroid levels, increased sex hormone-binding globulin (SHBG) and improved the hirsutism score of those women with PCOS who were unresponsive to traditional treatment with oral contraceptives. Acien et al[13] recently showed that the addition of a GnRH agonist did not significantly improve treatment results obtained with an oral contraceptive that contained cyproterone acetate; these investigators, however, suggested that the GnRH agonist regimen may be preferable in obese and severely hirsute patients because of its improved effects on 170HP and dehydroepiandrosterone sulphate (DHEA-S) levels and the hirsutism score.

Other studies[14,15] evaluated the combination of GnRH agonists, oestrogens (transdermal oestradiol or ethinyloestradiol) and medroxyprogesterone acetate (MPA) and found it to be effective and well tolerated for treatment periods of 6–12 months. Finally, Genazzani et al[16] found better results of GnRH agonist/oral contraceptive combined regimens in a 6-month, post-treatment, follow-up period, whereas Taskin et al[17] determined that these regimens are more effective than laparoscopic ovarian cauterization in restoring the optimal follicular environment in women with the PCOS.

In summary, GnRH agonists are an effective complement to more traditional steroids used for the management of hirsute patients with PCOS. Although these combined regimens may be indicated in specific subgroups of women with PCOS (for example, obese, severely hirsute), it is still questionable whether the added cost and inconvenience of GnRH agonist administration can result in significant therapeutic advantages over standard oestroprogestin therapy.

## OVULATION INDUCTION REGIMENS

GnRH agonists can be combined with different drugs and in various regimens to improve ovulation-induction planning and outcome.

Pre-treatment with a GnRH agonist permits optimal scheduling of patient candidates for menotrophin ovulation induction and minimization of patient variability. However, Gersak et al[18] showed no advantage in ovulation induction with human menopausal gonadotrophin (hMG) using GnRH agonist administration when compared with hMG treatment alone. Scheele et al[19] found that GnRH agonist supplementation of low-dose FSH regimens did not abolish patients' variability in their response to menotrophin and resulted in a lower incidence of monofolliculogenesis, possibly caused by postponed atresia. Conversely, reductions in spontaneous abortion rates (a common occurrence among PCOS patients) were reported when GnRH agonist and hMG regimens were compared with hMG alone[20] and clomiphene citrate.[21]

GnRH agonists can also be used instead of hCG to trigger the midcycle LH surge after menotrophin ovulation induction, with the goal of reducing the occurrence of ovarian hyperstimulation. Lanzone et al[22] found that this approach was associated with a reduced ovarian volume in the luteal phase, whereas ovulation and pregnancy rates were unaffected. Luteal phase support with exogenous steroids may be required in these patients to prevent luteal phase defects. Unfortunately, this approach cannot be employed in patients undergoing combined GnRH agonist and menotrophin ovulation induction for assisted reproduction, because pre-existing pituitary desensitization curtails GnRH agonist gonadotrophin response at midcycle. Nevertheless, the introduction of GnRH antagonists may in the future allow effective use of GnRH agonists to trigger ovulation at the end of follicular maturation.

GnRH agonists can also be employed to enhance responsivity of patients with PCOS to other ovulation-induction drugs such as pulsatile GnRH. In a large series of such patients we showed[23] that good ovulatory and pregnancy rates can be obtained with pulsatile GnRH (5 μg i.v. every 60 min) when such treatment is preceded by pituitary–ovarian suppression with a short-acting GnRH agonist (buserelin 300 μg, s.c. every 12 h, for 4–6 weeks). The improved outcome of pulsatile

GnRH in these patients probably results from the low serum LH and intraovarian androgen levels that are present after several weeks of GnRH agonist administration.[24] This approach to ovulation induction in PCOS is attractive because of the reduced incidence of complications of ovulation induction (ovarian hyperstimulation, multiple pregnancy) that are typical of this condition. Conversely, the long duration of this treatment regimen may limit practical use of this regimen in large numbers of patients with PCOS.

In summary, GnRH agonists can be used in association with various ovulation induction drugs to improve clinical results, reduce complications and optimize patient scheduling. The introduction of new gonadotrophin preparations and GnRH antagonists will certainly result in the development of new, potentially improved, treatment regimens.

## REFERENCES

1. Filicori M. Gonadotrophin-releasing hormone agonists. A guide to use and selection. *Drugs* 1994;**48**:41–58.
2. Filicori M, Cognigni GE, Arnone R, et al. Subcutaneous administration of a depot gonadotropin hormone-releasing hormone agonist induces profound reproductive axis suppression in women. *Fertil Steril* 1998; in press.
3. Sahin Y, Kelestimur F. 17-Hydroxyprogesterone response to buserelin testing in the polycystic ovary syndrome. *Clin Endocrinol* 1993;**39**:151–5.
4. Ibanez L, Hall JE, Potau N, Carrascosa A, Prat N, Taylor AE. Ovarian 17-hydroxyprogesterone hyperresponsiveness to gonadotropin-releasing hormone (GnRH) agonist challenge in women with polycystic ovary syndrome is not mediated by luteinizing hormone hypersecretion: evidence from GnRH agonist and human chorionic gonadotropin stimulation testing. *J Clin Endocrinol Metab* 1996;**81**:4103–7.
5. White D, Leigh A, Wilson C, Donaldson A, Franks S. Gonadotrophin and gonadal steroid response to a single dose of a long-acting agonist of gonadotrophin-releasing hormone in ovulatory and anovulatory women with polycystic ovary syndrome. *Clin Endocrinol* 1995;**42**:475–81.
6. Jakubowicz DJ, Nestler JE. 17alpha-Hydroxyprogesterone responses to leuprolide and serum androgens in obese women with and without polycystic ovary syndrome offer dietary weight loss. *J Clin Endocrinol Metab* 1997;**82**:556–60.
7. Nestler JE, Jakubowicz DJ. Decreases in ovarian cytochrome P450c17 alpha activity and serum free testosterone after reduction of insulin secretion in polycystic ovary syndrome. *N Engl J Med* 1996;**335**:617–23.
8. Escobar MH, Pazos F, Potau N, Garcia RR, Sancho JM, Varela C. Ovarian suppression with triptorelin and adrenal stimulation with adrenocorticotropin in functional hyperandrogenism: role of adrenal and ovarian cytochrome P450c17 alpha. *Fertil Steril* 1994;**62**:521–30.
9. Goni M, Markussis V, Tolis G. Efficacy of chronic therapy with the gonadotrophin releasing hormone agonist decapeptyl in patients with polycystic ovary syndrome. *Hum Reprod* 1994;**9**:1048–52.
10. Lasco A, Cucinotta D, Gigante A, et al. No changes of peripheral insulin resistance in polycystic ovary syndrome after long-term reduction of endogenous androgens with leuprolide. *Eur J Endocrinol* 1995;**133**:718–22.
11. Falsetti L, Pasinetti E. Treatment of moderate and severe hirsutism by gonadotropin-releasing hormone agonists in women with polycystic ovary syndrome and idiopathic hirsutism. *Fertil Steril* 1994;**61**:817–22.
12. Ciotta L, Cianci A, Giuffrida G, Marletta E, Agliano A, Palumbo G. Clinical and hormonal effects of gonadotropin-releasing hormone agonist plus an oral contraceptive in severely hirsute patients with polycystic ovary disease. *Fertil Steril* 1996;**65**:61–7.
13. Acien P, Mauri M, Gutierrez M. Clinical and hormonal effects of the combination gonadotrophin-releasing hormone agonist plus oral contraceptive pills containing ethinyl-oestradiol (EE) and cyproterone acetate (CPA) versus the EE-CPA pill alone on polycystic ovarian disease-related hyperandrogenisms. *Hum Reprod* 1997;**12**:423–9.
14. Lemay A, Faure N. Sequential estrogen–progestin addition to gonadotropin-releasing hormone agonist suppression for the chronic treatment of ovarian hyperandrogenism: a pilot

study. *J Clin Endocrinol Metab* 1994;**79:**1716–22.

15. Morcos RN, Abdul MM, Shikora E. Treatment of hirsutism with a gonadotropin-releasing hormone agonist and estrogen replacement therapy. *Fertil Steril* 1994;**61:**427–31.

16. Genazzani AD, Petraglia F, Battaglia C, Gamba O, Volpe A, Genazzani AR. A long-term treatment with gonadotropin-releasing hormone agonist plus a low-dose oral contraceptive improves the recovery of the ovulatory function in patients with polycystic ovary syndrome. *Fertil Steril* 1997;**67:**463–8.

17. Taskin O, Yalcinoglu AI, Kafkasli A, Burak F, Ozekici U. Comparison of the effects of ovarian cauterization and gonadotropin-releasing hormone agonist and oral contraceptive therapy combination on endocrine changes in women with polycystic ovary disease. *Fertil Steril* 1996;**65:**1115–18.

18. Gersak K, Meden VH, Tomazevic T. The effects of gonadotrophin-releasing hormone agonist on follicular development in patients with polycystic ovary syndrome in an in-vitro fertilization and embryo transfer programme. *Hum Reprod* 1994;**9:**1596–9.

19. Scheele F, Hompes PG, van der Meer M, Schoute E, Schoemaker J. The effects of a gonadotrophin-releasing hormone agonist on treatment with low dose follicle stimulating hormone in poly-

cystic ovary syndrome. *Hum Reprod* 1993; **8:**699–704.

20. Homburg R, Levy T, Berkovitz D, et al. Gonadotropin-releasing hormone agonist reduces the miscarriage rate for pregnancies achieved in women with polycystic ovary syndrome. *Fertil Steril* 1993;**59:**527–31.

21. Balen AH, Tan SL, MacDougall J, Jacobs HS. Miscarriage rates following in-vitro fertilization are increased in women with polycystic ovaries and reduced by pituitary desensitization with buserelin. *Hum Reprod* 1993;**8:**959–64.

22. Lanzone A, Fulghesu AM, Villa P, et al. Gonadotropin-releasing hormone agonist versus human chorionic gonadotropin as a trigger of ovulation in polycystic ovarian disease gonadotropin hyperstimulated cycles. *Fertil Steril* 1994;**62:**35–41.

23. Filicori M, Flamigni C, Dellai P, et al. Treatment of anovulation with pulsatile gonadotropin-releasing hormone: prognostic factors and clinical results in 600 cycles. *J Clin Endocrinol Metab* 1994;**79:**1215–20.

24. Filicori M, Campaniello E, Michelacci L, et al. Gonadotropin-releasing hormone (GnRH) analog suppression renders polycystic ovarian disease patients more susceptible to ovulation induction with pulsatile GnRH. *J Clin Endocrinol Metab* 1988;**66:**327–33.

# 7

# Optimizing protocols for ovulation induction

Nicholas S Macklon, Babek Imani, Bart CJM Fauser

**Clomiphene citrate** • **Gonadotrophin therapy** • **Monitoring** • **Preparations** • **Pulsatile gonadotrophin-releasing hormone therapy** • **Adjunctive therapies** • **Surgical ovulation induction** • **Conclusion**

The goal of ovulation induction is to induce monofollicular development and subsequent ovulation in anovulatory infertile women. This should be differentiated from stimulation of multiple follicle development in ovulatory women, as is done with assisted conception techniques. Women with the polycystic ovary syndrome (PCOS) have normogonadotrophic and normo-oestrogenic anovulation (WHO group 2) and constitute the largest group of anovulatory women encountered in clinical practice (60–85% of cases).[1] The heterogeneity of the PCOS[2] is reflected in the varying response exhibited to ovulation induction regimens. In this chapter, we review the methods by which monofollicular development and subsequent ovulation can be achieved, thus avoiding the two principal complications of ovulation induction in the PCOS: multiple pregnancy and the ovarian hyperstimulation syndrome (OHSS).

## CLOMIPHENE CITRATE

In most centres, the anti-oestrogen clomiphene citrate is the first-line treatment for ovulation induction in women with normogonadotrophic, normo-oestrogenic anovulation. Although clomiphene citrate has been in widespread clinical use for over 30 years, its mechanism of action remains unclear. It is thought to occupy oestrogen receptors in the hypothalamus and pituitary, thereby blocking oestradiol negative feedback. Thus, serum follicle-stimulating hormone (FSH) concentrations rise, resulting in stimulation of follicle growth and follicular oestradiol production. In addition other mechanisms of action may also operate.[3]

Clomiphene citrate consists of two isomers: the biologically active *trans*-isomer enclomiphene and the less active *cis*-isomer zuclomiphene.[4] Many organs have oestrogen receptors, and clomiphene citrate therefore acts at many sites. The end-organ response to its combined oestrogenic and anti-oestrogenic properties determines its effect on that particular organ. The usual starting dose of clomiphene citrate is 50 mg/day for 5 consecutive days. It is often started on day 3 to day 5 after the onset of spontaneous or progesterone-induced menstrual bleeding. If the woman does not ovulate, the dose should be increased to 100 mg/day for 5 days in the next cycle (again

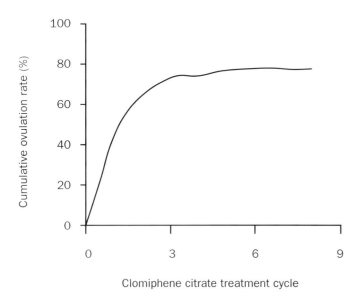

**Figure 1** Cumulative ovulation rates (first ovulation) with clomiphene citrate treatment: the initial dose was increased to 100 mg if ovulation did not occur with the first treatment cycle, and further increased to 150 mg if ovulation did not occur during the second treatment cycle.

after a spontaneous or progesterone-induced bleed). In case of absent ovarian response, the dose can be further increased to 150 mg/day for 5 days in the subsequent cycle. If ovulation occurs, a similar dose can be continued for 6–12 months or until pregnancy occurs. Retrospective cohort studies indicate that most women conceive after receiving clomiphene citrate within six cycles at doses no greater than 100 mg/day.[5] Higher doses (200 mg/day) or prolonged regimens may be successful in some resistant women.[6] The ovulatory response to clomiphene citrate can normally be assessed by means of a menstrual calendar. Regular menstruation every 4 weeks or so in a previously amenorrhoeic or oligomenorrhoeic woman suggests ovulatory cycles. A biphasic basal body temperature rise may provide further evidence of ovulation. Additional tests that can be performed to detect ovulation include ultrasonographic visualization of preovulatory follicular growth followed by collapse of the follicle, and the presence of an elevated serum progesterone concentration during the midluteal phase of the cycle. Although the beneficial effects of home luteinizing hormone (LH) monitoring remain

questionable, some patients may appreciate an early indicator of ovulation.

Employing the increase dose regimen of clomiphene citrate described above in 270 women, we have observed a cumulative ovulation rate over three cycles of more than 70%. Our data indicate that women who remain anovulatory after 3 months of treatment with a rising dose regimen to 150 mg are unlikely to respond to further treatment at this dosage (Figure 1). The reported rates of clinical pregnancy vary. In one series of 3022 women, for example, the pregnancy rate per cycle of treatment was 20%.[7] In another series of 70 women who ovulated after each of three treatment cycles, the cumulative pregnancy rate was 56%, similar to that occurring in the general population after 3 months of unprotected intercourse.[8] Our series of 210 women who ovulated with clomiphene citrate therapy demonstrates a cumulative pregnancy rate of 50% over six cycles, rising to 65% over eight cycles. Further treatment cycles did not lead to an increase in cumulative pregnancy rate (Figure 2). After 6 months of continuous treatment, the pregnancy rate per cycle has been shown to fall substan-

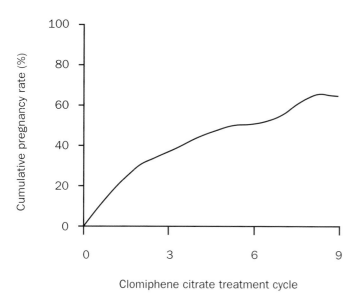

**Figure 2** Cumulative pregnancy rates among ovulatory women treated over nine cycles according to the clomiphene citrate regimen described in the text.

tially despite regular ovulation.[6] In planning therapy, consideration should be given to the possible association between clomiphene citrate, when used for more than 12 months, and ovarian cancer.[9] Pregnancy rates are lower among women who ovulate only after receiving higher doses of clomiphene citrate. This may relate to the deleterious effects of higher doses of clomiphene on the quality of cervical mucus and the endometrium.[10]

The means for identifying women who will remain resistant to clomiphene citrate induction of ovulation has until recently been restricted to clinical experience, which indicates obesity and hirsutism to be negative factors. Our group has recently identified clinical, ultrasonographic and endocrine factors associated with failure to ovulate in response to clomiphene citrate. We have developed a prediction model based on the free androgen index (FAI), body mass index (BMI), mean ovarian volume and the presence of oligomenorrhoea or amenorrhoea which, when combined to give a score, can be used to determine the probability of clomiphene resistance for an individual patient.[11] Analysis of the receiver operating characteristics (ROC) curve for the prediction model yields an area under

the curve of 0.82. Complications of clomiphene citrate therapy relate primarily to the risk of multiple pregnancy. Twin and triplet gestations occur in 9% and 0.3%, respectively, of clomiphene-induced pregnancies.[12] The incidence of birth defects appears to be similar to that in spontaneous pregnancies;[13] clomiphene is not associated with an increase in the rate of ectopic pregnancy.[14] The risk of the OHSS in patients is less than 1%. Contraindications to clomiphene citrate include liver disease and the presence of ovarian cysts.

Tamoxifen, like clomiphene, is an anti-oestrogen capable of inducing ovulation.[15] The usual starting dosage is 20 mg daily given for 5 days shortly after the initiation of a menstrual bleed. Tamoxifen has been used much less often than clomiphene for ovulation induction.

## GONADOTROPHIN THERAPY

Women with the PCOS who fail to respond to clomiphene citrate may be successfully made to ovulate with gonadotrophins. Since their introduction into clinical practice in 1961, gonadotrophins extracted from the urine of postmenopausal women (human menopausal gonadotrophins or hMG), in which the ratio of LH:FSH bioactivity is 1:1, have assumed a central role in ovulation induction. Refinement of the initially crude preparation procedure resulted in the availability of purified and highly purified urinary FSH. Since 1996, recombinant human FSH (rFSH, >99% purity) has been available in the clinic.[16]

The aim of ovulation induction with gonadotrophins, as with clomiphene citrate, is the formation of a single dominant follicle. In spontaneous cycles, this is achieved at the start of the cycle by a transient increase in serum FSH concentrations above the threshold value (Figure 3).[17] The concentrations then decrease, preventing more than one follicle from undergoing preovulatory development. To achieve development of a single follicle with exogenous gonadotrophin, specific treatment and monitoring protocols are needed. Although several approaches to ovulation induction with

gonadotrophins have been described, the two most frequently encountered in the literature and in clinical practice are the low-dose step-up protocol and, more recently, the step-down protocol.

## Dose regimens

### Step-up protocol

The conventional 'standard' step-up protocol has a starting dose of FSH 150 IU/day. However, this regimen is associated with a high complication rate. A multiple pregnancy rate of up to 36% has been reported, although ovarian hyperstimulation may occur in up to 14% of treatment cycles.[18] As a result, many centres abandoned this protocol in favour of a low-dose step-up protocol designed to allow the FSH threshold to be reached gradually, minimizing excessive stimulation and therefore the risk of development of multiple preovulatory follicles. In this protocol, the initial subcutaneous or intramuscular dose of FSH is 37.5–75 IU/day; the dose is increased only if, after 14 days, no response is documented on ultrasonography (and serum oestradiol monitoring). Increments of 37.5 IU are then given at weekly intervals up to a maximum of 225 IU/day. The detection of an ovarian response is an indication to continue the current dose until human chorionic gonadotrophin (hCG) can be given to stimulate ovulation, as described below (Figure 4). A recent series of 225 women with the PCOS treated over a 10-year period in one centre found rates of ovulation and pregnancy of 72% and 45%, respectively, after use of the low-dose step-up protocol.[19] Multiple folliculogenesis and hyperstimulation are less common than seen with the standard protocol[20] and pregnancy rates appear similar.[21] However, the results of the low-dose step-up protocol are negatively influenced by age, obesity and persistent raised serum LH concentrations.[19]

### Step-down protocol

The step-down protocol of ovulation induction mimics more closely the physiology of normal

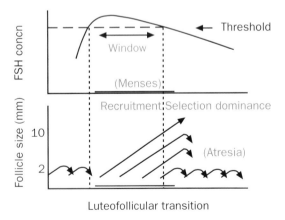

**Figure 3** The intercycle rise in serum FSH concentrations exceeds the threshold for recruitment of a cohort of follicles for further development. The number of follicles recruited is determined by the time ('window') in which the serum FSH is above the threshold at which recruitment occurs. (Adapted from Fauser and van Heusden.[17])

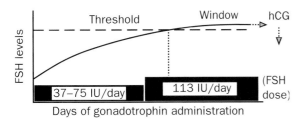

Dose increase: until 'ovarian response'

**Figure 4** Schematic representation of the low-dose step-up protocol of gonadotrophin administration for ovulation induction. The initial subcutaneous or intramuscular dose of FSH is 37.5–75 IU/day; the dose is increased only if, after 14 days, no response is documented on ultrasonography and serum oestradiol monitoring. Increments of 37.5 IU are then given at weekly intervals up to a maximum of 225 IU/day. Detection of an ovarian response is an indication to continue the current dose until hCG can be given to stimulate ovulation. (Adapted from Fauser et al.[18])

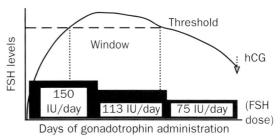

First dose reduction: transvaginal sonography
Second dose reduction: 3 days later

**Figure 5** Schematic representation of the step-down protocol (Rotterdam regimen) of gonadotrophin administration which is designed to bring about monofollicular development. This regimen mimics more closely the physiology of normal cycles. Therapy with FSH at 150 IU/day is started shortly after a spontaneous or progesterone-induced bleed and continued until a dominant follicle (≥10 mm) is seen on transvaginal ultrasonography. The dose is then decreased to 112.5 IU/day followed by a further decrease to 75 IU/day, which is continued until hCG is administered to induce ovulation. (Adapted from Fauser et al.[18])

cycles (Figure 5).[22] The underlying FSH window theory emphasizes the significance of decremental serum FSH levels for single dominant follicle development.[23] Therapy with 150 IU FSH/day is started shortly after a spontaneous or progesterone-induced bleed and continued until a dominant follicle (>10 mm) is seen on transvaginal ultrasonography. The dose is then decreased to 112.5 IU/day followed by a further decrease to 75 IU/day 3 days later, which is continued until hCG is administered to induce ovulation. The appropriate starting dose can be determined by using the low-dose step-up regimen for the first treatment cycle.

The low-dose step-up protocol is safe and effective but at the cost of an extended duration of treatment. Initial experience with the step-down protocol suggested that the duration of treatment and total gonadotrophin dosage were reduced compared with the low-dose step-up protocol, and that monofollicular growth was more frequently achieved.[22] These findings have recently been confirmed by a prospective randomized comparison of low-dose step-up and step-down regimens in 37 clomiphene-resistant women,[24] which demonstrated a higher incidence of monofollicular growth in women undergoing step-down ovulation induction, thereby reducing the risk of multiple pregnancy and hyperstimulation. Furthermore, principal complications of ovulation induction with gonadotrophins, ovarian hyperstimulation and multiple pregnancy may be reduced when the step-down protocol is used. However, the safety and efficacy of the step-down protocol in clinical practice should be confirmed through large multicentre studies.

## MONITORING

The ovarian response to gonadotrophin therapy is monitored using transvaginal ultrasonography to measure follicular diameter. The scans, usually performed every 2 or 4 days, should be focused on identifying follicles of intermediate size. Intramuscular hCG 5000–10 000 IU is given on the day that at least one follicle measures over 18 mm. If more than three follicles larger than 16 mm are present, stimulation should be stopped, hCG withheld, and use of a barrier contraceptive advised in order to prevent multiple pregnancies and ovarian hyperstimulation. Measurements of serum oestradiol may also be useful: preovulatory concentrations far above the normal range (14–40 ng/dl or 500–1500 pmol/l) may predict ovarian hyperstimulation.[25] However, it is unclear to what extent oestradiol levels add to information generated by ultrasonography alone.

The ovarian hyperstimulation syndrome is a potentially life-threatening complication characterized by ovarian enlargement, high serum sex steroids and, secondary to increased vascular permeability, accumulation of extravascular exudate primarily in the peritoneal cavity. Resultant haemoconcentration leads to a risk of thromboembolism.

## PREPARATIONS

A recent meta-analysis comparing the effectiveness of daily urinary FSH with daily hMG for inducing ovulation in women with the PCOS who had not responded to clomiphene demonstrated no difference in pregnancy rate per treatment.[26] However, the women given FSH were less likely to have moderately severe or severe OHSS.

With respect to rFSH, a recent multicentre prospective trial found that the cumulative ovulation rates were comparable with those achieved with purified urinary FSH (95% after three cycles).[27] The total dose of rFSH needed and the duration of treatment were less, and the complication rates were similar. Three prospective randomized trials comparing rFSH and urinary purified FSH in women receiving in vitro fertilization have recently been reported. One study of 123 women found that the two preparations were equally effective.[28] However, in

two larger trials of 981[29] and 235[30] women, the dose of a different rFSH preparation and the duration of rFSH treatment needed to stimulate follicle development were less, and more oocytes were recovered, implying greater efficacy for rFSH. Whether or not rFSH improves the clinical outcome in these women is not known.

Purified urinary FSH has some LH activity, but rFSH does not. The experience with rFSH in hypogonadotrophic hypogonadal women (WHO group 1) indicates that those women who have very low serum LH concentrations (< 0.5 IU/l) need exogenous hCG (or LH) to maintain adequate oestradiol biosynthesis and follicle development.[31]

## PULSATILE GONADOTROPHIN-RELEASING HORMONE THERAPY

The pulsatile administration of gonadotrophin-releasing hormone (GnRH) using an infusion pump stimulates the production of endogenous FSH and LH. The resulting serum FSH and LH concentrations remain within the normal range (because negative steroid feedback at the pituitary level remains intact) and the chances of multifollicular development and ovarian hyperstimulation are therefore low. Pulsatile GnRH administration is indicated for women with hypogonadotrophic hypogonadal anovulation (WHO group 1) who have normal pituitary function.[32] To mimic the normal pulsatile release of GnRH, a pulse interval of 60–90 min is used with a dose of 2.5–10 µg/pulse.[33,34]

Although ovulation rates of 90% and pregnancy rates of 80% have been reported in women with WHO group 1 anovulation, it is considerably less effective in women with the PCOS.[35] Cohort studies report varying results and there is still a lack of prospective randomized trials comparing pulsatile GnRH with gonadotrophin therapy in this group of patients. If it is to be used, prior suppression of endogenous hypophyseal gonadotrophins with GnRH agonists may improve the outcome.

## ADJUNCTIVE THERAPIES

Adjunctive treatment in addition to gonadotrophins may include dexamethasone suppression of adrenal androgen suppression, GnRH agonists to suppress high LH levels, dopamine agonists when hyperprolactinaemia is also present and growth hormone which has been hypothesized to improve ovarian responsiveness. However, none of these additional therapies has been shown to improve pregnancy rates in prospective randomized studies.

## SURGICAL OVULATION INDUCTION

The development of laparoscopic techniques has reawakened interest in surgical treatment for anovulation in those who fail to ovulate with medical therapy. Advocates of laparoscopic ovarian electrocautery, the most closely studied technique, point to its potential advantages over medical treatments: namely, the reduced risk of hyperstimulation and multiple pregnancies; the lack of monitoring required; and the fact that one treatment may result in many ovulatory cycles. Randomized controlled studies comparing the efficacy of laparoscopic treatments with established medical therapies have yet to be published, and our knowledge of the outcomes and potential complications of this form of therapy is limited to case series. In a recent review of the subject, Donesky and Adashi[36] analysed the outcomes in 947 patients from 28 reports. After treatment 82% ovulated spontaneously or with adjuvant medications (mostly clomiphene citrate) and of these 72% conceived. These figures compare with those reported for gonadotrophin ovulation induction.

The principal complication of the technique relates to pelvic adhesion formation. Studies employing second-look laparoscopy have indicated that adhesion formation occurs in more than 80% of women treated.[37,38] The significance of adhesions on subsequent fertility is unclear, however, because lysis does not appear to improve pregnancy rates.[39] Ovarian atrophy has also been associated with the procedure.[40] The mechanism by which ovarian electrocautery may induce ovulation remains speculative, although alteration of intraovarian feedback mechanisms on LH and androgen production, and subsequent circulating oestradiol levels, is likely to be a contributing factor, because ovulation rates are highest when LH levels are high preoperatively.[41] Given the possible long-term detrimental effects on fertility, however, ovarian electrocautery cannot be recommended over available medical therapies until its efficacy and safety have been demonstrated by well-designed, randomized, controlled studies.

## CONCLUSION

It is uncertain whether patients who do or do not ovulate but fail to conceive after clomiphene citrate therapy behave differently during gonadotrophin therapy. However, if the infertile patient with the PCOS is resistant to anti-oestrogen therapy, gonadotrophin treatment administered through low-dose protocols should be considered. Compared with conventional regimens, complication rates are reduced despite similar efficacy. It should be recognized that patients with the PCOS constitute a very heterogeneous group, so therapy outcome could benefit from improved classification. The identification of clinical characteristics that identify those women with anovulation unlikely to respond to clomiphene would permit earlier use of gonadotrophin therapy and potentially offer major health and economic benefits. Furthermore, if ovarian responsiveness to ovulation-induction therapy could be predicted for an individual patient, it might be possible to devise regimens that reduce the risk of ovarian hyperstimulation and multiple pregnancy.

## REFERENCES

1. Hull MGR. Epidemiology of infertility and polycystic ovarian disease: endocrinological and demographic studies. *Gynaecol Endocrinol* 1987;**1**:235–45.

2. Van Santbrink EJP, Hop WC, Fauser BCJM. Classification of normogonadotropic infertility: polycystic ovaries diagnosed by ultrasound versus endocrine characteristics of polycystic ovary syndrome. *Fertil Steril* 1997;**67**:452–8.

3. Butzow TL, Kettel LM, Yen SSC. Clomiphene citrate reduces serum insulin-like growth factor I and increases sex hormone binding globulin levels in women with polycystic ovary syndrome. *Fertil Steril* 1995;**63**:1200–3.

4. McDonough PG. The clomid twins: Waiting for a single isomer heaven (editorial). *Fertil Steril* 1997;**68**:186–7.

5. Adashi EY. Ovulation induction: Clomiphene citrate. In: *Reproductive Endocrinology, Surgery and Technology* (Adashi EY, Rock JA, Rosenwaks Z, eds). Philadelphia: Lippincott-Raven, 1995: 1196.

6. Fluker MR, Wang IY, Rowe TC. An extended 10-day course of clomiphene citrate (CC) in women with CC-resistant ovulatory disorders. *Fertil Steril* 1996;**66**:761–4.

7. Macgregor AH, Jonson JE, Bunde CA. Further clinical experience with clomiphene citrate. *Fertil Steril* 1968;**19**:616–22.

8. Gorlitsky GA, Kase NG, Speroff L. Ovulation and pregnancy rates with clomiphene citrate. *Obstet Gynecol* 1978;**51**:265–9.

9. Rossing MA, Dalling JR, Weiss NS, et al. Ovarian tumours in a cohort of infertile women. *N Engl J Med* 1994;**331**:335–9.

10. Dickey RP, Olar TT, Taylor SN, et al. Relationship of endometrial thickness and pattern to fecundity in ovulation induction cycles: Effect of clomiphene citrate alone and with human menopausal gonadotrophin. *Fertil Steril* 1993;**59**:756–60.

11. Imani B, Eikemans MJC, te Velde ER, Habbema JDF, Fauser BCJM. Predictors of patients remaining anovulatory during clomiphene citrate induction of ovulation in normogonadotrophic oligo-amenorrheic infertility. *J Clin Endocrinol Metab* 1998; in press.

12. Dickey RP, Holtkamp DE. Development, pharmacology and clinical experience with clomiphene citrate. *Hum Reprod Update* 1996; **2**:483–506.

13. Kurachi K, Aono T, Minagawa J, Miyake A. Congenital malformations of newborn infants after clomiphene-induced ovulation. *Fertil Steril* 1983;**40**:187.

14. Dickey RP, Matis R, Olar TT, et al. The occurrence of ectopic pregnancy with and without clomiphene citrate use in assisted and non-assisted reproductive technology. *J In Vitro Fertil Embryo Transf* 1989;**6**:294–7.

15. Messinis IE, Nillius SJ, Comparison between tamoxifen and clomiphene for induction of ovulation. *Acta Obstet Gynaecol Scand* 1982;**61**:377–81.

16. Fauser BCJM. Developments in human recombinant FSH technology: are we going in the right direction? *Hum Reprod* 1998; in press.

17. Fauser BCJM, van Heusden AM. Manipulation of human ovarian function: Physiological concepts and clinical consequences. *Endocrine Rev* 1997;**18**:71–106.

18. Fauser BCJM, Donderwinkel P, Schoot DC. The step-down principle in gonadotrophin treatment and the role of GnRH analogues. *Baillière's Clin Obstet Gynaecol* 1993;**7**:309–30.

19. White DM, Polson DW, Kiddy D, et al. Induction of ovulation with low dose gonadotrophins in polycystic ovary syndrome: An analysis of 109 pregnancies in 225 women. *J Clin Endocrinol Metab* 1996;**81**:3821–4.

20. Buvat J, Buvat HM, Marcolin G, et al. Purified follicle-stimulating hormone in polycystic ovary syndrome: slow administration is safer and more effective. *Fertil Steril* 1989;**52**:553–9.

21. Shoham Z, Patel A, Jacobs HS. Polycystic ovary syndrome: safety and effectiveness of a stepwise and low-dose administration of purified FSH. *Fertil Steril* 1991;**55**:1051–6.

22. van Santbrink EJP, Donderwinkel PFJ, van Dessel TJHM, et al. Gonadotrophin induction of ovulation using a step-down dose regimen: Single center clinical experience in 82 patients. *Hum Reprod* 1995;**10**:1048.

23. Schipper I, Hop WCJ, Fauser BCJM. The Follicle-Stimulating Hormone (FSH) threshold/window concept examined by differential interventions with exogenous FSH during the follicular phase of the normal menstrual cycle: duration rather than magnitude of FSH increase affects follicle development. *J Clin Endocrin Metab* 1998; in press.

24. van Santbrink EJP, Fauser BCJM. Urinary follicle hormone for normogonadotrophic clomiphene-resistant infertility: Prospective, randomized

comparison between low dose step-up and step-down dose regimens. *J Clin Endocrinol Metab* 1997;**82:**3597–602.

25. Haning RV, Austin CW, Carlston IH, et al. Plasma estradiol is superior to ultrasound and urinary estriol glucuronide as a predictor of ovarian hyperstimulation during induction of ovulation with menotropins. *Fertil Steril* 1983;**40:**31–6.

26. Hughes E, Collins J, Vanderkerkhove P. Ovulation induction with urinary follicle stimulating hormone vs human menopausal gonadotropin for clomiphene-resistant polycystic ovary syndrome. *The Cochrane Library* 1996;**3:**1–8.

27. Coelingh Bennink HJ, Fauser BCJM, Out HJ, et al. Recombinant FSH (Puregon) is more efficient than urinary FSH (Metrodin) in women with clomiphene-resistant normogonadotrophic chronic anovulatory: A prospective, multi-centre, assessor-blind, randomised clinical trial. *Fertil Steril* 1998;**69:**19–25.

28. Recombinant human FSH Study Group. Clinical assessment of recombinant human follicle-stimulating hormone in stimulating ovarian follicular development before in vitro fertilization. *Fertil Steril* 1995;**63:**77–86.

29. Out HJ, Mannaerts BMJL, Driessen SGAJ, et al. A randomized, assessor-blind, multicentre study comparing recombinant and urinary follicle-stimulating hormone (Puregon vs Metrodin) in in-vitro fertilization. *Hum Reprod* 1995;**10:**2534–40.

30. Begh C, Howles CM, Borg K, et al. Recombinant human follicle stimulating hormone (r-hFSH; Gonal F®) versus highly purified urinary FSH (Metrodin HP®): results of a randomized comparative study in women undergoing assisted reproductive techiques. *Hum Reprod* 1997; **12:**2133–9.

31. Kousta E, White DM, Piazzi A, et al. Successful induction of ovulation and completed pregnancy using recombinant human luteinizing hormone

and follicle stimulating hormone in a woman with Kallmann's syndrome. *Hum Reprod* 1996;**11:**70–1.

32. Martin KA, Hall JE, Adams JM, Crowley WFJ. Comparison of exogenous gonadotropins and pulsatile gonadotropin-releasing hormone for induction of ovulation in hypogonadotropic amenorrhea. *J Clin Endocrinol Metab* 1993; **77:**125–9.

33. Jansen RP. Pulsatile intravenous gonadotrophin releasing hormone for ovulation induction: determinants of follicular and luteal phase responses. *Hum Reprod* 1993;**2**(suppl):193–6.

34. Martin K, Santoro N, Hall J, et al. Management of ovulatory disorders with pulsatile gonadotropin-releasing hormone. *J Clin Endocrinol Metab* 1990;**71:**1081A–1081G.

35. Kelly AC, Jewelewicz R. Alternate regimens for ovulation induction in polycystic ovarian disease. *Fertil Steril* 1990;**54:**195–202.

36. Donesky BW, Adashi EY. Surgical ovulation induction: the role of ovarian diathermy in polycytic ovary syndrome. *Baillière's Clin Obstet Gynaecol* 1996;**10:**293–309.

37. Gürgan T, Kisnisci H, Yarali H. Evaluation of adhesion formation after laparoscopic treatment of polycystic ovarian disease. *Fertil Steril* 1991;**56:**1176–8.

38. Greenblaat EM, Casper RF. Adhesion formation after laparoscopic ovarian cautery for polycystic ovarian syndrome: lack of correlation with pregnancy rate. *Fertil Steril* 1993;**60:**766–70.

39. Gürgan T, Urman B, Aksu T. The effect of short-interval laparoscopic lysis of adhesions on pregnancy rates following Nd:Yag laser photocoagulation of polycystic ovaries. *Obstet Gynaecol* 1992;**80:**45–7.

40. Dabirashrafi H. Complications of laparoscopic ovarian cauterization. *Fertil Steril* 1989;**52:**878–9.

41. Abdel Gadir A, Khatim MS, Alnaser HMI. Ovarian electrocautery: responders versus non-responders. *Gynaecol Endocrinol* 1993;**7:**43–8.

# 8

# Detrimental effects of LH hypersecretion

Roy Homburg

**Clinical evidence • Contradictory evidence • Methods to reduce LH concentrations and their effect on treatment results • Mechanism of the adverse effects of elevated LH concentrations • Conclusions**

The polycystic ovary syndrome (PCOS) is a very heterogeneous syndrome and may present in a wide range of symptoms, varying from mild hirsutism or acne only with regular menstrual cycles to the full-blown syndrome of obesity, amenorrhoea, hirsutism and infertility. Biochemical changes are similarly heterogeneous. Hypersecretion of luteinizing hormone (LH) occurs in about 40% of women who have ultrasonographically diagnosed polycystic ovaries[1] and has been associated with an increased risk of infertility and miscarriage.[2]

The inappropriate secretion of LH that occurs in the PCOS is a tonic hypersecretion, and should be differentiated from a premature surge which may occur during either ovulation-induction regimens or superovulation for assisted conception procedures. Although women with normal or polycystic ovaries may have a spontaneous LH surge during ovulation-induction regimens, tonic hypersecretion of LH during the follicular phase of the cycle occurs, however, only in women with the PCOS.

## CLINICAL EVIDENCE

### Epidemiological data

In a study of 556 patients with ultrasonographically diagnosed polycystic ovaries (PCO), Conway et al[3] found that those who complained of infertility had significantly higher LH concentrations (mean = 11.3 IU/l) than those who did not complain (mean = 6.7 IU/l). Of these subjects, 44% had a serum LH concentration that exceeded 10 IU/l and in these infertility was significantly more prevalent (37%) than in the group with normal LH measurements (21%). Balen et al[1] compared the LH concentrations in groups of women with ultrasonographically diagnosed PCO who had primary infertility ($n = 228$), secondary infertility ($n = 121$) and proven fertility ($n = 116$). The mean serum LH concentration of those with primary infertility (11 IU/l) was significantly higher than that of women with secondary infertility (9 IU/l), and both were very significantly higher than in those with proven fertility (7.2 IU/l). The rate of infertility increased if the serum LH concentration was greater than 10 IU/l. These two studies illustrate not only the association of high concentrations of LH with a disturbance of fertility potential, but also demonstrate that this association is dependent on the LH concentrations rather than on the mere presence of PCO.

## During natural cycles

Two studies have associated elevated LH concentrations in the follicular phase of a natural cycle with a disturbance of fertility potential. Regan et al[4] studied 193 women with regular cycles who were planning to become pregnant and showed that raised midfollicular phase serum LH concentrations (> 10 IU/l) were associated with a lower conception rate over 1 year (61%) compared with those in women with normal concentrations (80%). This was a significant difference; even more striking, however, was the much higher miscarriage rate (65%) in women with high midfollicular LH concentrations compared with those with normal values (12%).[4] A study of women undergoing 'natural cycle in vitro fertilization', which does not incorporate any ovarian stimulation, found fertilization rates of 45–50% in women who had elevated serum LH concentrations in either the early follicular or midfollicular phase, compared with a fertilization rate of 87.5% in a control group with normal serum LH concentrations.[5]

## During ovulation induction

Shoham et al[6] demonstrated that, in women treated with clomiphene citrate, high levels of LH during the follicular phase were associated with a reduced conception rate, in spite of adequate follicular growth and corpus luteum function, as indicated by measurements of serum oestradiol concentrations in the follicular phase and of progesterone concentrations in the luteal phase. The main mode of action of clomiphene is to boost follicle-stimulating hormone (FSH) concentrations in the early follicular phase but, unfortunately, it also raises LH levels at this apparently critical stage; for those patients who already have a high baseline level, the additional discharge of LH may seriously prejudice their chances to conceive.

In our own study[2] of a large group of patients with PCOS undergoing treatment with pulsatile luteinizing hormone-releasing hormone (LHRH) for induction of ovulation, follicular phase serum LH concentrations were significantly higher in those who failed to conceive (19 IU/l), than in those who conceived (12.4 IU/l). In addition, those who conceived but miscarried had significantly higher follicular phase LH concentrations (17.9 IU/l) than those who delivered successfully (9.6 IU/l). Homburg et al[2] also found that the miscarriage rate was 33% in women with the PCOS, compared with 10.6% in those with hypogonadotrophic hypogonadism who were treated in a similar fashion and also had a much higher rate of conception. From this first study of LH in ovulation induction, it was thus very clear that, in women with the PCOS, there was a significantly reduced chance of conception, and there was an increased risk of miscarriage in those with an elevated follicular phase plasma LH concentration compared with those with the PCOS and normal follicular phase LH levels. Furthermore, this study demonstrated that LH was the true culprit because there were no significant differences of any other hormonal parameter measured (testosterone, dihydroepiandrosterone sulphate (DHEAS), androstenedione, FSH or prolactin) between those who conceived and those who did not, and between those who delivered and those who miscarried.

In 100 women with the PCOS who were treated with low-dose gonadotrophin therapy, the association of raised baseline and/or midfollicular phase plasma LH concentrations with a poor response to treatment was also demonstrated by Hamilton-Fairley et al.[7] In this series, the patients with an elevated LH concentration also had a higher rate of miscarriage than the women with POC and normal LH levels.

## During superovulation for IVF

Stanger and Yovich[8] were the first to suggest an association between LH levels and impaired fertility. They demonstrated, in 1985, that oocytes obtained from women undergoing in vitro fertilization (IVF) who had a serum LH value greater than 1 SD (standard deviation) above the mean on the day of administration of human chorionic gonadotrophin (hCG) had a significantly reduced rate of fertilization and cleavage.[8] This relationship was confirmed by Howles et al[9] in a series of 200 patients in whom elevated urinary LH excretion in the 2 days before hCG administration was associated with poor oocyte quality, poor embryo viability and reduced pregnancy rates.

Although, in the studies of women undergoing IVF by Stanger and Yovich[8] and Howles et al,[9] late follicular phase LH secretion was assessed making it difficult to distinguish clearly between tonic elevation of LH and the onset of the preovulatory LH surge, the study of Punnonen et al[10] differentiated between the effect on the outcome of IVF of a premature LH surge occurring within 12 hours of hCG administration (no effect) and the effect when the surge occurred more than 12 hours before hCG (embryo cleavage significantly reduced). They demonstrated the critical nature of the timing of the exposure to LH in determining the adverse outcome. The studies of Homburg et al[2] and Regan et al,[4] already noted, determined pretreatment and midfollicular concentrations and so provide convincing evidence that it is tonic hypersecretion of LH that is detrimental to reproductive health.

## Further evidence

In women attending a recurrent miscarriage clinic, Sagle et al[11] reported that 82% had polycystic ovaries, detected by ultrasonography; women attending that clinic were also found to have abnormalities of follicular phase LH secretion.[12] In a study of 538 patients undergoing IVF for conditions other than anovulatory infertility, it was significant that polycystic ovaries were detected by ultrasonography in 45% of those who miscarried compared with 31% of those with ongoing pregnancies.[13]

## CONTRADICTORY EVIDENCE

Although this large body of clinical evidence for a deleterious effect of high LH concentrations on fertility potential is convincing, two further studies contradict these findings. In a study of 596 women undergoing IVF, serum LH concentrations above either the 75th or 95th centile for more than 3 days had no significant effect on either fertilization or pregnancy rates.[14] Furthermore, another study found a closer relationship between an elevated serum progesterone concentration, but not LH concentration, with respect to failure of fertilization during IVF.[15] The discrepancies between these studies and those described above may be explained by different study populations or methodology but, on the whole, the answer is enigmatic.

## METHODS TO REDUCE LH CONCENTRATIONS AND THEIR EFFECT ON TREATMENT RESULTS

If the results of the studies presented above truly reflect a deleterious effect of high follicular phase concentrations of LH on rates of conception and miscarriage, then the converse should also be true, that is, treatment to reduce LH concentrations during the follicular phase should increase conception and reduce miscarriage rates. Three methods for reducing LH secretion and the results obtained are described.

### Progesterone pre-treatment

In the normal ovulatory cycle, it is progesterone that is responsible for the reduction of LH concentrations in the luteal phase and induction of ovulation by any means in the PCOS is often followed by a temporary reduction of LH levels. We administered micronized proges-terone for 5 days to 10 amenorrhoeic women with the PCOS who were clomiphene resistant. We demonstrated a slowing of LH pulse fre-quency and an increased pulse amplitude with a resultant reduction in serum LH concentra-tions in seven of the ten women.[16] All seven of these women then responded to clomiphene in the following cycle and three of them con-ceived. None of the three whose LH concentra-tions remained high became responsive to clomiphene.

## Combined GnRH agonist–gonadotrophin therapy

There is now mounting evidence that the ability of GnRH agonists to reduce the inordinately elevated concentrations of LH prevalent in some 40% of women with the PCOS serves to increase ovulation and pregnancy rates and to reduce the prevalence of early spontaneous miscarriage. A study from our group[17] looked at the performance of women with PCOS undergoing IVF/embryo transfer (ET) who had high mean LH concentrations, compared with a control group of normally cycling women with mechanical infertility. Pregnancy rates were similar in the two groups; although GnRH ago-nist treatment reduced the miscarriage rate by half compared with gonadotrophins alone in the PCOS group, its administration to the con-trol group had no such effect. In a further study from our centre,[18] 239 women with PCOS received human menopausal gonadotrophin (hMG) with or without an GnRH agonist for ovulation induction or superovulation for IVF/ET. Of pregnancies achieved with an GnRH agonist, 17.6% miscarried compared with 39% of those achieved with gonadotrophins alone. Cumulative live-birth rates after four cycles for GnRH agonists were 64% compared with 26% for gonadotrophins only. Similarly, Balen et al[13] analysed the out-come of treatment in 182 women with PCO detected ultrasonographically who conceived after IVF. They found a highly significant reduction in the rate of miscarriage when

buserelin was used to achieve pituitary desensi-tization followed by stimulation with hMG (15 of 74, 20%) compared with the use of clomiphene and hMG (51 of 108, 47%).

Unfortunately, a prospective, randomized study is not yet available to evaluate the effect of pituitary desensitization on miscarriage rates in women with the PCOS undergoing ovulation induction or IVF. Such a study is very difficult to perform because the number of pregnancies that would have to be attained to demonstrate a 30% difference in miscarriage rates between treatment protocols with and without the use of GnRH agonist is enormous. In addition, in view of the IVF data presented above, it may prove ethically difficult not to use an GnRH agonist for women with the PCOS undergoing super-ovulation for IVF. In a different population of 1537 women with recurrent miscarriage, 52% had PCO, of whom 13% had an elevated serum LH concentration and 57% an elevated urinary secretion of LH.[19] In a prospective, randomized study in this large heterogeneous group of women with recurrent miscarriage, the effect of a spontaneous cycle with or without luteal phase support and the use of an GnRH agonist and hMG with luteal phase support were exam-ined. No benefit was obtained from the use of the GnRH agonist. Taking into account the selection of cases in this series and the inaccura-cies inherent in the measurement of urinary LH, while providing food for thought and fur-ther more specific investigation, it is difficult to transpose these results to the data presented above.

## Laparoscopic ovarian puncture

The main endocrine change caused by laparo-scopic ovarian puncture for ovulation induction in women with the PCOS is a fall in serum LH concentration.[20–22] The patients who failed to ovulate postoperatively were the patients who did not experience a fall in LH levels.[21] In a small study by Balen and Jacobs,[23] five patients (50%) ovulated within 6 weeks of laparoscopic ovarian diathermy but the remaining five failed to ovulate by 12 weeks, although all subsequently ovulated in response to either clomiphene citrate or gonadotrophin therapy. There were no significant differences between the baseline hormone measurements of the responders and those of the non-responders. When the pre- and post-treatment values were compared, there were no differences in the serum FSH and testosterone concentrations in either the responders or the non-responders. In the responders, however, there was a significant fall of the serum LH concentration postoperatively, whereas in the non-responders there was no difference in the LH concentrations before and after treatment. In a continuation of the study by Gadir et al,[21] however, although those who ovulated but had an early resumption of the anovulatory state were found to return to preoperative LH concentrations, those who ovulated persistently maintained a normal LH level. Further, those patients with the highest preoperative LH concentrations were the most likely to ovulate spontaneously after the operation.[21]

The only significant report on miscarriage rates after laparoscopic ovarian diathermy so far[24] involved 58 pregnancies with a miscarriage rate of 14%, much lower than that usually experienced in women with the PCOS (30–40% – see above). A summary of the studies quoted above suggest that the best results from this operation have been obtained in clomipheneresistant women who are slim and have raised serum LH concentrations.

## MECHANISM OF THE ADVERSE EFFECTS OF ELEVATED LH CONCENTRATIONS

Whether the deleterious effects of high LH concentrations are a result of a direct influence on the oocyte or adversely affect the endometrium was the first question to be addressed by us.[25] This study attempted to answer the question by examining, in recipients, the performance of embryos derived from oocytes donated by women with the PCOS who underwent ovarian stimulation with gonadotrophins with or without an GnRH agonist. Thus, the endometrium of the recipients was a constant, whereas the donated oocytes were exposed (no GnRH agonist) or not exposed (with GnRH agonist) to high concentrations of LH during superovulation. A total of 79 patients with the PCOS, themselves undergoing IVF/ET, donated supernumerary oocytes to 145 patients (159 cycles) in an ovum donation programme. Of the 145 recipients, 70 received oocytes derived from non-GnRH agonist cycles and 75 from GnRH cycles. The implantation rate/embryo transferred from oocytes from donors given GnRH agonist and those who were not was 11.7% vs 6.6% ($p < 0.05$), the pregnancy rate/transfer was 28% vs 18% and the miscarriage rate 8.7% vs 21.4%. This implies that high LH concentrations affect the oocyte and not the endometrium.

Recent data in women undergoing the transfer of frozen embryos in natural cycles also failed to implicate the endometrium as the target of the effect of LH.[26] The embryos in this study had been generated in IVF cycles in which pituitary desensitization had been used to achieve suppression of LH levels. Thus, the elevated LH concentrations seen in the subsequent natural cycles of some of the women who received the frozen embryos could not have affected embryo quality and could only have exerted an effect by altering the endometrium. No effect on outcome was detected.

We therefore look to the oocyte as the target of LH effect and, first, to the influence of LH on the oocyte in a normal ovulatory cycle. Dekel et al[27] reported that LH leads to disruption of the processes that traverse the intercellular space between the cumulus granulosa cells and the oocyte, which then results in a fall of intraoocyte cAMP – and hence a reduction in the 'oocyte maturation inhibitor' – and the resumption of meiosis.[27] In the normal course of events, these changes occur as a consequence of the LH surge. The interval between ovulation and fertilization, that is, the exposure of the oocyte to high concentrations of LH and the consequent resumption of meiosis, is critical and, if this interval is exceeded, physiologically aged oocytes are produced which may be subject to reproductive failure. Thus, a possible explanation of the adverse effect of hypersecretion of LH on human fertility is that hypersecretion of LH during the follicular phase results in an elevated concentration of intrafollicular LH which, in turn, results in premature oocyte maturation, with subsequent ovulation of a prematurely matured egg. Thus inappropriate release of LH may profoundly affect the timing of oocyte maturation so that the released egg is either unable to be fertilized[2] or, even if it is fertilized, will tend to miscarry.[4]

## CONCLUSIONS

In addition to the difficulties involved in conceiving for women with the PCOS, the high incidence of spontaneous miscarriages when a conception is attained presents a further problem. The weight of evidence presented here implicates elevated concentrations of LH as an important factor in the causation of these distressing effects. The present hypothesis suggests that these adverse effects of high LH concentrations are a result of the induction of an early resumption of meiosis and, therefore, abnormal oocyte maturation, which is the main cause of reproductive failure in women who hypersecrete LH during the follicular phase of the ovulation cycle.

## REFERENCES

1. Balen AH, Conway GS, Kaltsas G, et al. Polycystic ovary syndrome: The spectrum of the disorder in 1741 patients. *Hum Reprod* 1995; **10**:2107–11.
2. Homburg R, Armar NA, Eshel A, et al. Influence of serum luteinising hormone concentrations on ovulation, conception and early pregnancy loss in polycystic ovary syndrome. *BMJ* 1988; **297**:1024–6.
3. Conway GS, Honour JW, Jacobs HS. Heterogeneity of the polycystic ovary syndrome: clinical, endocrine and ultrasound features in 556 patients. *Clin Endocrinol* 1989;**30**:459–70.
4. Regan L, Owen EJ, Jacobs HS. Hypersecretion of luteinising hormone, infertility and miscarriage. *Lancet* 1990;**336**:1141–4.
5. Verma S, Monks N, Turner K, et al. Influence of elevated LH during follicular phase on fertility as assessed in a natural IVF programme. *Seventh Annual Meeting of the ESHRE and the Seventh World Congress on IVF and Assisted Procreation*, Paris, July 1991, p. 68.
6. Shoham Z, Borenstein R, Lunenfeld B, Pariente C. Hormonal profiles following clomiphene citrate therapy in conception and nonconception cycles. *Clin Endocrinol* 1990;**33**:271–8.
7. Hamilton-Fairley D, Kiddy D, Watson H, et al. Association of moderate obesity with a poor pregnancy outcome in women with polycystic ovary syndrome treated with low dose gonadotrophin. *Br J Obstet Gynaecol* 1992;**99**:28–31.
8. Stanger JD, Yovich JL. Reduced in-vitro fertilisation of human oocyte from patients with raised basal luteinising hormone levels during the follicular phase. *Br J Obstet Gynaecol* 1985;**92**:385–93.
9. Howles CM, Macnamee MC, Edwards RG, et al. Effect of high tonic levels of luteinising hormone on outcome of in-vitro fertilisation. *Lancet* 1986;**i**:521–2.
10. Punnonen R, Ashorn R, Vilja P, et al. Spontaneous luteinizing hormone surge and cleavage of in vitro fertilized embryos. *Fertil Steril* 1988;**49**:479–82.
11. Sagle M, Bishop K, Alexander FM, et al. Recurrent early miscarriage and polycystic ovaries. *BMJ* 1988;**297**:1027–8.
12. Watson H, Hamilton-Fairley D, Kiddy D, et al. Abnormalities of follicular phase luteinising hormone secretion in women with recurrent early miscarriage. *J Endocrinol* 1989;**123**(suppl):abstract 25.
13. Balen AH, Tan SL, MacDougall J, Jacobs HS. Miscarriage rates following in-vitro fertilisation are increased in women with polycystic ovaries and reduced by pituitary desensitisation with buserelin. *Hum Reprod* 1993;**8**:959–64.
14. Thomas A, Okamoto S, O'Shea F, et al. Do raised serum luteinizing hormone levels during stimulation for in vitro fertilisation predict outcome? *Br J Obstet Gynaecol* 1989;**96**:1328–32.
15. Kagawa T, Yamano S, Nishida S, et al. Relationship among serum levels of luteinising hormone, estradiol and progesterone during follicle stimulation and results of in-vitro fertilisa-

tion and embryo transfer. *J Assisted Reprod Genetics* 1992;**9:**106–12.

16. Homburg R, Weisglass L, Goldman J. Improved treatment for anovulation in polycystic ovarian disease utilising the effect of progesterone on the inappropriate gonadotrophin release and clomiphene response. *Hum Reprod* 1988;**3:**285–8.

17. Homburg R, Berkovitz D, Levy T, et al. In-vitro fertilization and embryo transfer for the treatment of infertility associated with polycystic ovary syndrome. *Fertil Steril* 1993;**60:**858–63.

18. Homburg R, Levy T, Berkovitz D, et al. Gonadotropin-releasing hormone agonist reduces the miscarriage rate for pregnancies achieved in women with polycystic ovary syndrome. *Fertil Steril* 1993;**59:**527–31.

19. Clifford K, Rai R, Watson H, et al. Does suppressing LH secretion reduce the miscarriage rate? Results of a randomised controlled trial. *BMJ* 1996;**312:**1508–11.

20. Rossmanith WG, Keckstein J, Spatzier K, Lauritzen C. The impact of ovarian laser surgery on the gonadotrophin secretion in women with PCOS. *Clin Endocrinol* 1991;**34:**223–30.

21. Gadir AA, Khatim MS, Mowafi RS, et al. Hormonal changes in patients with polycystic ovarian disease after ovarian electrocautery or pituitary desensitization. *Clin Endocrinol* 1990;**32:**749–54.

22. Armar NA, McGarrigle HHG, Honour JW, et al. Laparoscopic ovarian diathermy in the management of anovulatory infertility in women with polycystic ovaries: endocrine changes and clinical outcome. *Fertil Steril* 1990;**53:**45–9.

23. Balen AH, Jacobs HS. A prospective study comparing unilateral and bilateral laparoscopic ovarian diathermy in women with the polycystic ovary syndrome. *Fertil Steril* 1994;**62:**921–5.

24. Armar NA, Lachelin GCL. Laparoscopic ovarian diathermy: an effective treatment for anti-oestrogen resistant anovulatory infertility in women with the polycystic ovary syndrome. *Br J Obstet Gynaecol* 1993;**100:**161–4.

25. Ashkenazi J, Farhi J, Orvieto R, et al. Polycystic ovary syndrome patients as oocyte donors: The effect of ovarian stimulation protocol on the implantation rate of the recipient. *Fertil Steril* 1995;**64:**564–7.

26. Polson DW, Chanda M, Bedi S, et al. The effect of serum luteinising hormone concentrations on success rates of frozen embryo replacement into natural cycles. *Br Congress Obstet Gynaecol* 1992;abstract 152.

27. Dekel N, Galiani D, Aberdam E. Regulation of rat oocyte maturation: involvement of protein kinases. In: *Fertilisation in Mammals* (Bavister BD, Cummins J, Roldan ERS, eds). Norwell: Serono Symposia, 1990: 17–24.

# Part IV
# Recombinant Drugs

# 9

# Basic knowledge about recombinant gonadotropic hormone production

Scott Chappel, Christine Kelton, Noreen Nugent

**Construction of vectors for the expression of the glycoprotein common α subunit in mammalian cells • Construction of the expression vector that encodes the human FSH β subunit gene • Construction of the expression vector that encodes the human LH β subunit gene • Expression and characterization of human recombinant LH • Recombinant LH in vitro bioactivity • Expression and purification of recombinant human FSH • In vitro and in vivo biological activity assessment of recombinant DNA-derived human FSH • The physiological significance of FSH isoforms**

Follicle-stimulating hormone (FSH) and luteinizing hormone (LH) belong to a family of glycoprotein hormones that includes human chorionic gonadotropin (hCG) and thyroid-stimulating hormone (TSH).[1] These hormones are heterodimers, consisting of an α subunit that is identical among all of them and a hormone-specific β subunit.[1,2] LH and FSH are required for normal reproductive function in both the male and female. These protein hormones play critical roles in both spermatogenesis and folliculogenesis. FSH alone or FSH in combination with LH is used clinically to stimulate follicular development. For the past 30 years, the source of human gonadotropins for this purpose has been the urine of postmenopausal women. As a result of the ever increasing demand for gonadotropins, and the concern over the use of products derived from human sources, an extensive effort was made to clone and express the genes that encode FSH and LH and express them in a mammalian cell.

Expression of the gonadotropins by recombinant DNA technology required the isolation and cloning of three different genes: the common α subunit and the hormone-specific β subunit for each hormone. The common α subunit for the gonadotropins contains two asparagine-linked oligosaccharides at residues 52 and 78.[3–5] The β subunit of FSH contains two asparagine-linked oligosaccharides at residues 7 and 24. The β subunit for LH contains one N-linked oligosaccharide attachment site at residue 30. These carbohydrate residues are essential for biological activity both in vitro and in vivo.[6–9] Therefore, a mammalian cell expression system was required. This chapter describes the cloning and engineering of these genes and their expression. These recombinant gonadotropins are now used clinically.

## CONSTRUCTION OF VECTORS FOR THE EXPRESSION OF THE GLYCOPROTEIN COMMON α SUBUNIT IN MAMMALIAN CELLS

To express human FSH and LH in a mammalian cell expression system, separate expression vectors that contained DNA encoding the α and β subunits were prepared as described.

The human α subunit genomic fragment used for expression purposes was 11 kilobase-pairs (kb) in length and was derived from a 17-kb genomic clone identical to that described previously.[10,11] The endogenous gene-promoter region was removed by cleavage at the unique *BamH*I site in exon I. The fragment that resulted included the remainder of exon I, all of the coding exons II, III, and IV, as well as the intervening sequences, and about 2 kb of the 3′-flanking sequence. The termini of the 11-kb fragment were converted to *Sal*I sites before its inser-

tion into the unique *Xho*I site of the CLH3AXSV2DHFR expression vector shown in Figure 1. In this construct, transcription of the α gene was directed by the mouse metallothionein-I (MMT-I) promoter and the endogenous α subunit gene polyadenylation signal was used for 3′ processing of the mRNA. The expression vector also contained the mouse dihydrofolate reductase (DHFR) gene. This gene was used as a selectable and amplifiable marker. A restriction endonuclease map of the complete human α subunit expression vector plasmid as shown in Figure 1.

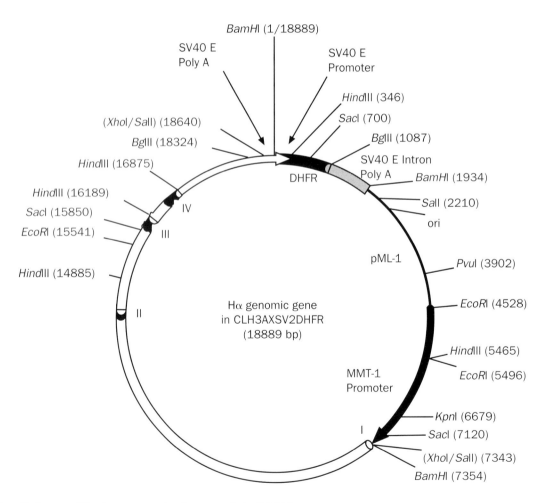

**Figure 1** A map of the human α subunit expression plasmid

## CONSTRUCTION OF THE EXPRESSION VECTOR THAT ENCODES THE HUMAN FSH β SUBUNIT GENE

The human FSH β coding region was obtained from a DdeI–Sau3AI subfragment of the genomic clone as described previously.[12,13] As the endogenous FSH β polyadenylation signal was removed during engineering, the SV40 early polyadenylation signal supplied by the vector was used for 3′ processing of the FSH β subunit transcript. The murine ornithine decarboxylase (ODC) transcriptional unit was also part of the vector. The ODC gene, like the DHFR gene, is a selectable and amplifiable marker. A restriction map of the complete human FSH β subunit expression vector as shown in Figure 2.

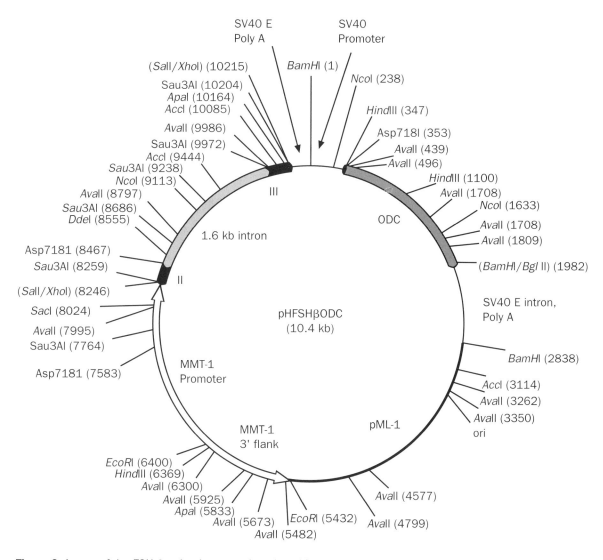

**Figure 2** A map of the FSH β subunit expression plasmid

## CONSTRUCTION OF THE EXPRESSION VECTOR THAT ENCODES THE HUMAN LH β SUBUNIT GENE

The human LH β DNA fragment was a 520-bp HindIII–BamHI composite clone. Two clones were isolated from a human pituitary cDNA library.[13] Neither clone was complete, but the combined sequence encoded 15 amino acids of the signal peptide, the entire mature peptide of 121 amino acids and the complete 3'-untranslated region of the mRNA. Sequences corresponding to the first four amino acids of the signal peptide, including the start ATG, were not contained in either clone.

To engineer a functional LH β subunit expression construct, about 60 base-pairs (bp) of the 5' end of hCG β cDNA was added at the first DdeI site to create a hybrid molecule that contained the start ATG sequence and a complete signal peptide. This resulted in a single amino acid difference between the recombinant LH β amino acid sequence and the natural LH β amino acid sequence. This change was from leucine (in the natural LH β) to phenylalanine (in the recombinant LH β) at the fourth amino acid in the signal peptide. The secretory signal is removed from the protein upon translocation across the endoplasmic reticulum and therefore no hCG-β-derived sequences are present in the mature recombinant LH β.

About 670 bp of the first intron of the mouse immunoglobulin κ chain was fused 5' to the LH β subunit expression construct. This piece of DNA was added to increase mRNA accumulation. The reconstructed LH β fragment was inserted into the same expression vector described for the FSH β gene so that transcription was directed by the MMT-1 promoter. As the endogenous LH β polyadenylation signal was removed during engineering, the SV40 early polyA signal supplied by the vector was used for 3' processing of the LH β subunit transcript.

## EXPRESSION AND CHARACTERIZATION OF HUMAN RECOMBINANT LH

The α and LH β constructs prepared as described above were transfected into Chinese hamster (CHO) cells using a 1:1 or 1:3 ratio (α:β). The α and β LH expression vector plasmids were co-transfected by the calcium phosphate precipitation method. Methotrexate was used for selection and amplification. As co-amplification of the α and LH β plasmids was a frequent occurrence when the cells are exposed to step-wise increases in methotrexate, the direct and separate amplification of the LH β plasmid using an ODC antagonist, was found to be unnecessary. A full amplification protocol was employed, with initial selection beginning at 0.02 μmol/l methotrexate up to 5.0 μmol/l. Four recombinant CHO cell lines expressing human LH were evaluated in T-flask culture. An optimized cloning protocol yielded a high number of clones which was either equal to or greater than the preclonal cell lines. Cells cloned under selective conditions displayed equivalent growth and expression characteristics as those derived under non-selective conditions. In addition, the stability of expression over 65 population doublings was not influenced by the different cloning conditions.

Recombinant DNA-derived human LH was purified by conventional methods (concentration, ion exchange, and size exclusion steps). The purified protein was analyzed by a variety of techniques. Reverse phase high-performance liquid chromatography (HPLC) of recombinant LH showed one α peak and several β peaks resulting from C-terminal length heterogeneity. Complete amino acid sequencing was carried out on the subunits. As with pituitary LH, some C-terminal variants of the β subunit were found with lengths of 116, 119, 120, and 121 residues.[19,20]

Multiple lots of recombinant human LH were analyzed to determine the monosaccharide content of the N-linked oligosaccharides. Twelve lots were derived from perfusion culture runs whereas three were derived from batch cultures. Batch cultures contained lower levels of sialic acid, containing approximately

1.0 mol sialic acid per 3 mol mannose. Perfusion cultures contained higher levels of sialic acid: about 2 mol sialic acid per 3 mol of mannose. All of the oligosaccharide chains on LH α and β contained sialic acid at the terminus with no sulfates.

By isoelectric focusing, the LH derived from perfusion culture contained isoforms with charges within the range 6–10. This was similar to the range and profile described by others for human, bovine, and ovine pituitary LH.[21,22]

## RECOMBINANT LH IN VITRO BIOACTIVITY

Some MA-10 cells were isolated from a mouse Leydig cell tumor. As MA-10 cells have a deficiency in 17α-hydroxylase activity, they respond to human LH and hCG stimulation by the production of progesterone in the media instead of the testosterone produced by normal Leydig cells. The degree of LH bioactivity is proportional to the level of progesterone production. Purified recombinant LH was tested by in vitro bioassay with MA-10 cells. All batches were shown to be biologically active and equivalent to a pituitary standard with this in vitro assay.

## EXPRESSION AND PURIFICATION OF RECOMBINANT HUMAN FSH

A DHFR-deficient CHO cell line (CHO-DUKX) was transfected with separate expression vectors containing the α and β FSH genes. Transfectants were selected after the addition of methotrexate. Colonies were selected and cultures were amplified with increasing amounts of methotrexate to obtain higher levels of FSH expression. Individual transfectants were screened by assaying culture supernatants for expressed human FSH by radioimmunoassay. The cell culture with the best expression was subcloned. The single cell clone with the highest expression was expanded for use in bioproduction. The recombinant human FSH expressed by this clonal cell line was purified by a three-step process which included anion exchange, immunoaffinity, and size exclusion chromatography. The FSH protein was shown to be more than 95% pure by several different methods (sodium dodecylsulfate–polyacrylamide gel electrophoresis or SDS-PAGE and silver staining) and the protein was sequenced to show correspondence to the predicted amino acid sequence derived from the DNA sequence.

The purified recombinant FSH was also analyzed for carbohydrate content and found to exhibit a content similar to that reported for other pituitary standards, as well as other recombinant DNA-derived FSH.

The oligosaccharides found on the α and β subunits of FSH are required for full biological activity and affect plasma half-life and therefore the overall potency of the molecule.[7–9,14] Variations in the glycosylation pattern at these sites results in the production of multiple forms of FSH produced by the anterior pituitary gland.[15,16] Likewise, FSH produced by recombinant DNA technology also exists in multiple forms as shown by isoelectric focusing which separates the molecules on the basis of overall charge.[17,18] Our studies have shown that the isoelectric focusing profile of FSH produced by recombinant DNA technology is similar to that found within the anterior pituitary gland and exhibits a preponderance of acidic isoforms. These forms have been shown by many authors to have the longest survival time in circulation and the greatest in vivo bioactivity.

## IN VITRO AND IN VIVO BIOLOGICAL ACTIVITY ASSESSMENT OF RECOMBINANT DNA-DERIVED HUMAN FSH

The granulosa cell bioassay was used to assess in vitro bioactivity.[23] In this assay, immature female rats treated with diethylstilbestrol were ovariectomized and granulosa cells were isolated and cultured in serum-free medium. After 24 h of culture, the medium was changed and fresh medium was added which contained an aromatizable androgen substrate. Several days later the medium was harvested and quantified for estradiol activity by a sensitive and specific radioimmunoassay. Estradiol production from the androgen substrate is proportional to the amount of the aromatase enzyme induced by FSH stimulation of the granulosa cells. Using conditioned medium from the clonal cell line that expresses FSH, as well as recombinant FSH after purification, dose–response curves parallel to that obtained with human pituitary FSH were obtained. Bioactivity of the recombinant human FSH was also demonstrated using a Y-1 FSH receptor-based bioassay.[24] In this assay, the gene for the human FSH receptor was expressed on the cell membrane of Y-1 cells, a murine adrenal tumor cell line. Activation of the FSH receptor in this cell line induces the expression of progesterone. Concentrations of progesterone in the cell culture medium is proportional to the amount of FSH present during the incubation period. Dose–response curves parallel to those obtained with human pituitary FSH standards were obtained using purified human recombinant FSH.

In vivo biological potency was also determined using the rat ovarian weight gain assay of Steelman and Pohley[25] and shown to be equivalent to urinary preparations of FSH. Thus, all biochemical, in vitro and in vivo bioassays demonstrated equivalence of the recombinant material to other human FSH preparations.

## THE PHYSIOLOGICAL SIGNIFICANCE OF FSH ISOFORMS

During the menstrual cycle, estrogens and androgens feed back to change the rate of secretion of FSH from the pituitary gland. It is clear that steroid hormone feedback affects not only the amount of FSH being released but also the type. It also affects not only how much hormone is secreted by the pituitary gland, but also the survival time of the FSH in circulation. Measurement of FSH concentration in blood during the menstrual cycle by both a bioassay and immunoassay and by analysis of the ratio does not always result in a constant number. This is thought to reflect differences in either the bioactivity or immunogenicity (structure?) of the FSH molecule released at different times during the cycle.[15,16]

In the complete absence of ovarian steroids (postmenopause), large amounts of FSH are secreted and this material has a much longer survival time in circulation. Women with functioning ovaries have much lower amounts of FSH circulating because of the completion of the negative feedback loop. FSH secreted by the pituitary of women with detectable levels of estradiol has a shorter plasma half-life.

These different forms of FSH could be identified not only by survival time but also by the technique of isoelectric focusing which separates proteins on the basis of charge. FSH forms with a longer half-life exhibit a more acidic isoelectric point as a result of the increased amount of the terminal sugar, sialic acid, within the molecule. Thus, the presence or absence of estradiol affected the biochemistry of the molecule, causing a shift in the overall charge of the molecule being produced by the anterior pituitary gland.[15]

It has been shown that, during the menstrual cycle, there is a change in the overall charge of FSH secreted by the anterior pituitary gland. At the time of the midcycle gonadotropin surge, there is a shift to more basic isoelectric forms. When sialic acid residues are removed from the FSH molecule, the terminal galactose binds to the asialoglycoprotein receptor on the liver or the kidneys to take it out of circulation.[14] So the fewer sialic acid molecules that are present on the FSH molecule, the more exposed are galactose residues and the more rapidly the molecule is removed from circulation.

In the early follicular phase of the menstrual cycle, we see that most of the FSH in the serum of women is of the acidic variety, at midcycle we see a shift to more basic forms. In the luteal phase, more acidic forms are predominant. During the periovulatory period, the plasma half-life of FSH is at its lowest point compared with during the follicular or luteal phase, again suggesting that the FSH stimulus has a shorter half-life and a more basic isoelectric point. We hypothesize the physiological basis for FSH heterogeneity as follows.

During the time of menstruation a lack of

negative feedback from the ovaries results in the pituitary producing larger amounts of FSH and this FSH is heavily sialylated. A long plasma half-life ensures that that message from the pituitary gland will arrive at the ovaries.

Once the ovaries begin responding to the long-acting FSH signal, it begins to secrete estradiol, inhibin, and other factors fed back to the pituitary gland, this causes not only a diminution in the total amount of FSH that is being secreted, but also a shift to more basic, shorter-acting forms. By limiting the amount and duration of the FSH stimulus provided to the developing cohort of follicles, only the most rapidly growing follicles continue to grow. This helps to select the dominant follicle. Injections of FSH with a longer half-life (such as that obtained from the urine of postmenopausal women) removes the mechanism for selection of the dominant follicle, and allows the development of multiple follicles.

As the isoform profile of recombinant human FSH is similar to that found in the pituitary gland, it may be possible to develop second-generation FSH products in which it is desirable to administer either a long-acting FSH stimulus (such as in IVF protocols) or shorter-acting forms to obtain moment-to-moment control over follicular developments (ovulation induction in patients with polycystic ovarian disease).

The use of recombinant DNA technology has created an unlimited supply of purified gonadotropins. Recombinant FSH exists as a heterogeneous population similar to that found within the anterior pituitary gland. The use of these separated recombinant human FSH isoforms (particularly the more basic isoforms) could allow a more physiologic approach, mimicking those seen in circulation during follicular development, and this might help in driving ovarian stimulation in cases where treatment is far from physiologic, although control is very important for obtaining multiple follicular growth and at the same time for avoiding the ovarian hyperstimulation syndrome.

## REFERENCES

1. Pierce JG, Parsons TF. Glycoprotein hormones: structure and functions. *Annu Rev Biochem* 1981;**50:**465–95.
2. Gray CJ. Glycoprotein gonadotropins. Structure and synthesis. *Acta Endocrinol* 1988;**288:**20–7.
3. Green ED, Baenziger JU. Asparagine-linked oligosaccharides on lutropin, follitropin and thyrotropin. Part I. *J Biol Chem* 1988;**263:**25–35.
4. Baenziger JU, Green ED. Pituitary glycoprotein hormone oligosaccharides: structure, synthesis and function of asparagine-linked oligosaccharides on lutropin, follitropin and thyrotropin. *Biochim Biophys Acta* 1988;**947:**287–306.
5. Green ED, Baenziger JU. Asparagine linked oligosaccharides on lutropin, follitropin and thyrotropin II. Distribution of sulfated and sialylated oligosaccharides on bovine, ovine and human pituitary glycoprotein hormones. *J Biol Chem* 1988;**263:**36–44.
6. Sairam MR. Deglycosylation of ovine pituitary lutropin subunits effects on subunit interaction and hormonal activity. *Arch Biochem Biophys* 1980;**204:**199–206.
7. Sairam MR, Bhargavi GN. A role for glycosylation of the alpha subunit in transduction of biological signal in glycoprotein hormones. *Science* 1985;**229:**65–7.
8. Keene J, Nishimori K, Galway AB, et al. Recombinant deglycosylated human FSH is an antagonist of human FSH action in cultured rat granulosa cells. *Endocrine J* 1994;**2:**175–80.
9. Bishop L, Robertson D, Cahir N, et al. Specific roles of the asparagine-linked carbohydrate residues of recombinant human follicle stimulating hormone in receptor binding and signal transduction. *Mol Endocrinol* 1994;**8:**722–31.
10. Fiddes JC, Goodman HM. Isolation, cloning and sequence analysis of the cDNA for the alpha subunit of human chorionic gonadotropin. *Nature* 1979;**281:**351–6.
11. Fiddes JC, Goodman H. The genes encoding the common alpha subunit of the four human gonadotropins. *J Mol Appl Genet* 1981;**1:**13–18.
12. Jameson JL, Becker CB, Lindell CM, et al. Human follicle stimulating hormone beta sub-

unit gene encodes multiple messenger ribonucleic acids. *Mol Endocrinol* 1988;**2**:806–15.

13. Chappel SC, Kelton C, Nugent N. Expression of human gonadotropins by recombinant DNA methods. In *Hormones in Gynecologic Endocrinology* (Genazzaini AR, Petrahlia F, eds). London: Parthenon Publishers, 1992: 179–84.

14. Ashwell G, Harford J. Carbohydrate-specific receptors of the liver. *Annu Rev Biochem* 1982;**51**:531–54.

15. Chappel SC. Heterogeneity of follicle stimulating hormone – control and physiological function. *Hum Reprod Update* 1995;**1**:479–87.

16. Ulloa-Aguirre A, Midgley AR Jr, Beitins IZ, Padmanabhan V. Follicle-stimulating isohormones: characterization and physiological relevance. *Endocrinol Rev* 1995;**16**:765–87.

17. Cerpa-Poljak A, Bishop LA, Hort YJ, et al. Isoelectric charge of recombinant human follicle stimulating hormone isoforms determines receptor affinity and in vitro bioactivity. *Endocrinology* 1993;**132**:351–6.

18. Robertson WR. Gonadotropin isoform pattern in different pharmaceutical preparations. In: *Gonadotrophin Isoforms Facts and Future* (Kahn JA, ed.). Serono Fertility Series, Volume 2. Copenhagen: Ciconia Foundation, 1997: 53–60.

19. Shome B, Parlow AF. The primary structure of the hormone specific beta subunit of human pituitary luteinizing hormone (hLH). *J Clin Endocrinol Metab* 1973;**6**:618.

20. Sairam MR, Li CH. Human pituitary lutrophin, isolation, properties and complete amino acid sequence of the beta subunit. *Biochim Biophys Acta* 1975:**412**:70–81.

21. Snyder PJ, Bashey HM, Montecinos A, et al. Secretion of multiple forms of human luteinizing hormone by cultured fetal human pituitary cells. *J Clin Endocrinol Metab* 1989;**68**:1033–8.

22. Zalesky DD, Grotjan HE. Comparison of intracellular and secreted isoforms of bovine and ovine luteinizing hormone. *Biol Reprod* 1991;**44**:1016–24.

23. Jia XC, Hsueh AJW. Granulosa cell aromatase bioassay for follicle-stimulating hormone: validation and application of the method. *Endocrinology* 1986;**119**:1570–7.

24. Kelton CA, Cheng SV, Nugent NP, et al. The cloning of the human follicle stimulating hormone receptor and its expression in COS-7 and CHO cells. *Mol Cell Endocrinol* 1992;**89**:141–51.

25. Steelman SL, Pohley FM. Assay of the follicle stimulating hormone based on the augmentation with human chorionic gonadotropin. *Endocrinology* 1953;**53**:604–16.

# 10

# The use of recombinant human FSH in in vitro fertilization

Colin M Howles, Matts Wikland

**Early studies in IVF • Recombinant versus urinary FSH in ART • Choice of regimen for superovulation induction • Conclusions**

The history of the use of exogenous gonado-trophin preparations to stimulate human ovar-ian activity goes back to the late 1930s (see Alberda et al[1] for a historical review of in vitro fertilization (IVF)). At that time, the gonadotrophins used were of animal origin, extracted from pig pituitaries or from pregnant horse serum. Although an ovarian response could be evoked, a laparotomy was required to establish follicle maturity and, with repeated use, the patient being treated became refrac-tory. It was hypothesized that an 'anti-hormone' was at work, which neutralized the effectiveness of the injected substance.[2,3] Despite these problems, animal extracts were used routinely for almost 30 years.

During the 1950s, other researchers turned to extracting human gonadotrophins either from pituitaries obtained from cadavers[4] or from human menopausal urines.[5–7] In fact, a process for the extraction of human menopausal gonadotrophin (hMG) from human meno-pausal urine had been devised as early as 1947 by an Italian, Pietro Donini, the senior chemist for Serono in Rome. However, the process was published in a relatively unknown journal[8] and languished in obscurity – along with the

authors' forecasts of the potential therapeutic utility of this product for the treatment of human infertility.

It was not until 1957 that a series of chance events led to the 'rediscovery' of Donini's results and the development of contacts between Serono and the members of the G- (or Gonadotrophin) Club. This club, an academic group dedicated to research on the therapeutic use of gonadotrophins in humans, seized the opportunity to obtain sufficient quantities of this urine-derived hMG, named Pergonal, for clinical research and to establish an interna-tional reference standard. The original Pergonal had a very low specific activity (8 IU/mg) and, even in current hMG preparations, only 1–2% of the protein present is gonadotrophin.

During the 1980s, especially after the devel-opment of IVF, there was a tremendous increase in the demand for urinary gon-adotrophins. Serono continued to develop a range of urinary follicle-stimulating hormone (FSH) products: first Metrodin (u-hFSH) in 1983, which still had a low specific activity (100–150 IU FSH/mg protein) but from which the luteinizing hormone (LH) had been removed by immunochromatography; then, in

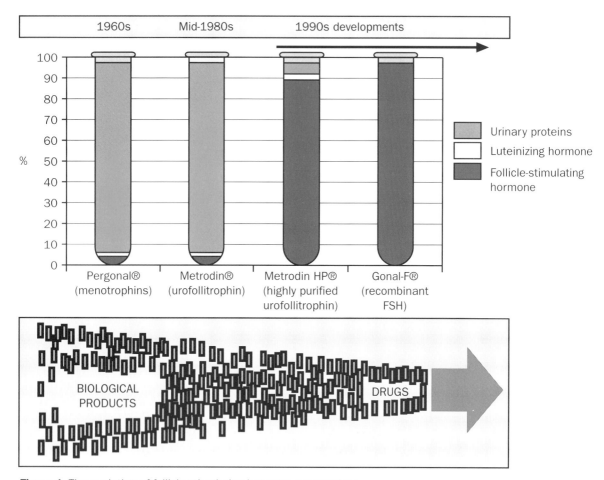

**Figure 1** The evolution of follicle-stimulating hormone preparations.

1993, highly purified urinary FSH (u-hFSH HP, Metrodin HP) with a specific activity of around 9000 IU FSH/mg protein (Fig. 1). Metrodin HP was the first highly pure biological extract that could be characterized by an assortment of physicochemical tests, thus offering improved batch-to-batch consistency. Furthermore, as a result of its high purity, it could be injected subcutaneously, unlike the earlier preparations which had to be administered intramuscularly. However, despite the high specific activity of

Metrodin HP, the starting material is heterogeneous and requires the collection of over 60 000 000 litres of urine from approximately 300 000 donors per year by Serono.

The final transition to a true drug, where the starting material and complete manufacture are under rigorous control, was made in 1995 with the first European approval of recombinant FSH (r-hFSH; Gonal-F) by the European Medicines Evaluation Agency. In the development of Gonal-F, the $\alpha$ and $\beta$ human FSH genes

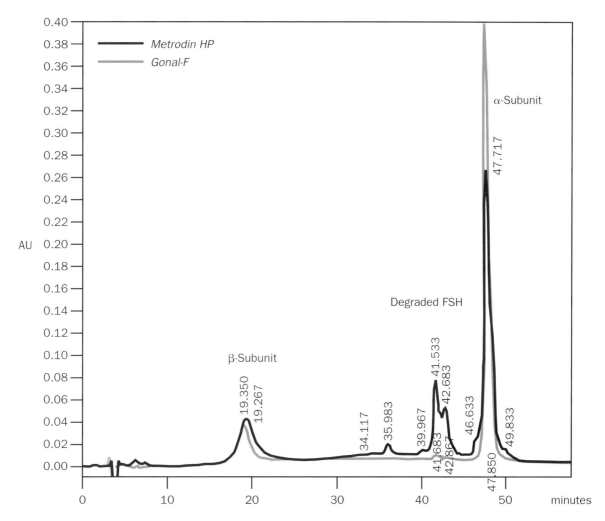

**Figure 2** Reverse phase high-pressure liquid chromatography shows that there are low levels of FSH degradation products in r-hFSH compared with u-hFSH HP.

were transfected into Chinese hamster ovary (CHO) cells.[9,10] A clonal CHO cell was selected on the basis of its ability to express biologically active FSH in quantities sufficient to make the production process viable. After a six-step purification procedure, the resulting r-hFSH is biochemically highly pure (> 99% FSH), with a high specific activity (in the region of 10 000 IU/mg protein). It is structurally identi-cal to native pituitary hFSH, demonstrating a range of FSH isoforms similar to those found during the natural menstrual cycle. However, unlike u-hFSH, r-hFSH shows a low level of degradation and/or oxidation (typically less than 10% versus 30–40% for the former) (Fig. 2).

Some evidence from clinical cases indicates the large amount of nonspecific human urinary proteins in urinary gonadotrophins may provoke adverse immune reactions. For instance, one report has detailed the successful use of recombinant FSH in establishing a clinical pregnancy without untoward events in a woman who had developed serious systemic reactions to urinary gonadotrophins.[11]

There are currently two recombinant human FSH preparations available: Gonal-F (Ares-Serono, Geneva, Switzerland) and Puregon/Follistim (NV Organon, Oss, The Netherlands). The two r-hFSH molecules are structurally and biochemically almost indistinguishable, except for some minor differences in isoform profile. Furthermore, clinical data have recently demonstrated that both preparations, if administered on an equivalent international unit basis, produce identical stimulation characteristics (Table 1),[12] although there is some evidence that, compared with Gonal-F, Puregon is less well tolerated after subcutaneous administration.[12,13] In view of their similarities in clinical effectiveness, data obtained from both preparations are discussed.

Although r-hFSH is approved for use in two main indications – anovulation in clomiphene-resistant World Health Organization group II patients and multiple follicular stimulation for normally ovulating women undergoing assisted reproductive techniques (ART) – the former indication is discussed elsewhere in this book (see Chapter 11). This chapter describes the use of r-hFSH in ART.

## EARLY STUDIES IN IVF

The clinical utility of r-hFSH was first demonstrated in 1992, when case reports confirmed that r-hFSH used in combination with a gonadotrophin-releasing hormone (GnRH) agonist could successfully stimulate multiple follicular development and oestradiol secretion, in patients undergoing IVF and embryo transfer.[14,15] The retrieved oocytes were fertilized and the first pregnancies were achieved.

Following these early case reports, the efficacy of r-hFSH in ART in combination with different GnRH agonists employed in a long protocol was investigated in a number of clinical trials.[16,17]

## RECOMBINANT VERSUS URINARY FSH IN ART

As part of the clinical development programme for both r-hFSH preparations, a number of key

---

**Table 1  Gonal-F versus Puregon in women undergoing IVF:[11] characteristics of patients receiving hCG (values are means ± SD)**

|  | Gonal-F® | Puregon® |
| --- | --- | --- |
| Patients | 22 | 22 |
| Total follicles | 13 ± 7 | 15 ± 10 |
| Oocytes retrieved | 12 ± 8 | 12 ± 8 |
| Days of FSH | 9 ± 1 | 9 ± 1 |
| Ampoules of FSH used (75 IU equivalent) | 17.8 ± 4.1 | 17.8 ± 4.5 |
| Embryos transferred | 2 ± 1 | 2 ± 1 |
| Clinical pregnancy/cycle (%) | 32 | 18 |
| Patients with injection reactions (%) | 36 | 57 |

studies have been carried out to document the safety and efficacy of r-hFSH in ART compared with urine-derived FSH. Most have involved protocols that include pituitary desensitization[18–22] and are discussed further in this chapter. Those studies that were designed with sufficient statistical power have clearly demonstrated that r-hFSH, at an ovarian level, is more effective than urinary gonadotrophins in promoting the process of follicular development – the primary physiological role for FSH in the female.

Although the few studies that have investigated the safety and efficacy of r-hFSH in non-down-regulated cycles in ART[23,24] are not considered here, they also confirm the superior effectiveness of the recombinant product compared with urinary extracts.

## Recombinant versus urinary FSH with a GnRH agonist in a long protocol

In 1995, the results were published of the first multicentre, prospective, randomized clinical trial comparing r-hFSH and u-hFSH in women undergoing IVF and embryo transfer (ET). In this small study, 60 patients were treated with r-hFSH (given subcutaneously) and 63 with u-hFSH (given intramuscularly) after down-regulation with intranasal buserelin in a long protocol. The results confirmed r-hFSH to be as safe and effective as u-hFSH in stimulating ovarian follicular development.

Another prospective, multicentre study compared r-hFSH with u-hFSH in an IVF-ET programme.[19] A total of 981 patients who received intranasal buserelin were randomized to treatment with r-hFSH or u-hFSH given intramuscularly. Among patients receiving the recombinant product ($n = 585$), a significantly higher number of oocytes (10.8 vs 8.9, adjusted for centre effect; $p < 0.0001$) were retrieved with a lower total dose of FSH (2138 vs 2385 IU; $p < 0.0001$) over a shorter treatment period (10.7 vs 11.3 days; $p < 0.0001$) compared with u-hFSH. The number of high-quality embryos was also significantly higher among those

receiving r-hFSH (3.1 vs 2.6 for u-hFSH; $p = 0.003$), but there were no differences between the two groups in implantation rates or clinical pregnancy rates per attempt and per transfer. However, more embryos were cryopreserved in the group receiving r-hFSH (mean 2.58 compared with 1.18 among the u-hFSH patients), reflecting the high number of mature oocytes and high-quality embryos obtained from these patients. When frozen embryo cycles were included in the analysis, ongoing pregnancy rates were significantly in favour of r-hFSH (25.5% with r-hFSH vs 20.4% with u-hFSH; $p < 0.05$). The incidence of the ovarian hyperstimulation syndrome (OHSS) was similar in the two treatment groups (3.2% with r-hFSH and 2.0% with u-hFSH) and no anti-FSH antibodies were detected in patients receiving the recombinant product.

In a further comparison of r-hFSH with u-hFSH in IFV-ET, down-regulation was with triptorelin given daily by subcutaneous injection.[20] A total of 99 women were included in this prospective, assessor-blind, multicentre study and were randomized in a ratio of 3:2 to receive r-hFSH ($n = 60$) or u-hFSH ($n = 39$) given intramuscularly. In this small study the differences between the r-hFSH and u-hFSH groups in this study were not statistically significant. Three patients (5%) who received r-hFSH were hospitalized for the OHSS, but there were no cases in the u-hFSH group.

These studies all confirmed the earlier observation that r-hFSH alone can successfully induce multiple follicular growth,[16] even in pituitary down-regulated cycles with very low endogenous LH activity. Furthermore, they indicated that r-hFSH was more effective than u-hFSH in inducing multiple ovulation for IVF-ET. Although the findings of these studies do not all show significant differences, it seems likely that this is a reflection of their lack of statistical power to detect small differences.[25]

That controlled ovarian stimulation with r-hFSH leads to statistically significantly higher ongoing pregnancy rates, compared with urinary FSH and hMG, was further substantiated by a meta-analysis of three prospective multicentre, randomized, comparative trials.[26] Such analyses are particularly useful when the results from several studies lack statistical significance yet appear to show effects with similar trends.[27] This meta-analysis found that the ongoing pregnancy rate at least 12 weeks after ET per started cycle was 22.9% for r-hFSH and 17.9% for urinary gonadotrophins. The 5% treatment difference was statistically significant in favour of r-hFSH ($p = 0.044$). Furthermore, when the replacement of cryopreserved embryos was also taken into account, the treatment difference increased to 6.4% ($p = 0.011$ in favour of r-hFSH).

## Comparison of recombinant with highly purified urinary FSH

The next question to be answered was: is the recombinant product any more effective in inducing multiple follicular development for ART than highly purified urinary FSH, a product with a specific activity that approaches r-hFSH and that can also be injected subcutaneously?

The results of a prospective, randomized, assessor-blind, two-centre study were published in the second half of 1997 (Table 2).[21] The study showed that r-hFSH (Gonal F) is more effective than highly purified urinary FSH (Metrodin HP, u-hFSH HP) in inducing multiple follicular development in women undergoing ovarian stimulation for IVF (including intracytoplasmic sperm injection or ICSI. Patients were down-regulated with intranasal buserelin in a long protocol, and were randomized to receive r-hFSH ($n = 119$) or u-hFSH HP ($n = 114$), both given subcutaneously. The mean number of oocytes retrieved, the primary endpoint of the study, was significantly higher among those given r-hFSH than in those receiving u-hFSH HP. Furthermore, the number of FSH treatment days and the number of 75 IU ampoules used were significantly less with r-hFSH than with u-hFSH HP. Among patients treated using ICSI (63 in each group) no difference in oocyte maturation was observed between the two groups.

However, the mean number of embryos obtained was over 70% higher among patients receiving r-hFSH. As a result of the lower oocyte yield in the u-hFSH HP group, a higher proportion of patients had only one embryo replaced (12.4% vs 1.8% of those in the r-hFSH group), whereas, in the majority of cases, two embryos were transferred. However, there were no significant differences between the r-hFSH and u-hFSH groups in the pregnancy rate per started cycle (45% and 37%, respectively) and per embryo transfer (48% and 47%, respectively). The authors of this study comment that differences in the pregnancy rate may become apparent after the addition of cryopreserved ET cycles. The number of cryopreserved embryos was significantly higher in the r-hFSH group than in the u-hFSH HP group ($3.2 \pm 3.0$ vs $1.7 \pm 2.5$; $p < 0.0001$), giving a potentially higher chance of conceiving from a single cycle. Both treatments were well tolerated, and the incidence of the OHSS was 5.1% and 1.7%, respectively, in the r-hFSH and u-hFSH HP groups.

Recently, the preliminary results of the first double-blind, randomized comparison of r-hFSH (Gonal-F) and u-hFSH HP (Metrodin HP) administered subcutaneously in women undergoing ART have been published (Table 3).[22] This study included 278 pituitary down-regulated patients and found that, among those treated with r-hFSH, there was a significantly higher mean number of oocytes recovered and embryos obtained. Furthermore, in the r-hFSH group, the treatment duration was significantly shorter than in the u-hFSH HP group and significantly fewer 75 IU ampoules were required. The study power was not sufficient to detect a difference in ongoing clinical pregnancy rates. The incidence of severe OHSS was <1% in both groups.

## Recombinant FSH is more effective than urine-derived FSH in superovulation induction for ART

Although all these studies differ in their design and in the regimens used, the overall conclu-

**Table 2 Recombinant versus highly purified urinary FSH in women undergoing ART:[21] characteristics of patients receiving hCG (values are means ± SD)**

|  | r-hFSH | u-hFSH HP | p value |
|---|---|---|---|
| Ampoules (75 IU) FSH | 21.9 ± 5.1 | 31.9 ± 13.4 | <0.0001 |
| FSH (days) | 11.0 ± 1.6 | 13.5 ± 3.7 | <0.001 |
| Oocytes retrieved | 12.2 ± 5.5 | 7.6 ± 4.4 | <0.0001 |
| Oestradiol on day of hCG (nmol/l) | 6.55 ± 5.75 | 3.95 ± 3.9 | <0.001 |
| Embryos cleaved on day 2 | 8.1 ± 4.2 | 4.7 ± 3.5 | <0.0001 |
| Embryos transferred | 2.0 ± 0.19 | 1.9 ± 0.4 | NS |
| Pregnancy/cycle (%) | 53/119 (45) | 42/114 (37) | NS |
| Twin pregnancies (%) | 17 (32) | 9 (25) | NS |
| Implantation rate (%) | 32 | 31 | NS |

**Table 3 Results of the first double-blind randomized comparison of r-hFSH and u-hFSH in women undergoing ART[22] (values are means ± SD)**

|  | r-hFSH ($n = 130$) | u-hFSH ($n = 116$) | p value |
|---|---|---|---|
| Oocytes retrieved | 11.0 ± 5.9 | 8.8 ± 4.8 | 0.0001 |
| Ampoules (75 IU) FSH | 27.6 ± 10.2 | 40.7 ± 13.6 | 0.0001 |
| FSH (days) | 11.7 ± 1.9 | 14.5 ± 3.3 | 0.001 |
| Embryos – day 2 | 5.0 ± 3.7 | 3.5 ± 2.9 | 0.0002 |
| Ongoing pregnancy rate/started cycle (%) | 25/139(18) | 25/139(18) | NS |

sion has to be that, compared with u-hFSH and u-hFSH HP, the use of r-hFSH to induce super-ovulation in women undergoing ART is associated with more embryos being obtained after the administration of a lower total FSH dose.

Furthermore, recent data demonstrate what has been suspected for many years: the number of embryos in culture is a major determinant in predicting pregnancy outcome. An analysis of data entered in the Human Embryology and Fertilisation Authority database has revealed that women who had more than four embryos in culture had a significantly higher chance of achieving a pregnancy than those with four or less embryos.[28] This was true for all age groups treated. Furthermore, among the women with more than four embryos in culture who subsequently had two or three embryos transferred (24.4% vs 23.4%), the incidence of pregnancy was similar irrespective of the number of embryos transferred. However, the chance of a multiple pregnancy increased from 6.6% with the replacement of two embryos vs 9.2% with the replacement of three.[29] Thus, among women with multiple embryos, fewer embryos should perhaps be replaced in order to reduce the incidence of multiple pregnancies.

Another line of evidence clearly demonstrates the importance of having a large number (>4) of gametes available for transfer. Scholtes and Zeilmaker,[30] who replaced blastocytes in 265 sequential transfers, found that the chance of having at least one blastocyte to transfer was significantly increased if the woman had more than four oocytes collected. If the woman had 10–15 oocytes (the current 'ideal' number), the chance of blastocyte transfer was 80%.

If, as is apparent from this review, the use of r-hFSH to stimulate superovulation results in a higher number of embryos than with urinary FSH products, the embryos that are not needed for immediate transfer can be cryopreserved.

For couples who have cryopreserved embryos available, the potential for subsequent pregnancy is only slightly less than that obtained after the transfer of fresh embryos (Table 4).[29,31,32] This is a significant benefit for the couple, providing them with an additional boost in their pregnancy potential per stimulated cycle.

## CHOICE OF REGIMEN FOR SUPEROVULATION INDUCTION

The variation in the detail of the regimens used in the studies outlined above reflects the fact that, even after almost 15 years of use of gonadotrophin preparations, there is still some controversy as to the most appropriate method of ovarian stimulation to promote the growth and development of a health cohort of follicles, and thus yield the optimum number of mature oocytes for fertilization in vitro.

The starting dose of FSH in normally ovulating women undergoing ovarian stimulation for IVF is usually between 150 and 225 IU/day FSH, depending on the patient's age or previous ovarian response. In a study by Habu-Heija

---

**Table 4 Live birth rates in IVF after transfer of fresh and cryopreserved embryos**

| | |
|---|---|
| *USA (~35 000 cycles)* | |
| IVF live birth rate/transfer (%) | 25.1 |
| Cryopreserved embryo replacement live birth/transfer (%) | 15.1 |
| | |
| *UK (~29 000 cycles)* | |
| IVF live birth rate (%) | 15.4 |
| Cryopreserved embryo replacement live birth/transfer (%) | 11.1 |
| | |
| *France (~35 000 cycles)* | |
| IVF pregnancy/cycle (%) | 17.2 |
| Cryopreserved embryo replacement live birth/transfer (%) | 11.6 |

Data for 1995 from National Registries in the US, UK and France.[29,31,32]

et al[33] using hMG, the lower starting dose was found to be inferior to 225 IU/day FSH. By contrast, data from two large multicentre studies using r-hFSH for ovarian stimulation in women undergoing IVF[34,35] indicate that the response to ovarian stimulation using a fixed starting dose of 150 IU r-hFSH was similar to that obtained with 225 IU. However, Devroey and colleagues, on the basis of a non-comparative study, have suggested recently that a starting dose of 100 IU r-hFSH may be sufficient.[36]

Apart from the starting doses of r-hFSH, the design of the Devroey study[36] (initial dose 100 IU Puregon for the first 4 days) was similar to that reported by Bergh et al in 1997[21] (initial dose 150 IU Gonal-F for the first 6 days). In both studies, patients were down-regulated with buserelin, given intranasally in a long agonist protocol. Human chorionic gonadotrophin (hCG) 10 000 IU was administered when there were three follicles of 17 mm or more diameter in the Devroey study, and when there was one follicle of 18 mm or more plus at least two of 16 mm in the Bergh study. It seems justifiable,

therefore, to compare the outcome data on ovarian responses in the two studies (Table 5). The comparison indicates that, with a 150 IU starting dose, a lower total dose of r-hFSH and a shorter treatment duration were required, and suggests that a starting dose of 100 IU is actually suboptimal in an unselected ART population. This is because increasing the dose in the late stimulation phase will not be effective if the same criteria for administering hCG are maintained. However, a comparative study is required to confirm this.

Another variable in the protocols is the dosing regimen of GnRH agonist (see Chapters 15 and 17). Recently, Frydman and colleagues have shown that the total dose of FSH required to reach their criteria for hCG administration (one follicle $\geq 18$ mm diameter and more than two follicles $\geq 16$ mm diameter) was affected by the type of pituitary down-regulation that patients were given.[22] In patients down-regulated by a GnRH agonist depot, the total dose of r-hFSH required was $28.4 \times 75$ IU ampoules whereas, in patients given daily

---

**Table 5 The effect of starting dose on ovarian response in ART patients: a comparison of data from Bergh et al[21] and Devroey et al[35]**

|  | Devroey et al 1998 (Puregon 100 IU) | Bergh et al 1997 (Gonal-F 150 IU) |
| --- | --- | --- |
| Patients | 43 | 119 |
| Age (years) | 31.7 | $32 \pm 3.5$[a] |
| BMI | 23.2 | $22.3 \pm 2.4$[a] |
| Total dose (IU) | 1807 | 1642.5[a] |
| Ampoules (75 IU equivalent) | 24.1 | $21.9 \pm 5.1$[a] |
| Days FSH | 13.3 | $11.0 \pm 1.6$[a] |
| Oocytes | 11.7 | $12.2 \pm 5.5$[a] |
| Embryos | 7.0 | 8.1 |
| Pregnancies/cycle (%) | 14/43 (32.6) | 53/119 (45) |

[a] Values are means $\pm$ SD.

GnRH agonists either subcutaneously or intranasally, only 20.1 and 20.9 ampoules, respectively, were used.[22] These results suggest that depot administration of the GnRH agonist should not be the route of choice.

Further studies in the future should help to clarify the optimum r-hFSH down-regulation regimen to be used in ART in order to maximize the cost-effectiveness of this treatment.

## CONCLUSIONS

There are a number of hypotheses as to why r-hFSH is more effective in stimulating follicular development than urinary gonadotrophins. It has been proposed that differences in the pharmaceutical formulation or the presence of FSH-inhibiting substances in urinary FSH may play a role. There has been much speculation on the role that certain FSH isoforms may play in determining in vivo bioactivity;[19] for example, recombinant h-FSH preparations certainly contain slightly more basic FSH isoforms than u-hFSH HP. What is probably more important is the higher degree of consistency of the FSH present between batches of r-hFSH compared to that found in urinary-derived gonadotrophin preparations, including u-hFSH HP: for example, in u-hFSH HP, the percentage of degraded/oxidized forms of FSH is around 30–40% (see Fig. 2). However, for Gonal-F the corresponding value is less than 10% and this variable is one of the many release specifications. Additionally, the variation in degraded FSH between batches is significantly higher in u-hFSH HP compared to Gonal-F.

Finally, gonadotrophin preparations are released for clinical use on the basis of the in vivo bioassay (Steelman Pohley), which has an inherent variability of ±20%. Studies using r-hFSH in an IVF population suggest that there may be a poor correlation with the clinical response.[19,21] A major advantage that r-hFSH has over urinary preparations is that eventually r-hFSH will be released on the basis of mass.

However, these hypotheses are purely speculative and further research is needed to examine their influence on the clinical effectiveness of r-hFSH.

The use of r-hFSH also offers a number of advantages over urine-derived FSH preparations. Clinical trials with r-hFSH continue to accumulate evidence that, compared with u-hFSH and u-hFSH HP, its use is associated with the need for a lower total dose of FSH, and with more embryos being obtained. The number of embryos in culture is a major determinant in predicting pregnancy outcome, and the cryopreservation of supernumerary embryos provides couples with an additional boost in their pregnancy potential per stimulated cycle. Furthermore, unlike u-hFSH or hMG, which are administered intramuscularly, highly pure r-hFSH can be injected subcutaneously, making it suitable for self-administration – a major advantage for the patient.

## REFERENCES

1. Alberda Ath, Gan RA, Vemer HM, eds. *Pioneers in in vitro fertilization.* Carnforth: Parthenon Publishing, 1993.
2. Ostergaard E. *Antigonadotrophic substances.* Copenhagen: E Munksgaard, 1942.
3. Zondek B, Sulman F. *The antigonadotrophic factor with consideration of the antihormone problem.* Baltimore: Williams & Wilkins Company, 1942.
4. Gemzell CA, Diczfalusy E, Tillinger G. Clinical effect of human pituitary follicle-stimulating hormone (FSH). *J Clin Endocrinol Metab* 1958; **18**:1333–48.
5. Borth R, Lunenfeld B, Watteville de H. Activité gonadotrope d'un extrait d'urines de femmes en menopause. *Experientia* 1954;**10**:266–70.
6. Borth R, Lunenfeld B, Riotton G, Watteville de

H. Activité gonadotrope d'un extrait d'urines de femmes en menopause 2me communication). *Experientia* 1957;**13**:115–21.

7. Benz F, Borth R, Brown PS, et al. Collaborative assay of two gonadotropin preparations from human post-menopausal urine. *J Endocrinol* 1959;**19**:158–63.

8. Donini P, Montezemolo R. *Rassegna di Clinica, Terapia e Scienze Affini. A publication of the Biologic Istituto Serono* 1949;**48**(143):3–28.

9. Chappel S, Kelton C, Nugent N. Expression of human gonadotropins by recombinant DNA methods. In: Genazzi AR, Petraglia F, eds. *Proceedings of the 3rd World Congress on Gynecological Endocrinology*. Carnforth: Parthenon Publishing, 1992:179–84.

10. Howles CM. Genetic engineering of human FSH (Gonal-F). *Hum Reprod Update* 1996;**2**:172–91.

11. Phipps WR, Holden D, Sheehan RD. Use of recombinant human FSH for IVF/ET after severe systemic immunoglobin E-mediated reaction to urofollitropin. *Fertil Steril* 1996;**66**:148–50.

12. Brinsden P, Akagbosu F, Gibbons L et al. Gonal-F vs Puregon: Results of a randomized, assessor-blind, comparative study in women undergoing ART. *14th Annual Meeting of the European Society for Human Reproduction and Embryology*, Gothenburg, 1998: Abstract.

13. Sargeant SD. A study to evaluate the ease of use and tolerability by patients of gonadotrophins old and new. *BFS Annual Meeting*, Sheffield 1998: Abstract F9.

14. Germond M, Dessole S, Senn A et al. Successful in-vitro fertilization and embryo transfer after treatment with recombinant human FSH. *Lancet* 1992;**339**:1170.

15. Devroey P, Van Steirteghem A, Mannaerts B, Coelingh Bennink H. Successful in-vitro fertilization and embryo transfer after treatment with recombinant human FSH. *Lancet* 1992; **339**:1170–1.

16. Devroey P, Mannaerts B, Smitz J et al. Clinical outcome of a pilot efficacy study on recombinant human follicle-stimulating hormone (Org 32489) combined with various gonadtrophin releasing hormone agonist regimens. *Hum Reprod* 1994; **9**:1064–9.

17. Reddy R, Al-Oum M, Ledger W, et al. An alternate day step-down regimen using Gonal-F® (r-hFSH) in IVF: a UK multicentre study. *Hum Reprod* 1996;**11**:130–1.

18. Recombinant Human FSH Study Group. Clinical assessment of recombinant human follicle-stimulating hormone in stimulating ovarian follicular development before *in vitro* fertilization. *Fertil Steril* 1995;**63**:77–86.

19. Out HJ, Mannaerts BMJL, Driessen SGAJ et al. A prospective, randomized, assessor-blind, multicentre study comparing recombinant and urinary follicle-stimulating hormone (Puregon versus Metrodin) in *in vitro* fertilization. *Hum Reprod* 1995;**10**:2534–40.

20. Hedon B, Out HJ, Hughes JN et al. Efficacy and safety of recombinant FSH (Puregon) in infertile women pituitary-suppressed with triptorelin undergoing *in vitro* fertilisation: a prospective, randomised, assessor-blind, multicentre trial. *Hum Reprod* 1995;**10**:3102–6.

21. Bergh C, Howles CM, Borg K et al. Recombinant human follicle stimulating hormone (r-hFSH; Gonal-F®) versus highly purified urinary FSH (Metrodin® HP): results of a randomized comparative study in women undergoing assisted reproductive techniques. *Hum Reprod* 1997; **12**:2133–39.

22. Frydman R, Avril C, Camier B, et al. A double-blind, randomised study comparing the efficacy of recombinant human follicle stimulating hormone (r-hFSH/Gonal-F®) and highly purified urinary FSH (u-hFSH HP/Metrodin® HP) in inducing superovulation in women undergoing Assisted Reproductive Techniques (ART). *14th Annual Meeting of the European Society for Human Reproduction and Embryology*, Gothenburg, 1998: Abstract.

23. Jansen CAM, Van Os MC. Puregon without analogs: an oxymoron. *Gynecol Endocrinol* 1996;**10**(suppl 1):34.

24. Strowitzki T, Kentenich H, Kiesel L et al. Ovarian stimulation in women undergoing in-vitro fertilization and embryo transfer using recombinant human follicle stimulating hormone (Gonal-F) in non-down-regulated cycles. *Hum Reprod* 1995;**10**:3097–101.

25. McDonough PG. The coming of wonders [Editorial comment]. *Fertil Steril* 1997;**67**:412–13.

26. Out HJ, Driessen SGAJ, Mannaerts BMJL, Coelingh Bennick HJT. Recombinant follicle-stimulating hormone (follitropin beta, Puregon®) yields higher pregnancy rates in in vitro fertilization than urinary gonadotropins. *Fertil Steril* 1997;**68**:138–42.

27. D'Agostinho RB, Weintraub M. Meta-analysis: a method for synthesizing research. *Clin Pharmacol Ther* 1995;**58**:605–16.

28. Templeton AA. The UK Registry of IVF treat-

ment cycles. What can we learn from the indications, techniques and results? Presented at the symposium on current opinions in the treatment of the infertile couple. XV FIGO World Congress, Copenhagen, 1997.

29. Human Fertilisation and Embryology Authority Sixth Annual Report 1997: Paxton House, 30 Artillery Lane, London E1 7LS.

30. Scholtes MCW, Zeilmaker GH. Blastocyst transfer in day-5 embryo transfer depends primarily on number of oocytes retrieved and not on age. *Fertil Steril* 1998;**69**:78–83.

31. FIVNAT, Bachelot A, Rossin-Amar B et al. Bilan FIVNAT 1195. *Contracept Fertil Sex* 1996;**24**:694–9.

32. Society for Assisted Reproductive Technology and American Society for Reproductive Medicine. Assisted reproductive technology in the US and Canada: *Fertil Steril* 1998;**69**:389–98.

33. Habu-Heija AT, Yates RWS, Barrett T, et al. A comparison of two starting doses of human menopausal gonadotrophin for follicle stimulation in unselected patients for in-vitro fertilization. *Hum Reprod* 1995;**10**:801–3.

34. Thornton SJ. Starting doses in IVF and effects on outcome. *Hum Reprod* 1996;**11**:104 (Abstract).

35. Camier B, The French multicentre trialists, Howles CM, Truong. A multicentre, prospective, randomised study to compare low dose protocol versus conventional administration of recombinant human follicle stimulating hormone (Gonal-F®) in normo-responder women undergoing IVF/ICSI. *14th Annual Meeting of the European Society for Human Reproduction and Embryology*, Gothenburg, 1998: Abstract.

36. Devroey P, Tournaye H, Van Steirteghem A et al. The use of a 100 IU starting dose of recombinant follicle stimulating hormone (Puregon) in in-vitro fertilization. *Hum Reprod* 1998;**13**:565–6.

# 11

# The use of recombinant human FSH in ovulation induction

Jean Noel Hugues

**Clinical experiences with rhFSH** • **Conclusions**

Human gonadotrophin preparations have been used extensively over the last three decades for the successful treatment of human infertility. Initially, human gonadotrophin preparations were developed to restore fertility in anovulatory patients by stimulating normal follicular development. The first pregnancy was obtained with extracts from human pituitary glands containing follicle-stimulating hormone (FSH) and luteinizing hormone (LH).[1] Soon afterwards, gonadotrophins extracted from postmenopausal urine (human menopausal gonadotrophin, hMG) were available, also proved to be effective[2] and became the standard gonadotrophin preparation for about three decades. Human menopausal gonadotrophin contains a mixture of FSH (75 IU) and LH (75 IU) (in vivo bioactivity ratio = 1) and is of low specific activity. A successive supplementary purification step substantially decreased LH-like activity leading to a novel commercial purified FSH (pFSH) preparation. Besides obtaining a more purified product, the rationale of developing pFSH was that, in every clinical situation, FSH alone is sufficient to increase folliculogenesis and the LH compound in hMG preparations could be responsible for the high incidence of treatment complications, especially

in patients with increased endogenous LH levels.[3] Although pFSH has been shown to be at least as effective as hMG for stimulating follicular development, the production of these hormones depends on the collection of huge amounts of urine. The use of urine sources implies limited product consistency with varying amounts of LH and human chorionic gonadotrophin (hCG).[4] Other disadvantages of urinary preparations are the theoretical risk of contamination and the limited purity of the product.

Through the application of recombinant DNA technology, it is now possible to produce FSH for therapeutic use without the need for extraction from human fluids. To achieve production of a human FSH dimer, genomic clones containing the complete FSH $\alpha$ and $\beta$ subunit coding sequences were transfected into Chinese hamster ovary (CHO) cells.[5] Subsequently, stable cell lines synthesizing the FSH dimer were selected.[6] CHO cells appeared able to assemble the subunits and to glycosylate the molecule. As a result of the capacity of CHO cell lines to grow in a serum-free medium, high purity of the glycoprotein product was ensured. Selected cell lines demonstrated a high number of plasmid copies which remained well integrated during culturing of the cells for a period of 3 months. In addition, the isohormone profile remained stable during this interval. Hence, the batch-to-batch consistency of the product is complete. The biological activity of recombinant human FSH (rhFSH) was ascertained using rat granulosa cell cultures and intact immature rats.[7,8] Human rFSH appears to be very similar to pituitary and urinary FSH, although it shows minor differences in the structure of the carbohydrate side chains and contains more basic isohormones than the hormone from both natural sources.[9]

The first clinical studies using rhFSH as a therapeutic agent were published in 1992. Case reports indicated that rhFSH alone stimulates multiple ovarian follicular growth and oestradiol secretion in patients undergoing IVF with embryo transfer who were pre-treated with a gonadotrophin-releasing hormone (GnRH) agonist. Retrieved oocytes were fertilized and viable pregnancies obtained.[10,11] Subsequently, several phase III clinical studies have been completed, including those for ovulation induction in chronic anovulatory patients. In 1995, the first rhFSH preparation (Gonal F, Ares-Serono, SA, Switzerland) was registered in the European community, while a second became available in 1996 (Puregon, NV Organon, the Netherlands). These are now currently available in most countries.

## CLINICAL EXPERIENCES WITH rhFSH

A large proportion of patients who suffer from infertility and anovulation exhibit insufficient response to antioestrogen medication and gonadotrophins represent an effective second-line treatment. According to the World Health Organization (WHO) classification of anovulation,[12] these patients are usually allocated to either group I characterized by low oestrogen production related to hypogonadotrophic hypogonadism or the group II with persistent oestrogen secretion. In both groups, the clinical challenge is to achieve the maturation and ovulation of a minimal number of follicles (and preferably only one) to obtain a singleton pregnancy and no ovarian hyperstimulation syndrome

(OHSS). Although it appears that this goal is mainly achieved by a careful manipulation of gonadotrophins rather than by the choice of the molecule itself, the recent introduction of rhFSH justifies addressing this important issue. Indeed, differences in carbohydrate moities of the glycoprotein may cause differences in metabolic clearance and biological activity.[13] Moreover, changes in isoform distribution represent a way of modulating FSH biopotency.[14] Therefore, the clinical efficacy and safety of rhFSH are examined in both WHO anovulatory groups.

## Clinical assessment in WHO group I anovulation

Although it is a rare cause of anovulation, patients of WHO group I have been particularly studied because the central failure to induce gonadotroph secretion leads to abnormally low serum gonadotrophin levels and ovarian oestrogen secretion is negligible. This unusual endocrine pattern provides a unique opportunity for both assessment of pharmacokinetic and pharmacodynamic properties of rhFSH and evaluation of the respective roles of FSH and LH in folliculogenesis.

### Pharmacokinetic properties of rhFSH
It was previously shown that the long half-life of purified FSH after intramuscular administration induces accumulating serum FSH levels. When serum immunoreactive FSH concentrations were compared in gonadotrophin-deficient women after the administration of rhFSH and urinary FSH, no difference was noted for the time interval to reach peak FSH concentrations, but the maximum concentration ($C_{max}$) and area under the curve (AUC) were lower after rhFSH than after urinary FSH injection.[15] The calculated half-life of rhFSH was 30–40 h with both treatments. Interestingly, a negative relationship between body weight and serum FSH concentrations was observed which corroborated the concept that body weight is a major determining factor for the dose and duration of gonadotrophin stimulation. Thus, adjustment of FSH dose in relation to body

weight can reduce ovarian response variability. As a result of its high purity (>99%), rhFSH is suitable for both intramuscular and subcutaneous administration. The latter route is more suitable for self-administration and reduces time and cost of medical staff. Comparison of both routes of administration in women whose pituitary was suppressed by the high-dose oral contraceptive Lyndiol (2.5 mg lynestrenol and 0.05 mg ethinyl oestradiol) showed that the absorption of rhFSH administered subcutaneously tended to be slower, resulting in lower serum FSH concentrations during the absorption phase and in higher concentrations thereafter. However, the bioavailability was almost equal and the intersubject variability for $C_{max}$ was reduced after subcutaneous injection. After administration of doses of rhFSH that increased weekly, serum FSH concentrations increased in a dose-dependent manner and steady-state levels were reached after about 3–5 days.[16,17] Other studies have been done in healthy female volunteers who were pituitary down-regulated by a GnRH agonist which confirmed that the pharmacokinetic characteristics of rhFSH are similar to those of urinary human FSH.[18,19] The important points that emerge from more studies and which are relevant to the induction of follicle growth are: (a) there is no correlation between the blood level of FSH and ovarian response; and (2) dose adjustments should be made at intervals of no less than 3–5 days.

*Role of rhFSH in folliculogenesis*
The hypothesis of gonadotrophin synergism, introduced almost half a century ago,[20] emphasized the importance of an interplay between FSH and LH for normal oestrogen production and follicular development. Subsequently, this concept was supported by observations that, in immature mice, injection of pure urinary FSH increased ovarian weight but uterine growth was unaffected, suggesting that FSH alone is able to promote follicular development without concomitant oestrogen production.[21] Similarly, administration of pituitary or pure FSH in hypogonadotrophic women resulted in normal follicular growth without oestrogen secretion.[22,23] On the basis of these observations, the two-cell, two-gonadotrophin theory of follicular steroidogenesis was raised. According to this hypothesis, the ovarian theca cells stimulated by LH secrete androgens that diffuse through the basal membrane into the granulosa cells, where the FSH-induced enzyme system converts them to oestrogens.[24,25]

A first case of hypogonadotrophic hypogonadism treated with rhFSH was reported by Schoot et al.[26] Multiple follicular development visualized by ultrasonography was achieved whereas the serum oestradiol concentrations remained very low. Moreover, follicular fluid oestradiol concentrations were about 1500 times lower than expected in normal preovulatory phase and serum progesterone showed no increase after hCG administration. This observation was confirmed in other studies including a larger number of patients[16,27] (Figure 1). They extended the previous observations which indicated that high intrafollicular oestradiol concentrations may not be mandatory for ongoing maturation of follicles in humans. Another intriguing observation was that serum immunoreactive inhibin increased a few days before a minor rise in serum oestradiol concentrations. Thus, there is speculation that inhibin produced by FSH-stimulated granulosa may act as a paracrine regulator to stimulate theca cell androgen production; this, in turn, provides some substrate for oestradiol synthesis by granulosa cells.[28] The absence of the increase in the serum progesterone level after injection of hCG may be explained by the low local oestradiol concentrations which are insufficient for the induction of LH receptors. Finally, serum androgen concentrations remained stable during stimulation, showing that rhFSH exhibits no intrinsic LH activity.

Altogether these data confirm the dissociation between the mitogenic and steroidogenic activity of FSH and emphasize that, if follicular development is dependent predominantly on FSH, steroidogenesis is mainly supported by the synergistic action of FSH and LH. This latter concept was recently re-evaluated in WHO group I patients treated with a fixed dose of rhFSH (150 IU/day) and rhLH at doses ranging from 25 to 225 IU/day[29] (Figure 2). The higher

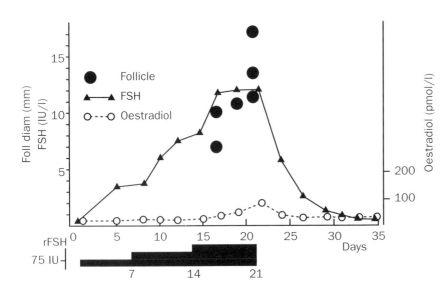

**Figure 1** Serum FSH and oestradiol (E$_2$) concentrations and follicular development during the weekly administration of increasing doses of human recombinant FSH for 21 days in a woman with hypogonadotrophic hypogonadism. (From Shoham et al,[27] with permission.)

doses of rhLH could promote optimal ovarian oestradiol secretion and enhance the ability of the follicle to luteinize after hCG administration. Thus, rhFSH is effective in stimulating follicular development in WHO group I anovulation, but co-administration of LH is mandatory in order to obtain adequate follicular steroidogenesis, as demonstrated by oestradiol secretion, endometrial growth and luteal phase progesterone secretion.

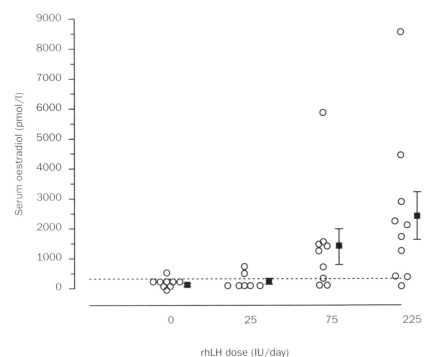

**Figure 2** Individual serum oestradiol concentrations in WHO group I women after administration of 150 IU rhFSH/day and a fixed dose of rhLH, that is 0, 25, 75 or 225 IU/day. (From Loumaye et al,[29] with permission.)

## Clinical assessment in WHO group II anovulation

The second indication for rhFSH to be evaluated is the stimulation of single follicular development in WHO group II anovulatory patients. The first case reports published[30,31] concerned women whose anovulation was related to the polycystic ovary syndrome (PCOS) resistant to clomiphene citrate. In both studies, a chronic low-dose protocol was used because it is a safe and effective regimen in those patients who had high level of sensitivity to gonadotrophins.[32–34] Administration of rhFSH resulted in an exponential rise in serum oestradiol and immunoreactive inhibin, showing that exposure to endogenous LH is sufficient to support FSH-induced follicular development in WHO group II anovulation (Figure 3). Pregnancies and births resulting from this therapy testify further to the normal follicular development.[35] Subsequently, another study, including a larger number of WHO group II patients who

did not have the PCOS, was reported.[36] It confirmed the effectiveness of rhFSH in inducing a mono- or bifollicular ovarian response in 89 of 107 cycles (83.2%), and the pregnancy rate was good (14% per ovulatory cycle).

Another approach for testing rFSH was to compare the efficacy and safety with those of urinary FSH (urofollitrophin or Metrodin; uhFSH). Indeed, data from superovulation for assisted reproductive technologies indicated that rhFSH appeared to be more efficacious than uhFSH, as assessed by significantly higher final oestradiol values and a larger number of follicles recruited, oocytes retrieved or embryos obtained.[37,38] Furthermore, the ongoing pregnancy rate was significantly higher in the rFSH-treated women.[37] These studies also demonstrated a higher efficiency in that the results were obtained using a significantly lower total dose in a shorter treatment period.

In a first series of studies,[39–41] rhFSH has been shown to be as effective and safe as uhFSH and

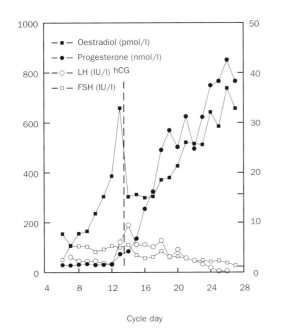

**Figure 3** Serum oestradiol, FSH, LH and progesterone concentrations during a cycle treated with rhFSH in a woman with WHO II anovulation. The day of hCG administration is marked by the dotted line. (From Van Dessel et al,[35] with permission.)

**Table 1** Comparative data from cycles treated with rhFSH (Puregon) or uhFSH (Metrodin) in women with WHO II anovulation.

| Parameter | Puregon (*n* = 105) | Metrodin (*n* = 67) | *p* value |
|---|---|---|---|
| Efficiency | | | |
| Median total dose (IU) | 750 | 1035 | < 0.001 |
| Median duration of treatment (days) | 10.0 | 13.0 | < 0.001 |
| Efficacy | | | |
| Median maximum estradiol (pmol/l) | 1400 | 1000 | NS |
| Number of follicles ≥ 12 mm | 3.6 | 2.6 | < 0.001 |
| Number of follicles ≥ 15 mm | 2.0 | 1.7 | NS |
| Cancellations (%) | 11.4 | 10.4 | NS |
| Cumulative ovulation rate (%) | 95 | 96 | NS |
| Cumulative pregnancy rate (%) | 27 | 24 | NS |

From Geurts et al,[42] with permission.

the rate of monofollicular development seemed to be higher with rhFSH.[41] More recently, a large prospective multicentre study, comparing the efficacy of rhFSH and uhFSH for three consecutive cycles in patients with normogonadotrophic chronic anovulation classified in WHO group II, demonstrated that rhFSH is more efficient, as illustrated by a significantly higher number of follicles with diameters of over 12 mm and a significantly higher median serum oestradiol concentration[42,43] (Table 1). Moreover, the median total dose needed to reach ovulation and the median treatment duration were significantly lower in rhFSH-treated patients. Differences between rFSH and uFSH which might explain this increased effectiveness include the isohormone profile,[44] the percentage of degraded FSH forms present,[38] the pharmaceutical formulation, contaminating proteins possibly with FSH-inhibiting activity in uFSH or small differences in the oligosaccharide structure.[45] Although the ratio of bioactive:immunoreactive rFSH has been shown to be higher than that of uFSH,[44] it is dangerous to draw conclusions about its significance because of the inaccuracies of these

assays.[46] It is noteworthy that serum immunoreactive FSH levels were lower after rhFSH administration, which is in good agreement with the more basic isohormone profile of rhFSH and its higher clearance rate. However, differences could also be related to the feedback effect of higher levels of serum oestradiol on endogenous FSH levels. Although the apparent higher activity of recombinant FSH did not correlate with an increased cancellation rate resulting from ovarian hyperstimulation, lower starting doses and careful increments in the daily dosage must be recommended.

However, it is still not clear whether rhFSH administration needs some special attention, particularly for patients with anovulatory infertility related to the PCOS. The 'FSH-threshold' concept initially put forward by Brown[47] has gained wide support. Based on clinical observations of gonadotrophin-stimulated cycles, it emphasized the narrow range of requirements for FSH to initiate follicular growth and led to advise a stepwise administration of increasing amounts of gonadotrophins (conventional 'step-up' protocol) until the ovarian response is considered to be sufficient, according to ultrasonography and hormone determinations. Later on, other authors[32–34] suggested a slower and less pronounced increase in gonadotrophin doses to reduce the incidence of ovarian hyperstimulation further. This 'chronic, low-dose, step-up' regimen is now widely used to induce ovulation in oligomenorrhoeic women who are infertile. However, to our knowledge, only a few publications have prospectively compared the efficiency of conventional and chronic low-dose administration of rhFSH. Homburg et al[48] included some patients treated with rhFSH in their comparative study of the two protocols, but pooled these data with those obtained after uhFSH administration. More recently, a comparative prospective study of a chronic low-dose versus a conventional ovulation regimen, which used rhFSH in anovulatory infertile women classified in WHO group II, showed that rhFSH is efficient and safe in both treatment protocols and confirmed that the chronic low-dose regimen is associated with a higher rate of mono- or bifollicular development.[49]

From these data, it may be concluded that the apparent higher efficiency of rhFSH justifies its preferential use in the chronic low-dose procedure for stimulation of ovulation in WHO II group patients. The starting dose must be chosen according to the clinical features of the patient and after a careful examination of some previous ovarian hyperstimulations; rhFSH 37.5 IU/day may be recommended in this later situation and small increments in doses (range 12.5–18.7 IU/day) may be sufficient to achieve the threshold value after a median treatment duration of 2 weeks.

We have previously shown,[50] using a sequential protocol, that combining an initial chronic low-dose administration of uhFSH followed by a step-down regimen after follicular selection is a safe and effective method in patients with the PCOS. Another study is in progress to evaluate the effectiveness of rhFSH with this regimen.

### Overall safety experience with rhFSH

Experience with rhFSH is quickly growing and all clinical studies performed world wide indicate that some observed serious adverse events (ovarian hyperstimulation) are related to the pharmacological property of the compound and that its local tolerance is good after both intramuscular and subcutaneous injection.[51] The fact that rhFSH can be injected subcutaneously led to voluntary self-administration in about 50% of cases, contrasting with less than 10% in the uhFSH group.[40] Moreover, in a patient with a history of a severe systemic immunoglobulin E-mediated reaction to uhFSH, presumably related to non-gonadotrophin proteins, rhFSH may be used successfully.[52] In addition, to date, no sera have been found to be positive for anti-FSH antibody.

### CONCLUSIONS

Human FSH is now produced in vitro by recombinant DNA technology and has been purified and formulated, leading to preparations that are suitable for therapeutic use in humans via subcutaneous administration. The rhFSH appears to be safe and effective for stimulating follicular development in WHO group II anovulation, whereas co-administration of exogenous LH is mandatory in order to obtain adequate follicular steroidogenesis in WHO group I anovulation. Although some reports indicate a higher efficiency for this new compound compared with previous urinary preparations, it deserves further confirmation in future studies in chronic anovulatory women. Differences in the isohormone profile and in the oligosaccharide structure seem to be too small to be considered relevant to the determination of therapeutic differences from uhFSH. The difference (30%) in the level of oxidized forms may be important; however, further studies are required to elucidate the mechanisms involved. Another challenge in the near future could be to determine which isoforms of FSH are the most adequate for a safe and effective induction of ovulation. Currently, both purity and batch-to-batch consistency make rhFSH the first choice of treatment in infertile women with WHO group II anovulation.

## REFERENCES

1. Gemzell CA, Diczfalusy E, Tillinger KG. Human pituitary follicle-stimulating hormone. 1. Clinical effect of a partly purified preparation. *Ciba Foundation Colloquia Endocrinol* 1960;**13**:191.

2. Lunenfeld B, Sulimovici S, Rabau E, Eshkol A. L'induction de l'ovulation dans les amenorrhées hypophysaires par un traitement combiné de gonadotrophines urinaires ménopausiques et de gonadotrophines chorioniques. *C R Soc Fr Gynécol* 1962;**5**:30–4.

3. Raj SG, Berger MJ, Grimes EM, Taymor MI. The use of gonadotropins for the induction of ovulation in women with polycystic ovarian disease. *Fertil Steril* 1977;**28**:1280–4.

4. Harlin J, Kahn SA, Diczfalusy E. Molecular composition of luteinizing hormone and follicle stimulating hormone in commercial gonadotropin preparations. *Fertil Steril* 1986;**46**:1055–60.

5. Boime I, Keene J, Matsuk MM, et al. Expression of recombinant human FSH and LH in mammalian cells: a source of potential agonists and antagonists for controlling fertility. In: *FSH Alone in Ovulation Induction* (Lunenfeld B, ed.). Carnforth: Parthenon Publishing, 1990: 45–62.

6. Keene JL, Matsuk MM, Otani T, et al. Expression of biologically active human follitropin in Chinese hamster ovary cells. *J Biol Chem* 1989;**246**:4769–75.

7. Galway AB, Hsueh AJW, Keene JL, et al. In vitro and in vivo bioactivity of recombinant follicle-stimulating hormone and partially deglycosylated variants secreted by transfected eukaryotic cell lines. *Endocrinology* 1990;**127**:93–9.

8. Mannaerts B, de Leeuw R, Geelen J, et al. Comparative in vitro and in vivo studies on the biological characteristics of recombinant human follicle stimulating hormone. *Endocrinology* 1991;**129**:2623–30.

9. Kloosterboer HJ. Biological characteristics of recombinant FSH isohormones. *Hum Reprod* 1994;**9**(suppl 4):52–3.

10. Germond M, Dessole S, Senn A, et al. Successful in-vitro fertilization and embryo transfer after treatment with recombinant human FSH. *Lancet* 1992;**339**:1170.

11. Devroey P, Van Steirteghem A, Mannaerts B, Coelingh Bennink H. Successful in-vitro fertilization and embryo transfer after treatment with recombinant human FSH. *Lancet* 1992; **339**:1170–1.

12. World Health Organization. Agents stimulating gonadal function in the human. Report of a WHO scientific group. *Wld Hlth Org Techn Rep Ser* 1973: 514.

13. Boime I, Fares F, Lapolt PA, et al. Structure–function studies of gonadotropins using site directed mutagenesis and gene transfer: design of a long-acting follitropin agonist. In: *GnRH, GnRH Analogs, Gonadotropins and Gonadal Peptides* (Bouchard P, et al, eds). Carnforth: Parthenon Publishing, 1992: 347–57.

14. Fauser BCJM, Soto D, Czekala NM, Hsueh AJW. Granulosa cell aromatase bioassays: changes of bioactive FSH levels in the female. *J Steroid Biochem* 1989;**33**:721–6.

15. Mannaerts B, Shoham Z, Schoot DC, et al. Single-dose pharmacokinetics and pharmacodynamics of recombinant human follicle-stimulating hormone (Org 32487) in gonadotropin deficient volunteers. *Fertil Steril* 1993;**59**:108–14.

16. Schoot DC, Harlin J, Shoham Z, et al. Recombinant human follicle-stimulating hormone and ovarian response in gonadotrophin-deficient women. *Hum Reprod* 1994;**9**:1237–42.

17. Mannaerts B, Fauser BCJM, Lalhou N, et al. Serum hormone concentrations during treatment with multiple rising doses of recombinant follicle stimulating hormone (Puregon) in men with hypogonadotropic hypogonadism. *Fertil Steril* 1996;**65**:406–10.

18. Le Cotonnec JY, Porchet HC, Beltrami V, et al. Clinical pharmacology of recombinant human follicle-stimulating hormone (FSH). I. Comparative pharmacokinetics with urinary human FSH. *Fertil Steril* 1994;**61**:669–78.

19. Le Cotonnec JY, Porchet HC, Beltrami V, et al. Clinical pharmacology of recombinant human follicle-stimulating hormone. II. Single doses and steady state pharmacokinetics. *Fertil Steril* 1994;**61**:679–86.

20. Fevold HL. Synergism of follicle stimulating and luteinizing hormone in producing estrogen secretion. *Endocrinology* 1941;**28**:33–6.

21. Eshkol A, Lunenfeld B. Purification and separation of follicle stimulating hormone (FSH) and luteinizing hormone from human menopausal gonadotrophin: III. Effects of a biologically apparently pure FSH preparation on ovaries and uteri of intact immature mice. *Acta Endocrinol (Copenh)* 1967;**54**:91–5.

22. Berger MJ, Taymor ML. The role of luteinizing hormone in human follicular maturation and

function. *Am J Obstet Gynecol* 1971;**111**:708–10.

23. Couzinet B, Lestrat N, Brailly S, et al. Stimulation of ovarian follicular maturation with pure follicle stimulating hormone in women with gonadotropin deficiency. *J Clin Endocrinol Metab* 1988;**66**:552–6.

24. Short RV. Steroids in the follicular fluid and the corpus luteum of the mare; a 'two-cell type' theory of ovarian steroid synthesis. *J Endocrinol* 1962;**24**:59–63.

25. Ryan KJ, Petro Z, Kaiser J. Steroid formation by isolated and recombinant ovarian and theca cells. *J Clin Endocrinol Metab* 1968:**28**:355–8.

26. Schoot DC, Coelingh Bennink HJT, Mannaerts B, et al. Human recombinant follicle-stimulating hormone induces growth of preovulatory follicles without concomitant increase in androgen and estrogen biosynthesis in a woman with isolated gonadotropin deficiency. *J Clin Endocrinol Metab* 1992;**74**:1471–3.

27. Shoham Z, Mannaerts B, Insler V, Coelingh Bennink HJT. Induction of follicular growth using recombinant human follicle-stimulating hormone in two volunteer women with hypogonadotropic hypogonadism. *Fertil Steril* 1993;**59**:738–42.

28. Hillier SG, Yong EL, Illingworth PJ, et al. Effect of recombinant inhibin on androgen synthesis in cultured human thecal cells. *Mol Cell Endocrinol* 1991;**75**:R1–6.

29. Shoham Z, Loumaye E, Piazzi A. A dose finding study to determine the effective dose of recombinant human luteinizing hormone to support FSH-induced follicular development in hypogonadotropic hypogonadal (HH) women. *51st Annual Meeting of the American Society for Reproductive Medicine*, Seattle, Washington DC, 1995: abstract 0–142.

30. Donderwinkel PFJ, Schoot DC, Coelingh Bennink HJT, Fauser BCJM. Pregnancy after induction of ovulation with recombinant human FSH in polycystic ovary syndrome. *Lancet* 1992;**340**:983.

31. Hornnes P, Giroud D, Howles C, Loumaye E. Recombinant human follicle-stimulating hormone treatment leads to normal follicular growth, oestradiol secretion, and pregnancy in a World Health Organization group II anovulatory woman. *Fertil Steril* 1993;**60**:724–6.

32. Seibel MM, Kamrava MM, McArdle C, Taymor ML. Treatment of polycystic ovarian disease with chronic low dose follicle stimulating hormone: biochemical changes and ultrasound correlation. *Int J Fertil* 1984;**29**:39–43.

33. Polson DW, Mason HD, Saldahna MB, Franks S. Ovulation of a single dominant follicle during treatment with low dose pulsatile follicle stimulating hormone in women with polycystic ovary syndrome. *Clin Endocrinol* 1987;**26**:205–12.

34. Buvat JB, Buvat-Herbaut M, Marcollin G, et al. Purified follicle-stimulating hormone in polycystic ovary syndrome: Slow administration is safer and more effective. *Fertil Steril* 1989;**52**:553–9.

35. Van Dessel HJHM, Donderwinkel PFJ, Coelingh Bennink HJT, Fauser BCJM. First established pregnancy and birth after induction of ovulation with recombinant human follicle-stimulating hormone in polycystic ovary syndrome. *Hum Reprod* 1994;**9**:55–6.

36. Wiedemann R, Katzorke Th, Schindler A, et al. Low-dose recombinant human follicle-stimulating hormone therapy in World Health Organization group II anovulatory women. *11th Annual Meeting of the European Society for Human Reproduction and Embryology*, Hamburg, 1995: abstract 224.

37. Out HJ, Driessen SGAJ, Mannaerts BMJL, Coelingh Bennink HJT. Recombinant follicle-stimulating hormone (follitropin beta, Puregon) yields higher pregnancy rates in in vitro fertilization than urinary gonadotropins. *Fertil Steril* 1997;**68**:38–42.

38. Bergh C, Howles CM, Borg K, et al. Recombinant human follicle stimulating hormone (r-hFSH; Gonal-F) versus highly purified urinary FSH (Metrodin HP): results of a randomized comparative study in women undergoing assisted reproductive techniques. *Hum Reprod* 1997;**12**:2133–9.

39. Jacobs H. Efficacy of recombinant human follicle stimulating hormone Gonal-F for inducing ovulation in WHO Group II anovulatory patients. Preliminary results of a comparative, multicentre study. *9th Annual Meeting of the European Society for Human Reproduction and Embryology*, Thessaloniki, 1993: abstract 241.

40. Loumaye E, Martineau I, Piazzi A, et al. Clinical assessment of human gonadotrophins produced by recombinant DNA technology. *Hum Reprod* 1996;**11**(suppl 1):95–107.

41. Gurgan T, Yarali H, Bukulmez O, et al. Treatment of clomiphene citrate-resistant polycystic ovarian syndrome with a 'low-dose step-up' protocol: prospective study comparing recombinant with pure FSH. *13th Annual Meeting of the European Society for Human Reproduction and*

*Embryology*, Edinburgh, 1997: abstract 0–173.

42. Geurts TBP, Peters MJH, van Bruggen JGC, et al. Puregon (Org 32489): human recombinant FSH. *Drugs Today* 1997;**33**(suppl 1/F):1–25.

43. White D, Fauser BCJM, Ohbrai M, et al. Recombinant FSH (Puregon) is more efficient than urinary FSH (Metrodin) in clomiphene-resistant normogonadotropic chronic anovulatory women: a prospective, multicenter, assessor-blind, randomised, clinical trial. *Fertil Steril* 1998; in press.

44. Matikainen T, de Leeuw R, Mannaerts B, Huhtaniemi I. Circulating bioactive and immunoreactive recombinant human follicle stimulating hormone (Org 32489) after administration to gonadotropin-deficient subjects. *Fertil Steril* 1994;**61**:62–9.

45. Hard K, Mekking A, Damm JBL, et al. Isolation and structure determination of the intact sialylated N-linked carbohydrate chains of recombinant human follitropin expressed in Chinese hamster ovary cells. *Eur J Biochem* 1990;**193**:263–71.

46. Chappel SC, Heterogeneity of follicle stimulating hormone: control and physiological function. *Hum Reprod Update* 1995;**1**:479–87.

47. Brown JB. Pituitary control of ovarian function – concepts derived from gonadotrophin therapy. *Aust NZ J Obstet Gynaecol* 1978;**18**:47–54.

48. Homburg R, Levy T, Ben-Rafael A. A comparative prospective study of conventional regimen with chronic low-dose administration of follicle-stimulating hormone for anovulation associated with polycystic ovary syndrome. *Fertil Steril* 1995;**63**:729–33.

49. Hedon B, Hugues JN, Emperaire JC, et al. A comparative prospective study of a chronic low dose versus a conventional ovulation stimulation regimen using recombinant human follicle-stimulating hormone (Gonal F) in WHO group II anovulatory infertile women. *13th Annual Meeting of the European Society for Human Reproduction and Embryology*, Edinburgh, 1997: abstract P 211.

50. Hugues JN, Cedrin-Durnerin I, Avril C, et al. Sequential step-up and step-down dose regimen: an alternative method for ovulation induction with follicle stimulating hormone in polycystic ovary syndrome. *Hum Reprod* 1996;**11**:2581–4.

51. Out HJ, Reimitz PE, Coelingh Bennink HJT. A prospective, randomized study to assess the tolerance and efficacy of intramuscular and subcutaneous administration of recombinant follicle-stimulating hormone (Puregon). *Fertil Steril* 1997;**67**:278–83.

52. Phipps WR, Holden D, Sheehan RK. Use of recombinant human follicle-stimulating hormone for in vitro fertilization–embryo transfer after severe systemic immunoglobulin E-mediated reaction to urofollitropin. *Fertil Steril* 1996;**66**:148–50.

# 12

# The use of recombinant luteinizing hormone, gonadotrophin-releasing hormone agonist or human chorionic gonadotrophin to trigger ovulation

Ernest Loumaye, Angela Piazzi, Patrick Engrand

**The need for a surrogate LH surge  •  The natural LH surge  •  The human chorionic gonadotrophin surge  •  Alternatives to the hCG surge  •  Conclusions**

The midcycle luteinizing hormone (LH) surge is a key event in the menstrual cycle. Appropriate timing and adequate duration and amplitude of this surge are prerequisites for human female fertility. An adequate surge will lead to several changes at the follicle level that are pivotal for obtaining a pregnancy. First, the surge induces the cumulus oophorus mucinification, allowing the oocyte to be released subsequently from the follicular wall. Second, it provokes the resumption of the oocyte meiosis, that is, from germinal vesicle stage to metaphase II. Reaching the metaphase II meiotic stage is a mandatory step for allowing proper fertilization of the oocyte and embryonic development. Third, the LH surge triggers follicular rupture, expelling the oocyte from the follicle and leading to its capture by the fallopian tube. Finally, it induces a shift in the granulosa cell steroidogenic process, changing it from a dominating oestradiol secretory process towards a progesterone secretory process, forming an active corpus luteum.

Three major regulatory factors have been identified as playing a role in the induction of the midcycle LH surge: the hypothalamic gonadotrophin-releasing hormone (GnRH), the ovarian steroids (oestradiol and progesterone), and some less well characterized peptide hormones (for example, gonadotrophin surge-attenuating factor).[1]

## THE NEED FOR A SURROGATE LH SURGE

In several clinical situations, a surrogate LH surge must be produced, because the endogenous feedback mechanisms that produce an endogenous LH surge are absent or impaired.

In anovulation resulting from severe gonadotrophin deficiency (WHO group 1 anovulation; hypogonadotrophic hypogonadism), follicular growth induced by a combined administration of follicle-stimulating hormone (FSH) and LH is usually not followed by a spontaneous LH surge. In anovulation resulting from a hypothalamic–pituitary dysfunction, which is characterized by residual gonadotrophin and oestradiol secretion (WHO group 2 anovulation; polycystic ovary syndrome or PCOS), the restoration of follicular growth by FSH administration does not usually lead to a correct timing and adequate amplitude of the LH surge.[2] Treatment of anovulation with gonadotrophins thus requires the production of a surrogate LH surge.

In ovulatory patients undergoing stimulation of multiple follicular development by administration of pharmacological doses of FSH before assisted reproductive technology (ART), it has been shown that feedback mechanisms are often disrupted. This leads to mistimed LH surges that are often also blunted.[3,4] The administration of a surrogate LH surge has therefore become a standard procedure in ART. Moreover, as mistimed LH surges have been regarded as a cause of failure of the ART treatment, most patients are now pre-treated with an GnRH agonist. This treatment abolishes pituitary responsiveness to endogenous GnRH, and prevents the occurrence of a spontaneous endogenous LH surge.[4] This has resulted in a significant improvement of ART treatment outcome.[5]

A third indication for a LH surge surrogate could be in patients undergoing intrauterine insemination with washed sperm (IUI); in such patients the probability of conception appears to be related to the duration of the spontaneous surge.[6] In this study, an LH surge lasting for one day was associated with a pregnancy rate three times lower than that obtained when the surge lasted for 2 days. It is, however, not established whether the abnormal surge is the primary defect or if, in these infertile patients, it is the consequence of an impaired follicular development or a mistimed feedback mechanism. Moreover, the clinical efficacy of administering a surrogate LH surge to prolong the LH signal remains to be established.

## THE NATURAL LH SURGE

The main characteristics of a natural LH surge as reported in the literature are summarized in Table 1. The natural surge lasts for about 2 days and is made up of an ascending phase, a plateau and a descending phase. LH serum levels, when measured by radio-immunoassay (RIA), are about 10–20 times the basal LH levels. Figure 1 shows mean values for serum immunoreactive LH concentrations, assayed with an immunoradiometric assay (IRMA) in four female volunteers who underwent

**Table 1 Summary of LH surge characteristics**

| LH surge characteristics | Natural midcycle LH surge | hCG (5000 IU i.m.) | GnRH agonist-induced surge |
|---|---|---|---|
| Surge duration (h) | 49 ± 9 | >96 | 24–48 |
| Ascending phase (h) | ≅14 | ≅20 | ≅4 |
| Plateau (h) | ≅14 | 0 | 0 |
| Descending phase (h) | ≅20 | >72 | 20–36 |
| LH peak value (IU/l) | 100–200 | – | 50–250 |
| Peak:baseline ratio | 10–20 | – | 10–20 |

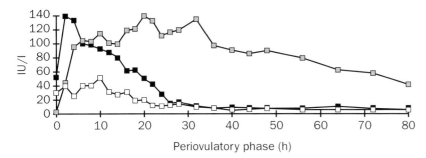

**Figure 1** Mean LH and hCG profiles of four female volunteers who were monitored during three cycles. A spontaneous LH surge was recorded during cycle A (□). An endogenous surge was triggered by one subcutaneous injection of 250 μg buserelin acetate when the dominant follicle reached a mean diameter of 18 mm in cycle B (■). During cycle C, hCG 5000 IU was administered when the leading follicle reached 18 mm (▨). Luteinizing hormone MAIAclone IRMA was used to measure serum LH levels in cycles A and B. Human chorionic gonadotrophin MAIAclone IRMA was used to measure serum hCG in cycle C (Serono study GF 6113, unpublished data).

frequent blood sampling around the midcycle period. In this study the mean peak value was $46 \pm 16$ IU/l. The absolute peak value was somewhat lower than that reported in the published data using an RIA, but the relative increase on baseline secretion was essentially similar (around tenfold). When frequent sampling is performed during the surge, a clearcut pulsatile pattern for the LH secretion is observed. The LH pulse frequency appears to be the same as that of the late follicular phase LH secretion. The amplitude of the pulse is, however, very significantly increased.[7]

Studies analysing the LH surges show relatively large variations between individuals in terms of duration and amplitude of the LH surge. This might result partially from insufficiently high sampling frequency. From a clinical point of view, this variation also suggests that patients may have different threshold levels for the LH surge, as is the case for FSH in terms of follicular development. This should be taken into account when designing a therapeutic regimen for inducing a surrogate LH surge that must be effective in most patients. Indeed,

in contrast to FSH therapy, no dose adjustment is possible.

In perfused rat ovaries, different thresholds have been identified for the different physiological roles of the surge.[8] Only 5% of the LH peak concentration is sufficient to trigger the resumption of oocyte meiosis. A significant dose–response relationship was recorded for the progesterone secretion, but 5% of the LH peak value concentration is also sufficient to trigger significant luteinization. By contrast, more than 85% of the LH surge peak concentration is required to trigger follicular rupture and ovulation. The practical consequence of this is that a regimen for inducing a surrogate surge needs to be designed based on the therapeutic objective. The regimen for provoking oocyte maturation and luteinization in patients for whom no follicular rupture is required (that is, before ovum pick-up [OPU] for ART), could be different from one aiming to provoke the full process of ovulation for in vivo conception.

In terms of steroid profiles at the time of the natural LH surge, progesterone has been shown to increase in two steps: an initial rise ending in a plateau at about 12 hours, followed by a second increase. Androstenedione and testosterone also surge at the time of the LH surge; their peak values are four times and two times higher than before their surges, respectively.[9]

## THE HUMAN CHORIONIC GONADOTROPHIN SURGE

Human chorionic gonadotrophin (hCG) shares with LH the common biological property of recognizing and activating the same receptor. It is, however, somewhat different from LH in terms of receptor affinity. The binding affinities of urinary hCG and of recombinant hCG are about two to four times higher than those of pituitary-derived human LH (hLH) and recombinant hLH (unpublished data). In addition, there are significant difference in terms of pharmacokinetic characteristics; hCG has a terminal half-life about three times longer than urinary hLH and recombinant hLH. Together these differences indicate that administration of an equal dose of LH and hCG (in terms of molarity), assuming all other pharmacokinetic properties to be similar (for example, rate and extent of absorption, distribution), will lead to a higher and more prolonged biological signal with hCG than with LH.

The use of urinary hCG instead of LH to mimic the preovulatory LH surge has been historically justified by the fact that urinary hCG was easier to obtain than LH. For the last 30 years, therapeutic preparations of hCG were extracted from the urine of pregnant women. Initially, having a preparation with a prolonged activity was an advantage, because ultrasonography was not available for timing the surge administration, and patients were generally WHO group 1 anovulators who require some luteal phase support. Recently, hCG produced in vitro by recombinant DNA technology has entered the clinical phase of evaluation (Ovidrel). The pharmacokinetic characteristics of the recombinant hCG are very similar to those of the urinary-derived hCG. Their terminal half-lives are about 30 h (unpublished data).

Based on extended experience with urinary hCG, its efficacy and its safety, it is anticipated that recombinant hCG will become the reference preparation for inducing a surrogate LH surge in most patients.

As mentioned earlier, the main characteristics of a standard hCG surge are summarized in Table 1 and Figure 1 shows mean values for immunoreactive hCG serum concentrations assayed with an IRMA in four female volunteers. These volunteers received 5000 IU hCG intramuscularly during a spontaneous cycle, when the dominant follicle reached a diameter of 18 mm. It should be noted that the units used for measuring hCG cannot be directly compared with the units used for LH serum concentrations, because assays are specific and do not use the same reference preparation. In addition, the units used to express the potency of a preparation (for example, of an ampoule of hCG for therapeutic use) cannot be directly converted into immunoactivity because they represent a biological activity in terms of in vivo activity, as determined by an in vivo bioassay (Van Hell assay).

The widely accepted dose range for hCG is 5000–10 000 IU as a single injection. One dose-finding study has indicated that 2000 IU is insufficient for the requirements of the in vitro fertilization (IVF) population, because no oocytes were retrieved at the OPU in 23% of patients receiving that dose. Successful oocyte retrieval was recorded in more than 95% of patients treated with 5000 and 10 000 IU hCG.[10]

The surge profile obtained after a single injection of hCG is more prolonged than the natural LH surge (see Figure 1 and Table 1). Practically, after an injection of 10 000 IU hCG, serum levels of the hormone were found to be above baseline in all patients up to day 10 after injection.[11]

The efficacy and safety of the surrogate hCG surge are well established and to date there are no arguments for questioning its use at least in most patients. However, the occurrence of the ovarian hyperstimulation syndrome (OHSS), multiple pregnancies and a somewhat low implantation rate after therapy with human menopausal gonadotrophin (hMG)–FSH/hCG has drawn clinicians' attention to the putative contribution of the prolonged activity of hCG to these adverse outcomes. It is well established that the amplitude of the response to FSH (that is, the number of growing follicles) will determine the risk of the OHSS and multiple pregnancy.[12] Therefore, the development of 'soft' protocols, which use the minimal effective dose of FSH with careful adjustment steps and monitoring of the ovarian response to the gonadotrophin, has led to a significant reduction in the incidence of these adverse outcomes. Using a 'chronic low dose protocol' for treating WHO group 2 anovulation, the incidence of significant OHSS is less than 1% and of multiple pregnancy around 5%.[13] Although these figures are low, and better than the figures obtained with standard regimens, a significant proportion of cycles still have to be cancelled, that is, in two large clinical trials using a strict, chronic, low-dose protocol, 24 of 513 cycles and 13 of 565 cycles were cancelled for risk of the OHSS before hCG administration (unpublished data). Therefore, further improvement of these figures would be medically relevant. In ART, severe OHSS is recorded in less than 0.5–2% of the treated cycles.[14] In this indication the incidence of multiple pregnancy is related to the number of embryos transferred.

In addition, in patients receiving hCG after controlled ovarian hyperstimulation (COH), preliminary data suggest that phase 4 progesterone rises more abruptly than in the natural cycle, which may accelerate the secretory changes in the endometrium to the point of phasing out endometrial receptivity, and thus in some cases impair the implantation process.[15] In this preliminary study, no significant changes in the androgen levels were recorded, contrasting with what is observed in the natural cycle. Further assessment of these differences in the steroid profiles between the natural surge and the hCG surge are needed to establish if they have a clinical relevance in terms of success rate after gonadotrophin therapy.

Finally, VEGF (vascular endothelium growth factor) has been proposed as a key factor of OHSS pathogenesis,[16] and hCG/LH directly stimulates VEGF synthesis by granulosa cells.[17]

## ALTERNATIVES TO THE HCG SURGE

The theoretical benefit of using LH instead of hCG, which provides a shorter, more physiological surrogate surge for those patients presenting a high risk of adverse outcome, has been addressed by clinicians since gonadotrophin therapy was first developed. In the early years, only pituitary-derived human LH was available, and very limited experience was gained. In the early 1980s, an attempt was made to reduce the hCG half-life by enzymatic desialylation of urine-derived hCG.[18] More recently, clinicians have used GnRH agonists as well as native GnRH for triggering an endogenous LH surge, and results from pilot works using hLH produced in vitro by recombinant DNA technology are available.

### Pituitary LH

Human LH preparations derived from cadaver pituitary glands were used in the 1960s to trigger final follicular maturation and ovulation in WHO class 1 anovulation treated with hMG. Repeated administrations of pituitary LH were used (that is, 800–1200 IU every 8 h for 24 h). Continuation of LH administration throughout the luteal phase was shown to be necessary to obtain a pregnancy.[19] This is not surprising considering that these patients are profoundly deficient in both LH and FSH. The pituitary-derived preparations are obviously no longer acceptable as therapeutic preparations because of the risk of infectious agent transmission.[20]

### GnRH agonists

The LH surge induced by GnRH agonists works through an indirect mechanism that relies on the patient's own pituitary response to GnRH. The main characteristics of a standard LH surge induced by an GnRH agonist, as reported in the literature, are summarised in Table 1. Published data suggest that multiple administrations of an GnRH agonist do not lead to a prolonged surge when compared with a single administration.[21,22] Figure 1 also shows the mean values for immunoreactive LH serum concentrations assayed with an immunoradio-metric assay in four female volunteers who received 250 µg buserelin subcutaneously dur-ing a spontaneous cycle, when the dominant follicle reached a diameter of 18 mm. In this study, the mean peak value was $127 \pm 55$ IU/l LH. The induced LH surge has a sharper profile and a higher peak value than the naturally occurring surge. Its duration is shorter than the natural surge and the hCG surge.

The efficacy and safety of the LH surge induced by an GnRH agonist have been investi-gated in three clinical situations. The first is WHO group 2/PCOS patients who are overre-sponding to hMG/FSH and therefore would, in most cases, have not received hCG because of the risk of the OHSS and multiple pregnancy. Table 2 summarizes these studies (those in which clomiphene citrate was used during the follicular phase were excluded, because an endogenous LH surge is consistently recorded during this treatment). Experience of this treat-ment is still limited; pregnancies can be obtained with a pregnancy rate of 17% per cycle. Some twins and triplets have been reported and the multiple pregnancy rate is around 10%. Some significant cases of the OHSS were reported after the GnRH agonist-induced surge, with an incidence of 2.5%. At least one case of the OHSS was reported in a cycle without conception.[23] Finally, a high inci-dence of luteal phase deficiency has been observed, which indicates luteal phase support when triggering an endogenous LH surge with an GnRH agonist.[24,25]

The second clinical indication in which GnRH agonist-induced surges have been used is to trigger final follicular maturation before ART. This applies to cycles that are not pre-treated with a GnRH agonist. These studies have recently been reviewed.[26] Contrasting with the WHO group 2 indication, studies have not been focused on patients who are overresponding. These studies suggest a reduction in the OHSS, but no definitive conclusions can be drawn in terms of differences from hCG surges.

The third indication is to trigger ovulation in ovulatory patients who underwent follicular growth stimulation with FSH before IUI. In a comparison between 416 cycles with FSH HP (highly purified)/hCG and 345 with FSH HP/GnRH agonist, the ovulation rate was simi-lar and the pregnancy rate was significantly higher in the GnRH agonist group.[27] No cases of the OHSS were reported in either group.

It is noteworthy that this indication has also been selected for a pilot study, in which five patients treated with ovarian stimulation and IUI were enrolled. In these patients pre-treated with an GnRH antagonist, a LH surge was suc-cessfully elicited with 0.1 mg triptorelin.[28] Luteinization was documented, but no preg-nancy was reported.

## Recombinant human LH

Human LH produced by DNA recombinant technology (LHadi, Serono) is now available as are human FSH and hCG.[29] Recombinant LH appears to have essentially similar pharmaco-kinetic characteristics to the pituitary-derived hLH. In monkeys, the distribution half-life ($t_\frac{1}{2}$), after intravenous administration was found to be less than 1 h, and the terminal $t_\frac{1}{2}$ to be $11.0 \pm 0.9$ h.[30] In humans, recombinant hLH was found to have a distribution $t_\frac{1}{2}$ of about 1 h and a terminal after intravenous administration of around 10 h.[31–33] This is similar to the urine-derived LH (hMG) terminal $t_\frac{1}{2}$, and contrasts with urine-derived hCG or recombinant hCG which have a distribution $t_\frac{1}{2}$ of about 5 h and a terminal $t_\frac{1}{2}$ of about 30 h. Hence, hCG will remain in the organism about three times longer than LH. Some experience with recombi-nant hLH for producing a surrogate LH surge has been gained in the monkey, the rabbit and, more recently, humans. In monkeys, recombi-nant hLH has been compared with pituitary LH and hCG in an IVF model.[34] Two injections of recombinant hLH 2500 IU at 18 h apart elicit LH surge levels for 36–48 h and induce peri-ovulatory events similar to those elicited by an hCG injection (1000 IU). Attenuated LH surges of 18–24 h reinitiate oocyte meiosis and

**Table 2  GnRH agonist-induced LH surge in WHO group 2/PCOS patients**

| Study | Year | Patient eligibility criteria | Analogue | Luteal support | No. of cycles | Moderate or severe OHSS | Pregnancy | Multiple pregnancy |
|---|---|---|---|---|---|---|---|---|
| Emperaire et al[21] | 1991 | $E_2$ > 1200 pg/ml and/or >3 follicles > 17 mm | Buserelin 3 × 200 μg i.n. | None | 48 | 0 | 8 | 1 |
| van der Meer et al[23] | 1993 | $E_2$ > 1200 pg/ml and/or >3 follicles > 18 mm | Buserelin 3 × 200 μg i.n. | Vaginal $P_4$ 300 mg/day | 27 | 3 | NA | – |
| Corson et al[37] | 1993 | ≥2 follicles > 17 mm | Nafarelin 1 or 2 × 400 μg i.n. | None | 22 | 0 | 3 | 0 |
| Lanzone et al[38] | 1994 | $E_2$ > 1200 pg/ml and/or >3 follicles > 15 mm | Buserelin 200 μg s.c. | $P_4$ 50 mg/day i.m. | 20 | 0 | 3 | 0 |
| Shalev et al[39] | 1994 | $E_2$ > 2500 pg/ml and/or ≥20 follicles > 14 mm | Decapeptyl 0.5 mg s.c. | $P_4$ 50 mg/day i.m. | 12 | 0 | 6 | 0 |
| Blumenfeld et al[40] | 1994 | $E_2$: 2800 ± 681 pg/ml ≥8 follicles ≥ 16 mm | GnRH 200 μg i.v. | hCG 2 × 2500 IU | 44 | 2 | 10 | 2 |
| Balasch et al[41] | 1994 | $E_2$ > 1000 pg/ml and/or ≥4 follicles ≥ 14 mm | Leuprolide 0.5 mg s.c. | None | 23 | 0 | 4 | 0 |
| **Total** | | | | | 196 | 5 (2.5%) | 34 (17%) | 3 (9%) |

$E_2$, oestradiol; $P_4$, progesterone; i.n., intranasal; s.c., subcutaneous; i.v., intravenous; i.m., intramuscular; NA, not applicable.

promote granulosa cell luteinization, but fail to promote corpus luteum development. In the rabbit, recombinant hLH 50 IU was compared with urinary hCG 50 IU for inducing ovulation.[35] In the recombinant hLH-treated group, the ovulation rate was lower but the implantation rate was higher than in the group treated with hCG.

In humans, recombinant hLH has been tested for triggering final follicular maturation before IVF–embryo transfer (ET). A first pregnancy has been reported.[36]

Recently, a large phase II study has been completed (unpublished data). This was a placebo-controlled, double-blind, multicentre study comparing different doses of recombinant hLH with urinary hCG in regular IVF patients. All patients were downregulated with an GnRH agonist using a long protocol. When downregulation was confirmed, stimulation was performed using recombinant FSH.

A comparison was made of recombinant hLH 5000, 15 000 or 30 000 IU, or recombinant LH 15 000 IU followed by 10 000 IU 2 days later, with urinary hCG 5000 IU. After final follicular maturation had been triggered, oocytes were retrieved and IVF or intracytoplasmic sperm injection (ICSI) was performed based on the indication. Embryo transfer was carried out on day 4, on average, after hCG or LH administration. All patients received the same luteal phase support (natural progesterone was administered vaginally from day 2 onwards). To assess the efficacy of recombinant hLH on final follicular maturation, four parameters were assessed: (1) the number of oocytes retrieved from follicles larger than 10 mm on the day of hCG/LH administration; (2) the cumulus oophorous maturity; (3) the oocyte nuclear maturity in some cases (eggs were classified as GV (germinal vesicle), metaphase I, metaphase II or atretic); and (4) the oocytes' potential for fertilization (proportion of two PN [pronuclei] oocytes in inseminated oocytes). (Note that patients from group 15 000 + 10 000 IU were pooled with those from group 15 000 IU.)

Two hundred and fifty-eight patients were enrolled in this study, of whom 250 received hCG or LH. The proportion of oocytes retrieved per follicle was 73% vs 74%, 76% vs 77% and 87% vs 74% for recombinant hLH 5000 IU, 15 000 IU and 30 000 IU versus urinary hCG, respectively. The proportion of 'mature' and 'very mature' oocytes was 82% vs 85%, 89% vs 88%, and 85% vs 90% for recombinant hLH 5000 IU, 15 000 IU and 30 000 IU versus urinary hCG, respectively.

About 58–91% of oocytes were in metaphase II, with the low dose of LH appearing to be as effective as hCG for triggering oocyte nuclear maturity. The proportion of inseminated oocytes resulting in 2PN fertilized oocytes was 54% vs 55%, 60% vs 54% and 61% vs 57% for recombinant hLH 5000 IU, 15 000 IU and 30 000 IU versus urinary hCG, respectively.

In this study, careful midluteal phase assessment of ovarian status and the OHSS was performed. Moderate OHSS was defined as (1) ovarian diameter over 5 cm, (2) ascites of ++ or more (in a semiquantitative scoring system ranging between 0 and ++++) and (3) abdominal symptoms lasting for 3 or more days.

Incidence of the OHSS was related to the level of ovarian response to FSH as well as to the treatment. Human chorionic gonadotrophin was more often associated with moderate OHSS than recombinant hLH (Table 3). Repeated administration of recombinant hLH led to a significant incidence of moderate OHSS, further confirming that the duration of the exposure to LH/hCG is a determinant for development of the OHSS.

## CONCLUSIONS

The LH surge at midcycle is a critical component in the process of ovulation and establishment of pregnancy.

Where exogenous gonadotrophins are employed for ovulation induction, for either COH or ART, the endogenous LH surge is often adversely affected by the altered dynamics of the cycle and a surrogate to ensure luteinization and/or follicular rupture is employed. Traditionally, the use of hCG has been standard

**Table 3  Clinically relevant OHSS (Serono study GF 7396, unpublished data)**

| Treatment | Serum oestradiol (pg/ml) | No. of follicles on hCG day | No. of patients | Moderate OHSS | Severe OHSS |
|---|---|---|---|---|---|
| Urinary hCG | ≤3000 | ≤20 | 69 | 4 (5.8%) | 0 |
| | >3000 | >20 | 52 | 8 (15.4%) | 1/52 (1.9%) |
| Recombinant hLH (one dose) | ≤3000 | ≤20 | 56 | 1 (1.8%) | 0 |
| | >3000 | >20 | 48 | 0 | 0 |
| Recombinant hLH (two doses) | ≤3000 | ≤20 | 17 | 1 (5.9%) | 0 |
| | >3000 | >20 | 8 | 3 (37.5%) | 0 |

practice in both of these indications, and its advantages and disadvantages have been well documented over the years. Patients at risk of adverse outcomes, such as the OHSS and multiple pregnancies, despite the use of an appropriate FSH administration regimen and careful treatment monitoring, could benefit from a more physiological LH surge. GnRH agonists have been employed for this purpose, but experience is limited and not all indications are suitable for its use. Most recently, recombinant LH had demonstrated promising results in inducing final follicular maturation and may offer some safety advantages in at-risk populations, as indicated by numbers of ovarian hyper-responsiveness. However, further work is necessary to elucidate and optimize dose, indications, efficacy and safety.

## REFERENCES

1. Fowler PA, Templeton A. The nature and function of putative gonadotropin surge-attenuating/inhibiting factor (GnSAF/IF). *Endocrine Rev* 1996;**17**:103–20.
2. Seibel MM, Kamrava MM, McArdle C, Taymor ML. Treatment of polycystic ovary disease with chronic low-dose follicle stimulating hormone: Biochemical changes and ultrasound correlation. *Int J Fertil* 1984:**29**:39–43.
3. Glasier A, Hillier SG, Thatcher SS, Baird DT, Wickings EJ. Superovulation with exogenous gonadotropins does not inhibit the luteinizing hormone surge. *Fertil Steril* 1988;**49**:81–5.
4. Loumaye E. The control of endogenous secretion of LH by gonadotropin-releasing hormone agonists during ovarian hyperstimulation for in-vitro fertilisation and embryo transfer. *Hum Reprod* 1990;**5**:357–76.
5. Hughes EG, Fedorkow DM, Daya S, Sagle MA, Van de Koppel P, Collins JA. The routine use of gonadotropin-releasing hormone agonists for IVF and gamete intrafallopian transfer: a meta-

analysis of randomised controlled trials. *Fertil Steril* 1992;**58**:888–96.

6. Cohlen BJ, te Velde ER, Scheffer G, van Kooij RJ, de Brouwer CPM, van Zonneveld P. The pattern of the luteinizing hormone surge in spontaneous cycles is related to the probability of conception. *Fertil Steril* 1993;**60**:413–17.

7. Adams JM, Taylor AE, Schoenfeld DA, Crowley WF, Hall JE. The midcycle gonadotropin surge in normal women occurs in the face of an unchanging gonadotropin-releasing hormone pulse frequency. *J Clin Endocrinol Metab* 1994;**79**:858–64.

8. Peluso JJ. Role of the amplitude of the gonadotropin surge in the rat. *Fertil Steril* 1990;**53**:150–4.

9. Hoff JD, Quigley M, Yen SSC. Hormonal dynamics at midcycle. A reevaluation. *J Clin Endocrinol Metab* 1983;**57**:792–6.

10. Abdalla HI, Ah-Moye M, Brinsden P, Howe DL, Okonofua F, Craft I. The effect of the dose of human chorionic gonadotropin and the type of gonadotropin stimulation on oocyte recovery rates in an in vitro fertilization program. *Fertil Steril* 1987;**6**:958–63.

11. Damewood MD, Shen W, Zacur HA, Wallach EE, Rock JA, Schlaff WD. Disappearance of exogenously administered human chorionic gonadotropin. *Fertil Steril* 1989;**52**:398–400.

12. Pride SM, James CSJ, Yuen BH. The ovarian hyperstimulation syndrome. *Semin Reprod Endocrinol* 1990;**8**:247–60.

13. Hamilton-Fairley D, Kiddy D, Watson H, Sagle M, Franks S. Low-dose gonadotrophin therapy for induction of ovulation in 100 women with polycystic ovary syndrome. *Hum Reprod* 1991;**6**:1095–9.

14. Rizk B, Smitz J. Ovarian hyperstimulation syndrome after superovulation using GnRH agonists for IVF and related procedures. *Hum Reprod* 1992;**7**:320–7.

15. Fanchin R, Castracane D, Taieb J, et al. The post-hCG hormonal profile in IVF-ET: plasma P increases 3 times more rapidly than in the menstrual cycle but androgens are unaffected. *Am Fertil Soc suppl* October 1993 [abstract].

16. Rizk B, Aboulghar M, Smitz J, Ron-El R. The role of vascular endothelial growth factor and interleukins in the pathogenesis of severe ovarian hyperstimulation syndrome. *Hum Reprod Update* 1997;**3**:255–66.

17. Christenson LK, Stouffer RL. Follicle-stimulating hormone and luteinizing hormone/chorionic gonadotropin stimulation of vascular endothelial growth factor production by macaque granulosa cells from pre and periovulatory follicles. *J Clin Endocrinol Metab* 1997;**82**:2135–42.

18. Crosignani PG, Donini P, Lombroso GC, Trojsi L. Preparation of partially desialylated hCG and its use for induction of ovulation after ovarian stimulation with human menopausal gonadotropin. *Acta Endocrinol* 1980;**95**:1–5.

19. Van de Wiele R, Bogumi J, Dyrenfurth I, Warren M, Jewelewich R, Ferin M. Mechanisms regulating the menstrual cycle in women. *Horm Res* 1970;**26**:63–103.

20. Cochius JI, Burns RJ, Blumbergs PC, Mack K, Alderman CP. Creutzfeldt–Jakob disease in a recipient of human pituitary-derived gonadotropin. *Aust NZ J Med* 1990;**20**:592–3.

21. Emperaire J, Ruffie A. Triggering ovulation with endogenous luteinizing hormone may prevent the ovarian hyperstimulation syndrome. *Hum Reprod* 1991;**6**:506–10.

22. Itskovitz J, Erlik Y, Boldes R, Levron J, Brandes JM. Induction of preovulatory luteinizing hormone surge and prevention of ovarian hyperstimulation syndrome by gonadotropin releasing hormone agonist. *Fertil Steril* 1991;**56**:213–20.

23. van der Meer S, Gerris J, Joostens M, Tas B. Triggering of ovulation using a gonadotrophin-releasing hormone agonist does not prevent ovarian hyperstimulation syndrome. *Hum Reprod* 1993;**8**:1628–31.

24. Balasch J, Fábregues F, Tur R, et al. Further characterization of the luteal phase inadequacy after gonadotrophin releasing hormone agonist induced ovulation in gonadotrophin stimulated cycles. *Fertil Steril* 1995;**10**:1377–81.

25. Gerris J, De Vits A, Joostens M, Van Royen E. Triggering of ovulation in human menopausal gonadotrophin-stimulated cycles: comparison between intravenously administered gonadotrophin-releasing hormone (100 and 500 µg), GnRH agonist (buserelin, 500 µg) and human chorionic gonadotrophin (10 000 IU). *Hum Reprod* 1995;**10**:56–62.

26. Gerris J. Prevention of ovarian hyperstimulation with preovulatory GnRH or GnRH agonists: does it work? In: *Ovulation Induction Update '98* (Filicori M, Flamigni C, eds). The Proceedings of the 2nd World Conference on Ovulation Induction held in Bologna, Italy, 12–13 September 1997. London: The Parthenon Publishing Group, 1998: 169–76.

27. Romeu A, Monzó A, Peiró T, Diez E, Peinado JA,

Quintero LA. Endogenous LH surge versus hCG as ovulation trigger after low-dose highly purified FSH in IUI: a comparison of 761 cycles. *J Ass Reprod Genet* 1997;**14**:518–24.

28. Olivennes F, Fanchin R, Bouchard P, Taieb J, Frydman R. Triggering of ovulation by a gonadotropin-releasing hormone (GnRH) agonist in patients pretreated with a GnRH antagonist. *Fertil Steril* 1996;**66**:151–3.

29. Agrawal R, West C, Conway GS, Page ML, Jacobs HS. Pregnancy after treatment with three recombinant gonadotropins. *Lancet* 1997;**349**: 29–30.

30. Porchet HC, Le Cotonnec J-Y, Neuteboom B, Canali S, Zanolo G. Pharmacokinetics of recombinant human luteinizing hormone after intravenous, intramuscular, and subcutaneous administration in monkeys and comparison with intravenous administration of pituitary human luteinizing hormone. *J Clin Endocrinol Metab* 1995;**80**:667–73.

31. Le Cotonnec J-Y, Porchet HC, Beltrami V, Munafo A. Clinical pharmacology of recombinant human luteinizing hormone. Part I. Pharmacokinetics after intravenous administration to healthy female volunteers and comparison with urinary human luteinizing hormone. *Fertil Steril* 1998;**69**:189–94.

32. Le Cotonnec J-Y, Porchet HC, Beltrami V, Munafo A. Clinical pharmacology of recombinant human luteinizing hormone. Part II. Bioavailability of recombinant human luteinizing hormone in humans assessed with an immunoassay and bioassay. *Fertil Steril* 1998;**69**:195–200.

33. Le Cotonnec J-Y, Loumaye E, Porchet HC, Beltrami V, Munafo A. Pharmacokinetic and pharmacodynamic interactions between recombinant human Luteinizing Hormone and recombinant human Follicle-Stimulating Hormone. *Fertil Steril* 1998;**69**:201–9.

34. Chandrasekher YA, Hutchison JS, Zelinski-Wooten MB, et al. Initiation of periovulatory events in primate follicles using recombinant and native human luteinizing hormone to mimic the midcycle gonadotropin surge. *J Clin Endocrinol Metab* 1994;**79**:298–306.

35. Romeu A, Molina I, Tresguerres JAF, Pla M, Peinado JA. Effect of recombinant human luteinizing hormone versus human chorionic gonadotrophin: effects on ovulation, embryo quality and transport, steroid balance and implantation in rabbits. *Hum Reprod* 1995;**10**:1290–6.

36. Imthurn B, Piazzi A, Loumaye E. Recombinant human luteinizing hormone to mimic mid-cycle LH surge. *Lancet* 1996;**248**:332–3.

37. Corson SL, Batzer FR, Gocial B, Maislin G. The luteal phase after ovulation induction with human menopausal gonadotropin and one versus two doses of a gonadotropin-releasing hormone agonist. *Fertil Steril* 1993;**59**:1251–6.

38. Lanzone A, Fulghesu AM, Villa P, et al. Gonadotropin-releasing hormone agonist versus human chorionic gonadotropin as a trigger of ovulation in polycystic ovarian disease gonadotropin hyperstimulated cycles. *Fertil Steril* 1994;**62**:35–41.

39. Shalev E, Geslevich Y, Ben-Ami M. Induction of pre-ovulatory luteinizing hormone surge by gonadotropin-releasing hormone agonist for women at risk for developing the ovarian hyperstimulation syndrome. *Hum Reprod* 1994;**9**:417–19.

40. Blumenfeld Z, Lang N, Amit A, Kahana L, Yoffe N. Native gonadotropin-releasing hormone for triggering follicular maturation in polycystic ovary syndrome patients undergoing human menopausal gonadotropin ovulation induction. *Fertil Steril* 1994;**62**:456–60.

41. Balasch J, Tur R, Creus M, et al. Triggering of ovulation by a gonadotropin releasing hormone agonist in gonadotropin-stimulated cycles for prevention of ovarian hyperstimulation syndrome and multiple pregnancy. *Gynecol Endocrinol* 1994;**8**:7–12.

# 13

# Ovarian stimulation with highly purified FSH and ovulation induction for IUI

Alberto Romeu, Ana Monzó, Luis Alberto Quintero, Eduardo Díez, Tomás Pieró

**Physiological basis of ovulation induction** • **Materials and methods** • **Results** • **Conclusion**

Intrauterine insemination (IUI) after ovarian stimulation and ovulation induction with gonadotrophins has been used for many years as an infertility treatment, although different aspects of its use are still being discussed.

As ovulation is induced after follicles have reached the preovulatory stage, and separated, fertile sperm are placed close to the oocyte, its practice should allow sufficiently good results to be obtained in terms of pregnancies in such different types of infertility as those involving male factors, cervical factors, minimal adhesions and endometriosis, non-obstructive tubal damage, anovulation, luteal phase defect and idiopathic infertility.

When IUI has been scheduled as an infertility treatment, induction of ovulation could be helpful in timing insemination in women who have normal ovulatory cycles and in anovulatory women.

This chapter presents the results of ovarian stimulation and ovulation induction for IUI using low-dose, highly purified follicle-stimulating hormone (HP-FSH) and triggering ovulation with either human chorionic gonadotrophin (hCG) or leuprolide acetate. Also, incidence of luteinized unruptured follicles (LUFs), luteal

phase support and complications of ovulation induction and IUI are discussed.

## PHYSIOLOGICAL BASIS OF OVULATION INDUCTION

From a physiological point of view, during the reproductive life of women, ovarian follicles have two possible destinations: (1) atresia as a consequence of granulosa cell apoptosis for most follicles and (2) development, maturation, ovulation and luteinization for just a few.[1]

The objectives of ovulation induction for IUI are: (1) to obtain at least one preovulatory follicle; (2) to trigger ovulation; (3) to induce a luteal phase which allows implantation if fertilization takes place; and (4) to prevent undesirable events such as ovarian hyperstimulation and multiple pregnancy.

Follicular development and maturation are imperfectly understood processes in which different factors of growth and tissue differentiation play different roles.[2,3]

The initial stages of folliculogenesis are not gonadotrophin dependent because hypophysectomy does not prevent follicular growth from primordial to early antral follicles.[4] Evidence in the literature supports the idea that activin represents a stimulus for preantral follicles and FSH is needed for the final development and differentiation of granulosa cells into a more mature phenotype.[5]

It is clear that FSH action is needed for the rescue of early antral follicles from apoptosis and for the development of complete maturation.[3,5,6] In fact, hypophysectomy increases apoptosis in antral follicles.[1,7] FSH action is probably mediated by insulin-like growth factor I (IGF-I), epidermal growth factor (EGF), fibroblast growth factor β (FGF-β) and others.[3] It has been proved that steroidogenesis can be maintained in follicles that have granulosa cells undergoing apoptosis[8] and increasing oestradiol levels could act synergistically with FSH in preventing follicular atresia.[9]

At the start of each menstrual cycle, early FSH-sensitive antral follicles can be recruited by elevated circulating levels of FSH. Such follicles have low aromatase activity and therefore relatively high levels of androgens in their microenvironment, resulting in potentiation of FSH action.[10] This may result, as demonstrated by Almahbobi et al,[11] because the binding of FSH to granulosa cells of hyperandrogenic ovaries is higher than that found in normal granulosa cells.

Nevertheless, the role played by intrafollicular high levels of androgens has been discussed because they have been characterized as apoptotic factors in the ovarian follicle.[2] It was also postulated that their elevated concentrations in follicular fluid from polycystic ovaries could play a role in abnormal steroidogenesis and proliferation of granulosa cells, as shown by Andreani et al.[12]

Once follicles have been recruited, a process of selection takes place. FSH plays an important role in this selection, although locally produced steroidal and non-steroidal factors modulate the FSH response.[13] At the same time, increasing levels of oestradiol and inhibin induce a decrease in circulating FSH levels.[14] As a result, the selected dominant follicle ensures its development to ovulation, that is, the number of follicles that ovulate is determined by the ovary–pituitary feedback as well as by locally produced steroids and non-steroidal agents.

Once the dominant follicle reaches preovulatory characteristics, the surge of luteinizing hormone (LH) is needed to trigger both ovulation and luteinization.[15,16] The lifespan of a corpus luteum is a process that is related to cell death by apoptosis. It has been shown that programmed cell death by apoptosis is involved in the luteal regression of women[17,18] and that other factors such as bcl-2[19] and hCG (either exogenous or of embryonic origin) could play a role in preventing apoptosis, rescuing the corpus luteum and maintaining its function in early pregnancy as shown in Figure 1 (unpublished data).

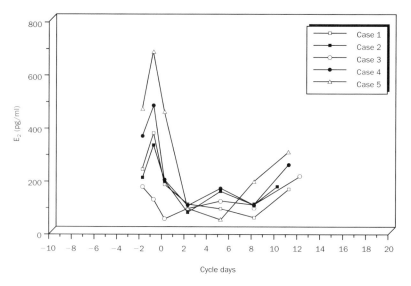

**Figure 1** Spontaneous rescue of corpus luteum function in 5 cases resulting in pregnancy after marked oestradiol (E₂) levels.

Therefore, pharmacologically conducted ovulation induction includes two different aspects: (1) development and maturation stimulation of the follicle which basically requires FSH and (2) induction of resumption of oocyte meiosis, granulosa cell luteinization and follicular wall rupture which also basically requires LH. Gonadotrophin-stimulated cycles can be achieved by giving human menopausal gonadotrophin (hMG) or FSH to stimulate follicular development and maturation, and by using hCG or gonadotrophin-releasing hormone (GnRH) agonists to trigger ovulation because they induce an endogenous surge of LH and FSH in women with normal pituitary gonadotrophin responsiveness.

In clinical practice, ovulation induction for IUI must be carried out on different categories of women: normogonadotrophic and hypogonadotrophic. Hypogonadic hypogonadotrophic women presenting both FSH and LH deficiency could need both hMG (FSH and LH action), to stimulate follicular development and steroidogenesis, and hCG (LH action), to trigger ovulation.

Luteal phase quality depends on the appropriate luteinization of a mature follicle, that is, hCG or LH may act on a preovulatory follicle with normal levels of LH receptors. Giving hCG when the dominant follicle is not mature could result in anovulation, LUFs or an inadequate luteal phase.[20] LUFs are frequently observed in stimulated cycles and cannot be prevented.[20] In terms of endocrine profiles and luteal phase duration, inadequate luteal phase could be avoided by giving either hCG or progesterone as luteal phase support.[21,22]

The establishment of a pregnancy is a possible beneficial outcome of inducing ovulation and practising IUI. Hyperstimulation syndrome, multiple pregnancy, abortion and ectopic pregnancy could all be undesirable events after such treatment.

## MATERIALS AND METHODS

### Infertility work-up

In the cases studied the diagnosis of male factor infertility was established from the WHO criteria after the following tests: semen bacteriology, computerized semen analysis (Cellsoft, CASA) and capacitation test (hamster test and hemizona assay if necessary), morphology test according to Kruger's criteria and an MAR test (serum antisperm antibodies if positive MAR test). The computerized semen analyser is included monthly in a quality control programme and shows good correlation with manual analysis.

The diagnosis of female factor infertility was established after the following tests: haematology and blood biochemistry, sexually transmitted disease serology, hormonal assessment of the cycle (FSH, LH, prolactin or PRL and serum hormone-binding globulin or SHBG in the early follicular phase, and oestradiol and progesterone in the midluteal phase), endometrial biopsy, determination of antisperm antibodies, hysterosalpingography (in all patients) and laparoscopy (in 838 patients, 81.21%).

The diagnosis of chronic hyperandrogenic anovulation (CHA) was established when patients showed oligomenorrhoea and/or hirsutism, ultrasonographic criteria (>10 follicles per ovary of size <10 mm and prominent stroma), progesterone levels lower than 4 ng/ml in the midluteal phase, abnormally low SHBG levels, LH/FSH ratio higher than 1.5 on cycle day 3, and/or abnormally high LH levels after the intravenous administration of 10 μg GnRH (>34 mU/ml, as assessed by a control group). In addition to these criteria, normal adrenal function assessed levels of serum dihydroepiandrosterone (SDHEA) and 17-hydroxyprogesterone after adrenocorticotrophin (ACTH) stimulation.

### Cycles

From September 1994 to October 1997, a total of 461 patients have been stimulated using

| Table 1 Main diagnosis and findings in the cycles included in the study | | |
|---|---|---|
| | **Number** | **Percentage** |
| Idiopathic | 35 | 3.39 |
| Immunological | 15 | 1.45 |
| Cervical | 35 | 3.39 |
| Chronic anovulation | 247 | 23.93 |
| Tubal damage | 180 | 17.44 |
| Endometriosis | 47 | 4.55 |
| Inadequate luteal phase | 117 | 11.34 |
| Uterine congenital anomaly | 3 | 0.29 |
| Other diagnosis (myoma) | 172 | 16.67 |
| Normal women | 181 | 17.54 |
| **Total** | **1032** | **99.99** |

HP-FSH in 1032 cycles and were included in this prospective non-randomized study (2.2 cycles per patient). The average age of the patients was $32.52 \pm 0.11$ years at the start of the cycle and their average body mass index (BMI) was $23.12 \pm 0.12$. Infertility was primary in 82.69% of the cases and secondary in the remainder (17.31%) with an average of $5.94 \pm 0.13$ years of infertility.

The primary diagnosis of the women is shown in Table 1 and the distribution of the cycles according to the total motile sperm recovered after capacitation is shown in Table 2.

From this sample, the following were identified and are described: 172 cycles stimulated in 74 patients who presented with normal reproductive function, 234 cycles stimulated in 113 patients who showed CHA and two cycles stimulated in two patients with hypogonadotrophic hypogonadism.

Intrauterine insemination was carried out using the husband's sperm in 724 cycles (70.4%)

| Table 2 Cycles classified according to the total number of motile sperm recovered after capacitation | | |
|---|---|---|
| **Motile sperm recovered (millions/ml)** | **Number** | **Percentage** |
| > 10 m | 480 | 46.5 |
| 5–10 m | 235 | 22.8 |
| 1–5 m | 282 | 27.2 |
| < 1 m | 35 | 3.4 |
| **Total** | **1032** | **99.9** |

and using frozen–thawed sperm from donors in 304 cycles (29.6%).

## Stimulation protocol

None of the patients had any treatment during the menstrual cycle previous to the stimulated cycle. After ultrasonography and oestradiol determination, ovarian stimulation started on day 3 of the cycle in those patients whose menstrual cycles usually lasted less than 35 days, and on day 5 of the cycle in those with a cycle usually lasting longer than 35 days.

Stimulation consisted of a daily subcutaneous injection of 75 IU HP-FSH (Neofertinorm, Laboratorios Serono SA, Madrid, Spain). In some cases of patients with CHA who presented a risk of hyperstimulation in a previous stimulated cycle, half an ampoule of FSH (37.5 IU) was administered daily at the start of the treatment. This dose could subsequently be increased or decreased by half an ampoule, depending on the ovarian response.

Four cycles in two hypogonadotrophic hypogonadic patients were stimulated with a combination of recombinant human FSH (rFSH) (Gonal-F, Lab. Serono, Madrid) and recombinant human LH (rLH) (Lhadi, Lab. Serono, Madrid).

The ovarian response to stimulation was controlled by measuring oestradiol serum levels using radio-immunoassay. The size of the ovaries, the number of follicles developed in each ovary and the largest diameter were all assessed by transvaginal ultrasonography. When considered necessary, the mean of 2 diameters of each follicle was evaluated. Endometrial development was also assessed.

## Ovulation induction

Ovulation was triggered by administering two subcutaneous doses of 1.5 mg leuprolide acetate (Procrin, Abbott, Madrid), 12 hours apart in 482 cycles or by the intramuscular administration of 7500–10 000 IU hCG (Profasi HP, Lab. Serono SA, Madrid) in 550 cycles. Leuprolide acetate and hCG were administered when at least one follicle with a diameter of 18 mm or more was observed, and circulating oestradiol levels reached the following values: 150 pg/ml per follicle $\geq$ 16 mm in diameter if only one follicle reached such a diameter; 120 pg/ml per follicle $\geq$ 16 mm in diameter if two follicles developed; and 100 pg/ml per follicle $\geq$ 16 mm in diameter if three follicles were present.

## Luteinized unruptured follicle evaluation

In 468 stimulated cycles of 244 patients aged 23–41 years (mean 32.8 $\pm$ 3.6), ultrasonography was carried out 24–30 hours after insemination in order to assess whether or not signs of follicular rupture were present. Infertility was primary in 68.34% of the cycles and secondary in 31.66%.

In 295 (62.93%) of these cycles, ovulation was triggered by hCG and, in the remaining 173 (37.07%), by leuprolide acetate.

Luteinized unruptured follicles were considered to occur if the dominant follicle was still present showing the same or longer diameter, and internal echoes and no liquid were seen in Douglas's cul-de-sac.

## Doppler Duplex Colour Assessment

Thirty-five stimulated cycles in 35 patients were evaluated using transvaginal colour Doppler ultrasonography (Aloka colour Doppler SSD-680, Aloka Co., Tokyo, Japan). A frequency of 5 MHz was used to derive the indices of blood flow and the high-pass filter was set at 100 MHz.

The intraovarian and uterine artery pulsatility index (PI) and resistance index (RI), as well as the maximum peak of systolic velocity (PSV) in vessels supplying the dominant follicle, were measured 20–22 hours after IUI.

## Semen preparation and IUI

For insemination, either fresh sperm obtained from the partner or frozen sperm from a semen bank was used. The cryopreserved samples were thawed at room temperature, and all the samples were capacitated by swim-up. Intrauterine insemination was carried out systematically 36 hours after the hCG injection or after the first leuprolide acetate injection. The day of ovulation induction was therefore on day 2, when considering day 0 to be the day of insemination (and ovulation).

## Cycle, ovulation, pregnancy and abortion

A cycle was defined as that in which hCG or an GnRH agonist was injected to trigger ovulation and insemination was carried out. Treatments cancelled before this occurred were not therefore considered for the study.

Ovulation was considered to have occurred whenever there was a pregnancy or when circulating progesterone levels exceeded 6 ng/ml during the luteal phase.

The existence of pregnancy was established whenever at least one embryo sac was present on the ultrasound scan obtained 14 days after a determination of a β-hCG plasma level higher than 20 mU/ml. Biochemical pregnancies were thus excluded from the pregnancy and abortion rates.

## Cancellation

Of the cycles, 123 (10.6%) were cancelled and not included in the study. The reasons for cancellation were: non-response (28 cycles); a drop in oestradiol levels that were 30% higher than the previous value before triggering ovulation (49 cycles); hyperstimulation risk (15 cycles); concomitant illness (12 cycles); and non-related treatment causes (18 cycles).

The risk of hyperstimulation was considered whenever more than four follicles with a diameter larger than 16 mm and/or oestradiol levels higher than 1500 pg/ml were observed.

## RESULTS

### Follicular development

*Total sample*
A total of 1032 consecutive HP-FSH-stimulated cycles in 461 patients were included. Data are presented as mean and standard error of mean unless signalled. Statistically significant differences were considered whenever $p$ is less than 0.05.

The main parameters of ovarian stimulation are shown in Table 3. Ovulation was triggered with hCG in 550 cycles (53.3%) and with leuprolide acetate in 482 cycles (46.7%).

*Normal ovulatory women (control group)*
From the total sample, 172 cycles corresponding to 74 patients (2.32 cycles per patient, on average) were identified as stimulated in women showing no abnormal findings. This series of cycles is considered as the control group and the results observed are compared with those observed in the CHA group.

The mean age of these patients was $32.85 \pm 0.24$ years and the BMI was $22.66 \pm 0.26$. Infertility was primary in 89% of the cycles and secondary in the remaining 11%. The duration of the infertility was $6.1 \pm 0.29$ years.

In 100 of these cycles, ovulation was triggered with hCG and in the remaining 72 leuprolide acetate was used.

Table 3 shows the main parameters that summarize the stimulation and Figures 13.2 and 13.3 show circulating levels of oestradiol and progesterone.

A monofollicular response was achieved in 32.6% of these cycles. In the remaining cycles a multifollicular response was observed, and the number of developed follicles was two to four.

*Chronic hyperandrogenic anovulation (WHO group II)*
In this group, 113 patients receiving 234 treatment cycles were evaluated. Three patients showed minimal endometriosis and 14 presented non-obstructive tubal damage as

**Table 3** Main parameters of the stimulation observed in the total number of cycles considered (*n* = 1032), in the group of normally cycling women (*n* = 172), and in the group of patients showing chronic hyperandrogenic anovulation (*n* = 234)

|  | Total sample | Normal cycle (CG) | Chronic anovulation (CHA) | *p* |
|---|---|---|---|---|
| Stimulation days | 8.79 ± 0.09 | 8.34 ± 0.18 | 10.44 ± 0.26 | 0.000 |
| FSH ampoules | 9.52 ± 0.14 | 8.66 ± 0.25 | 11.68 ± 0.36 | 0.000 |
| No. of follicles >16 mm | 2.98 ± 0.05 | 2.32 ± 0.11 | 3.04 ± 0.13 | 0.000 |
| Diameter of the largest follicle (mm) | 19.59 ± 0.05 | 19.60 ± 0.11 | 19.50 ± 0.09 | NS |
| Endometrium (mm) | 10.95 ± 0.06 | 10.75 ± 0.14 | 11.12 ± 0.12 | 0.046 |
| Motile sperm recovered (millions/ml) | 14.16 ± 0.53 | 21.45 ± 0.94 | 14.36 ± 1.08 | NS |
| Luteal phase days | 13.90 ± 0.07 | 14.14 ± 0.22 | 13.95 ± 0.15 | NS |

assessed by laparoscopy, but it was never considered as the main diagnosis.

The mean age of these patients was 32 ± 0.2 years and the BMI was 23.5 ± 0.3. Infertility was primary in 83.8% of the cycles and secondary in the remaining 16.2%; the duration of the infertility was 5.9 ± 0.3 years. There were no statistically significant differences when compared with the control group.

A summary of the ovarian stimulation characteristics is given in Table 3 and oestradiol and progesterone levels are shown in Figures 13.2 and 13.3. Ovulation was triggered with hCG in 126 cycles and with leuprolide acetate in 108 cycles.

The number of FSH ampoules required to achieve follicular maturation, as well as the number of days of stimulation and the total

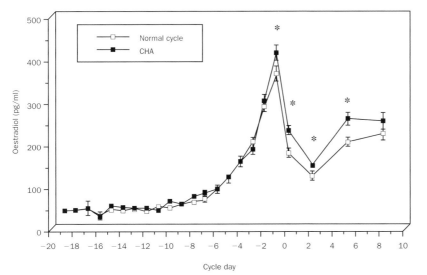

**Figure 2** Oestradiol peripheral levels in cycles stimulated to normal ovulatory patients and to patients showing chronic hyperandrogenic anovulation (CHA).
* $p < 0.05$.

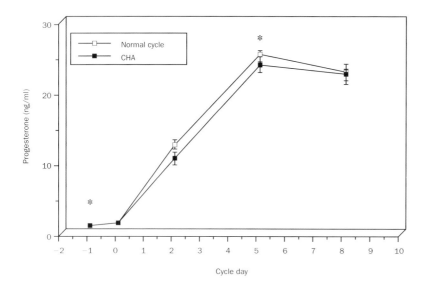

**Figure 3** Progesterone circulating levels in cycles stimulated to normal ovulatory patients and to patients showing chronic hyperandrogenic anovulation (CHA).
* $p < 0.05$.

number of mature follicles, were significantly higher in the CHA group compared with the control group.

A monofollicular response was achieved in 24.8% of these cycles. In the remaining cycles, a multifollicular response was observed, and the number of developed follicles was two to four.

Oestradiol circulating levels were significantly higher when compared with those of the control group on days −1, 0, +2 and +5 (see Figure 2). Peripheral progesterone levels were significantly higher on day −1 and significantly lower on day +5 when compared with those of the control group (see Figure 3). Oestradiol/progesterone ratios were significantly higher on cycle days −1, 0 and +5 when compared with those of the control group (Figure 4).

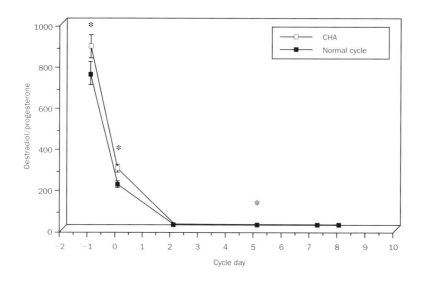

**Figure 4**
Oestradiol/progesterone ratios in cycles stimulated to normal ovulatory patients and to patients showing chronic hyperandrogenic anovulation (CHA).
* $p < 0.05$.

Twelve patients (six treated with hCG and six with leuprolide acetate) were evaluated using transvaginal colour Doppler ultrasonography as previously described. The intraovarian PI and RI were significantly lower in induced cycles with leuprolide acetate (PI: $0.67 \pm 0.1$ and $0.99 \pm 0.1$, respectively in leuprolide acetate and hCG cycles, $p = 0.02$; RI: $0.47 \pm 0$ and $0.58 \pm 0$ respectively in leuprolide acetate and hCG cycles, $p = 0.04$). When comparing Doppler parameters between cycles with ($n = 3$) and without pregnancy ($n = 9$), the maximum peak of systolic velocity in arterial vessels supplying the early corpus luteum was significantly higher in cycles in which a pregnancy was achieved ($29.7 \pm 4$ cm/s vs $15.7 \pm 2.4$ cm/s, respectively, $p = 0.04$).

*Hypogonadotrophic hypogonadism*
The diagnosis of hypogonadotrophic hypogonadism (anovulation WHO group I) was established in two patients with no abnormal findings and four treatment cycles were carried out. Obviously, it is not possible to compare them with other groups. Table 4 shows the main parameters summarizing the stimulation and Figure 5 shows the circulating levels of oestradiol and progesterone.

Ovarian stimulation and ovulation induction were successful and one pregnancy was established (one sac).

**LH and FSH-induced surge**

LH and FSH circulating levels were determined on cycle days $-2$, $-1$ and 0, before, 8 hours and 32 hours after the first injection of leuprolide acetate in 170 of the patients in whom ovulation was induced by an endogenous FSH and LH peak through the administration of leuprolide acetate (Figure 6).

**Ovulation, pregnancy and abortion rates**

Ovulation rates were 98.3% in the total sample, 100% in the control group, 97% in the CHA group, and 100% in four cycles corresponding to the women with hypogonadotrophic hypo-

**Table 4** Main parameters of the stimulation observed in the total number of cycles considered ($n = 1032$), in the group of normally cycling women ($n = 172$), and in the group with hypogonadotrophic hypogonadism ($n = 4$)

|  | Total sample | Normal cycle | hypogonadotrophic hypogonadism |
|---|---|---|---|
| Stimulation days | $8.79 \pm 0.09$ | $8.34 \pm 0.18$ | $11.75 \pm 1.44$ |
| FSH ampoules | $9.52 \pm 0.14$ | $8.66 \pm 0.25$ | $20.63 \pm 3.14*$ |
| rLH ampoules | 0 | 0 | 11.00 |
| No. of follicles >16 mm | $2.98 \pm 0.05$ | $2.32 \pm 0.11$ | $4.25 \pm 0.85$ |
| Diameter of the largest follicle (mm) | $19.59 \pm 0.05$ | $19.60 \pm 0.11$ | $19.50 \pm 0.65$ |
| Endometrium (mm) | $10.95 \pm 0.06$ | $10.75 \pm 0.14$ | $10.75 \pm 0.25$ |
| Motile sperm recovered (millions/ml) | $14.16 \pm 0.53$ | $21.45 \pm 0.94$ | $55.52 \pm 10.96$ |
| Luteal phase days | $21.65 \pm 0.80$ | $14.14 \pm 0.22$ | $11.33 \pm 2.31$ |

* In this group rFSH and rLH were used.

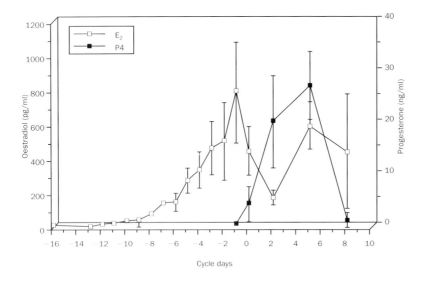

**Figure 5** Oestradiol ($E_2$) and progesterone (p) circulating levels observed in cycles stimulated to hypogonadotrophic hypogonadic patients ($n=4$).

gonadism. No statistically significant differences were observed between the groups.

The pregnancy rate in the total sample ($n = 1032$) was 20.8% ($n = 215$). The abortion rate of these pregnancies was 22.7% ($n = 49$). The cumulative pregnancy rate after four treatment cycles was 61%. As shown in Table 5, in our experience use of more than four IUI cycles did not significantly increase the cumulative pregnancy rate.

Pregnancy rates were 17.4% per cycle and 40.5% per patient in the control group ($n = 30$). In those cycles in which hCG was used to induce ovulation, the pregnancy rate was 11.1% ($n = 11$), whereas in cycles in which leuprolide acetate was administered to trigger ovulation, the pregnancy rate was 26.8% ($n = 19$). The difference reached statistical significance. No cases of multiple pregnancy were observed in this group and seven pregnancies (23.3%) ended in abortion before gestation week 12.

Pregnancy rates were 17.5% per cycle and

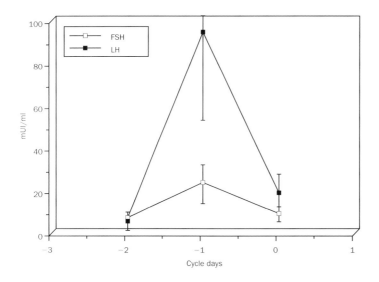

**Figure 6** FSH and LH preovulatory peripheral levels in cycles in which ovulation was triggered with leuprolide acetate.

| Table 5 Cumulative pregnancy rate | | | |
|---|---|---|---|
| Attempt | No. of cycles | No. of pregnancies | Cumulative pregnancy rate (%) |
| 1 | 263 | 70 | 27 |
| 2 | 218 | 51 | 44 |
| 3 | 156 | 26 | 53 |
| 4 | 113 | 20 | 61 |
| 5 | 67 | 7 | 65 |
| 6 | 32 | 1 | 66 |

36.3% per patient in the CHA group ($n = 41$). Eighteen pregnancies were achieved after ovulation induction with hCG (14.5% per cycle) and 23 pregnancies (21.3% per cycle) were obtained in patients treated with leuprolide acetate. The difference did not reach statistical significance. Three of 41 pregnancies (7.3%) showed two sacs. Eight pregnancies (19.5%) ended in abortion before gestation week 12.

One pregnancy was obtained from the treatment of the hypogonadic hypogonadotrophic patients.

## Luteal phase

To determine whether or not both the method of triggering ovulation and the different luteal support could play a role in the final outcome, 810 of the cycles were analysed in terms of pregnancy rates and hormonal profiles during the luteal phase. The distribution of these 810 cycles according to treatments used was as follows: in 339 cycles ovulation was triggered with leuprolide acetate and hCG was given as luteal support; in 48 cycles leuprolide acetate was used and progesterone was given as luteal support; in 312 cycles ovulation was triggered with hCG and hCG was also given as luteal support; and in 111 cycles ovulation was triggered with hCG and progesterone was given as luteal support.

When ovulation was triggered by leuprolide acetate, 2500 IU hCG was administered on cycle days 0, +2 and +5 or 200 mg vaginal progesterone was given daily from cycle day 0. When ovulation was triggered with hCG, 2500 IU hCG was injected on cycle days +2 and +5 or 200 mg vaginal progesterone was given daily from cycle day 0.

The pregnancy rate observed in each one of these series of treatment cycles, which depend on the ovulation induction and the luteal support, is shown in Table 6. A significantly higher pregnancy rate ($p = 0.0005$) was observed when ovulation was triggered with leuprolide acetate (27.65%) if compared with those cycles in which ovulation was triggered with hCG (17.49%). Slightly higher pregnancy rates were observed when hCG was used as luteal support but the differences did not reach statistical significance.

## Ectopic pregnancies

It has been reported that assisted reproduction procedures increase the incidence of ectopic pregnancies when compared with spontaneous pregnancies.[23,24] The outcome of 215 pregnancies obtained after IUI, using the stimulation protocol previously described, was reviewed in a retrospective study, and only two cases of ectopic pregnancy occurred; this supposes a rate of 0.9%, which is very similar to that

**Table 6 Pregnancy rate per cycle observed in each one of the groups according to the ovulation induction and the luteal phase support**

|  | Leuprolide acetate ($n = 387$) | hCG ($n = 423$) |
|---|---|---|
| Progesterone | 22.92 | 16.22 |
|  | ($n = 48$) | ($n = 111$) |
| hCG | 26.32 | 17.95 |
|  | ($n = 339$) | ($n = 312$) |

reported in spontaneous pregnancies. One of these patients had had a previous ectopic pregnancy in a spontaneous pregnancy, and the other was included in our IUI programme because of a male factor infertility with no evidence of tubal damage.

Neither the characteristics of ovarian stimulation nor the hormonal levels during the luteal phase showed statistical differences when compared with cycles achieved in viable pregnancies.

**Luteinized unruptured follicle**

Ninety-three pregnancies (19.71%) were obtained in the 498 cycles in which the occurrence of LUFs was assessed.

Luteinized unruptured follicles were considered to occur in 39 (8.33%) of these cycles (group I) and ovulation in 459 (91.67%) (group II). In 10% of the cases in which LUFs were diagnosed (four cycles), a pregnancy became evident later in the same cycle.

Ovulation was triggered with leuprolide acetate in 45.71% of the cycles in group I and in 36.36% of the cycles in group II; hCG was used in 54.29% of the cycles in group I and in 63.64% in group II. These differences did not reach statistical significance.

Five of the patients showed LUFs in two consecutive cycles. Three patients showed hyperandrogenic chronic anovulation, one patient

non-obstructive tubal damage and one endometriosis. Table 7 summarizes the main diagnosis in cycles assessing LUFs.

The incidence of endometriosis was significantly higher ($p = 0.004$) in group I than in group II. No other statistically significant differences were observed between groups in terms of both clinical aspects and stimulation parameters.

Peripheral levels of oestradiol were slightly lower in group I on cycle days +5 and +8 (Figure 7) and peripheral progesterone levels were significantly lower in group I when com-

**Table 7 Main diagnosis in patients in which LUF was assessed when stimulated in 498 cycles**

| Diagnosis | $n$ | % |
|---|---|---|
| Normal women | 69 | 28.15 |
| Anovulation | 57 | 23.53 |
| Tubal damage | 48 | 19.75 |
| ILP | 44 | 18.07 |
| Endometriosis | 18 | 7.14 |
| Cervical | 8 | 3.36 |
| **Total** | **244** | **100** |

ILP: inadequate luteal phase.

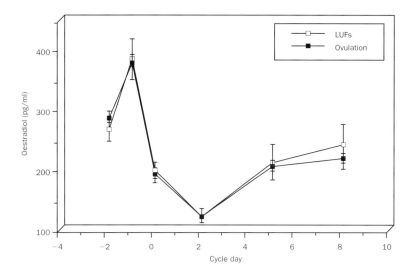

**Figure 7** Oestradiol circulating levels in ovulatory and LUF cycles.

pared with group II during the luteal phase (Figure 8).

## Comments

Infertility diagnosis and therapy in developed countries probably need to be more efficacious than in previous decades because the age of first pregnancy is higher than it was and, as a consequence, the age of patients consulting an infertility clinic is also higher.

On the other hand, even though infertile couples could benefit from consulting highly specialized clinics, gynaecologists not specifically trained in assisted reproduction techniques should know how to induce ovulation with gonadotrophins in a safe way and how to obtain good enough results to justify such practice.

It is generally admitted that IUI after ovarian stimulation and ovulation induction with gonadotrophins improves the results if compared with those observed after timed intercourse, as well as those after ovulation induction

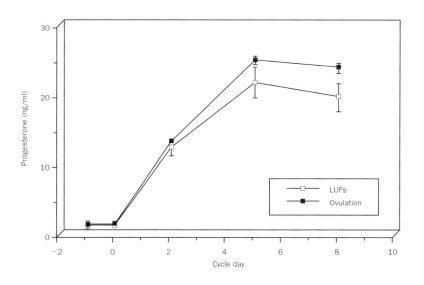

**Figure 8** Progesterone circulating levels in ovulatory and LUF cycles.

with clomiphene citrate.[25] Nevertheless, most of the authors point out that there is a non-negligible risk of ovarian hyperstimulation and there is concern about the risk of multiple pregnancies.[25,26]

The way of stimulating the ovary in order to induce ovulation plays an important role in determining the final outcome after insemination[24] in terms of pregnancy rate and incidence of both hyperstimulation and multiple pregnancy. Desirable stimulation can be reached by administering either FSH or hMG because LH does not seem to be necessary during stimulation[27,28] except in patients showing LH deficiency.[29]

To prevent hyperstimulation and multiple pregnancies, it was decided to stimulate with low subcutaneous doses of HP-FSH,[30,31] because 75 IU FSH has been proved to reach the threshold[32] that allows the development of a dominant follicle without inducing the growth of multiple follicles, that is, it was intended to mimic the natural cycle.

The results in terms of follicular development and oestradiol circulating levels agree with those in the literature.[33] The higher effectivity of low-dose FSH stimulation in preventing multifollicular development, compared with conventional protocols, has been proved.[34,35]

Particular comments are required concerning CHA. It is important to consider that: (1) deficient FSH activity could play an important role in the pathophysiology;[36] (2) FSH could prevent increased apoptosis in the follicles of hyperandrogenic ovaries;[11] (3) granulosa cells lack LH receptors at the start of the cycle;[37] and (4) LH action could only increase undesirable androgen production. From these considerations, it seems clear that FSH is the elective gonadotrophin for stimulation of follicular growth in patients showing CHA, as postulated by Birkhauser et al.[38]

The use of GnRH agonists was postulated to trigger ovulation in stimulated cycles for IUI.[39] Some authors postulated that its use could prevent hyperstimulation[40] and improve the results.[41] It was considered that a possible action of the induced FSH surge could play a role in improving the pregnancy rate.[15] Nevertheless, this FSH effect has been discussed from the findings in stimulated cycles for in vitro fertilization (IVF).[42]

Previous studies[43] have postulated that subtle changes in the endocrine environment when GnRH agonists were used to trigger ovulation could justify the improvement in the pregnancy rate. In this series changes in the vascularization of the corpus luteum have provided evidence of what could be improvements in luteal function and may justify the results in terms of higher pregnancy rates.

On the other hand, the very conservative use of FSH could justify the lack of cases of both ovarian hyperstimulation and multiple pregnancies. In fact other authors using GnRH agonists with higher doses of gonadotrophins observed higher rates of multiple pregnancies.[44]

It is interesting that a similar improvement in pregnancy rate was observed by Fuh et al;[45] in a series of cycles, in which hCG was given after the endogenous peak of LH occurred, the pregnancy rate was higher than in those cycles in which hCG was administered before the spontaneous LH peak.

Luteinized unruptured follicles have been considered as one of the factors that determine the lack of pregnancies in stimulated cycles when compared with the ovulation rate.[46] It is difficult to determine whether LUFs are present using either ultrasonography[47] or laparoscopy.[48] Nevertheless, it could be interesting to diagnose LUFs after ovulation induction in order to indicate IVF if considered necessary.

In the present series, LUFs were diagnosed in 8.3% of the cases with four cases being falsely positive. This is consistent with the rate encountered in other studies. Also, as postulated by Hamilton et al[20] and Donnez et al,[49] LUFs were more frequent in patients with endometriosis or previous pelvic inflammatory disease.

Endocrine changes were present in cycles with LUFs. As proved by Hamilton et al,[20] progesterone circulating levels were significantly lower in LUF cycles when compared with cycles with ovulation in the present series. Pregnancy rates obtained in this series of cycles was 20.8%, ranging between 11.1% and 26.8%, depending on the type of infertility, which is consistent with the results of other studies in the literature.[50,51] The lower pregnancy rate observed in normal women is most probably a result of the fact that a male infertility factor is present in all of these cases.

Significantly higher pregnancy rates were observed in cycles in which ovulation was triggered with leuprolide acetate. The differences in biological action between LH and hCG,[52] subtle endocrine changes and, as observed, improved vascularization of the corpus luteum may justify this finding.

There has been discussion[53] about whether there is any benefit in giving hCG or progesterone as luteal support. As all the cycles presented here underwent such treatments, it is not possible to obtain any conclusion on this particular aspect. Different studies in the literature, in which ovulation was triggered with leuprolide acetate and luteal support was not used, showed lower pregnancy rates.[40] In this study, in which hCG or progesterone was used as luteal support, a 27.65% pregnancy rate was achieved. As a consequence, we consider that when ovulation is triggered with leuprolide acetate luteal support is needed. A statistically significant difference in terms of pregnancy or abortion rates between the use of hCG and the use of progesterone was not observed.

No cases of the ovarian hyperstimulation syndrome were observed in this series which could be the result of a very conservative use of FSH, as similarly reported by other authors.[40] Abortion and ectopic pregnancy rates were consistent with the rates generally observed after ovulation induction and IUI.[50]

The rate of twins was low, as was expected from the low number of developed follicles already observed.[54] No multiple pregnancies with three or more sacs were obtained.

## CONCLUSION

We consider that stimulating ovarian follicular development with low doses of subcutaneous HP-FSH represents a safe way for triggering ovulation and performing IUI in normal ovulatory women as well as in cases of chronic anovulation. Such management of infertility does not require intensive monitoring and when indicated gives results that are good enough to encourage its practice. Even though more experience is needed, the combination of rFSH and rLH could offer similar results in cases of hypogonadotrophic hypogonadism.

There is probably a need to promote randomized studies and larger series to obtain definitive conclusions. From the present results, it seems reasonable to postulate that stimulating the ovary with low doses of FSH and triggering ovulation by inducing an endogenous peak of gonadotrophins with an GnRH agonist could improve the results if luteal support is used.

## REFERENCES

1. Nahum R, Beyth Y, Chun S-Y, Hsueh A, Tsafriri A. Early onset of deoxyribonucleic acid fragmentation during atresia of preovulatory ovarian follicles in rats. *Biol Reprod* 1996;**55**:1075–80.
2. Billig H, Chun S-Y, Eisenhauer K, Hsueh A. Gonadal cell apoptosis: hormone-regulated cell demise. *Hum Reprod Update* 1996;**2**:103–17.
3. Chun S-S, Eisenhauer K, Minami S, Billig H, Perlas E, Hsueh A. Hormonal regulation of apoptosis in early antral follicles: follicle-stimulating hormone as a major survival factor. *Endocrinology* 1996;**137**:1447–56.
4. Baird D. The ovarian cycle. In: *Ovarian Endocrinology* (Hillier S, ed.). London: Blackwell Science, 1991: 1–24.
5. Li R, Phillips D, Moore A, Mather J. Follicle-stimulating hormone induces terminal differentiation in a predifferentiated rat granulosa cell line (ROG). *Endocrinology* 1997;**138**:2648–57.
6. McGee E, Spears N, Minami S, et al. Preantral

ovarian follicles in serum-free culture: suppression of apoptosis after activation of the cyclic guanosine 3'5'-monophosphate pathway and stimulation of growth and differentiation by follicle-stimulating hormone. *Endocrinology* 1997;**138**:2417–24.

7. Hurwitz A, Ruutiainen-Altman K, Marzella L, Boero L, Dushnik MEY. Follicular atresia as an apoptotic process: atresia-associated increase in the ovarian expression of the putative apoptotic marker sulfated glycoprotein-2. *J Soc Gynecol Invest* 1996;**3**:199–208.

8. Jolly P, Tisdall D, Delath G, et al. Granulosa cell apoptosis, aromatase activity, cyclic adenosine 3',5'-monophosphate response to gonadotropins, and follicular fluid steroid levels during spontaneous and induced follicular atresia in ewes. *Biol Reprod* 1997;**56**:830–6.

9. Janz D, Van der Kraak G. Suppression of apoptosis by gonadotropin, 17β-estradiol, and epidermal growth factor in rainbow trout preovulatory ovarian follicles. *Gen Comp Endocrinol* 1997; **105**:186–93.

10. Hillier S. Sex steroid metabolism and follicular development in the ovary. *Oxf Rev Reprod Biol* 1985;**7**:168–222.

11. Almahbobi G, Anderiesz C, Hutchinson P, McFarlane J, Wood C, Trounson A. Functional integrity of granulosa cells from polycystic ovaries. *Clin Endocrinol* 1996;**44**:571–80.

12. Andreani C, Pierro E, Lazzarin N, Lanzone A, Caruso A, Mancuso S. Effect of follicular fluid on granulosa luteal cells from polycystic ovary. *Hum Reprod* 1996;**11**:2107–13.

13. Goodman A, Hodgen G. The ovarian triad of the primate menstrual cycle. *Rec Prog Horm Res* 1983;**9**:1–67.

14. Baird D. A model for follicular selection and ovulation: lessons from superovulation. *J Steroid Biochem* 1987;**27**:15–23.

15. Eppig J. FSH stimulates hyaluronic acid synthesis by oocytes – cumulus complexes from mouse preovulatory follicle. *Nature* 1979;**281**:483–6.

16. Stickland S, Beers W. Studies on the role of plasminogen activator in ovulation. In vitro response of granulosa cells to gonadotropins, cyclic nucleotides and prostaglandins. *J Biol Chem* 1976;**251**:5694–9.

17. Dharmarajan A, Goodman S, Tilly K, Tilly J. Apoptosis during functional corpus luteum regression: evidence of a role for chorionic gonadotropin in promoting luteal cell survival. *Endocrine J* 1994;**2**:295–303.

18. Shikone T, Yamoto M, Kokawa K, Yamashita K, Nishimori K, Nakano R. Apoptosis of human corpora lutea during cyclic luteal regression and early pregnancy. *J Clin Endocrinol Metab* 1996; **81**:2376–80.

19. Rodger F, Fraser H, Duncan W, Illingworth P. Immunolocalization of blc-2 in the human corpus luteum. *Hum Reprod* 1995;**10**:1566–70.

20. Hamilton C, Wetzels L, Eversd JLH, et al. Follicle growth curves and hormonal patterns in patients with the luteinized unruptured follicle syndrome. *Fertil Steril* 1985;**43**:541–8.

21. McDonough P. Progesterone therapy: benefit versus risk. *Fertil Steril* 1985;**44**:13–16.

22. Blumenfeld Z, Nahhas F. Luteal dysfunction in ovulation induction: the role of repetitive human chorionic gonadotropin supplementation during the luteal phase. *Fertil Steril* 1988;**50**:403–7.

23. Nachtigall R. Indications, techniques, and success rates for AIH. *Semin Reprod Med* 1987;**46**:13–15.

24. Lansac J, Thepot F, Mavaux M, et al. Pregnancy outcome after artificial insemination of IVF with frozen semen donor: a collaborative study of the French CECOS Federation on 21597 pregnancies. *Eur J Obstet Gynecol Reprod Biol* 1997;**74**:223–8.

25. Hughes E. The effectiveness of ovulation induction and intrauterine insemination in the treatment of persistent infertility: a meta-analysis. *Hum Reprod* 1997;**12**:1865–72.

26. Hurst B, Tiaden B, Kimball A, Schlaff W, Damewood M, Rock J. Superovulation with or without intrauterine insemination for the treatment of infertility. *J Reprod Med Obstet Gynecol* 1992;**37**:237–41.

27. Schenken R, William S, Hodgen G. Ovulation induction using 'pure' follicle stimulating hormone in monkeys. *Fertil Steril* 1984;**41**:629–34.

28. Gil F, Rodriguez-Ineba A, Micó J, Edo A, Galbis M, Romeu A. Inducción de la ovulación con FSH purificada en pacientes estériles afectas de anovulación crónica. *Revista Iberoamericana de Fertilidad* 1989;**6**:39–47.

29. Balasch J. Inducción de la ovulación: bases racionales para un esquema simplificado. *Actualidad Reproducción Humana* 1995;**5**:2–15.

30. Graf M, Freundl G. Klinische und endokrinologische Aspekte der Therapie mit reinum FSH. Ein Erfahrungsbericht. *Zentralbl Gynakol* 1990;**112**:81–90.

31. Remorgida V, Venturini P, Anserini P, Salerno E, De Cecco L. Use of combined exogenous gonadotropins and pulsatile gonadotropin-

releasing hormone in patients with polycystic ovarian disease. *Fertil Steril* 1991;**55**:61–5.

32. Brown J. Pituitary control of ovarian function – concepts derived from gonadotrophin therapy. *Aust N Z J Obstet Gynaecol* 1978;**18**:47–54.

33. Hamilton-Fairley D, Kiddy D, Watson H, Sagle M, Franks S. Low-dose gonadotrophin therapy for induction of ovulation in 100 women with polycystic ovary syndrome. *Hum Reprod* 1991;**6**:1095–9.

34. Homburg R, Levy T, Ben-Rafael Z. A comparative prospective study of conventional regimen with chronic low-dose administration of follicle-stimulating hormone for anovulation associated with polycystic ovary syndrome. *Fertil Steril* 1995;**63**:729–33.

35. Van der Meer M, Hompes P, Scheele F, Schoute E, Popp-Snijders C, Schomaker J. The importance of endogenous feedback for monofollicular growth in low-dose step-up ovulation induction with follicle-stimulating hormone in polycystic ovary syndrome: a randomized study. *Fertil Steril* 1996;**66**:571–6.

36. Hillier S. Follicular function in polycystic ovaries. In: *Chronic Hyperandrogenic Anovulation* (Coeling Bennink H, Vemer H, Van Keep P, eds). Carnforth: Parthenon, 1989: 27–35.

37. Hsueh A, Bicsak T, Jia X, Dahl K, Fauser B, Galway A. Granulosa cells as hormone targets: the role of biologically-active follicle-stimulating hormone in reproduction. *Rec Prog Horm Res* 1989;**45**:209–77.

38. Birkhauser M, Huber P, Neuenschwander E, Napflin S. Induktion der Follikelreifung mit 'reimen' FSH beim Polyzystischen Ovar-Syndrom. *Geburtshilfe Frauenheilkd* 1988;**48**:220–7.

39. Tulchinsky D, Nash H, Brown K, Paoletti-Falcone V, Poicaro J. A pilot study of the use of gonadotropin releasing hormone analog for triggering ovulation. *Fertil Steril* 1991;**55**:644–6.

40. Balasch J, Tur R, Creus M, et al. Triggering of ovulation by a gonadotropin releasing hormone agonist in gonadotropin-stimulated cycles for prevention of ovarian hyperstimulation syndrome and multiple pregnancy. *Gynecol Endocrinol* 1994;**8**:7–12.

41. Romeu A, Monzó A, Peiró T, Díez E, Peinado J, Quintero L. Endogenous LH surge versus hCG as ovulation trigger after low-dose highly purified FSH in IUI: a comparison of 761 cycles. *J Assisted Reprod Genet* 1997;**14**:439–45.

42. Vermeiden J, Roseboom T, Goverde A, et al. An artificially induced follicle stimulating hormone surge at the time of human chorionic gonadotrophin administration in controlled ovarian stimulation cycles has no effect on cumulus expansion, fertilization rate, embryo quality and implantation rate. *Hum Reprod* 1997;**12**:1399–402.

43. Romeu A, Molina I, Tresguerres J, Plá M, Peinado J. Effect of recombinant human luteinizing hormone versus human chorionic gonadotropin: effects on ovulation, embryo quality and transport, steroid balance and implantation in rabbits. *Hum Reprod* 1995;**10**:1290–6.

44. Balen A, Braat D, West C, Patel A, Jacobs H. Cumulative conception and live birth rates after the treatment of anovulatory infertility: safety and efficacy of ovulation induction in 200 patients. *Hum Reprod* 1994;**9**:1563–70.

45. Fuh K, Wang X, Tai A, Wong I, Norman R. Intrauterine insemination: effect of the temporal relationship between the luteinizing hormone surge, human chorionic gonadotrophin administration and insemination on pregnancy rates. *Hum Reprod* 1997;**12**:2162–6.

46. Townsend S, Brown J, Johnstone J. Induction of ovulation. *J Obstet Gynecol* 1966;**73**:529–34.

47. Check J, Adelson H, Dietterich C, Stern J. Pelvic sonography can predict ovum release in gonadotropin-treated patients as determined by pregnancy rate. *Hum Reprod* 1990;**5**:234–6.

48. Portuondo J, Pena J, Otaola C, Echanojauregui A. Absence of ovulation stigma in the conception cycle. *Int J Infertil* 1983;**28**:53–4.

49. Donnez J, Langercock S, Thomas K. Peritoneal fluid volume, 17 beta-oestradiol and progesterone concentrations in women with endometriosis and/or luteinized unruptured follicle syndrome. *Gynecol Obstet Invest* 1983;**16**:210–12.

50. Dodson W, Haney A. Controlled ovarian hyperstimulation and intrauterine insemination for treatment of infertility. *Fertil Steril* 1991;**55**:457–67.

51. Kemman E, Bohrer M, Shelden R, Fiasconaro G, Beardsley L. Active ovulation management increases the monthly probability of pregnancy occurrence in ovulatory women who receive intrauterine insemination. *Fertil Steril* 1987;**48**:916–20.

52. Conbarnous Y. *Comparative Approach of Structure Function Relationships of Gonadotropins*. Serono Symposia, vol 65. New York: Raven Press, 1989: 82–93.

53. Reshef E, Segars J, Hill GA, et al. Endometrial inadequacy after treatment with human

menopausal gonadotropin/human chorionic gonadotropin. *Fertil Steril* 1990;**54:**1012–16.

54. Dodson W, Hughes CJ, Haney A. Multiple pregnancies conceived with intrauterine insemination during superovulation: an evaluation of clinical characteristics and monitored parameters of conception cycles. *Am J Obstet Gynecol* 1988;**159:**382–5.

# Part V

# GnRH Agonists and Antagonists

# 14

# GnRH and its agonistic analogues: basic knowledge

Ariel Weissman, Zeev Shoham

**GnRH receptors and signal transduction** • **Pulsatile GnRH secretion** • **Agonistic and antagonist analogues of GnRH: mechanism of action** • **GnRH: metabolic pathways** • **Biosynthesis of GnRH analogues** • **Bioactivity and relative potency of GnRH agonistic analogues** • **Routes of administration** • **GnRH agonistic analogues: clinical applications**

Gonadotrophin-releasing hormone (GnRH) is the primary hypothalamic regulator of reproductive function. It was first isolated, characterized and synthesized independently in 1971 by Andrew Schally and Roger Guillemin, who were subsequently awarded the Nobel prize for their achievement. GnRH is a decapeptide which, like several other brain peptides, is synthesized as part of a much larger precursor peptide, the GnRH-associated peptide (GAP), which is made up of a sequence of 56 amino acids. The structure of GnRH is common to all mammals, including humans, and its action is similar in both the male and the female. GnRH is produced and released from a group of loosely connected neurons located in the medial basal hypothalamus, primarily within the arcuate nucleus, and in the preoptic area of the ventral hypothalamus. It is released by axonal transport and in a pulsatile fashion into the complex capillary net of the portal system, and binds to specific receptors in the plasma membrane of the anterior pituitary gonadotrophs, where it stimulates synthesis, storage and release of luteinizing hormone (LH) and follicle-stimulating hormone (FSH).

## GnRH RECEPTORS AND SIGNAL TRANSDUCTION

Binding of GnRH to its receptor in the phospholipid bilayer of the gonadotroph initiates an explosive cascade of intracellular events and responses. The GnRH receptor complementary DNA (cDNA) has recently been cloned:[1–3] and found to consist of 327 amino acids with a special configuration of seven transmembrane channel-like regions which traverse the plasma membrane back and forth. Each one of the seven transmembrane domains acts as a cell-surface receptor, which binds GnRH with high affinity. The signal transduction pathway includes coupling of the GnRH receptor to guanosine triphosphate (GTP)-regulating protein, or G-protein, and conversion of GTP to guanosine diphosphate (GDP). This step provides the energy for activation of several intracellular second messenger systems, consisting mainly of cytoplasmic calcium ions that interact with protein kinase C (PKC), as well as inositol triphosphate, diacylglycerol, arachidonic acid and its metabolites, and the leukotrienes.[4–6] The increased intracellular calcium concentration and activation of the PKC system lead to the release of gonadotrophins from the gonadotroph by exocytosis. Different mechanisms, which have not been fully elucidated, govern the GnRH-induced biosynthesis of gonadotrophins. GnRH regulates gene transcription through distinct GnRH-responsive DNA sequences. It has been demonstrated, for example, that normal production of the LH β subunit requires stimulation by GnRH, and that this process is mediated by the PKC system, calcium ions and calmodulin.[7]

## PULSATILE GnRH SECRETION

The maintenance of gonadotrophin secretion requires exposure of the pituitary to a pulsatile pattern of GnRH secretion, as was demonstrated in the classic series of experiments by Knobil and Hotchkiss.[8] GnRH pulses occur in association with electrical activities within the arcuate nucleus, an area of functionally interconnected GnRH neurons also known as the 'GnRH pulse generator'. As GnRH is released directly into the portal circulation, its short half-life, in the range of several minutes, does not allow for measurement and correlation between serum GnRH levels and its release pattern. Therefore, it was assumed, and subsequently validated in animal studies,[9] that the pulsatile fashion of LH secretion represents pulses of GnRH. The critical range of pulsatile release frequencies varies with the species and the physiological circumstances. In the human, it ranges from the shortest interpulse frequency of about 71 min in the late follicular phase to an interval of 216 min in the late luteal phase.[10–13] The quality of pulsatile gonadotrophin stimulation is of major importance to achieve ovulation. Even mild abnormalities in the frequency and/or amplitude of GnRH-induced LH pulses may interfere with regular ovulatory function.[14,15] Paradoxically, continuous or inappropriate high-frequency (>3 pulses/h) administration of GnRH or its agonistic analogues leads to desensitization of the pituitary gonadotroph, resulting in suppression of gonadotrophin release and subsequent blockade of ovarian or testicular function.[15] Thus, the gonadotroph is capable of adjusting its sensitivity to the degree of GnRH stimulus in a rapid and prominent way, which may be regarded as an endogenous safety mechanism, preventing hyperstimulation of the pituitary–gonadal axis.

## AGONISTIC AND ANTAGONIST ANALOGUES OF GnRH: MECHANISM OF ACTION

Although the exact cellular basis for desensitization of the gonadotroph has not been fully delineated, the extensive use of agonistic analogues of GnRH in research allowed for an explosive increase in information and knowledge. Upon acute administration, all GnRH agonistic analogues increase gonadotrophin secretion (the flare-up effect) and usually require 7–14 days to achieve a state of pituitary suppression. Prolonged administration of a GnRH agonist leads to down-regulation of GnRH receptors. The agonist-bound receptor is internalized via receptor-mediated endocytosis,[16] with kinetics determined by the potency of the analogue. The internalized complex subsequently undergoes dissociation, followed by degradation of the ligand and partial recycling of the receptors.[17] Thus, the number of GnRH receptors decreases. As receptors return to normal and then to supranormal levels, desensitization is maintained as a result of postreceptor mechanisms, including loss and impairment of functional GnRH receptor-linked calcium ion channels, as well as loss of the ability to transfer gonadotrophins from a non-releasable to a releasable pool[18] (Figure 1).

Antagonist analogues of GnRH have a direct inhibitory effect on gonadotrophin secretion. Antagonist molecules compete for and occupy pituitary GnRH receptors thus competitively blocking the access of endogenous GnRH, and precluding substantial receptor occupation and stimulation. Suppression attained by GnRH antagonists is immediate (no flare-up effect) and, as receptor loss does not occur, it requires a constant supply of antagonist to the gonadotroph so that all GnRH receptors are continuously occupied. Consequently, compared with agonistic analogues, a higher dose range of

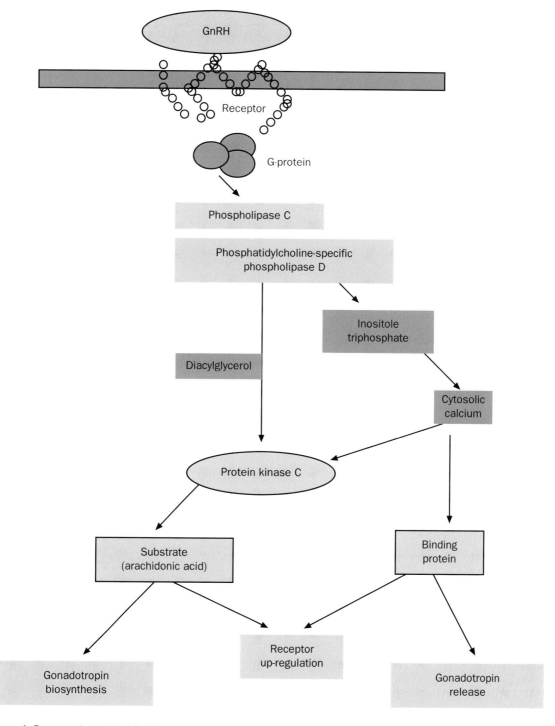

**Figure 1** Proposed model of GnRH receptor activation. Binding of GnRH to its receptor activates the G-protein. Thereafter phospholipase C and phosphatidylcholine-specific phospholipase D are activated. This causes the production of diacylglycerol and inositol triphosphate which mobilize calcium. Protein kinase is then being activated leading to gonadotrophin biosynthesis and release.

antagonists is required for effective pituitary suppression (micrograms versus milligrams, respectively).

## GnRH: METABOLIC PATHWAYS

Being a small peptide molecule that does not bind to circulating plasma proteins, GnRH is rapidly degraded by endopeptidases and cleared by glomerular filtration.[19,20] Its half-life in the peripheral circulation is only 2–8 min.[21,22] Although the biological activity of GnRH seems to be related to the amino acids at both ends of the molecule, its structural stability appears to depend mainly on the amino acid at the sixth position. Degradation of GnRH at the $Tyr^5$–$Gly^6$ position by a neutral endopeptidase splits the molecule into two biologically inactive residues. Additional degradation occurs by pyroglutamate aminopeptidase at the $Pyr$–$Glu^1$ position or cleavage at the carboxyl side of $Pro^9$ by a postproline-cleaving enzyme.[23,24]

## BIOSYNTHESIS OF GnRH ANALOGUES

The elucidation of the structure, function and metabolic pathways of native GnRH has prompted an intense effort by research laboratories and the pharmaceutical industry to synthesize potent and longer-acting agonist and antagonist analogues.[25] Over the past three decades, thousands of analogues of GnRH, both agonists and antagonists, have been synthesized. Only six of the agonistic analogues have become approved and clinically used drugs. The first generation of antagonist analogues had marked systemic side effects mediated by histamine release which slowed their further clinical development. At present, several third-generation antagonists with fewer side effects are at advanced stages of clinical trials and are expected to be approved for use in the near future.

The first major step in increasing the potency of GnRH was made with substitutions of glycine number 10 at the C-terminus. Although 90% of the biological activity is lost with splitting of glycine number 10, most of it is restored with the attachment of $NH_2$-ethylamide to the $Pro^9$.[26] The second major modification was the replacement of the glycine residue at position 6 by D-amino acids, which decreases enzymatic degradation. The combination of these two modifications was found to have synergistic biological activity, and agonistic analogues with D-amino acids at position 6 and $NH_2$-ethylamide substituting the $Gly^{10}$ amide not only are better protected against enzymatic degradation, but also have a higher receptor-binding affinity. The affinity can be increased further by introduction of larger, hydrophobic and more lipophilic D-amino acids at amino acid position number 6. The increased lipophilicity of the agonist is associated with a prolonged half-life, which may be attributed to reduced renal excretion through increased plasma protein binding, or fat tissue storage of non-ionized fat-soluble compounds.[26] Thus, all the clinically available GnRH agonists contain a D-amino acid at position 6 (Table 1). The agonists leuprolide [D-$Leu^6$, $Pro^9$-NEt] an buserelin [D-$Ser(O^tBu)^6$,$Pro^9$-NEt] contain an ethylamide, and goserelin [D-$Ser(O^tBu)^6$,$Pro^9$-AzaGly-$NH_2$] and histrelin [$N^t$-Bzl-D-$His^6$,$Pro^9$-AzaGly-$NH_2$] contain azaglycine at position 10 and are therefore nonapeptides. Nafarelin [D-$Nal(2)^6$] and triptorelin [D-$Trp^6$] contain the original $Gly^{10}$ amide, and are therefore decapeptides.

## BIOACTIVITY AND RELATIVE POTENCY OF GnRH AGONISTIC ANALOGUES

Various biological assays and animal models have been employed for testing the activity and potency of GnRH agonist preparations.[22,26] Commonly used in vitro assays have been measurement of LH and FSH secretion by dispersed pituitary cells, and receptor binding assay using purified pituitary membrane fractions. In vivo bioassays that were widely employed included oestrus suppression in normally cycling rats, induction of ovulation, stimulation of uterine growth, inhibition of pregnancy and stimulation of LH release in ovariectomized rats, and

**Table 1 The structure of GnRH and GnRH agonistic analogues**

| Compound | | | | | | Position 6 | | | | Position 10 |
|---|---|---|---|---|---|---|---|---|---|---|
| Amino acid (no.) | 1 | 2 | 3 | 4 | 5 | 6 | 7 | 8 | 9 | 10 |
| Native GnRH | Glu | His | Trp | Ser | Tyr | Gly | Leu | Arg | Pro | Gly-NH$_2$ |
| **Nonapeptides** | | | | | | | | | | |
| Leuprolide | | | | | | Leu | | | | NH-Et |
| Buserelin | | | | | | Ser(O$^t$Bu) | | | | NH-Et |
| Goserelin | | | | | | Ser(O$^t$Bu) | | | | AzaGly-NH$_2$ |
| Histrelin | | | | | | D-His(Bzl) | | | | AzaGly-NH$_2$ |
| **Decapeptides** | | | | | | | | | | |
| Nafarelin | | | | | | 2Nal | | | | Gly-NH$_2$ |
| Triptorelin | | | | | | Trp | | | | Gly-NH$_2$ |

stimulation of LH/FSH release in immature rats using infusion techniques. The available data usually describe the relative potency of a certain GnRH agonist compared with native GnRH (Table 2). Direct comparison between the clinically available GnRH agonists, under identical conditions, has never been undertaken. Therefore, translation of data from these models to humans should be done with caution. Leuprolide acetate, for example, was 50–80 times more potent than GnRH in the ovulation-induction test in rats,[27] and only 15 times more potent than the parent hormone in the test of increase in circulating LH levels in male rats. Nafarelin acetate, the most potent of currently available agonistic analogues, was 200 times more active than the endogenous hormone in suppressing oestrus in rats.[28,29]

As a result of specific pituitary uptake, lack of plasma protein binding[19,20] and the vast dilution of GnRH as it empties from the hypothalamic–pituitary portal system into the peripheral circulation, biologically significant amounts of GnRH are probably present only in the portal system.[30] Although extrapituitary receptors with nanomolar binding affinities have been reported in various organs, it is unlikely that hypothalamic GnRH reaches concentrations in the periphery sufficient to stimulate them. This is not the case with the administration of exogenous GnRH or its agonistic analogues, because they are widely distributed into the extracellular fluid. Although plasma protein binding of GnRH is negligible,[19,20] the stabilizing effect of the position 6 hydrophobic modifications in agonistic analogues allows for plasma protein binding with prolonged half-lives. Repeated or continuous administration of GnRH agonists leads to their accumulation and establishment of sustained concentrations in the peripheral circulation with potential extrapituitary effects.

## ROUTES OF ADMINISTRATION

As with many other peptides, the pharmacokinetics of plasma GnRH after single bolus intravenous administration shows two phases with

**Table 2** Trade names, plasma half-lives, relative potency, route of administration and recommended dose for the clinically available gonadotrophins

| Generic name | Trade name | Half-life | Relative potency | Administration route | Recommended dose |
|---|---|---|---|---|---|
| Native GnRH | | | 1 | i.v., s.c. | |
| **Nonapeptides** | | | | | |
| Leuprolide | Lupron | 90 min | 50–80 | s.c. | 500–1000 µg/day |
| | | | 20–30 | i.m. depot | 3.75–7.5 mg/month |
| Buserelin | Superfact, Supercur | 80 min | 20–40 | s.c., i.n. | 200–500 µg/day |
| | | | | | 300–400 three to four times daily |
| Histrelin | Supprelin | <60 min | 100 | s.c. | 100 µg/day |
| Goserelin | Zoladex | 4.5 h | 50–100 | s.c. implant | 3.6 mg/month |
| **Decapeptides** | | | | | |
| Nafarelin | Synarel | 3–4 h | 200 | i.n. | 200–400 twice daily |
| Triptorelin | Decapeptyl | 3–4.2 h | 36–144 | s.c., | 100–500 µg/day |
| | | | | i.m. depot | 3.75 mg/month |

typical half-lives of 2–8 min for the fast and 15–60 min for the slower phase. The pharmacokinetics and biological efficacy of GnRH agonistic analogues are related to their formulation and route of administration, which directly affect their absorption, metabolic clearance, bioavailability and affinity for the GnRH receptor. Efforts have been made to provide the most effective and practical route of administration for GnRH agonists. All GnRH agonistic analogues are small polypeptide molecules that need to be administered parenterally because they would otherwise be susceptible to gastrointestinal proteolysis. The oral and rectal administration of analogues is associated with a very low biopotency (0.01–1% vs parenteral administration). Rectal administration of leuprolide acetate in rats resulted in a low bioavailability of 16% and an even lower biopo-

tency of 0.6%.[31] Substantially higher absorption than through any other mucosal surface (56–85%) was obtained with vaginal administration of leuprolide acetate in rats, with biopotency comparable to the subcutaneous route and considerably better than the intranasal or rectal routes.[31] Absolute bioavailability, as determined by plasma leuprolide concentrations, was disappointingly low.

### The subcutaneous route

The subcutaneous route of GnRH agonist administration is currently most commonly used for a variety of clinical indications. It is characterized by high bioavailability (75–90%) and low interindividual variation. Subcutaneous doses of GnRH are associated with depot-like effects, resulting in prolonged and delayed absorption compared with intravenous administration.[32] These depot-like effects may be enhanced in GnRH agonists by their hydrophobic nature. After subcutaneous injection, the agonist is rapidly absorbed and blood concentrations remain elevated for many hours. Consequently, these agonists are effective when administered as single daily subcutaneous injections. Subcutaneous preparations are commercially available for buserelin, leuprolide, triptorelin and histrelin, with wide geographical variations in drug registration and use. Trade names and recommended daily doses are shown in Table 2.

## The intranasal route

Administration by nasal spray is now being widely used as a convenient alternative to parenteral administration with nasal preparations of buserelin and nafarelin available. Transnasal absorption has been enhanced with the development of more hydrophobic analogues and with the addition of absorption enhancers such as surfactant.[33] However, the intranasal route has several disadvantages, including marked interindividual variation in absorption and considerable losses of the peptide by proteolysis and swallowing.[34,35] In children with central precocious puberty, absolute serum buserelin concentrations after subcutaneous therapy were 100-fold higher than those after intranasal administration, and intranasal absorption was much more variable.[35] It was estimated that only 2.5–6% of the metered intranasal buserelin dose was absorbed into the systemic circulation.[35] Persistence of drugs in the nasal mucosa for up to 24 h is consistent with depot-like absorption effects which have been described for this tissue.[36] The prolonged release through the intranasal route makes this form of administration useful when lengthy GnRH receptor occupation is required, but nasal doses need to be administered two to four times daily to maintain an effective drug serum concentration. Moreover, the frequency of analogue administration may be a more important factor in

achieving pituitary down-regulation than the absolute serum concentration achieved. Suppression by single daily subcutaneous injections of buserelin required a minimum dose range of 10–30 μg/kg, yet intranasal buserelin produced the desired biological effect when provided three times daily in a concentration of 10 μg/dose (allowing for 5% absorption by nasal mucosa).[35]

## Depot formulations

Suppression of the pituitary–gonadal axis is more profound with continuous infusion than with intermittent administration of GnRH agonists in primates and humans.[37] Therefore, sustained or continuous release formulations have been developed allowing continuous exposure to agonistic analogues, with potentially improved efficacy and consistency of pituitary and gonadal suppression, and enhanced convenience and compliance offered to patients by reducing the frequency of drug administration. Depot preparations are especially convenient and useful in conditions where long-term pituitary desensitization is required (for example, prostatic cancer, endometriosis, fibroids), but have also been successfully used in the context of controlled ovarian hyperstimulation. Currently, available preparations include a suspension of 3.75 mg triptorelin or leuprolide in microcapsules injected intramuscularly once a month (a 7.5 mg preparation of leuprolide is available as well) or, alternatively, 3.6 mg goserelin dispersed in a biodegradable polymeric matrix of polyactide–coglycolide as a cylindrical rod implant injected subcutaneously every 4 weeks. The pharmacokinetics of the two sustained release systems are different. The microcapsule formulation induces an initial fast release of the agonist which slowly decreases thereafter during the following weeks, whereas blood concentrations from the goserelin implant progressively increase during the first 2 weeks before decreasing in an identical fashion in the following 2 weeks.[38,39] After administration of triptorelin, it is slowly released from the microcapsules into the circulation to give a plasma concentration of 200–500 pg/ml. The half-life during the distribution phase is 4.2 hours and 13.6 days during the elimination period. This therapeutic concentration is maintained for 4 weeks and, after a repeat injection, the steady-state concentration remains at about 400 pg/ml.[39] Plasma concentrations of the agonist during the delivery period of the depot are related to the total dose of the agonist dispersed in the polymer.[40,41]

Dose-finding studies in which the minimal effective dose for the different GnRH agonist formulations was evaluated are almost entirely absent. For example, the single administration of half-dose triptorelin depot (1.87 mg) appears to create an initial endocrine response which is similar to the one obtained by the full-dose depot.[42] Moreover, the duration of pituitary and ovarian suppression seems to be unaltered by the dose reduction. This may imply that, for certain clinical indications, the amount of agonist present in the standard depot preparations is much higher than what is actually needed to achieve the endocrine and clinical aims.

## GnRH AGONISTIC ANALOGUES: CLINICAL APPLICATIONS

The original incentive for development of agonistic analogues of GnRH was that they would eventually be used for the treatment of anovulation. However, soon after elucidation of the structure of GnRH, the 'paradoxical' ability of agonistic analogues to inhibit reproductive function in experimental animals was demonstrated.[43] Thus, the most important clinical applications of the potent GnRH agonists, or superagonists, were derived from their capacity to cause rapid desensitization of the gonadotrophs during prolonged administration, with a resultant reduction in serum gonadotrophin concentrations and constant inhibition of ovarian steroidogenesis. The potential for reversibly inducing a state of hypogonadotrophic hypogonadism, which was also termed 'medical gonadectomy' or 'medical hypophysectomy', allowed for the relatively rapid wide-scale introduction of GnRH agonists into clinical practice for a variety of indications, when complete abolishment of gonadotrophin secretion with subsequent suppression of gonadal steroids to the levels of castrated subjects was considered beneficial. This therapeutic approach has already had its efficacy and merits proved in the treatment of metastatic prostatic cancer, central precocious puberty, endometriosis, uterine fibroids, hirsutism and other conditions.[44]

Since the first report on the use of the combination of the GnRH agonist buserelin and gonadotrophins for ovarian stimulation for in vitro fertilization back in 1984,[45] numerous studies have demonstrated the efficacy of this concept. Subsequently, the use of GnRH agonists has gained widespread popularity, and an increasing number of assisted reproductive technology (ART) programmes use this approach nowadays as the predominant method of ovarian stimulation. The major advantage initially offered by the agonists was the efficient abolishment of the spontaneous LH surge. The incidence of premature LH surge and luteinization in cycles with exogenous gonadotrophin stimulation was noted by various investigators to range between 30% and 50%,[46] and, because it has been shown to affect both fertilization and pregnancy rates adversely, these cycles usually had to be cancelled. A meta-analysis of randomized controlled trials has shown that the use of GnRH agonists has not only reduced cancellation rates, but also increased the number of oocytes recovered, and improved clinical pregnancy rates per cycle commenced and per embryo transfer.[47]

A number of controversial issues remain concerning the use of GnRH agonists in assisted reproduction. The problems of which agonist should be used, what is the optimal dose, and which delivery system and protocol of administration would yield the best response and results have not been resolved. In addition, the future role of GnRH antagonists in ART has not been clearly defined yet. Many aspects of these relevant issues will be examined in the other chapters in this book.

## REFERENCES

1. Tsutsumi M, Zhou W, Millar RP, et al. Cloning and functional expression of a mouse gonado-tropin-releasing hormone receptor. *Mol Endocrinol* 1992;**6**:1163–9.
2. Kakar SS, Musgrove LC, Devor DC, et al. Cloning, sequencing, and expression of human gonadotropin releasing hormone (GnRH) receptor. *Biochem Biophys Res Commun* 1992;**189**:289–95.
3. Reinhart J, Mertz LM, Catt KJ. Molecular cloning and expression of cDNA encoding the murine gonadotropin-releasing hormone receptor. *J Biol Chem* 1992;**267**:21281–4.
4. Naor Z. Signal transduction mechanisms of $Ca^{2+}$ mobilizing hormones: the case of gonadotropin-releasing hormone. *Endocr Rev* 1990;**11**:326–53.
5. Kiesel L. Molecular mechanisms of gonado-trophin releasing hormone-stimulated gonadotro-phin secretion. *Hum Reprod* 1993;**8**(suppl 2):23–8.
6. Stojilkovic SS, Reinhart J, Catt KJ. Gonadotropin-releasing hormone receptors: structure and signal transduction pathways. *Endocr Rev* 1994;**15**:462–99.
7. Crowley WF, Conn PM (eds). *Modes of Action of GnRH and GnRH Analogs.* New York: Springer-Verlag, 1992: 26–54.
8. Knobil E, Hotchkiss J. The menstrual cycle and its neuroendocrine control. In: *The Physiology of Reproduction, 1971–94* (Knobil E, Neill J, eds). New York: Raven Press, 1988.
9. Levine JE, Duffy MT. Simultaneous measurement of luteinizing hormone (LH)-releasing hormone, LH and follicle-stimulating hormone release in intact and short-term castrate rats. *Endocrinology* 1988;**122**:2211–21.
10. Yen SS, Tsai CC, Naftolin F, et al. Pulsatile patterns of gonadotropin release in subjects with and without ovarian function. *J Clin Endocrinol Metab* 1972;**34**:671–5.
11. Backstorm CT, McNeilly AS, Leask RM, Baird DT. Pulsatile secretion of LH, FSH, prolactin, oestradiol and progesterone during the human menstrual cycle. *Clin Endocrinol* 1982;**17**:29–42.
12. Reame N, Sauder SE, Kelch RP, Marshall JC. Pulsatile gonadotropin secretion during the human menstrual cycle: evidence for altered frequency of gonadotropin-releasing hormone secretion. *J Clin Endocrinol Metab* 1984;**59**:328–37.
13. Crowley WF Jr, Filicori M, Spratt DI, Santoro NF. The physiology of gonadotropin-releasing hormone (GnRH) secretion in men and women. *Recent Prog Horm Res* 1985;**41**:473–531.
14. Knobil E. The neuroendocrine control of the menstrual cycle. *Recent Prog Horm Res* 1980; **36**:53–88.
15. Knobil E. The neuroendocrine control of ovulation. *Hum Reprod* 1988;**3**:469–72.
16. Suarez-Quian CA, Wynn PC, Catt KJ. Receptor-mediated endocytosis of GnRH analogs: differential processing of gold-labeled agonist and antagonist derivatives. *J Steroid Biochem* 1986; **24**:183–92.
17. Schvartz I, Hazum E. Internalization and recycling of receptor-bound gonadotropin-releasing hormone agonist in pituitary gonadotropes. *J Biol Chem* 1987;**262**:17046–50.
18. Stojilkovic SS, Rojas E, Stutzin A, et al. Desensitization of pituitary gonadotropin secretion by agonist-induced inactivation of voltage-sensitive calcium channels. *J Biol Chem* 1989;**264**:10939–42.
19. Tharandt L, Schulte H, Benker G, et al. Binding of luteinizing hormone releasing hormone to human serum proteins – influence of a chronic treatment with a more potent analogue of LH-RH. *Horm Metab Res* 1979;**11**:391–4.
20. Chan RL, Chaplin MD. Plasma binding of LHRH and nafareline acetate, a highly potent LHRH agonist. *Biochem Biophys Res Commun* 1985; **127**:673–9.
21. Jeffcoate SL, Greenwood RH, Holland DT. Blood and urine clearance of luteinizing hormone releasing hormone in man measured by radioimmunoassay. *J Endocrinol* 1974;**60**:305–14.
22. Handelsman DJ, Swerdloff RS. Pharmacokinetics of gonadotropin-releasing hormone and its analogs. *Endocr Rev* 1986;**7**:95–105.
23. Griffiths EC, McDermott JR. Enzymatic activation of hypothalmic regulatory hormones. *Mol Cell Endocrinol* 1983;**33**:1–25.
24. Conn PM, McArdle CA, Andrews WV, Huckle WR. The molecular basis of gonadotropin-releasing hormone (GnRH) action in the pituitary gonadotrope. *Biol Reprod* 1987;**36**:17–35.
25. Nestor JJ Jr. Development of agonistic LHRH analogs. In: *LHRH and its Analogs* (Vickery BH, Nestor JJ Jr, Hafez ESE, eds). Lancaster: MTP Press, 1984: 3–15.
26. Karten MJ, Rivier JE. Gonadotropin-releasing hormone analog design. Structure–function studies toward the development of agonists and antagonists: rationale and perspective. *Endocr Rev* 1986;**7**:44–66.

27. Rippel RH, Johnson ES, White WF, et al. Ovulation and gonadotropin-releasing activity of [p-Leu⁶,desGlyNH₂10, Pro-ethylamide⁹] GnRH. *Proc Soc Exp Biol Med* 1975;**148**:1193–7.

28. Nestor JJK, Ho TL, Simpson RA, et al. Synthesis and biological activity of some very hydrophobic superagonistic analogues of luteinizing hormone-releasing hormone. *J Med Chem* 1982;**25**:795–801.

29. Chan RL, Henzl MR, LePage ME, et al. Absorption and metabolism of nafarelin, a potent agonist of gonadotropin-releasing hormone. *Clin Pharmacol Ther* 1988;**44**:275–82.

30. Nett TM, Akbar AM, Niswender GD. Serum levels of luteinizing hormone and gonadotropin-releasing hormone in cycling, castrated and anestrous ewes. *Endocrinology* 1974;**94**:713–18.

31. Yamazaki I. Differences in pregnancy-terminating effectiveness of an LH-RH analogue by subcutaneous, vaginal, rectal and nasal routes in rats. *Endocrinol Jpn* 1982;**29**:415–21.

32. Handelsman DJ, Jansen RP, Boylan LM, et al. Pharmacokinetics of gonadotropin-releasing hormone: comparison of subcutaneous and intravenous routes. *J Clin Endocrinol Metab* 1984; **59**:739–46.

33. Okeda H, Yamazaki I, Ogawa Y, et al. Vaginal absorption of a potent luteinizing hormone-releasing hormone analog (leuprolide) in rats. I. Absorption by various routes and absorption enhancement. *J Pharm Sci* 1982;**71**:1367–71.

34. Anik ST, McRae G, Nerenberg C, et al. Nasal absorption of nafarelin acetate, the decapeptide [D-Nal(2)6]LHRH, in rhesus monkeys. *J Pharm Sci* 1984;**73**:684–5.

35. Holland FJ, Fishman L, Costigan DC, et al. Pharmacokinetic characteristics of the gonadotropin-releasing hormone analog D-Ser(TBU)-6EA10 Luteinizing hormone-releasing hormone (Buserelin) after subcutaneous and intranasal administration in children with central precocious puberty. *J Clin Endocrinol Metab* 1986;**63**:1065–70.

36. Aoki FY, Crawley JC. Distribution and removal of human serum albumin–technetium 99m instilled intranasally. *Br J Clin Pharmacol* 1976; **3**:869–78.

37. Bhasin S, Steiner B, Swerdloff R. Does constant infusion of gonadotropin-releasing hormone agonist lead to greater suppression of gonadal function in man than intermittent administration? *Fertil Steril* 1985;**44**:96–101.

38. Clayton RN, Bailey LC, Cottam J, et al. A radioimmunoassay for GnRH agonist analogue in serum of patients with prostate cancer treated with D-Ser (Tbu)⁶ AZA Gly¹⁰ GnRH. *Clin Endocrinol* 1985;**22**:453–62.

39. Happ J, Schultheiss H, Jacobi GH. Pharmacodynamics, pharmacokinetics and bioavailability of the prolonged LH-RH agonist Decapeptyl-SR. In: *Hormonal Manipulation of Cancer: Peptides, growth factors and new (anti) steroidal agents* (Klijn JGM, et al, eds). New York: Raven Press, 1987: 249–53.

40. Beck LR, Cowsar DR, Lewis DH, et al. New long-acting injectable microcapsule contraceptive system. *Am J Obstet Gynecol* 1979;**135**:419–26.

41. Zorn JR, Barata M, Brami C, et al. Ovarian stimulation for in vitro fertilization and GIFT combining administration of gonadotrophins and blockade of the pituitary with D-Trp6-LH-RH. *Eur J Obstet Gynecol Reprod Biol* 1988;**28**:116–20.

42. Balasch J, Gomez F, Casamitjana R, et al. Pituitary–ovarian suppression by the standard and half-doses of D-Trp-6 luteinizing hormone-releasing hormone depot. *Hum Reprod* 1992;**7**:1230–4.

43. Corbin A, Beattie CW. Post-coital contraceptive and uterotrophic effects of luteinizing hormone releasing hormone. *Endocr Res Commun* 1975;**2**: 445–8.

44. Conn PM, Crowley WF Jr. Gonadotropin-releasing hormone and its analogues. *N Engl J Med* 1991;**324**:93–103.

45. Porter RN, Smith W, Craft IL, et al. Induction of ovulation for in vitro fertilisation using buserelin and gonadotropins. *Lancet* 1984;**ii**:1284–5.

46. Fleming R, Coutts JR. Induction of multiple follicular growth in normally menstruating women with endogenous gonadotropin suppression. *Fertil Steril* 1986;**45**:226–30.

47. Hughes EG, Fedorkow DM, Daya S, et al. The routine use of gonadotropin-releasing hormone agonists prior to in vitro fertilization and gamete intrafallopian transfer: a meta-analysis of randomized controlled trials. *Fertil Steril* 1992;**58**:888–96.

# 15

# GnRH agonists: to dose or to overdose?

Joop Schoemaker, Fedde Scheele, Frank Broekmans, Ruth Janssens

**Preliminary studies** • **Suppressing the LH surge in controlled ovarian stimulation** • **Treatment of uterine myomas** • **Conclusions** • **Acknowledgments**

Finding the right dose of medication used in the treatment of infertility disorders has, for one reason or another, been notoriously difficult. Proper dose-finding studies in the use of gonadotrophins are lacking and it therefore took until the middle of the 1980s before the proper treatment protocol, with a maximum of effect and a minimum of side effects, was introduced by Polson and the group working with Stephen Franks.[1] The dose finding in pulsatile gonadotrophin-releasing hormone (GnRH) for hypogonadotrophic amenorrhoea was performed in a much better way by Crowley and his co-workers,[2] but the introduction of GnRH analogues again was not an example of excellent pharmaceutical research.

The impact of the addition of GnRH agonists to the armamentarium of gynaecologists has been enormous and has greatly influenced their daily practice. Stimulation of follicle growth in assisted reproduction, and the final maturation and induction of actual ovulation in ovulation-induction protocols, as well as the treatment of endometriosis and uterine leiomyomas, are major indications for these drugs.

GnRH-agonists have primarily been developed for the treatment of prostate cancer, in which it is mandatory for patients to have absolute suppression at least of luteinizing hormone (LH) to obtain the required effect, that is, cessation of the detrimental effect of androgens on the course of the disease. When other indications, such as those mentioned above, came into being, it was automatically assumed that the same dose would suffice for different indications. This, however, may not be the case.

In assisted reproduction, the aim of the use of GnRH analogues is to suppress an early appearance of the LH surge, caused by a precocious rise of oestradiol as a result of multiple follicle development. In this indication it may be enough to suppress gonadotrophin secretion only partially. In the treatment of endometriosis and uterine myomas, full suppression of oestrogen should, in theory, be obtained. However, Maheux and co-workers[3] showed that, in the treatment for uterine myomas, once a reduction in the size of the myoma has been obtained, a small amount of oestrogen could be administered to cope with the side effects of oestrogen deprivation, without stimulating regrowth of the myomas. This suggests that, instead of adding oestrogens to the therapy ('add back'), the dose of agonists could be reduced as well ('draw back'), resulting in the same effect. If this approach were to work in the treatment of myomas, it could also work in the treatment of endometriosis.

To address these issues a series of clinical experiments was conducted by our group. Intravenous infusions with different doses of native GnRH provided a standard by which the extent of pituitary suppression could be measured,[4] pharmacodynamic studies answered questions about the duration of action of subcutaneously administered GnRH[5–7] and different dose-finding studies, both in the suppression of the premature LH surge[8,9] and in the treatment of leiomyomas,[10] concluded the studies.

## PRELIMINARY STUDIES

In the mid-1980s the first investigations into the dose dependency of pituitary suppression by GnRH and its agonists were carried out. Native GnRH was infused intravenously in pulses every 8 min as a substitute for continuous infusion, in doses of 0.25, 0.5 or 1 µg/min for a duration of 4 weeks. The results are shown in Figure 1 for a representative volunteer. At that time, however, as a result of the cross-reactivity of the polyclonal antibody assays with free α subunits, neither full suppression nor dose dependency of LH secretion could be demonstrated.

With the arrival of monoclonal antibody assays changes occurred and we asked ourselves whether it would be possible to develop a measure by which pituitary suppression could be quantified. Such studies were performed by Scheele et al.[4] In this respect they addressed three basic questions:

1.  Is the degree of pituitary desensitization dependent on the dose of agonist used?
2.  What is the optimal way to measure the degree of pituitary desensitization?
3.  Is it possible to create a standard to express the degree of pituitary desensitization?

Twenty-four women were randomized into four groups of six women. To achieve pituitary desensitization, the four groups received 0.1,

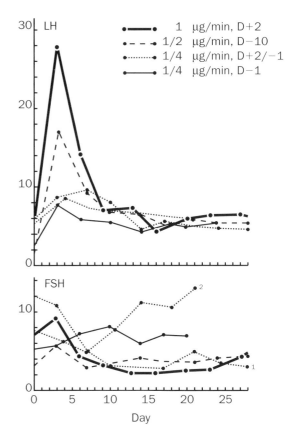

**Figure 1** Pituitary desensitization during intravenous infusion with different doses of native GnRH.

0.25, 0.5 or 1.0 µg/min GnRH intravenously for 6 weeks. Pituitary desensitization was measured by gonadotrophin levels as such, by responses to a 100 µg bolus of GnRH and by an oestradiol benzoate challenge test.[11] The level of LH and the responses of LH and follicle-stimulating hormone (FSH) to the GnRH challenge showed significant dose-dependent suppression. Multiple regression analysis indicated that the LH response to the GnRH challenge was the best way to measure pituitary desensitization. From the LH responses to the GnRH challenge a 'standard curve' was established for the assessment of the degree of pituitary desensitization (Figure 2). However, the

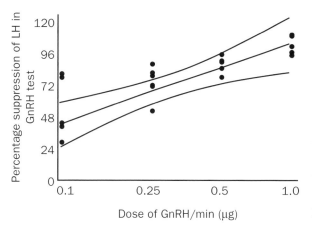

**Figure 2** The mean suppression, with 95% confidence limits, of the LH response to the GnRH challenge in the third week of GnRH infusion, plotted against the dose of GnRH infused. (Reproduced, with permission of the editor, from Scheele et al.[4])

cance for LH. When expressed as the proportion of the responses in the control group, even the LH response under suppression with 25 µg/day was less than 25%. The dose–response relationship persisted after discontinuation, the responses in the 25 µg group restoring the fastest. Also, even after 6 days, the response in this group had not surpassed the 50% of controls yet.

This study shows that not only is the response to native GnRH dependent on the suppression dose, but so is the response to long-acting GnRH agonists, such as triptorelin. The recovery from pituitary desensitization is also slow, indicating that in addition to, or instead of, decreasing the dose of agonists it might be appropriate to increase the interval between doses or discontinue the administration of the agonist at an earlier time.

## SUPPRESSING THE LH SURGE IN CONTROLLED OVARIAN STIMULATION

The use of a GnRH agonist in ovarian stimulation during ovulation induction was first advocated by Fleming and co-workers in 1985[12] and in assisted reproduction by Neveu et al[13] in 1987. The main goal of this additional treatment is to prevent spontaneous LH surges occurring and thus reduce the number of cancelled cycles. Different protocols have since been designed. Tan et al,[14,15] in both prospective and retrospective studies, showed that the so-called 'long protocol', particularly when started at the beginning of a menstrual cycle, yielded the best results with respect to cumulative pregnancy rates.

The dose used for desensitization in in vitro fertilization (IVF) has been derived from protocols, originally designed for use in the treatment of prostate cancer. The use of a lower dose of a GnRH agonist than commonly used has not been investigated in the literature for the suppression of a premature LH surge and only sporadically for other indications, but never in a clear dose-finding study.[16–18] Using lower dosages could, however, have a number of advantages, such as avoidance of a direct effect

relatively large confidence interval of the estimated regression line is a serious limitation for the accuracy of this unit of suppression. Subsequently, similar studies were carried out by Broekmans[5] to measure the degree of suppression after desensitization by different doses of triptorelin (Decapeptyl).

Thirty-two women with regular menstrual cycles were randomly divided into four groups of eight, each group receiving 25, 50, 100 or 200 µg triptorelin subcutaneously in a double-blind fashion. Treatment with triptorelin was started in the middle of the luteal phase and was continued for 18 days. Thirty-four women, who also had regular menstrual cycles, acted as a control group, having their pituitary function evaluated during the early follicular phase in the same way as in the treatment groups. Pituitary suppression was evaluated by GnRH challenge tests: 100 µg i.v. at day 17 of treatment and 2, 4 and 6 days after discontinuation of treatment. The LH and FSH responses, expressed as areas under the curve above baseline, correlated with the dose of triptorelin administered, again with the highest signifi-

of agonists on the ovary and/or oocyte at a time when the latter would be the most vulnerable for exogenous hazards (chemicals, radiation etc), that is, at the time of conception. Also, a better cost–benefit ratio might be achieved, not only because of a reduced dose of agonist, but also because of a reduced dose of FSH resulting from a less pronounced desensitization.

To investigate whether a lower dose of GnRH agonist would be adequate to suppress pituitary activity to such an extent that no spontaneous LH surge could be expected, Janssens et al[8] carried out a prospective, randomized, double-blind, dose-finding study, during regular ovarian stimulation for IVF, in which pituitary suppression was tested by a GnRH challenge test (500 µg GnRH) 1.5 hours before hCG was given.

Forty-eight patients were randomly divided into four groups of 12 patients each. Each group was treated with a different dose of triptorelin, that is, 5, 15, 50 or 100 µg per day, starting in the middle of the luteal phase of a cycle as determined by basal body temperature (BTC) readings. Ovarian stimulation was started on the third day of the subsequent menstrual bleeding with FSH (Metrodin), with either two or three ampoules, depending on age: two ampoules for women under 36 years and three ampoules for those over 35 years of age. Stimulation was continued until three follicles larger than 16 mm were present with at least one of them being 18 mm and a 17β-oestradiol level of at least 1500 pmol/l. Morning urinary LH (uLH) was determined daily until a follicle of at least 14 mm was observed. From then on uLH was determined three times each day in order to detect a possible premature LH surge. Such a surge was defined as two successive increasing uLH values of which the first value was twice or more that of the baseline uLH concentration (that is, the average uLH values between day 7 and the moment the largest follicle was 14 mm).

One and a half hours before the hCG was given, a GnRH challenge test was performed with an intravenous dose of 500 µg. Blood was sampled at 0, 30, 60 and 90 min after GnRH for LH and FSH determination. Subsequently, hCG

was given and oocyte retrieval followed according to standard procedures. Six patients, one from the 5-µg group, two from the 15-µg group, two from the 50-µg group and one from the 100-µg group, were dropped from the study because of either excessive (three patients) or insufficient (three patients) response.

The response appeared to be dose dependent, although no statistically significant difference was apparent between the 50 and the 100 µg dose. None of the patients exhibited a spontaneous LH surge but three patients, all from the 5-µg group, appeared to have ovulated, as evidenced by the disappearance of the follicles, between the GnRH challenge test and ovum pick-up, probably as the result of the LH increase brought about by the GnRH dose itself. There was no significant difference between the dose groups in number of oocyte/cumulus complexes retrieved, the fertilization rate or the number of pregnancies. However, the number of patients per group was indeed too small to draw conclusions with respect to clinical results under the different dosages. The study showed, however, that adequate suppression could be obtained under a 50-µg dose and possibly also under a 15-µg dose. Further studies with a larger number of patients were necessary to investigate whether the clinical results of IVF would be influenced by using a lower dose of a GnRH agonist.

To this extent a new prospective, randomized, double-blind, placebo-controlled study was undertaken to find the minimal daily dose necessary to suppress the pituitary to such an extent that no significant premature LH surge would occur.[9] Two hundred and forty patients were randomized over four groups, 60 in each arm, to receive either placebo or one of three different dose groups of triptorelin, that is, 15, 50 or 100 µg daily. Ovarian stimulation was performed as described above.

No spontaneous premature LH surge occurred in either of the GnRH agonist-treated patient groups. On the contrary, a premature LH surge occurred in 23% of the patients who were treated by placebo. A statistically significant dose–response was observed for the number of oocytes, fertilization rate, number of embryos and implantation rate. No such clear dose–response was seen with respect to (ongoing) pregnancy rate and live birth rate, but both items were highest in the 50-μg group. The higher number of oocytes and embryos, as well as the increase in fertilization and implantation rate, is paid for by the need for a higher total dose of FSH and a longer stimulation phase.

It is concluded that 15 μg triptorelin daily is sufficient for suppression of premature LH surges, but in order to obtain the better clinical results, as described in the literature, a dose of 50 μg seems to be the optimal dose.

## TREATMENT OF UTERINE MYOMAS

Uterine leiomyomas have been treated with GnRH agonists ever since the first publications by Filicori et al in 1983.[19] GnRH agonists suppress pituitary function by desensitizing the pituitary to GnRH such that secretion of LH and FSH is suppressed and, through the absence of ovarian stimulation, a hypo-oestrogenic state is induced. Using the regular dose for desensitization, that is, either using a depot preparation of 3.6 mg once a month or using 100 μg triptorelin per day, complete desensitization and complete hypo-oestrogenism are attained, leading to a decrease in size of both the myomas and the uterus itself. Several studies have shown now that, once reduction of the myomas has been achieved, a small daily dose of oestrogens will minimize the complaints of hypo-oestrogenism, such as hot flushes, dry vagina and recurrent cystitis, without inducing regrowth of the myomas.[3,20,21] These findings brought up the question of whether it would be possible, instead of adding oestrogens to reduce the side effects (add-back therapy), just to reduce the agonist dose (draw-back therapy), inducing partial instead of complete desensitization. To explore this the following experiment was carried out.

Twenty-four women with symptomatic uterine leiomyomas of such a size that the total uterine volume exceeded 300 ml, as measured by abdominal ultrasonography, were evaluated, after being treated with triptorelin 500 μg/day for one week, followed by 100 μg/day for 7 weeks. After this initial treatment of 8 weeks, the women were randomized double blindly to receive 5, 20 or 100 μg triptorelin per day for the next 18 weeks.

The hormone status of the patients was monitored by weekly LH, FSH, oestradiol, testosterone and androstenedione, and triptorelin measurements, as well as by GnRH challenge tests at weeks 0, 8, 14, 18, 22 and 26. Uterine and myoma size, where possible, were determined by magnetic resonance imaging (MRI) before treatment and after 8 and 26 weeks of treatment. Bone mineral density (BMD) was determined by dual X-ray absorptiometry (DXA) and bone turnover was assessed by calcium, phosphorus, albumin, total alkaline phosphatase (tAP), total acid phosphatase (tAcP), hydroxyproline (Hp) and creatinine (Cr) determinations, again before treatment and after 8 and 26 weeks of treatment.

During the standard dose treatment all women experienced hot flushes for some time. After the start of the randomized dose treatment, 80% of the patients continued having flushes although some changes in intensity were experienced. The frequency of spotting during treatment was 37.5%, and the appearance of spotting and hot flushes were equally distributed in the three dose groups. Intermittent menstrual-like bleeding occurred in 21% of the patients during randomized treatment, the bleeding being more frequent in the lowest dose group.

During the first 8 weeks, uterine volume and myoma volume have decreased by about 30%, as shown in Figure 3. Additional treatment with the different dosages gave a further, dose-related decrease in uterine and myoma size. However, at the end of 26 weeks of treatment there still was no difference in uterine and myoma size between the three groups.

Hormone assessment of pituitary suppression during treatment revealed that, after the 8 initial weeks of treatment, optimal suppression had been obtained. Between weeks 8 and 26 there was a dose-dependent change in the serum concentrations of LH, oestradiol and triptorelin, as well as a dose–response relation-

(a)

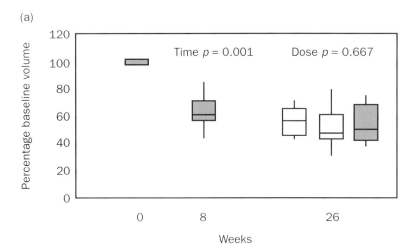

(b)

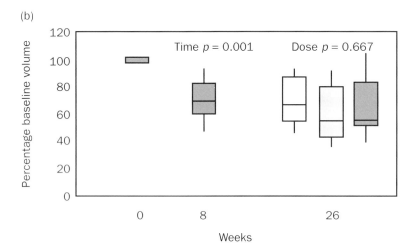

(c)

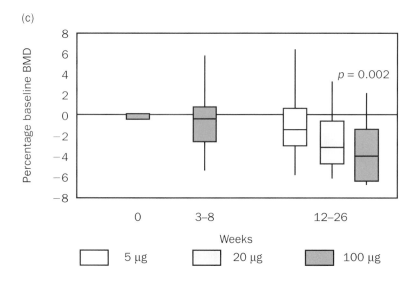

**Figure 3** Box and whisker plots of proportional change in (a) uterine volume, (b) myoma volume and (c) bone mineral density (BMD) after standard and randomized dose triptorelin treatment. (Reproduced, with permission of the editor, from Broekmans et al.[10])

ship of the LH response and the FSH response during the GnRH challenge tests (Figure 4).

By the end of the first 8 weeks of treatment, plasma phosphorus and tAP were significantly elevated and so was the Hp:Cr ratio. During weeks 8–26, calcium, phosphorus tAP and tAcP rose further in the 100 µg/day group. In the other two groups, these parameters were not

different from the baseline and 8-week values. The Hp:Cr ratio did not change further in any of the groups.

None of the measurements showed a dose dependency. After 8 weeks of treatment a 0.5% median reduction in BMD was observed for the group as a whole, but this was not a significantly different change. After 26 weeks of

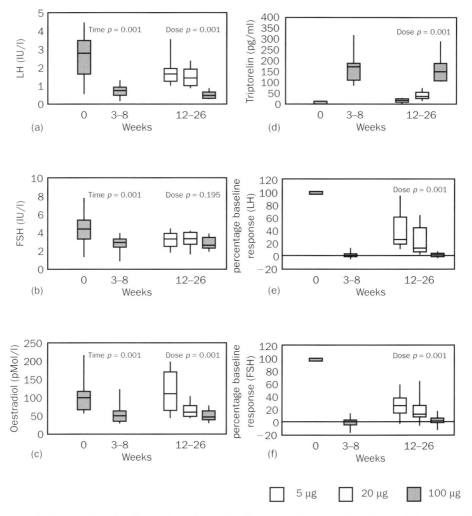

**Figure 4** Box and whisker plots (a–d) steady-state oestradiol and LH, FSH, triptorelin, and the proportional responses of (e) LH and (f) FSH to the GnRH challenge at baseline (0), 3–8 weeks and 12–26 weeks. (Reproduced and modified with permission of the editor from Broekmans et al.[10])

treatment in the 100-μg group the reduction was 3.7%, which was a significant deviation from baseline ($p = 0.002$). In the 5- and 20-μg groups, no significant deviation from baseline or 8-week values was observed. No dose dependency was present (see Figure 3).

This study shows that, after an initial treatment of leiomyomas with triptorelin for 8 weeks with the usual dose, a reduction of the dose can be made to at least 20 μg triptorelin, without jeopardizing the reduction obtained in uterine and myoma size during the first 8 weeks. BMD does not show a further decline during such continued treatment in contrast to continued treatment with 100 μg/day.

## CONCLUSIONS

Our studies have clearly shown that the usual dose of GnRH for treatment of uterine leiomyomas or for prevention of a premature LH surge in IVF is too high. The dosage for the latter indication can be reduced by at least 50% and for the former probably by 80% after the first 8 weeks of treatment with the usual dose.

As triptorelin comes in ampoules of 100 μg, the cost–benefit ratio will not improve if only half or even one-fifth of an ampoule is used per day, because nobody likes to keep open ampoules, or even filled syringes, overnight. Therefore other approaches should be looked for to reduce the dose. Such possibilities would include increasing the time between two applications or, particularly for the suppression of premature LH surges, discontinuing GnRH agonists a few days before a possible expected LH surge. Such strategies require development of new treatment protocols.

## ACKNOWLEDGMENTS

We would like to thank Ferring BV, the Netherlands, for the continuous financial and moral support for these studies. Despite the fact that studies such as ours might finally lead to reduced sales, they took the attitude that a proper dose was in the interest of the patient and therefore these studies should be performed.

## REFERENCES

1. Polson DW, Mason HD, Saldahna MB, Franks S. Ovulation of a single dominant follicle during treatment with low-dose pulsatile follicle stimulating hormone in women with polycystic ovary syndrome. *Clin Endocrinol (Oxf)* 1987;**26**:205–12.
2. Santoro N, Wierman ME, Filicori M, Waldstreicher J, Crowley WFJ. Intravenous administration of pulsatile gonadotropin-releasing hormone in hypothalamic amenorrhea: effects of dosage. *J Clin Endocrinol Metab* 1986;**62**:109–16.
3. Maheux R, Lemay A, Blanchet P, Friede J, Pratt X. Maintained reduction of uterine leiomyoma following addition of hormonal replacement therapy to a monthly luteinizing hormone-releasing hormone agonist implant: a pilot study. *Hum Reprod* 1991;**6**:500–5.
4. Scheele F, Hompes PG, Lambalk CB, Schoute E, Broekmans FJ, Schoemaker J. The GnRH challenge test: a quantitative measure of pituitary desensitization during GnRH agonist administration. *Clin Endocrinol (Oxf)* 1996;**44**:581–6.
5. Broekmans FJ, Hompes PG, Lambalk CB, Schoute E, Broeders A, Schoemaker J. Short term pituitary desensitization: effects of different doses of the gonadotrophin-releasing hormone agonist triptorelin. *Hum Reprod* 1996;**11**:55–60.
6. Broekmans FJ, Bernardus RE, Broeders A, Berkhout G, Schoemaker J. Pituitary responsiveness after administration of a GnRH agonist depot formulation: Decapeptyl CR. *Clin Endocrinol (Oxf)* 1993;**38**:579–87.
7. Broekmans FJ, Bernardus RE, Berkhout G, Schoemaker J. Pituitary and ovarian suppression after early follicular and mid-luteal administration of a LHRH agonist in a depot formulation: Decapeptyl CR. *Gynecol Endocrinol* 1992;**6**:153–61.
8. Janssens RMJ, Vermeiden JPW, Lambalk CB, Schats R, Schoemaker J. GnRH-agonist dose dependency of pituitary desensitization during

controlled ovarian hyperstimulation in IVF. *Hum Reprod* 1998; in press.

9. Janssens RMJ, Lambalk CB, Vermeiden JPW, Schats R, Schoemaker J. Dose-finding study of triptorelin-acetate for prevention of premature LH surge: a prospective, randomised, double blind, placebo controlled study. *Hum Reprod* 1998;**14**(suppl 1).

10. Broekmans FJ, Hompes PG, Heitbrink MA, et al. Two-step gonadotropin-releasing hormone agonist treatment of uterine leiomyomas: standard-dose therapy followed by reduced-dose therapy. *Am J Obstet Gynecol* 1996;**175**:1208–16.

11. Chang RJ, Jaffe RB. Progesterone effects on gonadotropin release in women pretreated with estradiol. *J Clin Endocrinol Metab* 1978;**47**:119–25.

12. Fleming R, Haxton MJ, Hamilton MP, et al. Successful treatment of infertile women with oligomenorrhoea using a combination of an LHRH agonist and exogenous gonadotrophins. *Br J Obstet Gynaecol* 1985;**92**:369–73.

13. Neveu S, Hedon B, Bringer J, et al. Ovarian stimulation by a combination of a gonadotropin-releasing hormone agonist and gonadotropins for in vitro fertilization. *Fertil Steril* 1987;**47**:639–43.

14. Tan SL, Maconochie N, Doyle P, et al. Cumulative conception and live-birth rates after in vitro fertilization with and without the use of long, short, and ultrashort regimens of the gonadotropin-releasing hormone agonist buserelin. *Am J Obstet Gynecol* 1994;**171**:513–20.

15. Tan SL, Kingsland C, Campbell S, et al. The long protocol of administration of gonadotropin-releasing hormone agonist is superior to the short protocol for ovarian stimulation for in vitro fertilization. *Fertil Steril* 1992;**57**:810–14.

16. Monroe SE, Blumenfeld Z, Andreyko JL, Schriock E, Henzl MR, Jaffe RB. Dose-dependent inhibition of pituitary-ovarian function during administration of a gonadotropin-releasing hormone agonistic analog (nafarelin). *J Clin Endocrinol Metab* 1986;**63**:1334–41.

17. Watanabe Y, Nakamura G. Effects of two different doses of leuprolide acetate depot on uterine cavity area in patients with uterine leiomyomata. *Fertil Steril* 1995;**63**:487–90.

18. Balasch J, Gomez F, Casamitjana R, Carmona F, Rivera F, Vanrell JA. Pituitary-ovarian suppression by the standard and half-doses of D-Trp-6-luteinizing hormone-releasing hormone depot. *Hum Reprod* 1992;**7**:1230–4.

19. Filicori M, Hall DA, Loughlin JS, Rivier S, Vale W, Crowley WF. A conservative approach to the management of uterine leiomyomata: pituitary desensitization by a luteinizing hormone-releasing hormone analogue. *Am J Obstet Gynecol* 1983;**147**:726–9.

20. Adashi EY. Long-term gonadotrophin-releasing hormone agonist therapy: the evolving issue of steroidal 'add-back' paradigms. *Hum Reprod* 1994;**9**:1380–97.

21. Friedman AJ, Daly M, Juneau Norcross M, et al. A prospective, randomized trial of gonadotropin-releasing hormone agonist plus estrogen-progestin or progestin 'add-back' regimens for women with leiomyomata uteri. *J Clin Endocrinol Metab* 1993;**76**:1439–45.

# 16

# The role of meta-analysis in determining which gonadotropin to use for ovarian stimulation

Salim Daya

**Systematic review and meta-analysis • Identification of studies • Study inclusion • Data summarization • Graphic display • Assessment of statistical heterogeneity in the effect of treatment • Estimating the combined effect of treatment • Sensitivity analysis • Methodologic quality • Subgroup analysis • Publication bias • Cumulative meta-analysis • Sequential monitoring boundaries • Conclusions**

Decision-making in clinical medicine involves the integration of clinical expertise with the best available external evidence. The field of reproductive medicine is witnessing rapid developments, especially in the area of assisted reproductive technology (ART). For example, the gonadotropin preparations available for ovarian stimulation have evolved over a relatively short time span from urinary-derived human menopausal gonadotropin (hMG) to genetically engineered follicle-stimulating hormone (FSH) using recombinant DNA technology. Such advances generate numerous questions involving treatment efficacy, diagnostic test accuracy, effect of exposure to various agents, course and prognosis of disease, and cost-effectiveness of new interventions.

Although recombinant FSH is gradually becoming available, the gonadotropins that are currently in use for ovarian stimulation are preparations extracted from the urine of postmenopausal women. Urinary-derived FSH and hMG are both effective in inducing follicular growth and maturation. However, the relative importance of FSH and luteinizing hormone (LH) in this process is still being investigated in light of evidence that LH plays only a minor role in folliculogenesis, and the fact that too much LH during follicular development and in the periovulatory phase may have detrimental effects on fertilization, cleavage, and embryo quality. Despite these observations, physicians are still undecided on which gonadotropin preparation to use for their patients. The ideal method of resolving this dilemma is to compare the two preparations in a randomized trial. There have been several such studies published since 1986, but in none of them has a statistically significant result been obtained, largely because of small sample sizes. The results of an interim analysis of a much larger study were published a few years ago demonstrating weak evidence in favor of FSH.[1] However, in the absence of a sufficiently large randomized trial, the question of which gonadotropin preparation is more efficacious has remained unresolved.

An alternative approach to deal with this

problem of an equipose is to review the evidence systematically and pool the data using meta-analysis, a strategy that is becoming increasingly popular. The principles of meta-analysis are described in this chapter by applying them to the question of the comparative efficacy of FSH and hMG.

## SYSTEMATIC REVIEW AND META-ANALYSIS

A systematic review is a structured process involving the assembly of information from a complete literature search on a subject and its reduction into a concise summary. The review establishes whether the scientific findings are consistent and can be generalized across populations, settings, and treatment variations, or whether the findings vary significantly by particular subgroups.[2]

The importance of power in a study to detect clinically important differences in outcome events between two interventions is not an intuitively obvious concept to many clinicians. Consequently, many of the studies that are undertaken have inadequate sample sizes to allow inferences to be made with confidence. The following arithmetic calculation highlights the difficulty faced with conducting trials of sufficient power to test the efficacy of interventions in ART. To detect a clinically important absolute difference in clinical pregnancy rate per cycle of 5% between the group with the new intervention and the control group (with expected pregnancy rates per cycle of 20% and 15%, respectively), a sample of approximately 1450 subjects will be required (with $\alpha = 0.05$ and $\beta = 0.2$ in a two-tailed analysis). Average clinics, with an annual volume of 200–300 cycles, will need to run the trial for at least 5–7 years before accrual is complete and conclusive evidence can be obtained. Clearly, it may not be feasible to conduct a trial of this size in a single centre because its duration is likely to be prohibitive unless it is undertaken as a multi-center task. Instead, investigators run smaller studies (in the hope of detecting large differences in event rates) and, when the magnitude of the effect size detectable by such studies is not observed, they erroneously conclude that no difference exists between the two interventions (as has been the case in the FSH and hMG comparison). By referring to a systematic review, one is likely to avoid making premature (and often incorrect) conclusions about the benefit (or lack thereof) of a particular intervention.

There are several steps that are important and necessary in conducting a good systematic review. These steps include: clearly specifying a research question; outlining a search strategy to identify and select relevant studies; assessing the validity of each study; extracting and pooling the data; and summarizing the results so that appropriate inferences can be made. Thus, the final common pathway for a systematic review is a quantitative summary of the data, or meta-analysis, which is a statistical procedure that integrates the results of several independent studies deemed on predefined criteria to be eligible for pooling.

The purpose of the statistical methods involved is simple and is geared towards answering four basic questions:

1. Are the results of the different studies similar?
2. To the extent that they are similar, what is the best overall estimate of the effect size?
3. How precise and robust is this estimate?
4. Can dissimilarities be explained?[3]

## IDENTIFICATION OF STUDIES

The search for studies should be comprehensive and involve several sources. The MEDLINE database is an important first step, but even the most thorough MEDLINE search is likely to miss many studies. Therefore, the search should include other databases such as Embase, Citation Index and the Cochrane Controlled Clinical Trials register. Scanning the reference list of selected publications and review articles often yields useful papers not identified in the initial search. Another important source of relevant studies is the 'gray' literature which includes theses, internal reports, non-peer-reviewed journals, and pharmaceutical industry files. Abstracts of major scientific meetings should be scanned for trials that have recently been completed. Authors of primary studies may be contacted for more information and further clarification and details of their studies. Finally, peer consultation should be sought for any remaining articles.

The search for studies comparing FSH and hMG involved all these strategies, including scanning the MEDLINE database covering the period 1983–98.

## STUDY INCLUSION

The method for selecting studies should be reliable and reproducible so that it can be replicated by others who wish to confirm the findings. The process starts with a clearly focused clinical question that outlines the population being studied, the active and control interventions being compared, and the outcome event that is of interest to the investigators. Selection criteria are then established that are sensible and reflect the clinical question, and provide direction for an efficient and comprehensive search of the literature. The criteria for including studies in the review can be narrow or fairly broad. With narrow inclusion criteria the risk for false-positive or false-negative results is increased because the number of data in the review are limited. Such criteria also preclude the study of appropriate and clinically important subgroups. In contrast, broad inclusion criteria increase the likelihood of finding wide variation in the results of the different studies (that is, heterogeneity), making analysis and interpretation of the results more challenging. As such a search will usually identify more studies than are relevant to the clinical question, a process for sorting through the materials is required so that the relevant studies can be retrieved. The specificity of the retrieval process will depend on the explicit nature of the criteria established; any ambiguity will result in errors and consequently a reduction in the accuracy of this process.

The selection criteria should be specific in several categories. The type of patient to be studied should include a clear description of the disease or condition and its severity, and the setting from which the population is drawn (for example, community or hospital). The main and control interventions should be specified with respect to the timing, dose, duration, and route of administration for medical therapies or the exact details if the intervention is surgical. The outcomes of interest should be unambiguous, clinically relevant, and defined clearly to avoid confusion while allowing generalization of the findings. The type of design will depend on the clinical question being asked and can be in the experimental or descriptive domains.

Although publication of studies in languages other than English may create problems with retrieval and translation, the decision must be made before beginning the search process about whether non-English literature sources should be accessed.

Meta-analysts can simplify the task of selecting articles from a large sample of studies by first reviewing all of the titles, then the abstracts, and then the complete articles, excluding studies at each step that do not meet one or more selection criteria. Although this process is quite efficient, there is a risk of missing relevant articles, the content of which may not be clearly specified in the title or abstract.

Only randomized or quasi-randomized controlled studies of hMG versus FSH in in vitro fertilization (IVF) or intracytoplasmic sperm injection (ICSI) were included. Studies were considered whether or not the ovarian stimulation regimen included gonadotropin-releasing hormone agonists (GnRH agonists). Studies using the short, flare-up protocol, in which GnRH agonists were started in the follicular phase of the treatment cycle, or the long suppression protocol, in which GnRH agonists were started in either the follicular phase of the treatment cycle or the luteal phase of the preceding cycle, were included.

Studies in which clomiphene citrate was used together with gonadotropins were excluded, because the mechanism of action of clomiphene citrate involves an increase in endogenous LH production. Also excluded were studies from which the data could not be extracted separately for each of the two treatment arms. Studies in which embryo transfer was performed more than 2 days after oocyte retrieval were excluded, because the effect of LH on the oocyte/embryo may be nullified by selecting only those embryos that have developed in vitro beyond 48 hours.

The primary outcome of interest was the clinical pregnancy rate per cycle commenced.

## DATA SUMMARIZATION

The data to be combined in a meta-analysis can be classified as either categorical or continuous in type. Categorical data are usually in binary format involving a yes/no categorization (for example, pregnancy or no pregnancy). Continuous data are expressed over a range of values (for example, serum progesterone levels after administration of vaginal progesterone suppositories). Binary data can be summarized by using several measures of treatment effect, including risk ratio (RR) and odds ratio (OR), both of which provide estimates of the relative efficacy of an intervention, and risk difference, which describes the absolute benefit of the intervention.

Continuous data can be summarized by the raw mean difference between the two groups if measured on the same scale (for example, serum progesterone), by the standardized mean difference when different scales are used (for example, different pain scales), or by the correlation coefficient between two continuous variables.[3]

## GRAPHIC DISPLAY

Results from each study are displayed graphically as point estimates and their confidence intervals. The odds ratio tree shown in Figure 1 displays the results summarized by the odds ratios and their 95% confidence intervals (95%CI) from the 11 studies[4–14] that met the inclusion criteria. The 95%CI indicates that, if the study were repeated 100 times, the interval would contain the true (but unknown) effect of

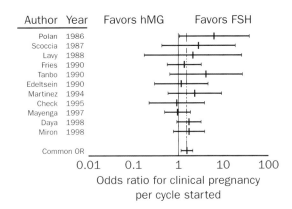

**Figure 1** Odds ratios for clinical pregnancy per IVF cycle started in studies comparing FSH with hMG. Breslow–Day test for homogeneity of treatment effect: $\chi^2 = 7.68$; $p = 0.660$. (See refs 4–14.)

the intervention on 95 occasions. The solid vertical line representing an OR of unity represents a null effect. If the 95%CI includes this odds ratio (that is, the horizontal line representing the confidence interval crosses the vertical line at OR = 1.0), then the observed effect of the experimental manoeuvre is not statistically significant at the conventional level of $p < 0.05$. The confidence interval in 10 of the 11 studies crossed the vertical line, indicating that the estimates of treatment effect were not statistically significant in these studies. A logarithmic scale is used for plotting the ORs, as shown in Figure 1, so that the confidence interval will extend symmetrically around the point estimate.

## ASSESSMENT OF STATISTICAL HETEROGENEITY IN THE EFFECT OF TREATMENT

Before the data from the studies can be combined, it is necessary to determine whether the effect of treatment is homogeneous across all studies. This assessment of homogeneity involves calculating the magnitude of statistical diversity that exists in the effect of treatment among the different studies.

Statistical heterogeneity may be attributable to two sources. First, study results can differ because of random sampling error; in other words, even if the true (but known) effect is the same in each study, the observed effect size will vary randomly around this true, fixed effect (that is, within study variance). Second, each study sample may have been drawn from a different population and, even if each enrolled a large number of subjects, the effect size would vary as a consequence. These results differ because of between-study variation and are called random effects. By examining the degree of homogeneity in the outcomes of the studies, using a statistical test based on the $\chi^2$ distribution, it can be determined whether the results of the study reflect a single underlying effect or a distribution of effects. If the test shows that significant heterogeneity is not present, then the differences among studies can be assumed to be a consequence of sampling variation and the data can be combined using a fixed effects model. On the other hand, in the presence of significant heterogeneity of treatment effect, a random effects model for combining the data is advocated.

In most of the gonadotropin studies an effect in favor of FSH was observed. The test of homogeneity of treatment effect performed using the method of Breslow and Day[15] was not significant ($\chi^2 = 7.68$; $p = 0.660$) indicating that no study had a statistically significant OR that was worse or better than the overall pooled OR. In Figure 1, the dashed vertical line plotted through the combined OR crosses the horizontal lines of all individual studies, indicating that this set of studies is homogeneous from the treatment effect point of view.

## ESTIMATING THE COMBINED EFFECT OF TREATMENT

The results of the different studies can be pooled by statistically combining them into an overall summary estimate. A simple arithmetic average of the results from all the studies would give misleading results depending on the relative contributions of small and large studies. The results of the smaller studies are more likely to be influenced by chance and, therefore, should be given less weight in the combined estimate. The methods employed in a meta-analysis take this fact into consideration by using a weighted average of the results, whereby the larger studies have more influence than the smaller ones. In general, in the fixed effects model, which considers all variability to be the result of random variation, each study is weighted by the inverse of its own variance, which is a function of the study size and the number of events in the study. The random effects model includes the between-study variance with the within-study variance because it assumes that there is a different underlying effect for each study. Consequently, the confidence interval around the combined effect is wider than with the fixed effects model.

Pooling the results of the gonadotropin studies using the fixed effects model produced a combined OR of 1.55 (95%CI = 1.15–2.10; $p = 0.004$). Thus, the meta-analysis indicated that the use of FSH for ovarian stimulation was associated with a significantly higher clinical pregnancy rate per cycle commenced.

## SENSITIVITY ANALYSIS

A sensitivity analysis is a useful method to assess the robustness of the findings by calculating the combined effect using both the fixed and random effects models. In situations where there is very little variation among studies, the combined effect will be virtually identical, although the confidence interval will be slightly wider with the random effects model.

In the gonadotropin example, the combined OR using the random effects model was 1.54 and the 95%CI was 1.13–2.09, an estimate that was very similar to that obtained with the fixed effects model. Thus, the sensitivity analysis demonstrates that the results from this meta-analysis are robust.

## METHODOLOGIC QUALITY

The methodologic quality of each study can be rated according to several predetermined criteria, such as method of randomization, concealment of treatment allocation, blinding of patients and investigators, completeness of follow-up of study subjects, and so on. It has been suggested that such quality scores should be incorporated into the meta-analysis so that the validity of the studies can be evaluated and ranked by methodologic rigor.[16-19] Combined effect estimates can then be calculated for studies of similar quality, thereby providing another type of sensitivity analysis. Theoretically, the better quality studies should provide more reliable effect size estimates. Although such an approach to meta-analysis seems logical, to date no scale or scoring system has been shown to correlate consistently with treatment efficacy.[20] Nevertheless, there is some evidence to suggest that studies of poor quality may overestimate the effect of treatment.[21,22]

## SUBGROUP ANALYSIS

Subgroup analysis is a useful method to address supplementary questions but requires the data for the subgroups to be available for each study. This approach may also provide insight into the sources of clinical heterogeneity (that is, variability resulting from clinical factors associated with the medical disorder being studied). However, it should be recognized that the power of subgroup analyses is reduced because the sample sizes are much smaller in the subgroups. Consequently, the results should be interpreted with caution, although they may be used as tools to generate hypotheses worthy of further testing.

In the gonadotropin example, there were three studies in which GnRH agonists were not used. A subgroup analysis was undertaken to calculate effect sizes with and without the use of GnRH agonists. The magnitude of the combined effect size was much larger when GnRH agonists were not used (OR = 3.65; 95%CI = 1.25–10.66) compared with when GnRH agonists were used (OR = 1.44; 95%CI = 1.06–1.97). One interpretation of this finding is that, in the absence of GnRH agonists, exogenous LH from hMG administration supplements the endogenous secretion of LH, thereby substantially increasing the total amount of LH present during follicular development with hMG. Consequently, the proposed deleterious effect of excessive LH on the likelihood of pregnancy would be enhanced, whereas in the presence of GnRH agonists, because only exogenously administered LH from the hMG preparation is present, the extent of the adverse effect would be lower.

## PUBLICATION BIAS

Publication bias occurs when completed studies are unavailable for analysis. In some situations, studies may not be retrieved despite a thorough search of potential databases. However, the amount of bias resulting from this problem has not been quantified. Another potential source of bias stems from the fact that studies with 'negative' results or a null effect are less likely to be published because either the investigators are not willing to submit them for publication, or the peer reviewers and editors are not sufficiently impressed by the findings to warrant their publication.[23,24] Using a questionnaire survey of a sample of reviewers and authors of a journal in social psychology, it was determined that approximately half the researchers whose work rejected the null hypothesis of no treatment effect would submit their results for publication, compared with only 6% of researchers whose work failed to reject the null hypothesis.[25] Furthermore, results of 'positive' studies are sometimes reported more than once, increasing the probability that they will be located in a search (that is, multiple publication bias).[26] These findings suggest that the published literature is likely to be biased with reports of 'positive' findings, the bias affecting smaller studies to a greater degree than larger studies. Although publication bias is difficult to eliminate, its presence may be suggested by two diagnostic techniques.

The first technique, which is called the 'fail-safe $n$' method, is a statistical calculation that allows the estimation of the number of 'negative' unpublished studies that would have to exist to nullify the significance of the pooled estimate of the effect size. This procedure, which is based on a method of combining $Z$ values, can estimate the number of such studies that have been tucked away in file-drawers in investigators' offices.[27] From this information the meta-analyst has to make a judgment whether the 'fail-safe $n$' is sufficiently large to render the possibility unlikely that this number of unpublished studies exists, or the number is so small that there is concern about the reliability of the combined results which should be interpreted cautiously.

For the gonadotropin studies, the 'fail-safe $n$' was found to be 10, a number that is relatively large and obviates the concern of publication bias being present (considering that the search to date has only identified 11 relevant studies for inclusion in the meta-analysis).

The second technique involves a visual exploration of the data using an inverted funnel plot.[28] In this method, a scatterplot is used to display the relationship between the effect estimate of each study and its sample size. The funnel plot is based on the fact that precision in estimating the underlying treatment effect will increase as the sample size of the study increases. Thus, one could plot the precision of the study (calculated as the inverse of the standard error) against the effect measure (for example, OR, RR, etc), as shown in Figure 2 for the gonadotropin studies. The results from smaller studies would be expected to be widely scattered along the bottom of the graph, whereas the spread from larger studies would be narrower. Therefore, in the absence of bias, the plot will have the appearance of a symmetrical inverted funnel, whereas, in the presence of bias, the funnel plot will be skewed and asymmetrical.

Applying the funnel plot test to the data from the gonadotropin studies, it can be seen quite readily from Figure 2 that the scatterplot follows a symmetrical, inverted funnel distribution. This graphic display provides reassuring

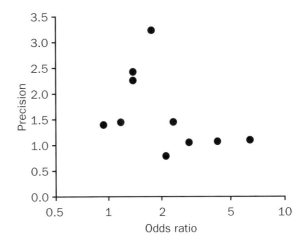

**Figure 2** Funnel plot for studies comparing FSH with hMG.

evidence that the meta-analysis is likely to be free from publication bias.

Although funnel plot asymmetry increases the likelihood of publication bias, it should be acknowledged that there may be other reasons for the asymmetry. For example, the 'negative' studies may end up being published in languages other than English and, if the search is limited only to the English literature, these studies will be missed (that is, English language bias).[29] 'Negative' studies are likely to be cited infrequently and, therefore, are more likely to be missed in the search for relevant studies (that is, citation bias).[30,31] Multiple publication bias will make it more likely that 'positive' studies will be located.[26] The methodologic rigor with which the study is conducted may affect the outcome, with lower quality studies showing larger effects.[22,32,33] The statistic used to measure the effect of the intervention may affect funnel plot symmetry, as is seen with high event rates, in which the use of the OR will be associated with an overestimation of the relative reduction, or increase, in risk.[34] Thus, in high-risk patients, if smaller studies are undertaken rather than larger studies, then the effect estimate may be large thereby producing a skewed funnel plot. Finally, the observed asymmetry may rise purely by chance.

The funnel plot is a useful simple visual test for the likelihood of bias in meta-analyses. However, the capacity to detect bias is limited when the assessment is based on only a few small studies. The results of such meta-analyses should be interpreted cautiously.

## CUMULATIVE META-ANALYSIS

Cumulative meta-analysis is a good method for assessing the effect of each study.[35] It is defined as the repeated performance of meta-analysis to calculate an updated pooled effect each time a new study becomes eligible for inclusion in the previously collected series of studies. The accumulation of studies may proceed according to the year of completion or publication of the study, the event rate in the control group, the size of the study, the size of the difference between the treated and control groups in the study, some quality score that has been assigned to the study, or other co-variates such as drug dosage or time to treatment.[35] The sequential pooling may be undertaken in ascending or descending order.

Cumulative meta-analysis is best interpreted in the Bayesian framework. The prior probability (that is, the prior belief) is generated by the pooled results of all prior studies, and the posterior probability is derived by adding the results of the new study to those of the others. This posterior probability then becomes the new prior probability for more data to be added when they become available.

Advantages of a cumulative meta-analysis include the determination of whether the pooled estimate has been robust over time and the point in time when statistical significance of the pooled result is reached. In this way, the benefit (or harm) of an intervention can be identified as early as possible by routinely updating the meta-analysis with each new study, thereby guiding clinical decisions in an efficient manner.

The cumulative meta-analysis of the gonadotropin data is shown in Figure 3. It can

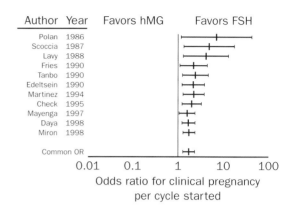

**Figure 3** Cumulative meta-analysis of studies comparing FSH with hMG. (See refs 4–14.)

be seen that, although a statistically significant difference was observed from the outset, the pooled effect was consistently significant from 1990 onwards (that is, after 285 patients had been enrolled). The magnitude of the pooled effect did not change much from 1995 onwards; the addition of more studies merely improved the precision of this estimate. Consequently, any further studies comparing FSH with hMG may now be superfluous and unnecessarily costly, if not unethical,[36] given that a significant treatment effect is evident from the meta-analysis.

## SEQUENTIAL MONITORING BOUNDARIES

There are no guidelines for assessing whether or not the statistical evidence from a meta-analysis is conclusive, other than the conventional interpretation of the $p$ value obtained after each new study is added to the analysis. However, the amount of information or the number of patients studied in the analysis are not fully accounted for by the $p$ value, that is, the same weight is assigned to the $p$ value whether it is based on a few data or on substantially greater numbers of data. There is no pre-defined sample size established before the analysis is commissioned. Furthermore, the repeated assessment of the accumulating evidence raises a methodologic concern regarding multiple testing and the overall *p* value for significance assigned to the cumulative meta-analysis.

The calculation of the optimal information size (OIS) to establish monitoring boundaries has been proposed as a strategy to introduce rules for the interpretation of evidence that is accumulated prospectively.[37] The concept of the OIS is that it provides a reference point for monitoring the progress of the cumulative meta-analysis by applying techniques adapted from those used to monitor individual clinical trials. The OIS can be calculated by first outlining the conditions for an optimal cumulative meta-analysis. These conditions include: the assumed control event rate for the outcome of interest; the treatment effect size expected; and the type I and type II error rates. As with a single trial that is designed to be definitive in answering a specific research question, so too must a cumulative meta-analysis be convincing by expecting it to contain enough information to have a high probability of detecting a clear effect of the intervention being studied.[37] This effect size proposed should be biologically plausible and medically worthy, while at the same time minimizing the possibility that false-positive results may occur from premature conclusions. Thus, the meta-analysis of the results of the series of studies should be so clear that further studies of the question would be redundant and unnecessary. Consequently, the type I error rate (α level) may be set at a more stringent level than the conventionally used level of 0.05 (for example, 0.01 or 0.001). Similarly, the power level may be set much higher than the conventional one of 80% (for example, 90% or 95%). These more conservative conditions can then be applied to any standard formula for sample size calculation to derive the OIS.

Various types of monitoring boundaries have been developed for the assessment of the strength of the accumulating evidence when multiple interim analyses are performed on the data from single trials. However, with meta-analyses one cannot be certain that one will become aware of all the studies ever to be conducted on any specific question. Therefore, similar interim analysis methods should be applied to cumulative meta-analyses. The α spending function provides one method that can be readily adapted for monitoring cumulative meta-analysis.[38] The boundary is characterized by the rate at which α is spent and by past decision times, but is independent of the number of future decision times.[37] The function itself is monotonously non-decreasing and is indexed by the accumulating information, with the information index representing the proportion of the maximum achieved.[37] The maximum amount of information is achieved when the OIS that has been calculated for the cumulative meta-analysis is reached. As mentioned above, the OIS is deliberately inflated by using more extreme α and β levels to account for any potential heterogeneity in the effect of treatment. The monitoring boundaries so developed provide a more robust approach compared with nominal *p* values for viewing the statistical evidence from a meta-analysis.[37] Upon crossing these statistical boundaries with the accumulated evidence, it can be concluded that future studies may not be needed for a particular intervention because convincing results have been achieved with the existing studies. Until this point is reached, however, further information from randomized trials would still be required.

This approach has been applied to the gonadotropin trials by assuming a clinical pregnancy rate per cycle with hMG of 15% and a relative improvement of 25% with FSH (to a clinical pregnancy rate of 18.5%). Using these event rates, the OIS required was calculated to be 2470 patients. It can be seen from Figure 4 that the monitoring boundary was crossed after the tenth consecutive trial, demonstrating that convincing evidence for the preference of FSH was available with the existing studies. It should be remembered that the difference in clinical pregnancy rate between FSH and hMG which was used for the OIS calculation was

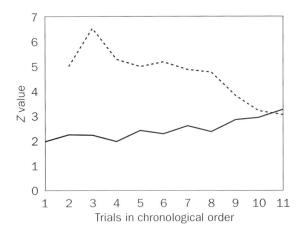

**Figure 4** Sequential monitoring boundary for cumulative meta-analysis of studies comparing FSH with hMG. Assumptions are: clinical pregnancy rate of 15% with hMG and 20% with FSH (that is, a relative treatment effect of 33%), two-sided $\alpha$ value of 0.05, and power of 90%. The cumulative Z value (solid line) crosses the sequential monitoring boundary (dotted line) after the tenth trial, demonstrating convincing evidence of the higher efficacy of FSH.

much smaller than that observed. Thus, the superiority of FSH for ovarian stimulation in IVF cycles has been unequivocally established.

## CONCLUSIONS

The ideal method of evaluating efficacy of a therapeutic intervention is by conducting a randomized trial with sufficient power to detect a clinically important effect size and with ad hoc stratification for the co-variates that influence outcome. However, in the field of reproductive medicine the size of the effect that is generally observed is relatively small, making it necessary to conduct large trials, a requirement that is often not feasible in single centers. Consequently, smaller studies are undertaken leading investigators to make premature and often incorrect inferences about the value of the interventions. A solution to this problem of underpowered studies is to perform a systematic review with meta-analysis of the data, so that the role of treatment can be ascertained and any factors leading to heterogeneity in the effect of treatment can be explored. By combining data from several studies, the statistical power is increased, thereby reducing the probability of false-negative results.

Meta-analyses provide robust estimates of treatment effect with enhanced precision and can help answer questions that single trials may have been unable to answer because of insufficient power. However, despite this advantage, there has been much criticism about the validity of the technique as a result of bias. The elements that are necessary to carry out a proper systematic review and meta-analysis are detailed in this chapter and illustrated using the example of comparing the efficacy of FSH with hMG for ovarian stimulation in IVF cycles. The major strength of a meta-analysis is in its ability to promote critical thinking. If done properly, the results of a meta-analysis can be very useful in influencing clinical decisions.

## REFERENCES

1. Daya S, Gunby J, Hughes EG, Collins JA, Sagle MA. Randomized controlled trial of follicle stimulating hormone versus human menopausal gonadotropin in in-vitro fertilization. *Hum Reprod* 1995;**10**:1392–96.
2. Mulrow CD. Rationale for systematic reviews. *BMJ* 1994;**309**:597–9.
3. Lau J, Ioannidis JPA, Schmid CH. Quantitative synthesis in systematic reviews. *Ann Intern Med* 1997;**127**:820–6.
4. Polan ML, Daniele A, Russell JB, DeCherney AL. Ovulation induction with human menopausal gonadotropin compared to human urinary follicle-stimulating hormone results in a significant shift in follicular fluid androgen levels without discernible differences in granulosa–luteal cell function. *J Clin Endocrinol Metab* 1986;**63**:1284–91.
5. Scoccia B, Blumenthal P, Wagner C, Prins G, Scommegna A, Marut EL. Comparison of uri-

nary human follicle-stimulating hormone and human menopausal gonadotropins for ovarian stimulation in an in vitro fertilization program. *Fertil Steril* 1987;**48**:446–9.

6. Lavy G, Pellicer A, Diamond MP, DeCherney AH. Ovarian stimulation for in vitro fertilization and embryo transfer, human menopausal gonadotropin versus pure human follicle simulating hormone: a randomized prospective study. *Fertil Steril* 1988;**50**:74–8.

7. Fries N, Hedon B, Eld J, et al. Etude randomisée FSH pure/hMG dans les stimulations ovariennes sous agonistes (Protocole Long) (abstract). *Contraception-fertilité-sexualité* 1990;**18**:670.

8. Tanbo T, Dale PO, Ejekshus E, Haug E, Abyholm T. Stimulation with human menopausal gonadotropin versus follicle-stimulation hormone after pituitary suppression in polycystic ovarian syndrome. *Fertil Steril* 1990;**53**:798–803.

9. Edelstein MC, Brzyski RG, Jones GS, Simonetti S, Muasher SJ. Equivalence of human menopausal gonadotropin and follicle-stimulating hormone stimulation after gonadotropin-releasing hormone agonist suppression. *Fertil Steril* 1990;**53**:103–6.

10. Martinez F, Coroleu B, Torello MJ, Maristany P, Parera N, Barri PN. Estudio comparative de estimulacion con FSH frente a hMG bajo analogos de la GnRH en fecundacion in vitro. *Actualidid en Reproduccion Humana* 1994;**3**:16–21.

11. Check JH, O'Shaughnessy A, Nazari A, Hoover L. Comparison of efficacy of high-dose pure follicle-stimulating hormone versus human menopausal gonadotropins for in vitro fertilization. *Gynecol Obstet Invest* 1995;**40**:117–19.

12. Mayenga JM, Belaisch-Allart J, Chouraqui A, Tesquier L, Serkine AM, Cohen J, Plachot M, Mandelbaum J. Essai controle randomise comparatif entre l'hormone folliculostimulante humaine (FSH-HP) et les gonadotrophines menopausiques humaines (hMG) en focondation in vitro. *Contracept Fertil Sex* 1997;**25**:371–4.

13. Daya S. hMG versus FSH: is there any difference. In: *Ovulation Induction Update '98* (Filcori M, Flamigni C, eds). Proceedings of the 2nd World Conference on Ovulation Induction, Bologna, Italy, 12–13 September 1997. New York: The Parthenon Publishing Group, 1998: 183–92.

14. Miron P, Casper R. Comparison between highly purified-FSH and hMG for superovulation in women undergoing in vitro fertilization. *J Soc Obstet Gynecol Canada* 1998;**20**:283–8.

15. Breslow NE, Day NE. *Statistical Methods in Cancer Research*, Vol 1. *Analysis of data from retrospective studies of disease.* Lyon: AIRC Scientific Publications, 1980.

16. Chalmers TC, Smith H Jr, Blackburn B, et al. A method for assessing the quality of a randomized control trial. *Controlled Clin Trials* 1981; **2**:31–49.

17. Mulrow CD, Linn WD, Gaul MK, Pugh JA. Assessing quality of a diagnostic test evaluation. *J Gen Intern Med* 1989;**4**:288–95.

18. Detsky AS, Naylor CD, O'Rourke K, McGreer AJ, L'Abbe KA. Incorporating variations in the quality of individual randomized trials into meta-analysis. *J Clin Epidemiol* 1992;**45**:255–65.

19. Moher D, Jadad AR, Nichol G, Penman M, Tugwell P, Walsh S. Assessing the quality of randomized controlled trials: an annotated bibliography of scales and checklists. *Controlled Clin Trials* 1995;**16**:62–73.

20. Emerson JD, Burdick E, Hoaglin DC, Mosteller F, Chalmers TC. An empirical study of the possible relation of treatment differences to quality scores in controlled randomized clinical trials. *Controlled Clin Trials* 1990;**11**:339–52.

21. Jadad AR, McQuay HJ. Meta-analyses to evaluate analgesic interventions: a systematic qualitative review of their methodology. *J Clin Epidemiol* 1996;**49**:235–43.

22. Schultz KF, Chalmers I, Hayes RJ, Altman DG. Empirical evidence of bias. Dimension of methodologic quality associated with estimates of treatment effects in controlled trials. *JAMA* 1995;**273**:408–12.

23. Dickersin K, Chan S, Chalmers JC, Sacks HS, Smith H Jr. Publication bias in clinical trials. *Controlled Clin Trials* 1987;**8**:343–53.

24. Dickersin K. The existence of publication bias and risk factors for its recurrence. *JAMA.* 1990; **263**:1385–9.

25. Greenwald AG. Consequences of prejudice against the null hypothesis. *Psychol Bull* 1975; **82**:1–20.

26. Huston P, Moher D. Redundancy, disaggregation, and the integrity of medical research. *Lancet* 1996;**347**:1024–6.

27. Rosenthal R. The 'File Drawer Problem' and tolerance for null results. *Psychol Bull* 1979; **86**:638–41.

28. Egger M, Smith GD, Schneider M, Minder C. Bias in meta-analysis detected by a simple, graphical test. *BMJ* 1997;**315**:629–34.

29. Egger M, Zelleweger-Zähner T, Schneider M, Junker C, Lengeler C, Antes G. Language bias in

randomized controlled trials published in English and German. *Lancet* 1997;**350:**326–9.

30. Gotzsche PC. Reference bias in reports of drug trials. *BMJ* 1987;**295:**654–6.

31. Ravnskov U. Cholesterol lowering trials in coronary heart disease: frequency of citation and outcome. *BMJ* 1992;**305:**15–19.

32. Chalmers TC, Celano P, Sacks HS, Smith H. Bias in treatment assignment in controlled clinical trials. *N Engl J Med* 1983;**309:**1358–61.

33. Altman DG. The scandal of poor medical research. *BMJ* 1994;**308:**283–4.

34. Egger M, Smith GD, Phillips AN. Meta-analysis. Principles and procedures. *BMJ* 1997;**315:**1533–7.

35. Lau J, Schmid CH, Chalmers TC. Cumulative meta-analysis of clinical trials builds evidence for exemplary medical care. *J Clin Epidemiol* 1995;**48:**45–57.

36. Murphy DJ, Povar GJ, Pawlson LG. Setting limits in clinical medicine. *Arch Intern Med* 1994;**154:**505–12.

37. Pogue JM, Yusuf S. Cumulating evidence from randomized trials: utilizing sequential monitoring boundaries for cumulative meta-analysis. *Controlled Clin Trials* 1997;**18:**580–93.

38. Lau KKG, De Mets DL. Discrete sequential boundaries for clinical trials. *Biometrika* 1983;**70:**659–63.

# 17

# GnRH agonist protocols: which one to use?

Juan Balasch, Colin M Howles

Use of GnRH agonists in in vitro fertilization • Use of GnRH agonists in COH and intrauterine insemination • Conclusions

Until the early 1980s, there was little need for the use of ovulation-inducing drugs in normally ovulating women. However, this viewpoint has dramatically changed as a result of assisted reproduction technologies (ART), which are being increasingly used for the treatment of both female and male infertility. It is now universally accepted that multiple follicular development is a prerequisite for a successful assisted reproduction technique. The reasons for this are based on abundant clinical evidence from most assisted reproduction centres of the world which indicate the benefits, in terms of pregnancy outcome, of having multiple gametes and embryos available.

Two major groups of normal ovulatory women became candidates for augmented follicular development: women undergoing ART treatment cycles, and women receiving controlled ovarian stimulation (COS) cycles, usually in association with artificial insemination, to overcome non-tubal infertility. In both of these circumstances, gonadotrophin-releasing hormone (GnRH) agonist analogues have been used and developed as adjuncts in the process of control and augmentation of folliculogenesis and ovulation.[1] However, although the use of

GnRH agonists together with gonadotrophins has gained widespread popularity and is the sole method of ovarian stimulation in many ART programmes today, a number of controversial issues remain concerning their mode of use. Different GnRH agonist drugs, routes of administration and protocols have been used for in vitro fertilization (IVF). This chapter analyses these aspects of GnRH agonist therapy.

## USE OF GnRH AGONISTS IN IN VITRO FERTILIZATION

### Rationale for use in IVF

Although the initial IVF success was achieved through the laborious monitoring of a natural cycle,[2] at present (almost) all IVF programmes use some form of ovarian stimulation to induce multiple follicular growth. This is because it increases the chances of having at least one embryo to transfer and also because, in general, the more oocytes that are retrieved, the more embryos will be available for transfer and cryopreservation, with an associated increase in pregnancy rates. Initially, most programmes used a combination of gonadotrophins, with or without the addition of clomiphene citrate. However, the vast majority of patients undergoing IVF treatment have a normal ovulatory cycle and therefore controlled ovarian hyperstimulation (COH) must be superimposed upon this cycle. This means that these ovarian stimulation regimens require close monitoring of follicular growth and are associated with a high incidence (5–25%) of premature luteinizing hormone (LH) surge, which has negative consequences on the IVF success rate, the convenience of treatment for the patient and the cost of the procedure. Some patients have even had inadvertent spontaneous ovulation immediately before oocyte recovery.[3,4] Consequently, gonadotrophin-only regimens are associated with a high cancellation rate, often approaching 30%.[5,6]

In 1984, the use of the GnRH agonist buserelin, in association with human menopausal gonadotrophin (hMG) was first reported for ovarian stimulation in IVF.[7] Since then, numerous reports have suggested that the use of GnRH agonists prevents spontaneous LH surges, and improves follicular response, fertilization and implantation rates, leading to a net increase in the pregnancy rate per cycle.[3,8] In addition, GnRH agonists are also currently used in virtually every ART programme to simplify patient scheduling. According to the World Collaborative Report on IVF of 1995,[9] the stimulation regimen most frequently used (85% of reported cycles) was the combination of GnRH agonists and gonadotrophins whereas clomiphene citrate (alone or associated with gonadotrophins) was used in only 7.5% of IVF cycles. The use of hMG or follicle-stimulating hormone (FSH) was reported in 12.5% of cycles, and spontaneous cycles were mentioned in 1.1% of cases.

The general principles of combined pituitary suppression/gonadotrophin ovarian stimulation therapy have been presented by Insler and Lunenfeld (Figure 1).[10] It is important to note that the combined therapy consists of two distinctive elements: pituitary suppression and ovarian stimulation. Each element exerts specific positive and adverse effects, and only the combination of all the corollaries produces the desired end result. Much of the early experience with the use of this combined therapy was focused on women defined by various criteria

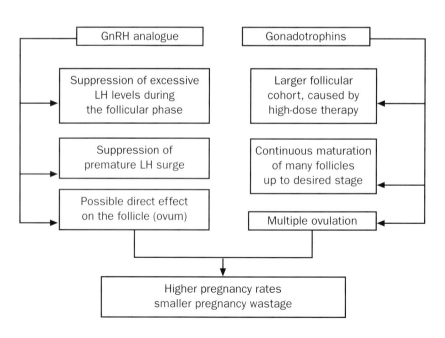

**Figure 1** General principles of combined pituitary suppression/ovarian stimulation therapy. (From Insler and Lunenfeld.[10])

as 'poor responders', but application was soon extended to all women entering cycles of ART.[1] However, although the advantage of using GnRH agonists in patients who were poor or abnormal responders in previous treatment cycles using gonadotrophins alone or in combination with clomiphene citrate was unquestionable,[3,11–13] what became a contentious issue was whether GnRH agonists should be routinely used for all patients undergoing IVF treatment.[4,14] In this regard, the clinician should ask two questions (1) Is there a benefit to using GnRH agonists in combination with gonadotrophins? and (2) if an GnRH agonist is to be used, what is the preferred GnRH agonist regimen?

## Routine use of GnRH agonists for all patients undergoing IVF

There are numerous studies (several of which were prospective, randomized, clinical trials) comparing the use of GnRH agonists with treatment cycles without analogues (reviewed in the literature[1,3,15]). However, as previously stressed[1,5] it is difficult to make a direct comparison of studies because these trials differ in the specific GnRH agonist used, the type of stimulation, the regimen received by the control population, and the entry criteria, with some controlling for prior IVF attempts, diagnosis and fertility history, and others examining patients who have failed prior IVF attempts. Many of these studies suffer from small sample size, adding to the problem of statistical significance in the interpretation of the results.[5] One of the difficulties in comparing outcomes of these reports is the correction needed for numbers of embryos transferred and number of implantations. Only a few studies have included implantation rate in the comparison of outcomes. In addition, outcomes need to be corrected for the additional benefit experienced or anticipated with transfer of cryopreserved embryos, and this is seldom included in the calculation of outcomes compared per cycle.[1] It was not, therefore, surprising that there was no uniform consensus among different IVF programmes as to which stimulation regimen was superior.[16–19]

In an attempt to resolve the GnRH agonist debate, a meta-analysis of randomized and quasi-randomized studies was reported in 1992 by Hughes et al.[20] This review concluded that pregnancy rates per cycle were increased with the use of GnRH agonists by a factor of 80–127%. The spontaneous abortion rate was similar with and without GnRH agonist use. Cancellation rate was decreased (largely as a result of an abolition of spontaneous LH surges), and the number of oocytes retrieved was increased with use of analogues. However, significantly more gonadotrophin was given, adding to cycle cost. Similarly, in a later study[21] involving 2893 women and designed to investigate the effect of ovarian stimulation regimens on cumulative conception and livebirth rates after IVF, the superiority of GnRH agonist/ gonadotrophin treatment over gonadotrophin alone or in combination with clomiphene citrate was confirmed. Tan et al[21] suggested two possible reasons for the significantly better results afforded by the GnRH agonist treatment. First, premature LH surges requiring cancellation of the treatment cycle, and premature ovulation before oocyte recovery was scheduled, were avoided. Moreover, although pituitary desensitization does not prevent asynchronous follicular growth, if it does occur, ovarian stimulation can be safely continued until there are an adequate number of follicles that reach the optimal size for egg recovery.

If the meta-analysis conclusions are to be accepted and pregnancy rates appear higher with GnRH agonist use, one must then ask which is the preferred GnRH agonist regimen for an IVF general programme.

## Protocols for GnRH agonist use in ovarian stimulation for IVF

GnRH agonists are used in several different superovulation protocols, including ultrashort protocol; short (flare) protocol; long protocols; and a long-term down-regulation (ultralong) protocol (Figure 2) – a topic that has recently

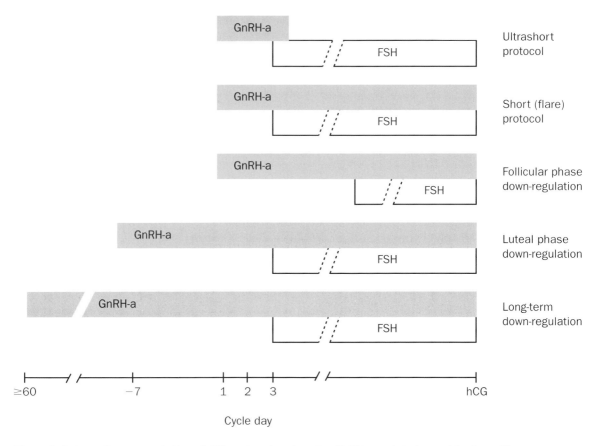

**Figure 2** Schematic representation of different protocols using GnRH agonists in combination with gonadotrophins for ovarian stimulation in IVF.

been reviewed.[5,22,23] The ultrashort and short protocols make use of the initial stimulatory effect of gonadotrophin secretion to promote follicular development before pituitary desensitization occurs. The GnRH agonist is usually given from cycle day 1 for 3 days in the ultrashort protocol or until injection of human chorionic gonadotrophin (hCG) in the flare protocol. Gonadotrophin stimulation is started 2–3 days after initiation of the GnRH agonist administration. Some have recommended starting both the GnRH agonist and FSH on cycle day 3 when using the short protocol, in order to enhance follicular recruitment and growth.[24] The short regimens have the advantage of a shorter dura-

tion of stimulation, with fewer ampoules of gonadotrophins used and lower costs. Accurate timing of hCG administration remains critical, however, when the short protocol is used, although there is no significant advantage in the precise timing of hCG injection after pituitary desensitization with the GnRH agonist which has led to the notion that IVF therapy can be greatly simplified.[4]

In the long protocols, the intent is to achieve pituitary down-regulation with suppression of endogenous gonadotrophins, before stimulation with exogenous FSH. There are two regimens of the long protocol: the long follicular protocol involves the administration of

GnRH agonists from cycle day 1 for approximately 12–14 days, whereas the long luteal protocol involves the administration of GnRH agonists from the midluteal phase of the previous cycle. The timing of GnRH agonist administration during the menstrual cycle may influence the time course of ovarian suppression, but results in the literature are contradictory when midluteal and early follicular phase protocols are compared regarding treatment time and effectiveness to obtain ovarian areas.[11,25-28] Thus, within-patient studies are needed to clarify this subject. Luteal start makes GnRH agonist use more practical, allows a more flexible timing of the IVF cycle and simplifies IVF therapy.[29] Despite early concerns regarding inadvertent exposure of concept to GnRH agonists when the midluteal phase initiation is used,[30] a condition that occurs in around 1% of IVF cycles,[31] later studies suggested that the occurrence of these pregnancies is not merely coincidental and that GnRH agonists may even have a positive role in fecundity through the mechanisms of LH action in the corpus luteum.[31] The rates of spontaneous abortion and ectopic pregnancy are not increased and nor is the rate of congenital anomalies.[31] The follicular regimen has the advantage that it does not require confirmation of the luteal phase and is preferable in oligo-ovulatory patients. However, some patients receiving daily follicular GnRH agonist treatment respond with a pronounced agonist response, stimulation of follicular cysts and persistently elevated oestradiol levels.[5]

Recently, an ultralong protocol was proposed for use in women with endometriosis undergoing IVF, on the basis of high pregnancy rates observed in a non-randomized study in which patients with severe endometriosis underwent 4 months of GnRH agonist induced amenorrhoea before IVF.[32] However, we have found that the use of long-term (4 months) down-regulation does not improve pregnancy rates in an IVF general programme, although it increased the total dose of gonadotrophins used.[33]

Although the recipes for each of the above protocols are easy to understand, the decision about which protocol to use in an IVF general programme becomes more complex and has prompted different comparative studies, each with their own biases. Very recently, Daya[23] reviewed the evidence to determine whether there are any systematic differences among the various protocols and methods of administration of GnRH agonists. Only randomized or quasi-randomized trials comparing the different GnRH agonist protocols were identified for review. The outcome measure was clinical pregnancy per cycle started and the typical odds ratio (OR) was calculated as the weighted estimate of the treatment effect across studies. A second analysis was carried out after including all valid studies comparing different doses and methods of administration of the GnRH agonist. Logistic regression was used to identify predictors of pregnancy.

Nineteen trials (comprising 2061 cycles) were selected that compared the long with the short protocol, four trials (comprising 648 cycles) comparing long with ultrashort protocols, and five trials (comprising 497 cycles) comparing follicular and luteal phase long protocols. In addition, there were 10 trials (comprising 1253 cycles) comparing depot versus daily administration of the GnRH agonist. These trials were subjected to a meta-analysis and the overall results are shown in Figure 3.[23]

The comparison between the long protocol and short/ultrashort protocols of GnRH agonist administration clearly shows that the former significantly increases the probabilities of conception and live birth after IVF. When long versus ultrashort protocols were compared, the overall combined OR (with its 95% confidence interval or CI) was 1.47 (1.02–2.12; $p = 0.039$), representing an absolute treatment effect of 6.7% (0.8–13.2%) and a relative treatment effect of 32.6% in favour of the long protocol. Similarly, the comparison between the long and short protocols showed that the overall combined OR was 1.26 (1.10–1.56; $p = 0.036$). This result represented an absolute treatment effect of 3.6% (0.5–7.3%) and a relative treatment effect of 18.8% in favour of the long protocol. Subgroup analyses of each of the two different types of long protocol compared with the short

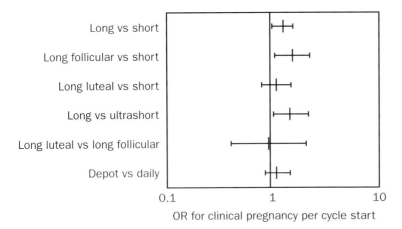

**Figure 3** Overall results of different meta-analyses of GnRH agonist protocols in IVF. (From Daya.[23])

protocol demonstrated a significant preference for the long follicular protocol. There were six trials using the long follicular protocol (comprising 758 cycles). The combined OR was 1.53 (1.06–2.22; $p = 0.008$), representing an absolute treatment effect of 6.3% and a relative treatment effect of 42.6% in favour of the long follicular protocol. The comparison of long luteal versus short protocols involved 11 trials (comprising 986 cycles) and produced a combined OR of 1.10 (0.82–1.49; $p = 0.51$), representing an absolute treatment effect of 0.5% and a relative treatment effect of 2.1%; this indicates that there was no significant difference between these two protocols. However, it should be noted that no significant differences were found in the meta-analysis when the long luteal and long follicular protocols were compared (relative risk, $R = 0.93$ [0.41–2.11] representing an absolute treatment effect of 0.52% [−7.07–8.11%] and relative treatment effect of 2.1%).

There are a number of possible reasons for the superiority of the long protocol.[4,23] It has been shown that the initial agonist action of the GnRH agonist (as seen with the ultrashort and short protocols) cause a rise in LH concentrations. This may lead to corpus luteum stimulation ('rescue') and an increase in thecal androgen levels which may impair folliculogenesis.[34] The degree of LH suppression is variable with the short protocol and it has been pointed out that 5–10% of cycles may be complicated by a premature LH surge.[4,23] Exposure of the developing follicle to inappropriately high levels of LH may adversely affect the reproductive process[35,36] and this may be particularly evident in patients in whom the return to baseline levels of LH takes longer than average, for example, in those who have polycystic ovaries or in whom cysts form as a result of GnRH agonist administration.[4]

In his exploratory analysis, Daya[23] included 42 trials (and a total of 4491 cycles) in which various protocols, routes of administration, type and dose of GnRH agonists were used. Several univariate analyses were performed. As no difference was observed between the long follicular and long luteal protocols, these groups were combined for all subsequent analyses. The overall crude pregnancy rates (shown in Figure 4) demonstrated a statistically significant linear trend ($p = 0.002$), with the long protocol being the best.

Improved outcome of IVF when the long GnRH agonist regimen is employed has also been reported in the French IVF Registry results for 1995 (FIVNAT)[37] (Table 1). The long protocol consistently resulted in a significantly higher pregnancy rate compared with either the short protocol or no agonist. Also the data demonstrated that adding exogenous LH (in the form of human menopausal gonadotrophin

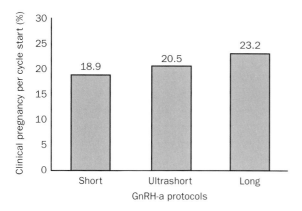

**Figure 4** Crude pregnancy rates using different GnRH agonist protocols in IVF. $\chi^2 = 9.60$; $p = 0.008$; $\chi^2$ for linear trend $= 9.54$; $p = 0.002$. (From Daya.[23])

[hMG]) was of no benefit in terms of pregnancy outcome. On the contrary, significantly more embryos were obtained after FSH stimulation whatever the agonist regimen used.

Finally, it should be noted that the meta-analysis by Daya[23] showed no difference between depot and daily administration of GnRH agonists. However, when the standard form (daily subcutaneous injections) and long-acting formulation (depot injection) of the same GnRH agonists have been compared for IVF, or cross-over studies were performed comparing short-acting and long-acting analogues in the same woman, better results have been shown in patients using the standard release formulation, including significantly higher implantation rates.[38,39] The concentration of the GnRH agonist in the follicular fluid increases with the duration of treatment and the longer ovarian exposure to higher doses of the analogue associated with the use of depot preparations exposes maturing oocytes and, later, young embryos to the peptide.[40] In addition, it should be stressed that, in a suppressed pituitary gland, the dose of the GnRH agonist needed to maintain suppression gradually decreases with the length of treatment;[25] the current practice of reducing the daily dose once ovarian suppression is evident is obviously possible with stan-

**Table 1 Outcome results according to type of protocol and gonadotrophin used ($n = 13\ 426$)[37]**

| Agonist protocol | Gonadotrophin | Embryos | Pregnancy/Oocyte recovery (%) |
|---|---|---|---|
| Short[a] | hMG | $3.8 \pm 3.5^c$ | 19.9 |
| | FSH | $4.7 \pm 4.3^d$ | 30.5 |
| | FSH/hMG | $3.3 \pm 3.1^c$ | 12.7 |
| Long[b] | hMG | $5.1 \pm 4.4^c$ | 24.9 |
| | FSH | $5.8 \pm 4.5^d$ | 28.3 |
| | FSH/hMG | $4.8 \pm 4.0^c$ | 24.1 |
| No agonist[a] | hMG | $2.8 \pm 2.6^c$ | 20.8 |
| | FSH | $3.9 \pm 3.1^d$ | 25.0 |
| | FSH/hMG | $3.3 \pm 2.8^c$ | 26.3 |

[b] vs [a] $p < 0.001$.
[d] vs [c] $p < 0.001$.

dard but not with depot formulations of GnRH agonists.

As reviewed by Daya in Chapter 16, GnRH agonists have an extrapituitary action including a direct inhibitory effect on steroidogenesis in human ovaries, and clinical studies have shown the usefulness of daily microdoses of GnRH agonists in enhancing follicular growth during ovulation induction with gonadotrophins in poor responders.[22,29] In fact, oversuppression of women with diminished ovarian reserve, and increased risk of the ovarian hyperstimulation syndrome (OHSS) in high responders, are potential disadvantages of adjunctive GnRH agonists in IVF stimulation protocols, mainly when the long protocol is used. Risk of the OHSS has to be taken into account, because a meta-analysis of the role of luteal phase support in IVF treatment concluded that the use of hCG is particularly beneficial in IVF cycles under pituitary suppression and appears to be superior to progesterone in this respect; however, the risk of the OHSS was significantly elevated when hCG was used.[41] The flare protocol has been advocated as a useful tool for patients who are poor responders to ovarian stimulation,[22] although others disagree.[4]

## Use of different GnRH agonists in IVF

A number of GnRH agonists have been approved for use in different countries. Previous studies have shown that different GnRH agonists are similarly effective in their ability to down-regulate the pituitary–ovarian axis function;[42] similar protocols using different GnRH agonists have yielded satisfactory results in IVF patients.[1,3,5] However, in vitro studies suggest that the inhibitory effect on ovarian steroidogenesis varies depending on the relative potency of the analogue used.[43] For hydrophobic GnRH agonists, there is a correlation between the hydrophobicity of substituents in position 6 and potency; in general, the potency increases with increasing hydrophobicity (Table 2).[44] Thus, they may have different effects on different human cells.

Comparisons have been made between different GnRH agonists for use in IVF cycles.

**Table 2 Structure and relative potency of GnRH agonist analogues**

| Name | Relative potency | \multicolumn{10}{c}{Amino acid sequence} | | | | | | | | | |
|------|------------------|---|---|---|---|---|---|---|---|---|----|
| | | 1 | 2 | 3 | 4 | 5 | 6 | 7 | 8 | 9 | 10 |
| | | Pyro-Glu | His | Trp | Ser | Tyr | Gly | Leu | Arg | Pro | Gly-NH$_2$ |
| GnRH | 1 | | | | | | | | | | |
| | 4 | | | | | | | | | | N-Et-NH$_2$ |
| | 4 | | | | | | D-Ala | | | | |
| | 14 | | | | | | D-Ala | | | | N-Et-NH$_2$ |
| Triptorelin | | | | | | | D-Trp | | | | |
| Leuprolide | 15 | | | | | | D-Leu | | | | N-Et-NH$_2$ |
| Buserelin | 20 | | | | | | D-Ser (tBu) | | | | N-Et-NH$_2$ |
| Nafarelin | | | | | | | D-Nal(2) | | | | N–Et-NH$_2$ |
| Deslorelin | 144 | | | | | | D-Trp | | | | N–Et-NH$_2$ |
| Histrelin | 210 | | | | | | D-His (ImBzl) | | | | N–Et-NH$_2$ |

Table 3 summarizes prospective randomized studies on the subject.[45–55] It is difficult to compare these studies directly because of differences in the selection of populations of patients, the specific GnRH agonist used with its appropriate route of administration, the treatment protocol used (both for GnRH agonists and gonadotrophin, including timing and dose) and the statistical significance of the study. No definite consensus of superiority is apparent from studies in Table 3; clearly, however, depot agonists have a more profound suppressive effect than daily injections. Intranasally administered GnRH agonists have a reduced absorption of 3–21% relative to subcutaneous and intravenous doses.[56] These differences may explain some of the results of the studies in Table 3.

## USE OF GnRH AGONISTS IN COH AND INTRAUTERINE INSEMINATION

As protocols using COH and intrauterine insemination (IUI) are used for women with non-tubal causes of infertility before progression to the more expensive and aggressive ART procedures, and because the addition of GnRH agonists to COH for IVF cycles improves the quality and/or quantity of oocytes obtained, especially in poor responders, it has been suggested that the addition of GnRH agonists for in vivo fertilization in COH/IUI cycles may also offer improved efficacy. However, the studies exploring this hypothesis are rather scanty and contradictory.

In the only prospective randomized study on the subject, including an 'unselected' subfertile population of normal ovulatory women initially presenting for hMG with IUI therapy, no significant differences were observed in subsequent cycle fecundity or live-birth rates between cycles treated with hMG alone or in conjunction with GnRH agonists (midluteal phase initiation).[57] In contrast, the retrospective work of Gagliardi et al[58] demonstrated a significant enhancement in both cycle fecundity and live births when GnRH agonist therapy was used. However, unlike the previous investigation,[57] in Gagliardi's study a 'selected' population was treated with GnRH agonists; the benefit of GnRH agonist therapy was evaluated in a preselected 'recalcitrant' subfertile population who had previously failed to conceive after several cycles (on average 3.2 cycles per patient) of hMG with IUI treatment. Finally, according to Manzi et al[59] only the selective use of GnRH agonists in those ('preselected') individuals who demonstrate premature luteinization during COH/IUI cycles results in a significant increase in the percentage of women conceiving a viable fetus.

When considering GnRH agonist adjunctive therapy in COH/IUI cycles, it should be remembered that most of these patients are women who ovulate normally, and augmented follicular development in such patients in cycles with no oocyte retrieval raise concerns about the development of the OHSS and high-order multiple pregnancies. For these reasons, analogues have been used much less commonly in COH/IUI cycles in normally ovulating women. On the other hand, in gonadotrophin ovulation-induction cycles at risk for the OHSS and multiple pregnancy, and where pituitary suppression is not used, a single subcutaneous injection of leuprolide acetate 0.5 mg may be an effective substitute for hCG as the ovulation inducing agent preventing those complications.[60]

## CONCLUSIONS

The widespread use of the GnRH agonists to control endogenous LH output and achieve augmentation of follicular development in most normally ovulating women has been the most exciting development of ovarian stimulation for IVF. Disadvantages, such as the requirement of additional medication and increased gonadotrophin dose and cycle cost, appear to be outweighed by the observed increase in ability to control the cycle, achievement of higher number of oocytes and embryos and improvement in pregnancy rates for most women. The long protocol of GnRH agonist administration not only increases pregnancy and live-birth rates, but also allows flexible timing for oocyte

**Table 3 Summary of prospective randomized studies comparing different GnRH agonists used in combination with gonadotrophins in ovarian stimulation for IVF**

| Author | Year | No. of patients | GnRH agonists compared | Treatment protocol | Results |
|---|---|---|---|---|---|
| Balasch et al[45] | 1992 | 70 | Buserelin s.c. Leuprolide s.c. | Long (midluteal) | Higher number of follicles punctured, oocytes retrieved, mature oocytes and embryos in group L |
| Parinaud et al[46] | 1992 | 246 | Buserelin s.c. Triptorelin s.c. Leuprolide s.c. | Long (cycle day 1) | E2 response lower in group B. Slightly higher pregnancy in group L |
| Penzias et al[47] | 1992 | 42 | Nafarelin i.n. Leuprolide s.c. | Long (cycle day 1) | Less ampoules of hMG used and more embryos frozen in group N |
| Tapanainen et al[48] | 1993 | 100 | Goserelin depot s.c. Buserelin i.n. | Long (midluteal) | More ampoules of hMG used and more side effects in group B |
| Dantas et al[49] | 1994 | 24 | Nafarelin i.n. Leuprolide s.c. | Long (midluteal) | E2 suppression level greater than 50 pg/ml in group N |
| Goldman et al[50] | 1994 | 108 | Buserelin i.n. Nafarelin i.n. | Long (midluteal) | Fewer ampoules of hMG used in group N |
| Lockwood et al[51] | 1995 | 240 | Buserelin i.n. Nafarelin i.n. | Long (midluteal) | Lower E2 levels on suppression and hCG days, and longer hMG treatment in group B. Time for down-regulation longer in group N |
| Oyensaya et al[52] | 1995 | 142 | Buserelin s.c. Goserelin depot s.c. | Long (cycle day 1–2) | Quicker pituitary suppression and higher pregnancy rate in group G |
| Tanos et al[53] | 1995 | 40 | Triptorelin s.c. Nafarelin i.n. | Long (midluteal) | Lower E2 suppression level and higher hMG dose, fertilization rate and extra embryos in group T |
| Avrech et al[54] | 1996 | 22 | Buserelin i.n. Nafarelin i.n. | Short | Higher plasma progesterone on hCG day in group N |
| Corson et al[55] | 1996 | 39 | Nafarelin i.n. Leuprolide s.c. | Long (midluteal) | No differences between groups. Pregnancy rate not reported |

(B), buserelin group; (L), leuprolide group; (T), triptorelin group; (N), nafarelin group; (G), goserelin depot group. s.c., subcutaneous; i.n., intranasal.

recovery and greatly simplifies IVF treatment. Most programmes reporting GnRH agonist use for IVF relied on midluteal phase initiation despite the lack of established data for superiority of this protocol (over early follicular start), but it is considered a more flexible and convenient way of programming the cycle because the start of gonadotrophin therapy is independent of the onset of menstruation. When selecting for the type of GnRH agonist to be used, the most favourable option seems to be single subcutaneous daily injections of the available GnRH agonist that has fewer effects on the ovary.

GnRH agonists have also been explored as adjunctive therapy in COH/IUI cycles, but their role is clearly of much less benefit when oocyte retrieval is not intended.

## REFERENCES

1.  Martin MC. Ovulation augmentation in the normally ovulatory woman. *Semin Reprod Endocrinol* 1993;**11:**209–16.
2.  Steptoe PC, Edwards RG. Birth after reimplantation of a human embryo. *Lancet* 1978;**ii:**366.
3.  Loumaye E. The control of endogenous secretion of LH by gonadotrophin-releasing hormone agonists during ovarian hyperstimulation for in-vitro fertilization and embryo transfer. *Hum Reprod* 1990;**5:**357–76.
4.  Tan SL. Gonadotrophin-releasing hormone agonists in assisted reproductive therapy. *Hum Reprod* 1996;**11**(suppl):137–42.
5.  Hardy RI, Hornstein MD. Ovulation induction with gonadotropin releasing hormone agonists. *Semin Reprod Endocrinol* 1995;**13:**22–31.
6.  Fleming R, Coutts JRT. Induction of multiple follicular development for IVF. *Br Med Bull* 1990;**46:**596–615.
7.  Porter RN, Smith W, Craft IL, et al. Induction of ovulation for in vitro fertilization using buserelin and gonadotrophins. *Lancet* 1984;**ii:**1284–5.
8.  Hughes EG, Fedorkow DM, Daya S, Sagle MA, Van de Koppel P, Collins JA. The routine use of gonadotropin-releasing hormone agonists prior to in vitro fertilization and gamete intrafallopian transfer: a meta-analysis of randomized controlled trials. *Fertil Steril* 1992;**58:**888–96.
9.  de Mouzon J, Lancaster P. World Collaborative Report on in vitro fertilization – 1993. *XVth World Congress on Fertility and Sterility*, Montpellier, September 17–22, 1995.
10. Insler V, Lunenfeld B. Application of GnRH analogues in the treatment of female infertility. In: *GnRH Analogues: The state of the art, 1993* (Lunenfeld B, Insler V, eds). Casterton Hall, Carnforth: The Parthenon Publishing Group, 1993: 37–48.
11. Serafini P, Stone B, Kerin J, Batzolin J, Quinn P, Marrs RP. An alternate approach to controlled ovarian hyperstimulation in 'poor responders': pretreatment with a gonadotropin-releasing hormone agonist. *Fertil Steril* 1988;**49:**90–5.
12. Sharma V, Williams J, Collins W, Riddle A, Mason B, Whitehead M. The sequential use of a luteinizing hormone-releasing hormone (LH-RH) agonist and human menopausal gonadotropins to stimulate folliculogenesis in patients with resistant ovaries. *J In Vitro Fertil Embryo Transfer* 1988;**5:**38–42.
13. Cummins JM, Yovich JM, Edinsinghe WR, Yovich JL. Pituitary down-regulation using leuprolide for the intensive ovulation management of poor prognosis patients having in vitro fertilization (IVF) related treatments. *J In Vitro Fert Embryo Transfer* 1989;**6:**345–52.
14. Tan SL, Dodds JE. Gonadotropin-releasing hormone agonists in ovulation induction. In: *The Ovary: Regulation, dysfunction and treatment* (Filicori M, Flamigni C, eds). Amsterdam: Elsevier Science, 1996: 403–12.
15. Schmidt-Sarosi C. GnRH agonists in in vitro fertilization and embryo transfer. *Infertil Reprod Med Clin North Am* 1993;**4:**83–98.
16. Antoine JM, Salat-Baroux J, Alvarez S, et al. Ovarian stimulation using human menopausal gonadotrophins with or without LHRH analogues in a long protocol for in vitro fertilization: a prospective randomized comparison. *Hum Reprod* 1990;**5:**565–9.
17. Lejeune B, Barlow P, Puissant F, Delvigne A, Vanrusselberge M, Leroy F. Use of buserelin acetate in an in vitro fertilization program: A comparison with classical clomiphene citrate-human menopausal gonadotropin therapy. *Fertil Steril* 1990;**54:**475–81.
18. Ferrier A, Rasweiler J, Bedford JM, Prey K, Berkeley AS. Evaluation of leuprolide acetate

and gonadotropins for in vitro fertilization or gamete intrafallopian transfer. *Fertil Steril* 1990;**54:**90–5.

19. Dor J, Ben-Shlomo I, Levran D, Rudak E, Yunish M, Mashiach S. The relative success of gonadotropin-releasing hormone analogue, clomiphene citrate, and gonadotropin in 1099 cycles of in vitro fertilization. *Fertil Steril* 1992;**58:**986–90.

20. Hughes EG, Federkow DM, Daya S, Sagle M, de Koppel P, Collins J. The routine use of gonadotropin-releasing hormone agonists prior to in vitro fertilization and gamete intrafallopian transfer: a meta-analysis of randomized controlled trials. *Fertil Steril* 1992;**58:**888–96.

21. Tan SL, Maconochie N, Doyle P, et al. Cumulative conception and live-birth rates after in vitro fertilization with and without the use of long, short, and ultrashort regimens of the gonadotropin-releasing hormone agonist buserelin. *Am J Obstet Gynecol* 1994;**171:**513–20.

22. Kowalik A, Barmat L. Gonadotropin-releasing hormone agonists as adjuncts to gonadotropins in follicular stimulation for in vitro fertilization. *Assist Reprod Rev* 1997;**7:**128–33.

23. Daya S. Optimal protocol for gonadotropin releasing hormone agonist use in ovarian stimulation. In: *In Vitro Fertilization and Assisted Reproduction* (Gomel V, Cheung PCK, eds). Bologna (Italy): Monduzzi Editore, 1997: 405–15.

24. Benavida CA, Blasco L, Tureck R, Mastroianni L, Flickinger GL. Comparison of different regimens of a gonadotropin-releasing hormone analog during ovarian stimulation for in vitro fertilization. *Fertil Steril* 1990;**53:**479–85.

25. Balasch J, Gómez F, Casamitjana R, Carmona F, Rivera F, Vanrell JA. Pituitary-ovarian suppression by the standard and half-doses of D-Trp-6-luteinizing hormone-releasing hormone depot. *Hum Reprod* 1992;**7:**1230–4.

26. Meldrum DR, Wisot A, Hamilton F, Gutlay AL, Huynh D, Kempton W. Timing of initiation and dose schedule of leuprolide influence the time course of ovarian suppression. *Fertil Steril* 1988;**50:**400–7.

27. Pellicer A, Simón C, Miró F, et al. Ovarian response and outcome of in-vitro fertilization in patients treated with gonadotrophin-releasing hormone analogues in different phases of the menstrual cycle. *Hum Reprod* 1989;**4:**285–9.

28. Ron-El R, Herman A, Golan A, van der Ven H, Caspi E, Diedrich K. The comparison of early follicular and midluteal administration of long-acting gonadotropin-releasing hormone agonist. *Fertil Steril* 1990;**54:**233–7.

29. Meldrum DR. Ovarian stimulation for assisted reproductive technology. *Infertil Reprod Med Clin North Am* 1993;**4:**643–52.

30. Serafini P, Batozofin J, Kerin J, Marrs R. Pregnancy: a risk to initiation of leuprolide acetate during the luteal phase before controlled ovarian hyperstimulation. *Fertil Steril* 1988; **50:**371–2.

31. Balasch J, Martinez F, Jové I, et al. Inadvertent gonadotrophin-releasing hormone agonist (GnRHa) administration in the luteal phase may improve fecundity in in-vitro fertilization patients. *Hum Reprod* 1993;**8:**1148–51.

32. Marcus SF, Edwards RG. High rates of pregnancy after long-term down-regulation of women with severe endometriosis. *Am J Obstet Gynecol* 1994;**171:**812–17.

33. Fabregues F, Balasch J, Creus M, et al. Long-term down-regulation does not improve pregnancy rates in an in-vitro fertilization program. *Fertil Steril* 1998; in press.

34. Filicori M, Flamigni C, Cognigni GE, et al. Different gonadotropin and leuprorelin ovulation induction regimens markedly affect follicular hormone levels and folliculogenesis. *Fertil Steril* 1996;**65:**387–93.

35. Howles C, Macnamee MC, Edwards RG, Goswamy R, Steptoe PC. Effect of high tonic levels of luteinizing hormone on outcome of in-vitro fertilization. *Lancet* 1986;**ii:**521–2.

36. Balen A, Tan SL, Jacobs HS. Hypersecretion of luteinizing hormone: a significant cause of infertility and miscarriage. *Br J Obstet Gynaecol* 1993;**100:**1082–9.

37. FIVNAT. Stimulation de l'ovulation. *Contracept Fertil Sex* 1996;**24:**710–12.

38. Vauthier D, Lefebvre G. The use of gonadotropin-releasing hormone analogs for in vitro ferilization: comparison between the standard form and long-acting formulation of D-Trp-6-luteinizing hormone-releasing hormone. *Fertil Steril* 1989;**51:**100–4.

39. Devreker F, Govaerts I, Bertrand E, Van den Bergh M, Gervy C, Englert Y. The long-acting gonadotropin-releasing hormone analogues impaired the implantation rate. *Fertil Steril* 1996;**65:**122–6.

40. Loumaye E, Coen G, Pampfer S, Vankrieken L, Thomas K. Use of gonadotropin-releasing hormone agonist during ovarian stimulation leads

to significant concentration of peptide in follicular fluids. *Fertil Steril* 1989;**52**:256–63.

41. Soliman S, Daya S, Collins J, Hughes EG. The role of luteal phase support in infertility treatment: a meta-analysis of randomized trials. *Fertil Steril* 1994;**61**:1068–76.

42. Insler V, Lunenfeld B, Potashnik G, Levy J. The effect of different LH-RH agonists on the levels of immunoreactive gonadotropins. *Gynecol Endocrinol* 1988;**2**:305–12.

43. Miró F, Sampaio MC, Tarín JJ, Pellicer A. Steroidogenesis in vitro of human granulosaluteal cells pretreated in vivo with two gonadotropin releasing hormone analogs employing different protocols. *Gynecol Endocrinol* 1992;**6**:77–84.

44. Conn PM, Crowley WF. Gonadotropin-releasing hormone and its analogues. *N Engl J Med* 1991;**324**:93–103.

45. Balasch J, Jové I, Moreno V, Civico S, Puerto B, Vanrell JA. The comparison of two gonadotropin-releasing hormone agonists in an in vitro fertilization program. *Fertil Steril* 1992;**58**:991–4.

46. Parinaud J, Oustry P, Perineau M, Rème JM, Monroziès X, Pontonnier G. Randomized trial of three luteinizing hormone-releasing hormone analogues used for ovarian stimulation in an in vitro fertilization program. *Fertil Steril* 1992;**57**:1265–8.

47. Penzias AS, Shamma FN, Gutmann JN, Jones EE, DeCherney AH, Lavy G. Nafarelin versus leuprolide in ovulation induction for in vitro fertilization: a randomized clinical trial. *Obstet Gynecol* 1992;**79**:739–42.

48. Tapanaienen J, Hovatta O, Juntunen K, et al. Subcutaneous goserelin versus intranasal buserelin for pituitary down-regulation in patients undergoing IVF: a randomized comparative study. *Hum Reprod* 1993;**8**:2052–5.

49. Dantas ZN, Vicino M, Balmaceda JP, Asch RH, Stone SC. Comparison between nafarelin and leuprolide acetate for in vitro fertilization: preliminary clinical study. *Fertil Steril* 1994;**61**:705–8.

50. Goldman JA, Dicker D, Feldberg D, Ashkenazi J, Voliowich I. A prospective randomized comparison of two gonadotrophin-releasing hormone agonists, nafarelin acetate and buserelin acetate, in in-vitro fertilization-embryo transfer. *Hum Reprod* 1994;**9**:226–8.

51. Lockwood GM, Pinkerton SM, Barlow DH. A prospective randomized single-blind compara-

tive trial of nafarelin acetate with buserelin in long-protocol gonadotrophin-releasing hormone analogue controlled in-vitro fertilization cycles. *Hum Reprod* 1995;**10**:293–8.

52. Oyensaya OA, Teo SK, Quah E, Abdurazak N, Lee FY, Cheng WC. Pituitary down-regulation prior to in-vitro fertilization and embryo transfer: a comparison between a single dose of Zoladex depot and multiple daily doses of Suprefact. *Hum Reprod* 1995;**10**:1042–4.

53. Tanos V, Friedler S, Shushan A, Strauss N, Hetsroni I, Lewin A. Comparison between nafarelin acetate and D-Trp-6-LHRH for temporary pituitary suppression in in vitro fertilization (IVF) patients: a prospective study. *J Assist Reprod Genet* 1995;**12**:715–19.

54. Avrech OM, Goldman GA, Pinkas H, et al. Intranasal nafarelin versus buserelin (short protocol) for controlled ovarian hyperstimulation before in vitro fertilization: a prospective clinical trial. *Gynecol Endocrinol* 1996;**10**:165–70.

55. Corson SL, Gutmann JN, Batzer FR, Gocial B. A double blind comparison of nafarelin and leuprolide acetate for down-regulation in IVF cycles. *Int J Fertil Menopausal Stud* 1996;**41**:446–9.

56. Chrisp P, Goa KL. Nafarelin – A review of its pharmacodynamic and pharmacokinetic properties, and clinical potential in sex hormone-related conditions. *Drugs* 1990;**39**:523–51.

57. Dodson WC, Walmer DK, Hughes CL, Yancy SE, Haney AF. Adjunctive leuprolide therapy does not improve cycle fecundity in controlled ovarian hyperstimulation and intrauterine insemination of subfertile women. *Obstet Gynecol* 1991;**78**:187–90.

58. Gagliardi CL, Emmi AM, Weiss G, Schmidt CL. Gonadotropin-releasing hormone agonist improves the efficiency of controlled ovarian hyperstimulation/intrauterine insemination. *Fertil Steril* 1991;**55**:939–44.

59. Manzi DL, Dumez S, Scott LB, Nulsen JC. Selective use of leuprolide acetate in women undergoing superovulation with intrauterine insemination results in significant improvement in pregnancy outcome. *Fertil Steril* 1995;**63**:866–73.

60. Balasch J, Tur R, Creus M, et al. Triggering of ovulation by a gonadotropin releasing agonist in gonadotropin-stimulated cycles for prevention of ovarian hyperstimulation syndrome and multiple pregnancy. *Gynecol Endocrinol* 1994;**8**:7–12.

# 18

# The use of GnRH antagonists in IVF

Ricardo Felberbaum, Klaus Diedrich

**GnRH antagonists** • **GnRH antagonists within controlled ovarian hyperstimulation** • **Direct effects on ovarian gonadal steroid secretion** • **On the verge of a new era in ART** • **Conclusions**

The use of gonadotrophin-releasing hormone (GnRH) agonists for the purposes of ovarian stimulation marks the start of modern management of assisted reproduction. Premature surges of luteinizing hormone (LH) were responsible for a reduced effectiveness of ovarian stimulation by human menopausal gonadotrophin (hMG) in an in vitro fertilization (IVF) programme. At the same time they had a negative effect on oocyte and embryo quality, and as a result of this on the pregnancy rates obtained.[1,2] The introduction of agonist treatment has remedied most of these difficulties and drawbacks, and the rate of stimulated cycles that have to be terminated has been reduced to about 2%. It has become possible to plan ovulation induction, with the result that the psychological pressure on patients and physicians has been eased to some extent. Suppression of endogenous hormone production by GnRH analogues, followed by gonadotrophin stimulation, has developed from second-line into first-line therapy.

Different treatment schedules are applied today, including the so-called 'long protocol', which aims at complete pituitary suppression, and the 'short' and 'ultrashort' protocols, in which attempts are made to harvest the initial 'flare-up' of gonadotrophins for ovarian stimulation.[3,4] Among these protocols the 'long protocol' is generally the most effective and is currently used most often. In Germany, for instance, more than 70% of all performed stimulated cycles for assisted reproduction technique (ART) are carried out according to the long protocol (Deutsches IVF Register 1996, Bundesgeschäftsstelle Ärztekammer Schleswig-Holstein, Bad Segeberg). However, this treatment modality has the disadvantage of a long treatment period up to desensitization as well as an increased requirement for gonadotrophins.[5] As a result of their different pharmacological mode of action GnRH antagonists have opened new avenues to controlled ovarian hyperstimulation for IVF, avoiding the disadvantages of agonists.

## GnRH ANTAGONISTS

In parallel with the development of GnRH agonists, other analogues were synthesized that also bind to the pituitary GnRH receptors but are not functional in inducing the release of

| | 1 | 2 | 3 | 4 | 5 | 6 | 7 | 8 | 9 | 10 |
|---|---|---|---|---|---|---|---|---|---|---|
| Cetrorelix | Ac-D-Nal(2) | D-Phe(4Cl) | D/Pal | Ser | Tyr | D/Cit | Leu | Arg | Pro | D-Ala-NH$_2$ |
| Ganirelix | Ac-D-Nal(2) | D-Phe(4Cl) | D/Pal | Ser | Tyr | D-hArg(Et$_2$) | Leu | L-hArg | Pro | D-Ala-NH$_2$ |

**Figure 1** GnRH antagonists of the newest generation: cetrorelix and ganirelix.

gonadotrophins. These compounds are far more complex than GnRH agonists, with modifications of the molecular structure not only at positions 6 and 10, but also at positions 1, 2, 3 and 8. In comparison to the GnRH agonists, the pharmacological mechanism by which GnRH antagonists suppress the liberation of gonadotrophins is completely different. Although the agonists act through down-regulation of receptors and desensitization of the gonadotrophic cells, the antagonists bind competitively to the receptors and thereby prevent the endogenous GnRH from exerting its stimulatory effects on the pituitary cells. Without any intrinsic activity of these compounds, the initial 'flare-up' that is common in agonist treatment is completely avoided and within hours the secretion of gonadotrophins decreases. This mechanism of action is dependent on the equilibrium between endogenous GnRH and the applied antagonist. As a result of this, the effect of antagonists is highly dose dependent, in contrast to that of the agonists.[6,7]

Although in the first generation of GnRH antagonists allergic side effects resulting from an induced histamine release hampered their clinical development, modern GnRH antagonists such as cetrorelix (ASTA-Medica, Frankfurt/Main, Germany) or ganirelix (Organon, Oss, the Netherlands) seem to have solved these problems and thus may become available medically in the near future; they have been used at our department (Figure 1).

## GnRH ANTAGONISTS WITHIN CONTROLLED OVARIAN HYPERSTIMULATION

### Multiple dose application: the 'Lübeck protocol'

In 1991 Dittkoff et al[8] demonstrated that an GnRH antagonist applied for a short period in the midcycle phase is capable of suppressing the ovulation-inducing LH peak. They administered 50 µg Nal-Glu [AcD-Nal[1]-DPhe[2]-D-Pal[3]-Arg[5]-D-Glu[6]-D-Ala[10]]/kg body weight per day for 4 days in the midcycle phase of 10 healthy, normally cycling women. The LH peak failed to occur, oestradiol production came to a halt and follicular growth was interrupted. After discontinuing the antagonists, gonadal function normalized within days. Apparently the antagonists neither depleted the FSH and LH stores of gonadotrophic cells nor inhibited gonadotrophin synthesis.

Transferring these results into a protocol of controlled ovarian hyperstimulation with gonadotrophins for avoiding the onset of premature luteinization, the premature LH surge seems to be abolished by the daily administration of the GnRH antagonist cetrorelix from day

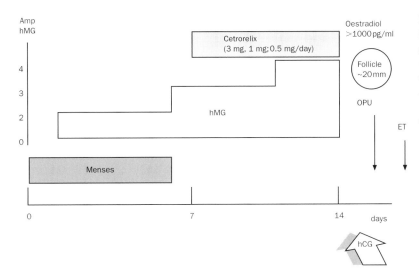

**Figure 2** Controlled ovarian hyperstimulation with gonadotrophins (hMG or recombinant FSH) and concomitant midcyclic GnRH antagonist treatment: the Lübeck protocol. ET, embryo transfer; OPU, oocyte pick up.

7 onwards up to ovulation induction: the 'Lübeck protocol' (Figure 2).

Starting on cycle day 2, patients have been treated with 150 IU hMG or, more recently, recombinant human FSH (rFSH) per day. From cycle day 7 until ovulation induction, patients were treated in the early stages of the development of this protocol with the rather high dosage of 3 mg cetrorelix/day, administered subcutaneously. On day 5 the dose of hMG was adjusted according to the individual ovarian response of the patient to the stimulation, assessed by oestradiol values and measurement of follicles. This treatment was continued until induction of ovulation with 10 000 IU hCG i.m., given when the leading follicle reached a diameter of 18–20 mm, measured by transvaginal ultrasonography, and when oestradiol values indicated a satisfactory follicular response.

To elucidate the question of the dosage necessary for sufficient suppression of the pituitary gland, three dosages were administered in two subsequent open phase II studies in accordance with the Lübeck protocol; the hormone profiles obtained, the number of oocytes retrieved, the fertilization rates and the consumption of hMG were compared. Thirty-five patients, all of whom had tubal infertility and no other infertility factors, were treated as described. No premature LH surge was observed (Figure 3). All

cycles could be evaluated. In the three dosage groups of FSH and LH, the course was similar with a profound suppression of LH and a less pronounced suppression of FSH; the latter probably resulted from the longer plasma half-life of the injected FSH. In the case of oestradiol there was a distinctly higher increase in concentration in the group treated with 0.5 mg cetrorelix/day, reaching an average maximum of 2165 pg/ml on cycle day 10, compared with 852 pg/ml in the 3-mg group and 1023 pg/ml in the 1-mg group. Although not significant, these differences seemed to indicate a slightly more sensitive reaction to stimulation with hMG in the group treated with the lowest dosage of antagonist compared with the others.

The fertilization rates of the recovered oocytes after conventional IVF were 45.3% in the 3-mg group, 53.2% in the 1-mg group and 67.7% in the 0.5-mg group, showing a clear tendency towards better results in the lower dosages. In the 3-mg group, 106 oocytes were recovered and 30 embryos were obtained, 36.7% of them being excellent according to morphological microscopic criteria. In the 1-mg group, 94 oocytes were collected and 28 embryos obtained, 53.6% being excellent. In the 0.5-mg group 127 oocytes were recovered and 27 embryos were obtained, 37% of them being excellent (Table 1).

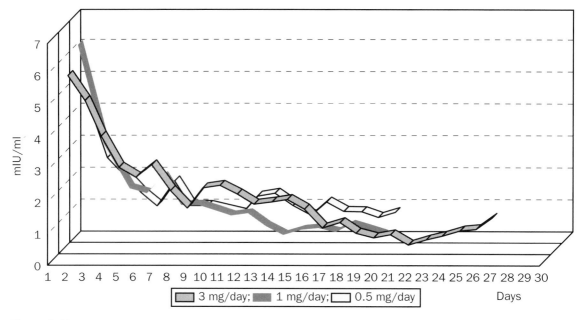

**Figure 3** Mean serum concentrations of LH (mIU/ml) under controlled ovarian hyperstimulation with hMG and concomitant cetrorelix administration at various dosages (series 1: 3 mg/day; series 2: 1 mg/day; series 3: 0.5 mg/day).

The average number of hMG ampoules used was 30 in the 3-mg group, 27 in the 1-mg group and 26 in the 0.5-mg group. These differences were not significant, and compare favourably with the number of ampoules used in an agonist 'long protocol'.[9]

Subsequent dose-finding studies also using 0.5 mg cetrorelix/day, 0.25 mg cetrorelix/day and 0.1 mg cetrorelix/day proved the efficacy and safety of 0.25 mg cetrorelix/day in avoiding premature LH surges, whereas at 0.1 mg cetrorelix/day premature LH surges could be observed.[10,11] In these studies intracytoplasmic sperm injection (ICSI) treatment of male subfertility of the partner was allowed, leading to fertilization rates within the range expected after

**Table 1** Recovered oocytes, fertilization rate, number and quality of embryos after controlled ovarian hyperstimulation with hMG and concomitant GnRH antagonist treatment in different dosages

|  | 3 mg | GnRH antagonist 1 mg | 0.5 mg |
|---|---|---|---|
| No. of oocytes | 106 | 94 | 127 |
| Fertilization rate (%) | 45.3 | 53.2 | 67.7 |
| No. of embryos | 30 | 28 | 27 |
| Excellent embryos (%) | 36.7 | 53.6 | 37 |

**Table 2 Stimulation and ICSI outcome in patients treated with hMG and concomitant midcyclic GnRH antagonist (cetrorelix) administration at 0.5 and 0.25 mg/day**

| | Cetrorelix | |
| | 0.5 mg/day | 0.25 mg/day |
| --- | --- | --- |
| No. of patients | 32 | 30 |
| No. of hMG ampoules | 35 | 33 |
| Duration of hMG treatment (days) | 11 | 10 |
| No. of follicles >15 mm the day of hCG | 10 | 10 |
| Estradiol the day of hCG (pg/ml) | 2122 | 2491 |
| Fertilization rate (%) | 55 | 59 |
| Cleavage rate (%) | 78 | 76 |
| Clinical pregnancy rate (%) | 31 | 30 |

From Albano et al.[11]
ICSI, intracytoplasmic sperm injection. hMG, human menopausal gonadotrophin; hCG, human chorionic gonadotrophin.

normal oocyte maturation. There were no significant differences regarding fertilization rates with two pronuclei, increase in oestradiol values, cleavage rate, clinical pregnancy rate per embryo transfer (ET) and implantation rate between the group treated with 0.5 mg cetrorelix/day and those treated with only 0.25 mg cetrorelix/day (Table 2). The clinical pregnancy rates per transfer were 30.7% in the 0.5-mg group and 29.6% in the 0.25-mg group. Interestingly, about 16% of the patients treated in this study with 0.5 mg cetrorelix/day and 10% of those treated with only 0.25 mg cetrorelix/day showed a significant rise in LH concentrations during the follicular phase, whereas progesterone concentrations remained low. These patients showed a significantly lower cleavage rate and no pregnancy occurred in this subgroup of patients. As these patients showed higher oestradiol concentrations than patients who did not have an increase in LH levels, these findings may suggest that an earlier administration of the antagonist may be necessary in high responders to avoid this LH increase, which may compromise the quality and maturity of the recovered oocytes.[11]

Up to now over 500 patients have been treated according to the Lübeck protocol. Neither oestradiol secretion nor follicular development was compromised by the GnRH antagonist cetrorelix at its minimal effective dose when controlled ovarian hyperstimulation (COH) was performed with recombinant RSH (K Diedrich and P Devroey, unpublished work). However, extreme suppression of LH secretion by high doses of GnRH antagonists could cause problems according to the two-cell/two-gonadotrophin hypothesis of follicular oestrogen production.[12] However, at lower doses (0.25 mg), this is not envisaged as a problem from work carried out to date.[13]

Preliminary data of a prospective multicentre study, comparing the results of COH according to the Lübeck protocol using cetrorelix at its minimal effective dose (0.25 mg/day) with those of a 'long' agonist protocol using buserelin show a reduced incidence of the ovarian hyperstimulation syndrome (OHSS). The incidence of the OHSS with no regard to its severity was considerably greater after buserelin treatment (10 of 74 patients, 13.5%) than after administration of cetrorelix (7 of 171, 4.1%). Similarly, the OHSS of patients who were WHO grades II–III and requiring hospitalization was seen more frequently in the buserelin group (5.4%) than in the cetrorelix group (K Diedrich and P Devroey, unpublished work). This may be attributed to the higher levels of oestradiol and larger numbers of small and medium-size follicles in the buserelin group.

### The 'French' protocol: single or dual administration

In parallel with the multiple dose administration, a different protocol for administration of GnRH antagonists in COH was developed by the French investigators Bouchard, Frydman and Olivennes; in this protocol the compound is used in a dosage of 2 mg or 3 mg as single or dual administration around day 9. The antagonist is injected when oestradiol levels reach 150–200 pg/ml and the follicle size is greater than 14 mm, which is usually the case on day 8 or 9 of the cycle[14,15] (Figure 4). They did not observe premature LH increases in any of the cycles studied and published to date. The injection of 3 mg cetrorelix was capable of preventing LH surges in the patients treated, intro-

ducing a very simple treatment protocol. Clinical pregnancy rates of over 30% per transfer are reported, which sounds very promising.

### Which protocol is the best?

To date over 1000 patients have been treated with these two protocols and both have proved to be safe and effective. The discussion about advantages and disadvantages of the two possible methods of administration is still going on, although we favour the Lübeck protocol because of its stability, which preserves all the advantages of the long agonist protocols that we are used to.

### Preserved pituitary response under GnRH antagonist treatment

Based on the mechanism of competitive binding, it is possible to modulate the degree of hormone suppression by the dose of antagonist administered. This preservation of the pituitary response as a result of competitive mechanisms could be demonstrated clearly by using an GnRH test during treatment with an GnRH antagonist. Three hours before injecting human chorionic gonadotrophin (hCG) for ovulation induction, 25 µg GnRH was administered in patients treated with 1 mg cetrorelix/day or

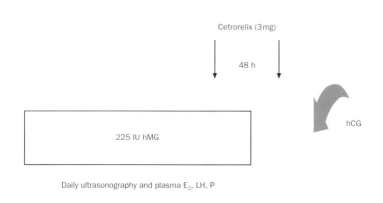

**Figure 4** Single or dual administration of the GnRH antagonist cetrorelix in COH around day 8: the 'French' protocol.[25]

Cetrorelix (3 mg)

48 h

hCG

225 IU hMG

Daily ultrasonography and plasma E$_2$, LH, P

0  1  2  3  4  5  6  7  8  9  10

3 mg cetrorelix/day. Blood samples for LH measurement were taken before and 30 min after GnRH treatment. The mean increase was 10 mIU/ml for the 3-mg group, whereas the average maximum concentration of serum LH in the 1-mg group was about 32.5 mIU/ml. These results were highly significant.[7] They could open new paths in the treatment of patients with higher risk of developing an OHSS, because it would allow the avoidance, in some cases, of deleterious effects of hCG administration. Ovulation induction is possible by GnRH agonists or native GnRH itself under antagonist treatment. This could help to lower the incidence rate of early onset OHSS.[16,17]

## DIRECT EFFECTS ON OVARIAN GONADAL STEROID SECRETION

Administered in a multidose fashion in the midcycle phase, the minimal effective daily dose of cetrorelix (0.25 mg/day) does not impair either oestradiol secretion in vivo or follicular development using hMG or recombinant FSH for COH. However, the importance of GnRH receptors on the granulosa lutein (GL) cells and the possible direct extrapituitary actions of the GnRH antagonists are still a matter of debate, although the function of these receptors remains unknown. It could be shown, in the rat, that GnRH antagonists are able to inhibit gonadal steroid secretion in vitro.[18] Thus

a negative impact of GnRH antagonists on gonadal steroid secretion during COH or in the luteal phase in IVF cycles could not be ruled out. We tried to evaluate the possible negative effect of the GnRH antagonist cetrorelix on the in vitro function of GL cells from IVF/ICSI patients in comparison to those GL cells obtained after COH according to a long agonist protocol. GL cells were obtained during oocyte pick-up in 22 patients, 11 of whom had been stimulated with hMG according to the long agonist protocol. Eleven patients had been treated with hMG and simultaneous administration of the GnRH antagonist cetrorelix at its minimal effective dose (0.25 mg/day). GL cells, separated and washed over 45% Percoll, were pooled and 100 000 cells/well were incubated in 1 ml Ham's F10 medium. After 24, 48 and 72 hours, basal secretion of oestradiol and progesterone was measured as well as gonadal steroid secretion stimulated by 20 IU hCG for 6 hours. The progesterone and oestradiol concentrations in the culture medium were measured in triplicate by an immunological assay. Continuous accumulation and stimulated secretion were compared in the two treatment groups. The GL cells from women treated with the GnRH antagonist showed no significant differences in either basal or stimulated gonadal steroid secretion in all cultures, compared with the GL cells obtained from women down-regulated by GnRH agonists (Figure 5). After 72 h of culture, the progesterone concentration in the medium

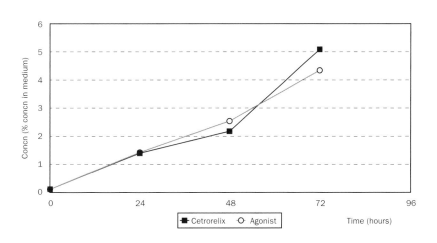

**Figure 5** Progesterone concentration in the medium of cultured granulosa lutein cells (100 000 per well in 1 ml Ham's F-10) after COH with hMG according to the 'long' agonist protocol and after COH according to the 'Lübeck' antagonist protocol. (Concentration as percentage of concentration in the medium after 1 hour of culture.)

had increased by 4326% in the agonist group and by 5063% in the cetrorelix group. Oestradiol concentration increases were 243% and 221%, respectively. Stimulation by hCG induced a twofold increase in progesterone concentration in the medium, compared with basal secretion, independent of the duration of culture. As a result it can be concluded that cetrorelix 0.25 mg/day, as used for COH in vivo, does not impair sexual steroid secretion of GL cells in vitro. It can therefore be assumed that the luteal phase in IVF cycles is not compromised by any direct effect of the GnRH antagonist. This is an important safety aspect of this new therapeutic approach to COH for IVF.

## ON THE VERGE OF A NEW ERA IN ART

Since 1992, we have experienced a veritable revolution in infertility treatment of the male as a consequence of the use of ICSI, with its excellent fertilization outcome irrespective of sperm morphology.[19,21] However, it seems timely to re-evaluate our therapeutic approach. Burden and risks for our patients have been put under the spotlight. The incidence of moderate and severe OHSS is still a serious problem. If the healthy single fetus pregnancy is the goal to aim for, a multiple pregnancy rate of over 20% demonstrates how often we fail in our attempt.

The development of recombinant gonadotrophins has marked an important scientific and therapeutic advance, and there is a hope that, through clinical use, there will be an overall improvement in the quality of stimulation[22] and final pregnancy rate.[23] After years of intensive clinical trials, GnRH antagonists are now to be introduced on to the market. They will probably replace GnRH agonists within COH for ART, because of the advantages that their mode of action have compared with agonist analogues.[24] However, the results are contradictory with regard to a possible reduction of gonadotrophins needed for sufficient ovarian stimulation.

Although the first studies to establish the dose for the multiple dose application, using 3 mg, 1 mg and 0.5 mg/day, seemed to show a clear tendency to lower amounts compared with the long agonist protocol, subsequent studies using 0.5 mg and 0.25 mg/day could not confirm these results. The French group, however, reported a reduction in gonadotrophins when compared with a long protocol of about 50%.[25]

Although our knowledge regarding oocyte and embryo quality after COH with concomitant GnRH antagonist treatment may still be limited, the rates of excellent embryos transferred seem to be satisfactory.[9,11] The long agonist protocol was regarded as advantageous because recruitment of a larger follicle cohort can be stimulated by exogenous gonadotrophins.[26] As in the short agonist protocol, this is not the case in protocols for COH using antagonists, where stimulation starts almost immediately after the follicular recruitment phase.[27]

The incidence of moderate and severe OHSS after COH with gonadotrophins and concomitant GnRH antagonist treatment seems to be favourable when compared with GnRH agonist long protocols (may be <2%) (K Diedrich and P Devroey, unpublished data). Overall, the most promising aspect of introducing GnRH antagonists into COH may be the possibility of making treatment duration shorter and more patient friendly. It may be possible to use a combination of clomiphene citrate with or without gonadotrophins. It has been shown that ovarian stimulation with clomiphene citrate only for the purpose of ICSI is perfectly feasible, applying the simplest and least aggressive form of stimulation.[28,29] The efficacy (in terms of pregnancy rates) would need to be assessed in large randomized clinical studies. However, such 'soft' protocols may be useful especially in patients who are at high risk of the OHSS. The first feasibility studies using cetrorelix for this purpose are in progress at the moment. Although the 'soft protocol' could be the safest method for COH in terms of patient burden and discomfort, it may be assumed that it could be compromised by a lower success rate in live births compared with long agonist protocol treatments, because it could reduce the number of embryos to be selected for transfer, therefore more stimulation cycles may be required.

However, in Germany this may be less of a problem since embryo selection is prohibited. Therefore, in Germany it is likely that these stimulation schemes will be the treatment of choice in the near future.

## CONCLUSIONS

It is still too early to speculate about the possible end of the agonist 'era'. GnRH agonists are valuable and safe pharmaceutical tools within controlled ovarian stimulation protocols. Safety and efficacy of the antagonists have still to be proven in long-term studies. Live births per stimulated cycle need to be documented in large series. However, from what has been discovered so far, the advantages of GnRH antagonists are evident. At some stage they will probably replace the agonists completely for this indication.

## REFERENCES

1. Loumaye E. The control of endogenous secretion of LH by gonadotrophin-releasing hormone agonists during ovarian hyperstimulation for in vitro fertilization and embryo transfer. *Hum Reprod* 1990;**5**:357–76.
2. Stanger JD, Yovich JL. Reduced in vitro fertilization of human oocytes from patients with raised basal luteinizing hormone levels during the follicular phase. *Br J Obstet Gynecol* 1985;**92**:385–93.
3. Macnamee MC, Howles CM, Edwards RG, Taylor PJ, Elder KT. Short term luteinizing hormone-releasing hormone agonist treatment: prospective trial of a novel ovarian stimulation regimen for in vitro fertilization. *Fertil Steril* 1989;**52**:264–9.
4. Loumaye E, de Cooman S, Anoma M, et al. Short term utilization of a gonadotrophin releasing hormone agonist (Buserelin) for induction of ovulation in an in-vitro fertilization program. *Ann NY Acad Sci* 1988;**541**:96–102.
5. Smitz J, Ron-El R, Tarlatzis BC. The use of gonadotrophin releasing hormone agonists for in vitro fertilization and other assisted procreation techniques: Experience from three centres. *Hum Reprod* 1992;**7**(suppl 1):49–66.
6. Reissmann T, Felberbaum R, Diedrich K, Engel J, Comaru-Schally AM, Schally AV. Development and applications of luteinizing hormone-releasing hormone antagonists in the treatment of infertility: an overview. *Hum Reprod* 1995;**10**:1974–81.
7. Felberbaum RE, Reissmann T, Küpker W, et al. Preserved pituitary response under ovarian stimulation with HMG and GnRH-antagonists (Cetrorelix) in women with tubal infertility. *Eur J Obstet Gynaecol Reprod Biol* 1995;**61**:151–5.

8. Dittkoff EC, Cassidenti DL, Paulson RJ, et al. The gonadotrophin-releasing hormone antagonist (Nal-Glu) acutely blocks the luteinizing hormone surge but allows for resumption of folliculogenesis in normal women. *Am J Obstet Gynecol* 1991;**165**:1811–17.
9. Felberbaum R, Reissmann T, Küpker W, et al. Hormone profiles under ovarian stimulation with human menopausal gonadotrophin (HMG) and concomitant administration of the gonadotrophin releasing hormone (GnRH)-antagonist Cetrorelix at different dosages. *J Assisted Reprod Genet* 1996;**13**:216–22.
10. Albano C, Smitz J, Camus M, et al. Hormonal profile during the follicular phase in cycles stimulated with a combination of human menopausal gonadotrophin and gonadotrophin-releasing hormone antagonist (Cetrorelix). *Hum Reprod* 1996;**11**:2114–18.
11. Albano C, Smitz J, Camus M, Riethmüller-Winzen H, Van Steirteghem A, Devroey P. Comparison of different doses of gonadotrophin-releasing hormone antagonist Cetrorelix during controlled ovarian hyperstimulation. *Fertil Steril* 1997;**67**:917–22.
12. Adashi EY. Endocrinology of the ovary. *Hum Reprod* 1994;**9**(suppl 2):36–51.
13. Loumaye E, Porchet HC, Beltrami V, et al. Ovulation induction with recombinant human follicle-stimulating hormone and luteinizing hormone. In: *Ovulation Induction. Basic science and clinical advances* (Filicori M, Flamigni C, eds). Amsterdam: Elsevier Science, 1994: 227–36.
14. Olivennes F, Fanchin R, Bouchard P. The single or dual administration of the gonadotrophin-releasing hormone antagonist Cetrorelix in an in

vitro fertilization – embryo transfer programme. *Fertil Steril* 1994;**62**:468–76.

15. Olivennes F, Fanchin R, Bouchard P, Taieb J, Selva J, Frydman R. Scheduled administration of a gonadotrophin-releasing hormone antagonist (Cetrorelix) on day 8 of in-vitro fertilization cycles: a pilot study. *Hum Reprod* 1995;**10**:1382–6.

16. Shalev E, Geslevich Y, Ben-Ami M. Induction of pre-ovulatory luteinizing hormone surge by gonadotrophin-releasing hormone agonist for women at risk for developing the ovarian hyperstimulation syndrome. *Hum Reprod* 1994;**9**:417–19.

17. Olivennes F, Fanchin R, Bouchard P, Taieb J, Frydman R. Triggering of ovulation by a gonadotrophin-releasing hormone (GnRH) agonist in patients pretreated with a GnRH antagonist. *Fertil Steril* 1996;**66**:151–3.

18. Spona J, Coy DH, Zatlasch E, Wakolbinger C. LHRH antagonist inhibits gonadal steroid secretion in vitro. *Peptides* 1985;**6**:379–82.

19. Palermo G, Joris H, Devroey P, Van Steirteghem AC. Pregnancies after intracytoplasmic injection of single spermatozoon into an oocyte. *Lancet* 1992;**340**:17–18.

20. Van Steirteghem AC. IVF and micromanipulation techniques for male-factor infertility. *Curr Opin Obstet Gynecol* 1994;**6**:173–7.

21. Küpker W, Al-Hasani S, Schulze W, et al. Morphology in intracytoplasmic sperm injection: preliminary results. *J Assisted Reprod Genet* 1995;**12**:620–6.

22. Bergh C, Howles CM, Borg K, Hamberger L, Josefsson B, Nilsson L, Wikland M. Recombinant human follicle stimulating hormone (r-FHS; Gonal-F) versus highly purified urinary FSH (Metrodin HP): results of a radomized comparative study in women undergoing assisted reproductive techniques. *Hum Reprod* 1997;**12**:2133–9.

23. Out HJ, Driessen SGAJ, Mannaerts BMJL, Coelingh Bennink HJT. Recombinant follicle-stimulation hormone (follitropin beta, Puregon) yields higher pregnancy rates in in vitro fertilization than urinary gonadotrophins. *Fertil Steril* 1998;**69**:suppl 1:40–4.

24. Bouchard P, Caraty A, Medalie D. Mechanism of action and clinical uses of GnRH-antagonist in women. In: *Recent Progress on GnRH and Gonadal Peptides* (Bouchard P, Haour F, Franchimont P, Schatz B, eds). Paris: Elsevier, 1990: 209–19.

25. Olivennes F, Bouchard P, Frydman R. The use of a new GnRH-antagonist (Cetrorelix) with a single dose protocol in IVF. *J Assisted Reprod Genet* 1997;**14**(suppl):15S.

26. Fleming R, Coutts JRT. Induction of multiple follicular growth in normally menstruating women with endogenous gonadotrophin suppression. *Fertil Steril* 1986;**45**:226–30.

27. Hillier SG. Current concepts of the role of FSH and LH in folliculogenesis. *Hum Reprod* 1994;**9**:188–91.

28. Felberbaum R, Montzka P, Küpker W, et al. High fertilization rate after ovarian stimulation with clomiphene citrate for ICSI. *Hum Reprod* 1997;**12**:abstract book 1:150.

29. Ludwig M, Montzka P, Felberbaum R, Al-Hasani S, Diedrich C, Diedrich K. Stimulation by clomifen in intracytoplasmic sperm injection (ICSI). *Geburtschilfe Frauenheilkd* 1997;**57**:561–5.

# Part VI
# In Vitro Fertilization and
# Micromanipulation

# 19

# Different treatment protocols for different indications

Paul Devroey

Human menopausal gonadotrophins alone or in association with clomiphene citrate • LHRH agonist cycles • LHRH antagonist and gonadotrophins

In women with regular menstrual cycles it could be argued that assisted reproduction has to be performed using the one available metaphase II oocyte.[1] The approach will allow repetition of the treatment every month, to avoid multiple pregnancies and to avoid the ovarian hyperstimulation syndrome. The use of the natural cycle, however, implies close monitoring of the cycle especially in relation to the occurrence of the luteinizing hormone (LH) surge. The close monitoring and the risk of losing the cycle have made the use of the natural cycle unacceptable. For this reason almost all centres for in vitro fertilization (IVF) and embryo transfer use stimulated regimens to control ovarian superovulation. So-called 'ovarian superovulation' is currently the standard procedure in IVF.[2] Different drugs are now used either on a routine basis or in a research protocol. The drugs available are human menopausal gonadotrophins (hMGs), human recombinant follicle-stimulating hormone (FSH), agonists and antagonists for LH-releasing hormone (LHRH) and anti-oestrogenic drugs.

## HUMAN MENOPAUSAL GONADOTROPHINS ALONE OR IN ASSOCIATION WITH CLOMIPHENE CITRATE

This protocol, when it has no kind of down-regulation, has an important negative effect on the cycle outcome as a result of the occurrence of LH surges.[3] In fact, there are different variations of follicular LH elevations, either relating to a premature LH elevation or rise, or being an endogenous, normally timed, LH surge. In both situations clinical management is extremely difficult. Either the cycle has to be cancelled, especially in the case of a premature LH rise associated with a rise in progesterone, or the oocyte retrieval has to be done 20 hours after the onset of the LH surge. This is only possible if the cycle is closely monitored. Moreover, the LH surge in hMG/clomid–hMG stimulated cycles is on the whole attenuated, which makes detection extremely difficult. Furthermore, it is impossible to predict the occurrence of a premature LH surge or of an endogenous one. For those reasons, currently few cycles are performed with clomiphene citrate/hMG or hMG alone.

## LHRH AGONIST CYCLES

An important step was taken when LHRH agonist treatment became available.[4] After an initially stimulatory phase, down-regulation is
achieved and no LH rise is detected.[5] This protocol has the important advantage that the
injection of human chorionic gonadotrophin
(hCG) can be performed within a certain window of days, as the LH surge is unlikely to
occur. The use of a LHRH agonist is now a standard procedure. Although the regimen leads to
fewer cancellations, refined analysis of the data
demonstrate clearly that, even in women
younger than 40 years, there is a variety of
ovarian responses. It has been clearly
demonstrated that, in order to achieve a 26%
ongoing pregnancy rate in women younger
than 40, a minimum of seven cumulus–oocyte
complexes has to be retrieved[6] (Table 1), that is,
seven follicles have to be present in agonist
hMG cycles. If fewer than seven cumulus
oocyte complexes are retrieved, the ongoing
pregnancy rate drops to 15% which is a significant reduction. The reason for this difference
could be related to the presence of a cohort of
responsive follicles containing a high number
of oocytes that can be fertilized. The ovarian
responsiveness decides the embryo quality. If

only three follicles are present the ongoing
pregnancy rate drops to 9%. This observation
indicates that only a reduced cohort of oocytes
can be stimulated and that fewer good quality
embryos are available for replacement. This
finding has been demonstrated on 3841 stimulated cycles. The number of ampoules needed is
significantly higher in the group with poor
response. More research is needed to predict
those who respond well or poorly. The best predictor is probably the antral follicle count using
vaginal ultrasonography.[7]

There are two important questions with
regard to this observation: what is the percentage of women with reduced ovarian responsiveness in agonist hMG-stimulated cycles and
what is the consequence in relation to the rate
of cancellation of oocyte retrievals? In our study
group of women younger than 40, 12.5% (478 of
3814) had a reduced chance of conception. Do
these cycles have to be cancelled and would
a different stimulation protocol give better
results? There has been no systematic research
so far to demonstrate that changing the stimulation protocol could improve the outcome. In a
limited group of 71 women younger than 40
with fewer than seven follicles, the mean number of ampoules of hMG needed was 44; in
women with more than seven follicles, only 30

**Table 1 Ongoing pregnancy rate and numbers of cumulus oocyte complexes retrieved in women younger than 40 years**

| Age (years) | Cumulus–oocyte complexes | Transfers (*n*) | Ongoing pregnancy rate (%) |
|---|---|---|---|
| <40 | <7 | 478 | 13* |
| <40 | >7 | 3336 | 29* |

*$p < 0.001$.
From Vandervorst et al.[6]

**Table 2** Analysis of 71 cycles in women younger than 40 years

| No. of patients | Age (years)* | FSH (U/l)* | Days (mean)** | No. of ampoules** | Oestradiol (ng/l)** | Cumulus–oocyte complexes** |
|---|---|---|---|---|---|---|
| 16 | 33 | 5.96 | 13.8 | 44 | 1419 | 4.9 |
| 55 | 31 | 5.67 | 11.8 | 30.1 | 2496 | 16.9 |

*p = NS; **p = 0.01.
From P Devroey, personal communication.

ampoules were needed (p = 0.007). The mean duration of stimulation was also significantly longer when fewer cumulus oocyte complexes were retrieved (Table 2).

These results have been obtained with LHRH agonist treatment associated with hMG. If monotherapy with human recombinant FSH is used, the amount of LH needed for follicular growth relies entirely on the presence of the remaining LH after down-regulation. We have clearly demonstrated that using different agonists with human recombinant FSH, a sufficient amount of LH is available.[8] It would be extremely interesting to analyse whether a similar relationship between ovarian responsiveness and pregnancy rate is observed after use of human recombinant FSH. Such an analysis of oocyte recovery rates could give different results, but this analysis has not yet been done.

The number of retrieved oocytes is crucially important in preimplantation genetic diagnosis. It has been clearly demonstrated that the number of transferred embryos is significantly increased in patients where nine or more cumulus oocyte complexes are retrieved (0.77 vs 1.94; p < 0.001).[9]

As demonstrated in Table 2 the number of ampoules needed in agonist hMG cycles is about 40 in poor responders and 30 in normal responders. In our phase II study using recombinant FSH in association with different ago-

nists the number of ampoules needed was also slightly above 30.8. Can this number be reduced using different stimulation protocols? In a multicentre study comparing human recombinant FSH with urofollitrophin (Metrodin High Purity) far fewer ampoules were used in the recombinant FSH group (28.5 vs 31.8)[10] (Table 3). Also, comparing human recombinant FSH with urofollitrophin fewer ampoules of recombinant FSH were needed (21.9 vs 31.9) (p < 0.0001)[11] (Table 4).

The consumption of gonadotrophins is closely related to the stimulation policy. It can be speculated that about 25 ampoules are needed in normal responders.

## LHRH ANTAGONIST AND GONADOTROPHINS

From a theoretical viewpoint there is a need to avoid the stimulatory effect of the agonist and to avoid the use of the long protocol. An LHRH antagonist provides a tool that is able to block immediately the output of LH.[12,13] Two compounds are under clinical investigation so far: Cetrorelix (ASTA, Frankfurt, Germany) and Ganirelix (Organon, Oss, The Netherlands). Dose-finding studies have demonstrated that the minimal effective dose is 0.25 mg for Cetrorelix[14] and 0.25 mg for Ganirelix.[15]

It has been clearly demonstrated that the

**Table 3 Comparative evaluation of women stimulated with recombinant FSH and urinary FSH in the long protocol for in vitro fertilization**

|  | Recombinant FSH group | Urinary FSH group | Significance |
|---|---|---|---|
| No. of patients | 585 | 396 |  |
| Total FSH Dose (IU) | 2138 | 2358 | <0.0001 |
| Duration of treatment (days) | 10.7 | 11.3 | <0.0001 |
| No. of follicles ≥17 mm on hCG day | 4.6 | 4.4 | 0.09 |
| No. of follicles ≥15 mm on hCG day | 7.5 | 6.7 | <0.001 |
| Oestradiol on hCG day (pmol/l) | 6084 | 5179 | <0.0001 |
| No. of oocytes retrieved | 10.8 | 9.0 | <0.0001 |
| No. of mature oocytes retrieved | 8.6 | 6.8 | <0.0001 |
| No. of high quality embryos | 3.1 | 2.6 | <0.01 |
| Ongoing pregnancy rate/attempt (%) | 22.2 | 18.2 | 0.13 |
| Ongoing pregnancy rate/transfer (%) | 26 | 22 | 0.19 |
| Total ongoing pregnancy rate/attempt (%)[a] | 25.6 | 20.4 | 0.05 |

[a]Including frozen embryos.
From Out et al.[10]

**Table 4 Stimulation characteristics of patients receiving human chorionic gonadotrophin (hCG; values are means ± SD)**

|  | Gonal-F | Metrodin HP | p value |
|---|---|---|---|
| No. of patients receiving hCG | 119 | 102 |  |
| No. of days of FSH treatment | 11.0 ± 1.6 | 13.5 ± 3.7 | <0.0001 |
| No. of ampoules FSH (75 IU equivalent) | 21.9 ± 5.1 | 31.9 ± 13.4 | <0.0001 |
| No. of follicles >10 mm in diameter on the day of hCG | 12.7 ± 4.9 | 8.4 ± 4.2 | <0.002 |
| Oestradiol concentration on the day of hCG (nmol/l) | 6.55 ± 5.75 | 3.95 ± 3.90 | <0.001 |
| No. of oocytes retrieved | 12.2 ± 5.5 | 7.6 ± 4.4 | <0.0001 |
| No. of oocytes retrieved/no. of follicles >10 mm in diameter on the day of hCG (%) | 92.6 ± 11.9 | 75.8 ± 29.0 | <0.004 |

From Bergh et al.[11]

association of LHRH antagonist with either hMG or recombinant FSH provides acceptable pregnancy rates. Several studies have been performed so far but the phase III data have not yet been published. The comparison between the use of hMG with Cetrorelix versus buserelin and between Puregon and Ganirelix versus buserelin is currently carried out in phase III trials. Several comparisons still need to be performed, for example, that between Ganirelix and Puregon versus hMG.

In a small randomized prospective study comparing Cetrorelix–hMG ($n = 15$) with Cetrorelix– Gonal-F ($n = 15$) we were unable to find any difference in outcome. The number of days of gonadotrophin stimulation and those of Cetrorelix administration were similar. No differences in metaphase II oocyte rates or implantation rates were observed.

It is also interesting to observe that the number of ampoules used was similar in both groups, that is, about 23. At this stage there is no reason to speculate that the number of ampoules used will decrease with the use of the antagonist. However, as this was a small study which lacked statistical power, we have to wait for the results of large studies before a definitive conclusion can be reached.

Several questions remain unsolved so far. An intriguing one is the evaluation of the luteal phase. Theoretically the antagonist should not have a deleterious effect on the luteal phase. In a phase II study performed with Cetrorelix in patients without luteal phase supplementation we observed a luteal phase defect in three of six cycles.[16] More research is needed to find out if there is any luteal phase defect and if there is

one the physiopathology has to be defined. The use of LHRH antagonist also opens new possibilities to investigate the role of human chorionic gonadotrophin (hCG) in the initiation of the ovarian hyperstimulation syndrome (OHSS). The question is whether there is any difference in the occurrence of the OHSS in patients treated with antagonist compared with treatment with the agonist. Of course the use of recombinant LH or the LHRH agonist to induce ovulation would be useful. Furthermore, by using recombinant LH or an LHRH agonist the analysis of the luteal phase will be informative.

An important question is related to the number of oocytes needed in assisted reproduction. By changing the stimulation protocols, the aim should be to obtain less fertilizable metaphase II oocytes. In a pilot study using anti-oestrogen therapy we obtain a fertilization rate of 84.2% (64 zygotes per 76 metaphase II oocytes) and a cleavage rate of 98.4% (63 per 64). In this study population the number of cumulus–oocyte complexes retrieved was only three. One of the future stimulation protocols could be the association of anti-oestrogen therapy, gonadotrophins and antagonists. However, the success of such a protocol would ultimately depend upon current pregnancy rates being at least maintained. If recombinant LH or an LHRH agonist is administered to induce ovulation, the occurrence of the OHSS could also be decreased.

In conclusion, in the near future different drugs will become available to obtain controlled ovarian hyperstimulation. It is of paramount importance to design stimulation protocols avoiding the OHSS.

## REFERENCES

1. Foulot H, Ranoux C, Dubuisson JB, et al. In vitro fertilization without ovarian stimulation: a simplified protocol applied in 80 cycles. *Fertil Steril* 1989;**52**:617–21.
2. Abdalla HI, Ahuja KK, Leonard T, et al. Comparative trial of luteinizing hormone-releasing hormone analog/human menopausal gonadotropin and clomiphene citrate/human menopausal gonadotropin in an assisted conception program. *Fertil Steril* 1990;**53**:473–8.
3. Devroey P, Naaktgeboren N, Traey E, et al. Hormonal evaluation of failed ovarian stimula-

tion in an in vitro fertilization program. *IV World Conference on In Vitro Fertilization*, Melbourne, Australia 1985; abstract p 6.

4. Porter RN, Smith W, Craft IL, et al. Induction of ovulation for in-vitro fertilization using Buserelin and gonadotropins. *Lancet* 1984; **ii:**1284–5.

5. Smitz J, Devroey P, Braeckmans P, et al. Management of failed cycles in an IVF/GIFT program with the combination of a GnRH analogue and HMG. *Hum Reprod* 1987;**2:**309–14.

6. Vandervorst M, Joris H, Van Steirteghem A, et al. Correlation between ongoing pregnancy rates and the number of cumulus–oocyte-complexes retrieved in agonist-hMG stimulated ICSI cycles. *Hum Reprod* 1997; **12**(suppl):168–9.

7. Broekmans FJ, Scheffer GJ, Dorland M, et al. Ovarian reserve tests in a normal fertile and IVF population. *Abstract Book of the British Fertility Society.* 1998;S2.

8. Devroey P, Mannaerts B, Smitz J, et al. Clinical outcome of a pilot study on recombinant human follicle-stimulating hormone (Org 32489) combined with various gonadotropin releasing hormone agonist regimens. *Hum Reprod* 1994; **9:**1064–9.

9. Vandervorst M, Liebaers I, Van Waesberghe L, et al. Is there a minimum number of cumulus–oocyte-complexes needed for successful PGD? *Abstracts from the Second International Symposium on Preimplantation Genetics*, Chicago, September 18–21, 1997;**14:**475.

10. Out JH, Mannaerts B, Driessen S, et al. A prospective, randomized, assessor-blind, multicenter study comparing recombinant and urinary follicle stimulating hormone (Puregon®

11. Bergh C, Howles CM, Borg K, et al. Recombinant human follicle stimulating hormone (r-hFSH; Gonal-F®) versus highly purified urinary FSH (Metrodin HP®): results of a randomized comparative study in women undergoing assisted reproductive techniques. *Hum Reprod* 1997; **12:**2133–9.

12. Reissmann TH, Felberbaum R, Diedrich K, et al. Development and applications of luteinizing hormone-releasing hormone antagonists in a treatment of infertility: an overview. *Hum Reprod* 1995;**10:**1974–81.

13. Albano C, Smitz J, Camus M, et al. Hormonal profile during the follicular phase in cycles stimulated with combination of human menopausal gonadotropin (HMG) and gonadotropin-releasing hormone antagonist (cetrorelix). *Hum Reprod* 1996;**11:**2114–18.

14. Albano C, Smitz J, Camus M, et al. Comparison of different doses of gonadotrophin-releasing hormone antagonist cetrorelix during controlled ovarian hyperstimulation. *Fertil Steril* 1997; **67:**917–22.

15. Mannaerts B, Recombinant FSH and GNRH antagonist: role of antagonist dose. In: *Abstracts of Ovulation Induction Update* 1997, Bologna, OR-20.

16. Albano C, Grimbizis G, Smitz J, et al. The luteal phase of non-supplemented cycles after ovarian superovulation with human menopausal gonadotropin and the gonadotropin-releasing hormone antagonist Cetrorelix. *Fertil Steril* 1998; in press.

versus Metrodin) in in vitro fertilization. *Hum Reprod* 1995;**10:**2534–40.

# 20

# The use of lasers for micromanipulation

Marc Germond, Marie-Pierre Primi, Alfred Senn, Klaus Rink, Guy Delacrétaz

**Micromanipulation methods • Biological and clinical applications of micromanipulations • The 1.48 µM diode laser • Conclusion • Acknowledgements**

The zona pellucida (ZP), the chemical and bio-physical properties of which have been extensively studied,[1,2] is a glycoprotein matrix surrounding mammalian oocytes. During fertilization, it represents a mechanical and selective barrier that only capacitated spermatozoa are able to cross.[3,4] Once gamete fusion has occurred, it serves as a confined shelter in which the embryo is protected from micro-organisms, viruses and immune cells, and where it can proceed up to morula compaction without blastomere loss. The ZP then needs to be broken up by the expanding blastocyst just before uterine implantation. Over the last 10 years, several micromanipulation techniques for the ZP have been reported by which it is opened, thinned, drilled or slit using mechanical or chemical methods in order to improve a specific biological process, such as fertilization or blastocyst hatching, or to allow embryonic biopsy.

Zona pellucida micromanipulation with lasers is more recent. The use of lasers is first compared from a methodological point of view with mechanical and chemical techniques, then the possible involvement of lasers in clinical situations are discussed with particular emphasis on the 1.48 µm diode laser.

## MICROMANIPULATION METHODS

### Mechanical and chemical methods

Mechanical[5] or chemical methods[6] have been used since the mid-1980s to create slits or holes in the ZP of mammalian oocytes or embryos.

The mechanical partial zona dissection (PZD) implies passing a sharpened pipette obliquely through the ZP and emerging on the opposite side without harming the oocyte, and then using it to rub the ZP against the holding pipette in order to produce a slit.[7] Even if this technique is easy to perform,[8] it results in breaches of variable sizes, which when they are too small may negatively affect the hatching process.[9]

The aptitude of the ZP proteinic structure to dissolve at low pH has led to the development of a second technique, based on the use of an acidic Tyrode's solution for drilling holes in the ZP[10,11] with the help of a micropipette. Holes of more regular sizes can be produced with this method, but successful handling of this technique needs expertise because of the reported toxicity of Tyrode's solution to human oocytes[12] and embryos during their early stages of development.[7,13]

## Laser methods

As the mechanical or chemical drilling procedures described above are unable to produce standardized holes or are hazardous for the embryos, drilling of the ZP by lasers has been proposed as an alternative.[14,15] In order to bring about a significant methodological improvement, micromanipulation of the ZP by lasers should (1) be accurately controlled and produce the ZP opening with no mechanical, thermal or mutagenic side effects, (2) provide a touch-free objective-delivered accessibility of laser light to the target with minimal absorption by the culture dish and the aqueous medium, and (3) be affordable and easily adapted to any existing inverted microscope. Keeping these requirements in mind, the various laser systems that have been proposed can be reviewed (Table 1).

An argon fluoride (ArF) excimer laser emitting at 193 nm was first reported to be successful in opening the ZP and helping fertilization of mouse oocytes.[16,17] As this ultraviolet radiation has a penetration depth of less than 1 μm in water, the laser beam has to be delivered in a contact mode with an air-filled micropipette acting as a hollow wave guide. Longer wavelengths (266, 308, 355, 366 and 532 nm), which are absorbed less by aqueous solutions and thus deliverable to the target in a non-touch mode through microscope obectives, were then investigated[18] and the xenon chloride (XeCl)

laser (308 nm) was shown to be suited for ZP microdrilling.[19] A commercially available 337-nm nitrogen laser (PALM) has also been proposed as a ZP opening tool or, in combination with optical tweezers, as a micromanipulation tool for the improvement of in vitro fertilization (IVF).[20] Use of the 308 and 337 nm radiations needs both a special high-power objective (100 ×) and quartz slides to focus the ultraviolet radiation properly and achieve ablation of the ZP matrix.

Infrared is another region of the light spectrum that exhibits strong light absorption bands by water and which is thus likely to interact successfully with the ZP. An Er:YAG (erbium:yttrium–aluminium–garnet) laser emitting at 2.94 μm was described as a ZP microdissection tool. As this radiation has a penetration depth of about 3 μm in water, the laser light has to be delivered perpendicularly to the ZP in a contact mode using laser optical fibres.[21] At shorter infrared wavelengths, a 1.48 μm InGaAsP (indium–gallium–arsenic–phosphorus) diode laser[22,23] and a 2.1 μm Ho:YSGG (holmium:yttrium–scandium–gallium–garnet)[24] laser were shown to produce holes in the ZP through microscope objectives in a non-contact mode. Of all the described laser approaches for ZP microdissection, the infrared lasers undoubtedly present a major advantage, because they are not likely to cause the harmful mutagenic effects that ultraviolet lasers do.[25]

**Table 1 Lasers proposed for ZP micromanipulation**

| Type of laser | Abbreviation | Wavelength (nm) | Mode of action |
| --- | --- | --- | --- |
| Argon fluoride excimer | ArF | 193 | Pulsed |
| Krypton fluoride excimer | KrF | 248 | Pulsed |
| Xenon chloride excimer | XeCl | 308 | Pulsed |
| Nitrogen | $N_2$ | 337 | Pulsed |
| Erbium:yttrium–aluminium–garnet | Er:YAG | 2940 | Pulsed |
| 1.48 μm diode laser | InGaAsP | 1480 | Continuous |
| Holmium:yttrium–scandium–gallium–garnet | Ho:YSGG | 2100 | Pulsed |

In the case of the 1.48 μm diode laser, drilling is accomplished by delivering a single laser pulse of less than 50 ms tangentially to the ZP. The drilling mechanism is explained by a thermal effect induced at the focal point by the absorption of the laser energy by water and/or ZP macromolecules, leading to a confined thermolysis of the ZP matrix.[23] This laser combines all the special requirements formulated above, which is not the case for the other lasers described. Indeed, oocytes or embryos can be maintained in their usual culture dish and medium during the drilling without requiring special optical equipment as they do for ultraviolet lasers,[20] a change of medium[26] or micromanipulators and sterilizable microfibres as for the 2.9 μm Er:YAG laser.[27]

## BIOLOGICAL AND CLINICAL APPLICATIONS OF MICROMANIPULATIONS

### Assisted fertilization

Mechanical or chemical methods for creating openings in the ZP were developed at first for the enhancement of the IVF rates when the mechanical barrier of the ZP was thought to act as a major impediment to gamete fusion. PZD was first reported as a technique for assisting fertilization.[28–30] This approach was soon challenged by subzonal insemination (SUZI), which consists of mechanically inserting one or several spermatozoa into the perivitelline space.[31]

More recently, intracytoplasmic sperm injection (ICSI), which involves the injection of a spermatozoon directly into the ooplasm,[32,33] proved to be so greatly superior to SUZI,[34] and therefore to PZD,[35] that it remains the only widely accepted method of assisted fertilization in the human.[36]

Besides their use in ZP dissection before IVF,[27,37] lasers have not been very useful in terms of assisted fertilization in humans. However, their remarkable electromagnetic properties have allowed optical tweezers to be designed for trapping small objects and moving them along the three axes.[15] Despite the report

of the effects of such laser tweezers on spermatozoon motility after capture in the trap for several minutes,[20,38] concern about the effects on sperm of a Nd:YAG (cw Nd:YAG laser, 1064 nm) trap has been raised after the observation of reduced motility for laser exposures of more than 30 seconds.[39] Later, a Ti-sapphire laser tuned at 760 nm enabled measurement of the power needed by human sperm for escaping from the trap and demonstration that this power increased in the presence of cumulus cells.[40]

Nevertheless, the use of optical tweezers for spermatozoon injection after zona dissection could be a logical step forward in the control of assisted fertilization procedures. First attempts, using a combined technique of an ultraviolet laser microbeam (PALM) and an Nd:YAG optical tweezer trap, have been reported in animals.[20,41,42] Before their use is extended to human applications, optical tweezers remain essentially a research tool for the study of the kinetic behavior of spermatozoa and of early membrane interactions during gamete fusion.

### Assisted hatching

Hatching of the blastocyst out of the ZP is an essential step which has to occur before uterine implantation. The poor implantation rate after transfer of apparently normal looking embryos is one of the unsolved problems encountered in IVF. Besides intrinsic embryo abnormalities or defective uterine receptivity, a hatching failure could partly explain the low implantation rate. Blastocyst hatching might be impaired in some patients when the ZP is too thick or hardened by in vitro culture,[43] hyaluronidase treatment for decoronization,[44] freezing,[45] or simply physiological ageing.[46] It has been hypothesized that assisted hatching may enhance embryo implantation not only by mechanically facilitating the hatching process but also by permitting earlier embryo– endometrium contact, because synchronization between embryo development and uterine receptivity is necessary for implantation efficiency.

Acid drilling or PZD has been used for

**Table 2 Summary of the clinical studies performed with various assisted hatching (AH) techniques and results obtained in terms of implantation (IR) and clinical pregnancy (CP) rates**

| Reference | Technique for AH | Patient selection | Other specification | IR/CP increased |
|---|---|---|---|---|
| Cohen et al[47] | Tyrode's | Normal FSH | | No/– |
| | | Poor prognosis ZP ≥ 15 μm | | Yes/– |
| Tucker et al[48] | Zona thinning with Tyrode's | Unselected or poor prognosis | Co-culture | No/no |
| Schoolcraft et al[53] | Tyrode's | Poor prognosis ≥39 years | | Yes/yes |
| Wiemer et al[73] | Tyrode's | Poor prognosis | Co-culture | Yes/yes |
| Stein et al[51] | PZD | 3 IVF failures | | –/no |
| | | ≥38 years | | –/yes |
| Schoolcraft et al[74] | Tyrode's | ≥40 years Routinely applied | | Yes/yes |
| Hellebaut et al[50] | PZD | Unselected | ±ICSI | No/no |
| Hu et al[49] | Tyrode's | Unselected | | Yes/yes |
| Check et al[54] | Tyrode's | Unselected | Thawed embryos 6–8 cell stage | Yes/yes |
| Tucker et al[52] | Tyrode's | Unselected ≥35 years | Co-culture + ICSI | No/no Yes/yes |
| Chao et al[55] | PZD | IVF failures | ET TET | Yes/yes No/no |
| Tao and Tamis[56] | Tyrode's | Poor prognosis ≥38 years | Thawed embryos 2–4 cell stage | Yes/yes |
| Obruca et al[27] | Er:YAG | IVF failures | | Yes/yes |
| Antinori et al[75] | Zona thinning with Er:YAG | 2–4 IVF failures First IVF | | Yes/yes Yes/yes |
| Antinori et al[57] | PALM UV | 2–4 failures | | Yes/yes |

ET, embryo transfer.

several years in clinical settings to improve pregnancy rates after embryo transfer (Table 2). Cohen et al[47] showed that the implantation rates of human embryos correlated with the ZP thickness. These authors also reported that 15% of IVF embryos presented a ZP more than 15 μm thick.[5] It has been demonstrated that zona thinning alone is not sufficient to promote implantation, which suggests that the inner layer of the human ZP has to be fully breached.[48] Apart from a single study,[49] all published reports have stated that implantation is not improved by assisted hatching in non-selected IVF patient populations.[47,50–52] However, in some subgroups of poor prognosis patients, that is with elevated basal FSH, repeated IVF failures, thick ZP or frozen–thawed embryo transfers, assisted hatching was repeatedly associated with higher implantation and pregnancy rates.[47,51–56]

These last conclusions were also reached when assisted hatching was performed with Er:YAG[27] or PALM[57] lasers. Lasers have an important advantage over other tools, because the drilling can be done at early stages of embryo development (from day 1 on), which means that shorter durations of in vitro culture are possible.

## Preimplantation genetic diagnosis

Preimplantation genetic diagnosis (PGD) requires performing biopsies on early stage embryos for further genetic analysis. All biopsies are obtained by micromanipulative removal of the target cells after microdissection of the ZP.[58] PGD is usually performed on one or two biopsied blastomeres from a six- to ten-cell embryo,[59] a situation similar to the loss of blastomeres after cryopreservation.[60] Usually, a hole is drilled in the ZP and the blastomere is simply extracted with an aspiration micropipette.[59]

Another method for PGD, developed experimentally, consists of excising tissue from blastocysts. In this case, a slit is made in the zona opposite to the inner cell mass and a hernia of trophoectoderm formed 18–24 hours later is biopsied.[61,62] The advantage of this method is associated with the number of cells available for the diagnostic procedure.

It appears that PGD can be reliably performed on the first (preconception diagnosis) or second polar bodies[63,64] without harming further development of the embryo. Until now, sharp aspiration needles have been necessary to penetrate the ZP and aspirate the polar body. The efficacy of this method depends on the ability to retrieve the polar body without damaging the oocyte and loosing chromosomal material.

Lasers have to date found little clinical applications in the biopsy of polar bodies, blastomeres or trophectoderm. Ease of use of the 1.48 µm diode laser has uncovered new possibilities in this field, so that experimental studies are currently being performed and are described below.

## Anucleated fragments removal

Micromanipulation techniques have also aimed at rescuing embryos that develop an excessive amount of degenerate material as a result of partial embryonic degeneration or fragmentation. Experimentally, in mice, it was shown that the hatching process of embryos, in which one or two blastomeres out of four cells had been destroyed and subsequently degenerated, is adversely affected. Removal of the extracellular material by micromanipulation potentially reverted the hatching and proved to be beneficial.[65] When removing small amounts of fragments from embryos during assisted hatching, the pregnancy rate in 36 patients with extracted fragments was shown to be relatively high (41%) considering the poor morphology of the embryos involved.[66]

Lasers could have another application here by simplifying the opening of the ZP in comparison to the usual method of acid drilling.

## THE 1.48 µM DIODE LASER

A collaboration between two academic centres in Lausanne (Institut d'Optique Appliquée, Ecole Polytechnique Fédérale de Lausanne, and Unité de Médecine de la Reproduction, Département de Gynécologie–Obstétrique, CHUV) has led to the concept and development of a non-touch microdissection system based on the use of a 1.48 µm diode laser.[22,23,67] This laser system is now commercially available as an individual unit (Figure 1) adaptable to almost any inverted microscope (Fertilase, Medical Technologies Montreux, Lausanne, Switzerland).

## Animal experimentation

### Safety studies
The efficacy and safety of the 1.48 µm diode laser has been investigated by determining the ability of mouse oocytes to fertilize in vitro and develop in vivo after ZP microdrilling.[68] Decoronization with hyaluronidase reduces both

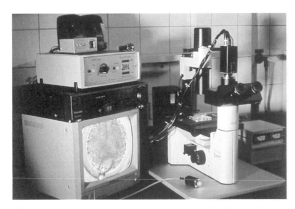

**Figure 1** Inverted microscope equipped with the laser microdrilling system (Fertilase, Medical Technologies, Montreux). A drilled bovine oocyte is shown on the video screen.

fertilization and implantation rates probably by hardening the ZP. After laser ZP drilling, the fertilization rates of oocytes treated with hyaluronidase were restored to those obtained in untreated oocytes. Birth rate was also found to be identical to that of the untreated group. Pups derived from ZP-drilled embryos were comparable, in terms of development and reproductive ability, to those from control embryos, confirming the lack of any long-term deleterious effect of laser treatment.

### Assisted hatching

Another study was performed in mouse embryos to test the impact of ZP drilling on in vitro and in vivo developments.[69] Hatching

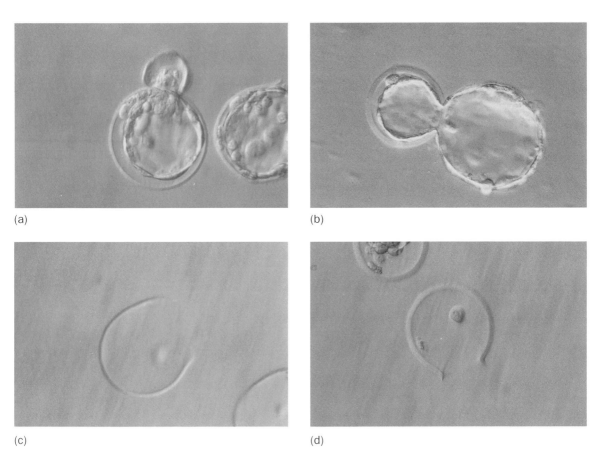

(a)       (b)

(c)       (d)

**Figure 2** Hatching of control (a) and laser-drilled (b) mouse blastocysts. Empty ZPs of hatched control (c) and laser-drilled (d) blastocysts. Notice the thinner ZP width in the control.

initiation, visualized by the appearance of a small herniation of the embryonic cells, occurred one day earlier in drilled embryos compared with undrilled controls. In laser-treated embryos, no thinning of the ZP was observed before hatching and the embryos were able to hatch by progressively extruding from the drilled hole (Figure 2). However, the hatching enhancement observed in vitro had no impact on the number of mice born per embryo transferred which was found to be close to that of the control (45%). There again, the development and reproductive capacity (up to generation F4) of the mice born from drilled embryos were comparable to controls.

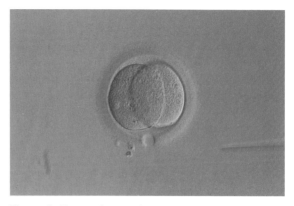

**Figure 3** Human frozen–thawed embryo just after laser microdrilling on day 2. The transfer led to a clinical pregnancy. The picture was taken on a different microscope and a micropipette (visible on the side) was needed to reorient the embryo in order to bring the hole into focus.

### Polar body biopsy

Second polar body biopsy is one approach to preimplantation genetic diagnosis. Montag et al[70] have developed a method in mice using laser microdissection of the ZP and aspiration of the polar bodies with flame-polished blunt needles. Although this laser system does not require any mechanical stabilization of the zygotes, micropipettes were used to allow polar body biopsy immediately after laser microdissection using the same microscope set-up. A hole of about 14–18 μm was drilled with a single laser irradiation of 12–16 ms (1.2–1.6 mJ) and the polar body was then gently sucked into the blunt-ended needle. Laser microdissection and polar body biopsy were accomplished within 1–2 mins. Consequently, the authors showed that in mice this procedure is safe because it can be applied very rapidly and with high precision, therefore reducing the possibility of misdiagnosis as a result of disintegration or lysis of the polar body.

## Clinical applications

### Assisted hatching

The effect of assisted hatching was evaluated on frozen–thawed embryos in patients who had experienced at least two previous unsuccessful transfers of cryopreserved embryos. Sixty-five patients were enrolled in the study and matched retrospectively with 70 control patients to whom undrilled cryopreserved embryos were transferred. The treatment period of the two groups overlapped partly, but the laboratory and transfer techniques remained identical. Drilling of the embryos was performed before the transfer with the 1.48 μm diode laser by exposing the ZP to up to three 20–50 ms laser pulses (Figure 3). The cumulated embryo score (CES, number of blastomeres × grade) was calculated at the time of embryo transfer. An immunosuppressive and antibiotic treatment was prescribed for 7 days, from 2 days before to 5 days after embryo transfer. Clinical pregnancies were recorded when a gestational sac with heart activity was visible on ultrasonography 28–35 days after embryo transfer.

Results are summarized in Table 3. For transfers with a low CES (< 20), assisted hatching did not improve the clinical pregnancy (CP) or implantation rates (IR) significantly. When the CES was 20 or more, both rates were increased significantly by assisted hatching, IR from 3.6% to 14.7% and CP from 10.5% to 29.6%. Sixteen deliveries were obtained with the birth of 22 healthy children in the assisted hatching group, compared with four deliveries and four children in the control group.

**Table 3** Clinical pregnancy rates and implantation rates in two groups of patients whose frozen–thawed embryos were (assisted hatching, AH) or were not (control) drilled with the 1.48 μm diode laser just before embryo transfer (day 2)

| CES | | Control | AH | p |
|---|---|---|---|---|
| <20 | Mean transferred embryos | 2.3 ± 0.8 | 2.9 ± 0.5 | NS |
| | Clinical pregnancies/transfers (%) | 1/28 (3.6) | 3/54 (5.6) | NS |
| | Implantation (sacs/embryos) (%) | 1/65 (1.5) | 3/111 (2.7) | NS |
| ≥20 | Mean transferred embryos | 2.9 ± 0.7 | 2.6 ± 0.5 | NS |
| | Clinical pregnancies/transfers (%) | 4/38 (10.5) | 16/54 (29.6) | 0.0287 |
| | Implantation (sacs/embryos) (%) | 4/110 (3.6) | 21/143 (14.7) | 0.0035 |

A multicentre study is presently being performed on four different groups of patients with the following main objectives: (1) to define more precisely the clinical indications for ZP drilling and assisted hatching; (2) to investigate the benefit of an immunosuppressive treatment associated with antibiotic therapy on the implantation of laser-drilled embryos; and (3) to demonstrate the safety of the technique. Four European IVF centres (M Germond, Lausanne; H van der Ven, Bonn; J Mandelbaum, Paris; P Barri, Barcelona) equipped with the Fertilase system are collaborating in this double-blind randomized study.

*Preimplantation genetic diagnosis*
Barri's group in Barcelona is now developing two approaches for PGD using the Fertilase system. Boada et al.[71] have performed blastomere biopsies on 13 embryos with four or more cells. The embryos were held by two micromanipulators and positioned so as to drill the ZP near the blastomere selected for biopsy. Depending on the ZP thickness of each embryo, two to four laser shots of 8–22 ms were applied to the ZP to make a trench. In a minimal period of time, one blastomere was aspirated for embryo sexing, which was indicated by a history of haemophilia. One pregnancy was obtained in

two transfers (three female embryos). The authors concluded that the methodology is simple, quick, safe and is the best method for blastomere biopsy.

Trophectoderm biopsies using the same apparatus have already brought encouraging results.[72] Non-transferable human blastocysts were selected for this study. The 1.48 μm diode laser was used for the whole procedure, that is, drilling of the ZP (8–10 ms single laser shot) and cutting of the herniated trophoectoderm cells that protrude out of the ZP (30 ms shot). The herniated portion held with a suction micropipette was thus detached from the blastocyst and processed for analysis. They measured the re-expansion of the blastocysts and their ability to hatch. They concluded from these preliminary results that the procedure shows promise with regard to its efficiency and the blastocyst recovery rate.

**CONCLUSION**

Laser beams can be focused through microscope objectives in spots of high energy which allow microsurgical operations to be performed at the subcellular level. Infrared lasers – which are the least likely to induce mutagenic side effects – have proved to be the best adapted tools for human applications. Among these lasers, the 1.48 μm diode laser will increasingly compete with the mechanical and chemical procedures, because it allows holes of reproducible sizes to be made rapidly and safely without manipulating the embryo. In the case of PGD, it will also offer an accurate and effective way of practising biopsies. Once large clinical randomized studies performed in different centres have definitely demonstrated the efficacy of assisted hatching in selected groups of patients, laser ZP microdrilling will become a commonly accepted clinical tool.

## ACKNOWLEDGEMENTS

The authors would like to thank Dr M Montag and Professor H van der Ven (Department of Gynecology and Obstetrics, University of Bonn, Germany), Dr A Veiga and Professor P Barri (Institut Dexeus, Barcelona, Spain), for providing us with their experimental results in process of publication, and Dr J Mandelbaum (Necker Hospital, Paris, France), as well as the two above-mentioned groups, for collaborating with us to the multicentre trial.

## REFERENCES

1. Wassarman PM, Liu C, Litscher ES. Constructing the mammalian egg zona pellucida: some new pieces of an old puzzle. *J Cell Sci* 1996; **109**:2001–4.

2. Topfer-Petersen E, Calvete JJ, Sanz L, et al. Carbohydrate- and heparin-binding proteins in mammalian fertilization. *Andrologia* 1995; **27**:303–24.

3. Chang MC. The meaning of sperm capacitation. A historical perspective. *J Androl* 1984; **5**:45–50.

4. Tesarik J, Testart J. Human sperm–egg interactions and their disorders: implications in the management of infertility. *Hum Reprod* 1989; **4**:729–41.

5. Cohen J, Elsner C, Kort H, et al. Impairment of the hatching process following IVF in the human and improvement of implantation by assisting hatching using micromanipulation. *Hum Reprod* 1990; **5**:7–13.

6. Gordon JW. Use of micromanipulation for increasing the efficiency of mammalian fertilization in vitro. *Ann N Y Acad Sci* 1988; **541**:601–13.

7. Malter HE, Cohen J. Partial zona dissection of the human oocyte: a nontraumatic method using micromanipulation to assist zona pellucida penetration. *Fertil Steril* 1989; **51**:139–48.

8. Mandelbaum J. The effects of assisted hatching on the hatching process and implantation. *Hum Reprod* 1996; **11**(suppl 1):43–50.

9. Cohen J, Feldberg D. Effects of the size and number of zona pellucida openings on hatching and trophoblast outgrowth in the mouse embryo. *Mol Reprod Dev* 1991; **30**:70–8.

10. Gordon JW, Grunfeld L, Garrisi GJ, et al. Fertilization of human oocytes by sperm from infertile males after zona pellucida drilling. *Fertil Steril* 1988; **50**:68–73.

11. Gordon JW, Laufer N. Applications of micromanipulation to human in vitro fertilization. *J In Vitro Fertil Embryo Transfer* 1988; **5**:57–60.

12. Gordon JW, Talansky BE. Assisted fertilization by zona drilling: a mouse model for correction of oligospermia. *J Exp Zool* 1986; **239**:347–54.

13. Garrisi GJ, Talansky BE, Grunfeld L, et al. Clinical evaluation of three approaches to micromanipulation-assisted fertilization. *Fertil Steril* 1990; **54**:671–7.

14. Welch AJ, Motamedi M, Rastegar S, et al. Laser thermal ablation. *Photochem Photobiol* 1991; **53**:815–23.

15. Tadir Y, Wright WH. Vafa O, et al. Micromanipulation of gametes using laser microbeams. *Hum Reprod* 1991; **6**:1011–16.

16. Palanker D, Ohad S, Lewis A, et al. Technique for cellular microsurgery using the 193-nm excimer laser. *Lasers Surg Med* 1991; **11**:580–6.

17. Laufer N, Palanker D, Shufaro Y, et al. The efficacy and safety of zona pellucida drilling by a 193-nm excimer laser. *Fertil Steril* 1993; **59**:889–95.

18. Neev J, Tadir Y, Ho P, et al. Microscope delivered ultraviolet laser zona dissection: principles and practices. *J Assist Reprod Genet* 1992; **9**:513–23.

19. el-Danasouri I, Westphal LM, Neev Y, et al. Zona opening with 308 nm XeCl excimer laser improves fertilization by spermatozoa from

long-term vasectomized mice. *Hum Reprod* 1993;**8**:464–6.

20. Schutze K, Clement-Sengewald A, Ashkin A. Zona drilling and sperm insertion with combined laser microbeam and optical tweezers. *Fertil Steril* 1994;**61**:783–6.

21. Strohmer H, Feichtinger W. Successful clinical application of laser for micromanipulation in an in vitro fertilization program. *Fertil Steril* 1992;**58**:212–14.

22. Rink K, Delacretaz G, Salathe RP, et al. 1.48 µm diode laser microdissection of the zona pellucida of mouse zygotes. *SPIE* 1994;**2134A**:412–22.

23. Rink K, Delacretaz G, Salathe RP, et al. Non-contact microdrilling of mouse zona pellucida with an objective-delivered 1.48 µm diode laser. *Lasers Surg Med* 1996;**18**:52–62.

24. Neev J, Schiewe MC, Sung VW, et al. Assisted hatching in mouse embryos using a noncontact Ho:YSGG laser system. *J Assist Reprod Genet* 1995;**12**:288–93.

25. Kochevar IE. Cytotoxicity and mutagenicity of excimer laser radiation. *Lasers Surg Med* 1989; **9**:440–5.

26. Blanchet GB, Russell JB, Fincher CR Jr, et al. Laser micromanipulation in the mouse embryo: a novel approach to zona drilling. *Fertil Steril* 1992;**57**:1337–41.

27. Obruca A, Strohmer H, Sakkas D, et al. Use of lasers in assisted fertilization and hatching. *Hum Reprod* 1994;**9**:1723–6.

28. Depypere HT, McLaughlin KJ, Seamark RF, et al. Comparison of zona cutting and zona drilling as techniques for assisted fertilization in the mouse. *J Reprod Fertil* 1988;**84**:205–11.

29. Odawara Y, Lopata A. A zona opening procedure for improving in vitro fertilization at low sperm concentrations: a mouse model. *Fertil Steril* 1989;**51**:699–704.

30. Cohen J, Malter H, Wright G, et al. Partial zona dissection of human oocytes when failure of zona pellucida penetration is anticipated. *Hum Reprod* 1989;**4**:435–42.

31. Sathananthan AH, Ng SC, Trounson A, et al. Human micro-insemination by injection of single or multiple sperm: ultrastructure. *Hum Reprod* 1989;**4**:574–83.

32. Lanzendorf SE, Maloney MK, Veeck LL, et al. A preclinical evaluation of pronuclear formation by microinjection of human spermatozoa into human oocytes. *Fertil Steril* 1988;**49**:835–42.

33. Van Steirteghem AC, Nagy Z, Joris H, et al. High fertilization and implantation rates after intra-cytoplasmic sperm injection. *Hum Reprod* 1993;**8**:1061–6.

34. Van Steirteghem AC, Liu J, Joris H, et al. Higher success rate by intracytoplasmic sperm injection than by subzonal insemination. Report of a second series of 300 consecutive treatment cycles. *Hum Reprod* 1993;**8**:1055–60.

35. Sakkas D, Gianaroli L, Diotallevi L, et al. IVF treatment of moderate male factor infertility: a comparison of mini-Percoll, partial zona dissection and sub-zonal sperm insertion techniques. *Hum Reprod* 1993;**8**:587–91.

36. Alikani M, Cohen J, Palermo GD. Enhancement of fertilization by micromanipulation. *Curr Opin Obstet Gynecol* 1995;**7**:182–7.

37. Antinori S, Versaci C, Fuhrberg P, et al. Seventeen live births after the use of an erbium–yttrium aluminum garnet laser in the treatment of male factor infertility. *Hum Reprod* 1994;**9**:1891–6.

38. Colon JM, Sarosi P, McGovern PG, et al. Controlled micromanipulation of human sperm in three dimensions with an infrared laser optical trap: effect on sperm velocity. *Fertil Steril* 1992;**57**:695–8.

39. Tadir Y, Wright WH, Vafa O, et al. Force generated by human sperm correlated to velocity and determined using a laser generated optical trap. *Fertil Steril* 1990;**53**:944–7.

40. Westphal LM, el-Danasouri I, Schimiziu S, et al. Exposure of human spermatozoa to the cumulus oophorus results in increased relative force as measured by a 760 nm laser optical trap. *Hum Reprod* 1993;**8**:1083–6.

41. Enginsu ME, Schutze K, Bellanca S, et al. Micromanipulation of mouse gametes with laser microbeam and optical tweezers. *Hum Reprod* 1995;**10**:1761–4.

42. Clement-Sengewald A, Schutze K, Ashkin A, et al. Fertilization of bovine oocytes induced solely with combined laser microbeam and optical tweezers. *J Assist Reprod Genet* 1996;**13**:259–65.

43. De Felici M, Siracusa G. Spontaneous hardening of the zona pellucida of mouse oocytes during in vitro culture. *Gam Res* 1982;**6**:107–13.

44. Drobnis EZ, Andrew JB, Katz DF. Biophysical properties of the zona pellucida measured by capillary suction: is zona hardening a mechanical phenomenon? *J Exp Zool* 1988;**245**:206–19.

45. Carroll J, Depypere H, Matthews CD. Freeze-thaw induced changes of the zona pellucida explains decreased rates of fertilization in

frozen-thawed mouse oocytes. *J Reprod Fert* 1990;**90**:547–53.

46. Loret De Mola JR, Garside WT, Bucci J, et al. Analysis of the human zona pellucida during culture: correlation with diagnosis and the preovulatory hormonal environment. *J Assist Reprod Genet* 1997;**14**:332–6.

47. Cohen J, Alikani M, Trowbridge J, et al. Implantation enhancement by selective assisted hatching using zona drilling of human embryos with poor prognosis. *Hum Reprod* 1992;**7**:685–91.

48. Tucker MJ, Luecke NM, Wiker SR, et al. Chemical removal of the outside of the zona pellucida of day 3 human embryos has no impact on implantation rate. *J Assist Reprod Genet* 1993;**10**:187–91.

49. Hu Y, Hoffman, DI, Maxson WS, et al. Clinical application of nonselective assisted hatching of human embryos. *Fertil Steril* 1996;**66**:991–4.

50. Hellebaut S, De Sutter P, Dozortsev D, et al. Does assisted hatching improve implantation rates after in vitro fertilization or intracytoplasmic sperm injection in all patients? A prospective randomized study. *J Assist Reprod Genet* 1996;**13**:19–22.

51. Stein A, Rufas O, Amit S, et al. Assisted hatching by partial zona dissection of human pre-embryos in patients with recurrent implantation failure after in vitro fertilization. *Fertil Steril* 1995;**63**:838–41.

52. Tucker MJ, Morton PC, Wright G, et al. Enhancement of outcome from intracytoplasmic sperm injection: does co-culture or assisted hatching improve implantation rates? *Hum Reprod* 1996;**11**:2434–7.

53. Schoolcraft WB, Schlenker T, Gee M, et al. Assisted hatching in the treatment of poor prognosis in vitro fertilization candidates. *Fertil Steril* 1994;**62**:551–4.

54. Check JH, Hoover L, Nazari A, et al. The effect of assisted hatching on pregnancy rates after frozen embryo transfer. *Fertil Steril* 1996;**65**:254–7.

55. Chao KH, Chen SU, Chen HF, et al. Assisted hatching increases the implantation and pregnancy rate of in vitro fertilization (IVF)-embryo transfer (ET), but not that of IVF–tubal ET in patients with repeated IVF failures. *Fertil Steril* 1997;**67**:904–8.

56. Tao J, Tamis R. Application of assisted hatching for 2-day-old, frozen-thawed embryo transfer in a poor-prognosis population. *J Assist Reprod Genet* 1997;**14**:128–30.

57. Antinori S, Selman HA, Caffa B, et al. Zona opening of human embryos using a non-contact UV laser for assisted hatching in patients with poor prognosis of pregnancy. *Hum Reprod* 1996;**11**:2488–92.

58. Tarin JJ, Handyside AH. Embryo biopsy strategies for preimplantation diagnosis. *Fertil Steril* 1993;**59**:943–52.

59. Hardy K, Martin KL, Leese HJ, et al. Human preimplantation development in vitro is not adversely affected by biopsy at the 8-cell stage. *Hum Reprod* 1990;**5**:708–14.

60. Hartshorne GM, Wick K, Elder K, et al. Effect of cell number at freezing upon survival and viability of cleaving embryos generated from stimulated IVF cycles. *Hum Reprod* 1990;**5**:857–61.

61. Dokras A, Sargent IL, Ross C, et al. Trophectoderm biopsy in human blastocysts. *Hum Reprod* 1990;**5**:821–5.

62. Dokras A, Sargent IL, Ross C, et al. The human blastocyst: morphology and human chorionic gonadotrophin secretion in vitro. *Hum Reprod* 1991;**6**:1143–51.

63. Verlinsky Y, Cieslak J, Freidine M, et al. Polar body diagnosis of common aneuploidies by FISH. *J Assist Reprod Genet* 1996;**13**:157–62.

64. Verlinsky Y, Kuliev A. Preimplantation polar body diagnosis. *Biochem Mol Med* 1996;**58**:13–17.

65. Alikani M, Olivennes F, Cohen J. Microsurgical correction of partially degenerate mouse embryos promotes hatching and restores their viability. *Hum Reprod* 1993;**8**:1723–8.

66. Cohen J, Alikani M, Reing AM, et al. Selective assisted hatching of human embryos. *Ann Acad Med, Singapore* 1992;**21**:565–70.

67. Rink K, Delacretaz G, Salathe RP, et al. Laser surgery at the micrometer scale: possibilities and limits. *Society of Photo-optical Instrumentation Engineers* 1994;**2323**:262–72.

68. Germond M, Nocera D, Senn A, et al. Improved fertilization and implantation rates after non-touch zona pellucida microdrilling of mouse oocytes with a 1.48-μm diode laser beam. *Hum Reprod* 1996;**11**:1043–8.

69. Germond M, Nocera D, Senn A, et al. Microdissection of mouse and human zona pellucida using a 1.48-μm diode laser beam: efficacy and safety of the procedure. *Fertil Steril* 1995;**64**:604–11.

70. Montag M, van der Ven K, Delacretaz G, et al. Laser-assisted microdissection of the zona pellucida facilitates polar body biopsy. *Fertil Steril* 1998; in press.

71. Boada M, Carrera M, De la Iglesia C, et al. Successful use of laser for human embryo biopsy in preimplantation genetic diagnosis: report of two cases. *J Assist Reprod Genet* 1998; in press.

72. Veiga A, Sandalinas M, Benkhalifa M, et al. Laser blastocyst biopsy for preimplantation genetic diagnosis in the human. *J Assist Reprod Genet* 1997;**14:**476 (abstract).

73. Wiemer K, Yunxia H, Cuervo M, et al. The combination of coculture and selective assisted hatching: results from their clinical application. *Fertil Steril* 1994;**61:**105–10.

74. Schoolcraft W, Schlenker T, Jones G, et al. In vitro fertilisation in women age 40 and older: the impact of assisted hatching. *J Assist Reprod Genet* 1995;**12:**581–4.

75. Antinori S, Panci C, Selman H, et al. Zona thinning with the use of laser: a new approach to assisted hatching in humans. *Hum Reprod* 1996;**11:**590–4.

# 21

# Cryopreservation of oocytes

Eleonora Porcu, Raffaella Fabbri, Stefano Venturoli, Carlo Flamigni

**Cryobiology • Variables involved in the outcome of cryopreservation • Cryodamage • Clinical results**

Cryopreservation was introduced in humans to face accumulation of excess embryos resulting from in vitro fertilization and embryo transfer (IVF-ET). Unfortunately, embryo storage has several implications because moral, legal and religious problems also involve patients and clinicians. Therefore, in some countries the application of this technique has been strictly limited, and in some places even prohibited.

Human oocyte cryopreservation could be an alternative solution to these problems, allowing several clinical applications. In fact, this is the only method for preserving the reproductive capacity for women at risk of losing it as a result of premature ovarian failure, pelvic diseases, surgery or antineoplastic treatments.

Oocyte storage has faced technical difficulties compared with sperm or embryo cryopreservation because of the specific features of female germinal cells, as documented by the low number of births achieved after oocyte cryoconservation.[1-4] Oocytes are, indeed, one of the largest human cells, with a low surface:volume ratio. At ovulation, meiosis stops at the second metaphase, with the 23 dichromatid chromosomes aligned on the equatorial axis bound to the microtubules in the meiotic spindle. This structure is extremely sensitive to temperature. In fact cryoprotectants or ice crystals derived from the freezing–thawing process may cause depolymerization of spindle microtubules. Then, at fertilization time, normal separation of chromatids could be prevented, resulting in aneuploidy after extrusion of the second polar body.

## CRYOBIOLOGY

In the cryoconservation procedure the main steps are: (1) preliminary exposure to the cryoprotectants, substances that reduce cell damages depending on ice crystals; (2) progressive temperature reduction down to $-196°C$; (3) storage; (4) subsequent thawing after a variable length of time; and (5) dilution and washing of the cryoprotectants to restore a physiological microenvironment and allow the following development.

The two most critical moments affecting cell survival are the phase of initial cooling and the return to physiological conditions. When reducing the temperature between $-5$ and $-15°C$, ice nucleation is first induced in the extracellular medium by a process called 'seeding'. As the temperature is gradually decreased, ice builds up and the solutes concentrate in the extracellular medium. This determines an osmotic gradient: water moves out of the cytoplasm and cells shrink from the dehydration. If freezing is carried out slowly, water diffusion from the cell does not allow the formation of large ice crystals inside the cytoplasm.

A detailed mathematical model has been developed to calculate the rate of modification of cell volume, as a function of the permeability, surface area and temperature.[5] For those cells with a low surface:volume ratio, as for the female gametes, it is necessary for a low cooling rate to allow the diffusion of a sufficient amount of water out of the cell. For each cell type, by increasing the rate of freezing, survival decreases.[6] On the other hand, survival rate decreases if the speed of thawing is too low because ice crystals in the cytosol have enough time to enlarge. Two events that occur during thawing can reduce cell survival: recrystallization and osmotic shock. Recrystallization means that water moves back inside the cell and solidifies around the small ice crystals already formed, increasing their size. The likelihood of recrystallization depends on both cooling and thawing rates. It is possible to avoid this by careful dehydration and rapid thawing of the cell. Osmotic shock may occur if, after thawing, the cryoprotectant that penetrated the cell during cooling cannot diffuse out quickly enough to prevent the influx of water and swelling of the cell.

A careful review of the literature points out contrasting information about the most suitable and the least harmful methods of preserving cell integrity.

## VARIABLES INVOLVED IN THE OUTCOME OF CRYOPRESERVATION

The main factors that seem to influence the outcome of cryopreservation concern the oocyte (size, quality, age, maturity, cumulus) and the technique (type, temperature, concentration and exposure time of cryoprotectants, freezing and thawing rates).

## Variables related to the oocyte

### Oocyte size

Oocyte size is a critical parameter in the freezing process and it may influence the probability of intracellular ice formation and overall survival rates. The spermatozoa offer a clear example of the influence of this factor on survival rate after storage: male gametes in human species are 180 times smaller than female ones because of their smaller quantities of cytosol, and their survival rates are considerably higher. Moreover, mouse oocytes, whose size is smaller than those of humans and rabbits, show a higher survival rate.[7]

### Oocyte quality

It is essential to have very good quality to guarantee oocyte survival after thawing. Usually, only extra oocytes are frozen. Their quality is often poor, explaining the low survival rate after thawing. For this reason, some authors have stored only the best quality oocytes, for example, Chen.[2] In our infertility and IVF centre we decided to cryopreserve all the oocytes retrieved, when possible.

### Oocyte age

The oocytes should be stored shortly after pickup, between 38 and 40 hours after administration of human chorionic gonadotrophin (hCG).[2] Cryopreservation of aged oocytes shows a considerable decrease in fertilization rate and an increase of abnormal fertilization and polyploidy.[8] The oocytes must be cryopreserved the same day of collection, possibly within 8 hours.[8]

### Maturation stage

Pregnancies reported in the literature after oocyte cryopreservation were achieved with mature female gametes, that is, those at metaphase II. As reported by Al-Hasani et al[7] oocytes that are considered mature at pick-up give the highest survival and fertilization rates.

An alternative approach to mature gamete storage is represented by the cryopreservation of oocytes at prophase I, when meioisis is arrested at diplotene, and chromosomes are within the membrane-bound nucleus. After the first disappointing results, Toth et al[9] reported interesting outcomes: prophase I oocytes, collected from thin slices of ovarian tissue, are able to survive cryopreservation and mature to metaphase II after thawing.

Hovatta and co-workers[10] recently proposed the storage of thin slices of human ovarian tissue, which is rich in primordial follicles. Thanks to the good survival rate shown by the follicles, the oocytes should be able to mature in vitro, and be fertilized. Other authors[11] have proposed implanting thawed ovarian tissue into the abdomen.

*Cumulus oophorus*

Another variable that seems to affect the outcome of the cryopreservation technique is the oophorus cumulus. Various authors have supported or criticized cumulus removal. Some have shown that the absence of this large cellular complex could facilitate the penetration of the cryoprotectants inside the cytoplasm: the first pregnancies were indeed achieved using this method.[1,3] Gook et al[12] also reported a higher survival rate of oocytes stored without cumulus (69% vs 48%). However, some studies suggest a role for the cumulus in obtaining higher cell survival after cryoconservation.[13,14] In 1992, Imoedehme and Sigue[15] found a higher survival rate in oocytes with cumulus compared with those without (54% vs 27%, respectively); in addition, gametes stored with the intact cumulus also showed a higher fertilization and cleavage rate. The authors hypothesized that the presence of cumulus may offer a sort of protection against the osmotic stress caused by rapid concentration or dilution of the cryoprotectants during equilibration steps and removal after thawing.

# Variables related to the cryoconservation technique

*Cryoprotectants*

### Type of cryoprotectant

Cryoprotectants are substances with different chemical composition characterized by a high water solubility and a toxicity proportional to their concentration and temperature.

Cryoprotectants can be put into two different categories based on their ability to penetrate into the cells: intracellular (permeating) and extracellular (not permeating) agents. According to their chemical structure, it is possible to distinguish three classes of cryoprotectants: alcohols (methanol, ethanol, propanol, 1,2-propanediol, glycerol), carbohydrates (glucose, lactose, sucrose, starch) and dimethyl-sulphoxide (DMSO).

Cryoprotectants exert a complex action, depending on several properties. First of all, their presence in the freezing medium decreases its cryoscopic point to almost −2 or −3°C. Their protective effect is related to the ability to form hydrogen bonds with water, reducing the size of the ice crystals.

Agents such as glycerol and propanediol, thanks to their hydroxyl groups, can establish hydrogen bonds with molecules of water, as DMSO does through its oxygen atom. Cryoprotectants reduce electrolyte concentrations in the non-frozen medium. In a two-phase system, such as water and ice, if pressure remains uniform, the overall solute concentration in the water is fixed at any temperature. Then the addition of cryoprotectants reduces the amount of water that crystallizes.[6]

### Exposure temperature and concentration of cryoprotectants

The efficacy of cryoprotectants depends on the temperature at which these compounds are added to the freezing medium. Pickering and co-workers[16] demonstrated that human oocytes exposed to DMSO at 37°C lose their potential to fertilize. The authors suggest that the addition of DMSO to the medium must be performed at a temperature lower than 10°C, to avoid impairment of the fertilization rate. The optimal concentration of the cryoprotectant depends on the cell and species type.[17]

### Duration of exposure to cryoprotectants

In 1988 Sathananthan et al[18] demonstrated that the duration of exposure to DMSO influences the level of damage to the meiotic spindle:

although after 10–20 min the spindle shows normal morphology, 60 min at 1.5 mol/l are sufficient to induce severe alterations, which are irreversible in most oocytes. Van Der Elst et al[19] reported that exposure of the oocyte to propanediol 1.5 mol/l at 0°C for a short time (12 min) is harmless. In our centre the time of exposure of oocytes to propanediol is 10 min.

### Removal of cryoprotectants

The removal from the cytoplasm of the permeating cryoprotectant by stepwise dilution is an important step in the freezing process.[16] In fact, if after thawing oocytes are placed directly in a medium with no cryoprotectant, they could swell and burst because of the osmotic effect exerted by permeants. At this step, the use of non-permeating molecules, such as sucrose, increases the osmotic pressure of the external medium, opposing the inflow of water into the cytosol and so preventing bursting of oocytes.

## Freezing–thawing rate

The freezing–thawing rate affects the diffusion of water through the cell membrane. The optimal rate of thawing depends on the freezing procedure because this step controls the amount of ice inside the oocyte. Generally, if slow cooling is arrested at a temperature that is not too low (−30 or −40°C), some water remains in the cell; thus, thawing must be rapid to avoid the development of large ice crystals in the cytoplasm. Instead, if dehydration continues until −80°C, thawing must be slower to guarantee a suitable rehydration: this allows the cell to restore its initial volume gradually. Thawing is actually the limiting step of the whole process.

Several protocols for oocyte cryopreservation have been used, based on different rates of freezing and thawing.

### Slow freezing–rapid thawing

Oocyte storage is often performed with a slow freeze–rapid thaw procedure. Chen[1] achieved the first pregnancy world wide using this protocol. The same strategy was adopted by Siebzehnruebl et al.[20]

### Slow freezing–slow thawing

Although uncommon and rarely reported in literature, this method was used to obtain the second pregnancy using a frozen oocyte.[3] The authors used DMSO 1.5 mol/l as cryoprotectant and oocyte thawing was performed at room temperature.

### Ultrarapid freezing–rapid thawing

This method avoids the formation of ice crystals and induces a glassy, amorphous medium using high concentrations of cryoprotectants. Trounson[21] first applied this strategy to human oocyte cryopreservation by direct immersion of ova in liquid nitrogen (ultrarapid freezing). Rapid thawing was performed at 37°C, in a water bath. Nine of 18 mature human ova so treated survived to thawing, but all of them degenerated in culture.

### Vitrification

Vitrification is a process in which a highly concentrated solution of cryoprotectants solidifies during freezing without the formation of ice crystals, in a supercooled, highly viscous fluid.

A high cooling rate (almost 1500°C/min) and high concentrations of cryoprotectants such as DMSO, acetamide, propyleneglycol and polyethyleneglycol, are needed for vitrification. The theoretical basis of vitrification was clearly shown by Rall and Fahy[22] as a technique for preserving the embryos. However, results are discordant and toxicity of the cryoprotectants is confirmed by experimental studies.[6] Trounson[21] reported acceptable survival and fertilization rates but low cleavage rates. The cleavage block may be related to the irreversible damage induced in the cytoskeleton by the association of cooling and vitrification.

## CRYODAMAGE

An intact oocyte appears shiny, with no cell disruption. A damaged oocyte presents zona fractures, and dark, contracted and pyknotic cytoplasm (Figure 1). Several cell structures can be damaged during the whole process of freezing–thawing and by the cryoprotectants (Figure 2). This damage can result in morphological and functional abnormalities.

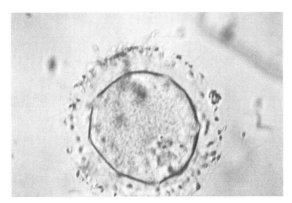

**Figure 1**   Damaged oocyte after cryopreservation.

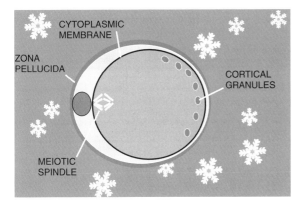

**Figure 2**   Possible sites of oocyte cryodamage.

## Meiotic spindle

Concern has been expressed about the possibility of inducing disarray in the meiotic spindle microtubules, because the oocyte cryopreserved at metaphase II presents the 23 dichromatid chromosomes strictly bound to the microtubules. This structure is extremely sensitive to temperature. According to the 'pushing body' theory, separation and movements of the chromatids are possible thanks to a proper polymerization and depolymerization of the microtubules constituting the meiotic spindle.

Any loss of these structures could spread the chromosomes out and cause aneuploidy.[6,14,18,19] It was demonstrated that, in mouse and rabbit oocytes, exposure to 1,2-propanediol depolymerizes the microfilaments.[23] Some authors postulated that, after thawing, the oocytes could repair some of the damage by the correct repolymerization of the spindle,[14,18] leading to the resumption of meiosis at fertilization and to subsequent events related to embryo cleavage and development. Van Blerkom and Davis[24] report that the rate of aneuploidy in human oocytes dehydrated by 1,2-propanediol and subsequently stored is about 4–5%. Gook et al[8,12] reported normal karyotypes and the absence of stray chromosomes in cryopreserved oocytes. They suggest that the meiotic spindle of human oocytes seems to be more resistant compared with that of murine gametes; they do not confirm in humans the results obtained in mice.

Another possible effect of cryopreservation is the untimely resumption of meiosis, with activation of parthenogenesis. This implies the risk of transferring an abnormal embryo, even if it is unable to go beyond the first cleavage stages.[25] Activation of parthenogenesis can be induced in a mammalian oocyte by a large number of chemical compounds containing a hydroxyl group, such as propanediol. In murine oocytes this event seems to depend on the concentration of the cryoprotectant, time of exposure and temperature at which the agent is added to the culture medium.[19]

Gook et al[26] demonstrated that only exposure to propanediol does not induce parthenogenesis, whereas the freezing process may cause it in 27–29% of the cases. In this study, parthenogenetic oocytes showed one pronucleus and extrusion of the second polar body in 18% of fresh oocytes and 5% of aged oocytes. On the contrary, two or more pronuclei probably derived from retention of the second polar body and the possible fragmentation into several subnuclei has been shown only in aged oocytes.

## Cytoskeleton

Another subcellular structure usually involved in cryopreservation damage is the cytoskeleton, the structures of which (microtubules, actin microfilaments and intermediate filaments) are extremely sensitive to low temperatures.

Hunter et al[27] suggest that the arrest of development in embryos derived from cryopreserved oocytes is related to subtle perturbations in their cytoarchitectonics, that is, cytoskeleton abnormalities may prevent the pronucleus membrane breakdown and the joining of maternal and paternal chromosomes. Alternatively, they can prevent the correct zygote cleavage or induce the formation of several endocytotic vacuoles in the cytoplasm after pronuclei formation.

## Cortical granules

During fertilization the exocytosis of the cortical granules (zona reaction) situated in the periphery of the oocyte prevents the entry of more than one spermatozoon (polyspermy block). A study of human and murine oocytes performed by electron microscopy detected reduction and morphological abnormalities of the granules after thawing.[28]

Van Blerkom and Davis,[24] reporting similar data, point out that the premature exocytosis of the cortical granules may lead to an untimely zona hardening and consequently affect the fertilization rates after conventional IVF. Probably the untimely release of the cortical granules is the result of the damage exerted by the cryoprotectants and the ice crystals on the actin microfilaments situated under the cell membrane.[17,23]

Al-Hasani and Diedrich[28] postulated that the high frequency of polyspermy in frozen–thawed oocytes is caused by the loss of the granules as a result of the freezing process. This allows the penetration of several spermatozoa. Sathananthan et al[14] noted that the cumulus may prevent exocytosis of the cortical granules.

In 1993, Gook et al[12] documented plenty of cortical granules in all the cryopreserved oocytes, postulating that the freezing process does not affect the release of these structures. Gook et al[8] also demonstrated that the high percentage of abnormal fertilizations is related to the protracted in vitro culture of the oocytes, rather than to the cooling procedure. In vitro culture and ageing of the oocytes could lead to cortical granular damage.

## Zona pellucida

Several researchers pointed out the risk of damage to the zona pellucida[29,30] in oocyte cryopreservation. Zona damage is believed to be caused either by the formation of fracture planes in the ice or by the ice crystals being able to trap or pierce the cell. The addition of polymers such as dextran and polyvinylpyrrolidone (PVP) reduce the size of the ice crystals and exert cryoprotective properties.[29]

## CLINICAL RESULTS

### Survival

The survival rate of cryopreserved oocytes varies considerably from less than 25% to more than 80%. Chen[2] reported one of the best survival rates cited in the literature (76%). He froze only mature (metaphase II) oocytes of very good quality.

Lower survival rates (25%) are reported by Al-Hasani et al[7] who, however, used only excess oocytes of IVF patients, which were usually immature and of poor quality. They compare DMSO and propanediol, achieving 28% of the survival rate with the first cryoprotectant (40 of 144) and 32% with the second (12 of 38).

Low survival rates were also reported by Kazem et al[30] (34.4%) and Tucker et al.[31] Both teams used propanediol.

Gook et al[26,32] reported a survival rate varying from 48% to 95%. They used propanediol and obtained better results with denuded oocytes (69% vs 48%). In addition, they found that aged oocytes survived better than fresh oocytes but had a low fertilization rate.

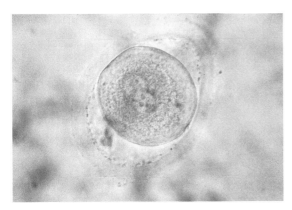

**Figure 3** Zygote of the first child conceived with the intracytoplasmic sperm injection of a frozen-thawed oocyte.

One reason for the wide variability of survival rate reported in literature may be the generally low number of frozen eggs evaluated in most studies.

Our centre has the largest series of frozen–thawed oocytes reported so far and our mean survival rate, about 57–58%,[33] probably represents the actual efficiency of this technique today. In our experience, the cumulus complex does not seem to condition oocyte survival significantly, in agreement with Mandelbaum's experience.[34]

## Fertilization

The fertilization rate of cryopreserved oocytes with IVF is extremely variable ranging from 13%[30] to 71%.[2] However, in most studies, variability is between 30% and 55%, being on average lower than the fertilization rate obtained with fresh oocytes.

Abnormal fertilization, usually polyploidy, ranges from 5%[32] to 10.8%[30] and 15.3%.[7] The often reduced fertilization rate and sometimes increased abnormal fertilization have been related to possible damage of the zona pellucida and the cortical granules, which would prevent interaction with spermatozoa.

Intracytoplasmic sperm injection (ICSI) has recently been proposed as a solution to these problems. With this technique, Gook's team[32] obtained 50% of normal fertilization together with 21% of abnormal fertilization. Compared with traditional IVF, embryos obtained with ICSI showed a better development. Similar experiences have been found by Kazem et al[30] who documented 43.2% of normal fertilization and by Tucker et al[31] who achieved a 65% fertilization rate and three pregnancies, all of which ended in abortion.

After a preliminary experience with IVF of frozen oocytes, which gave a 46% fertilization rate, our centre also undertook a study linking ICSI and oocyte cryopreservation. Superovulation was induced with a combination of a gonadotrophin-releasing hormone (GnRH) analogue and gonadotrophins.[35] Oocytes were cryopreserved with a slow freezing–fast thawing protocol using propanediol and sucrose as cryoprotectants[4] and inseminated using ICSI.[36] ICSI damage was 7%, much lower than that reported by Kazem et al[30] (32%) and Gook et al[32] (26.3%).

Our normal fertilization rate is 64.3%, similar to that obtained by Tucker et al.[31] Our abnormal fertilization rate (7.2%) resembles that found in IVF and ICSI of fresh oocytes. Most embryos have been of good quality with regular cleavage. In 1997 we reported the birth of a healthy female from ICSI of frozen oocytes (Figure 3).[4] We have currently achieved nine pregnancies and the birth of six healthy children.

The best results were obtained with embryo transfer in a hormone replacement cycle with pharmacological growth of the endometrium.

## Efficiency

Until recently, oocyte cryopreservation was considered a low efficiency technique because of low survival, fertilization and cleavage rates. With the introduction of ICSI, the results, in terms of fertilization, embryo cleavage and implantation, approach those obtained with fresh oocytes. The only limiting step seems to be oocyte survival which should be improved further.

## Safety

Safety of oocyte cryopreservation has been extensively debated. As previously discussed, the main concern is related to the possible damage of the meiotic spindle and the induction of aneuploidy. However, the investigations of Gook's team[8,12,26] are reassuring, showing normal karyotypes and absence of stray chromosomes in cryopreserved oocytes. It is likely that the cryopreservation processes expose oocytes to a rigid selection, allowing only the strongest cells to survive.

Our group have managed to transfer the encouraging results achieved in basic research into the clinical sphere and, with the use of two novel techniques such as ICSI and oocyte cryopreservation, have achieved the birth of six healthy children. Together with the four normal children born in Australia[1,2] and Germany[3] more than 10 years ago, these new births may be a significant and a long-awaited advance in fertility treatment.

## REFERENCES

1.  Chen C. Pregnancy after human oocyte cryopreservation. *Lancet* 1986;**i:**884–6.
2.  Chen C. Pregnancies after human oocyte cryopreservation. *Ann NY Acad Sci* 1987;**541:**541–9.
3.  Van Uem JFHM, Siebzehnruebl ER, Schun B, Koch R, Trotnow S, Lang N. Birth after cryopreservation of unfertilized oocytes. *Lancet* 1987;**i:**752–3.
4.  Porcu E, Fabbri R, Seracchioli R, Ciotti PM, Magrini O, Flamigni C. Birth of a healthy female after intracytoplasmic sperm injection of cryopreserved human oocytes. *Fertil Steril* 1997;**4:**724–6.
5.  Mazur P. Limits to life at low temperatures and at reduced water activities. *Orig Life* 1980;**10:**137.
6.  Friedler S, Giudice L, Lamb E. Cryopreservation of embryos and ova. *Feril Steril* 1988;**49:**743–64.
7.  Al Hasani S, Diedrich K, van der Ven H, Reinecke A, Hartje M, Krebs D. Cryopreservation of human oocytes. *Hum Reprod* 1987;**2:**695–700.
8.  Gook D, Osborn S, Bourne H, Johnston W. Fertilization of human oocytes following cryopreservation; normal karyotipes and absence of stray chromosomes. *Hum Reprod* 1994;**9:**684–91.
9.  Toth TL, Lazendorf SE, Sandow BA, et al. Cryopreservation of human prophase I oocytes collected from unstimulated follicles. *Fertil Steril* 1994;**61:**1077–82.
10. Hovatta O, Silye R, Krausz T, et al. Cryopreservation of human ovarian tissue using dimethylsulphoxide and propanediol-sucrose as cryoprotectants. *Hum Reprod* 1996;**11:**1268–72.
11. Newton H, Aubard Y, Rutherford A, Sharma V, Gosden R. Low temperature storage and grafting of human ovarian tissue. *Hum Reprod* 1996;**11:**1487–91.
12. Gook D, Osborn S, Johnston W. Cryopreservation of mouse and human oocytes using 1,2 propanediol and the configuration of the meiotic spindle. *Hum Reprod* 1993;**8:**1101–9.
13. Pellicer A, Lightman A, Parmer TG, Behrman HR, De Cherney AH. Morphologic and functional studies of immature rat oocyte-cumulus complexes after cryopreservation. *Fertil Steril* 1988;**50:**805–10.
14. Sathananthan AH, Kirby C, Trounson A, Philipatos D, Shaw J. The effects of cooling mouse oocytes. *J Assist Reprod Genet* 1992;**9:**139–48.
15. Imoedehme DG, Sigue AB. Survival of human oocytes cryopreserved with or without the cumulus in 1,2-propanediol. *J Assist Reprod Genet* 1992;**9:**323–7.
16. Pickering S, Braude P, Johnson M. Cryoprotection of human oocyte: inappropriate exposure to DMSO reduces fertilization rates. *Hum Reprod* 1991;**6:**142–3.
17. Vincent C, Pruliere G, Pajot-Augy E, Campion E, Garnier V, Renard JP. Effects of cryoprotectants on actin filaments during cryopreservation of one-cell rabbit embryos. *Cryobiology* 1990;**27:** 9–23.
18. Sathananthan AH, Trounson A, Freeman L, Brady T. The effects of cooling human oocytes. *Hum Reprod* 1988;**8:**968–77.

19. Van Der Elst J, Van Den Abbeel E, Nerinckx S, Van Steirteghem A. Parthenogenetic activation pattern and microtubular organization of the mouse oocyte after exposure to 1,2-propanediol. *Cryobiology* 1992;**29**:549–62.

20. Siebzehnruebl ER, Todorow S, Van Uem J, Koch R, Wildt L, Lang N. Cryopreservation of human and rabbit oocytes and one-cell embryos: a comparison of DMSO and propanediol. *Hum Reprod* 1989;**4**:312–17.

21. Trounson A. Freezing human eggs and embryos. *Fertil Steril* 1986;**46**:1–12.

22. Rall WF, Fahy GM. Ice free cryopreservation of mouse embryos at −196°C by vitrification. *Nature* 1985;**313**:573.

23. Vincent C, Pickering SJ, Johnson MH, Quick SJ. Dimethylsulfoxide affects the organization of microfilaments in the mouse oocyte. *Development* 1990;**26**:227–35.

24. Van Blerkom J, Davis P. Cytogenetic, cellular and developmental consequences of cryopreservation of immature and human oocytes. *Microscopy Res Tec* 1994;**27**:165–93.

25. Balakier H, Casper R. Experimentally induced parthenogenetic activation of human oocytes. *Hum Reprod* 1993;**5**:740–3.

26. Gook D, Osborn S, Johnston W. Parthenogenetic activation of human oocytes following cryopreservation using 1,2-propanediol. *Hum Reprod* 1995;**10**:654–8.

27. Hunter JE, Bernard A, Fuller B, Amso N, Shaw RW. Fertilization and development of the human oocyte following exposure to cryoprotectants, low temperatures and cryopreservation: a comparison of two techniques. *Hum Reprod* 1991;**6**:1460–5.

28. Al Hasani S, Diedrich K. Oocyte storage. In: *Gametes–The Oocyte* (Grudzinskas JG, Yovich JL, eds). Cambridge: Cambridge University Press, 1995: Chap 15, 376–95.

29. Dumoulin JCM, Bergers-Janssen JM, Pieters MH, Enginsu ME, Geraedts JPM, Evers JLH. The protective effects of polymers in the cryopreservation of human and mouse zonae pellucidae and embryos. *Fertil Steril* 1994;**62**:793–8.

30. Kazem R, Thompson LA, Srikantharajah A, Laing MA, Hamilton MPR, Templeton A. Cryopreservation of human oocytes and fertilization by two techniques: in-vitro fertilization and intracytoplasmic sperm injection. *Hum Reprod* 1995;**10**:2650–4.

31. Tucker M, Wright G, Morton P, Shanguo L, Massey J, Kort H. Preliminary experience with human oocyte cryopreservation using 1,2 propanediol and sucrose. *Hum Reprod* 1996;**11**:1513–15.

32. Gook D, Schiewe MC, Osborn S, Asch RH, Jansen RPS, Johnston WIH. Intracytoplasmic sperm injection and embryo development of human oocytes cryopreserved using 1,2-propanediol. *Hum Reprod* 1995;**10**:2637–41.

33. Porcu E, Fabbri R, Seracchioli R, et al. Birth and pregnancies after microinjection of cryopreserved human oocytes. *53rd Meeting of the American Society for Reproductive Medicine* 1997; abstr. 75.

34. Mandelbaum J, Junca AM, Plachot M, et al. Cryopreservation of human embryos and oocytes. *Hum Reprod* 1988;**3**:117–19.

35. Porcu E, Dal Prato L, Seracchioli R, Fabbri R, Longhi M, Flamigni C. Comparison between depot and standard release triptoreline in in vitro fertilization: pituitary sensitivity, luteal function, pregnancy outcome and perinatal results. *Fertil Steril* 1994;**62**:126–32.

36. Palermo G, Joris H, Devroey P, Van Steirteghem AC. Pregnancies after intracytoplasmic injection of a single spermatozoon into an oocyte. *Lancet* 1992;**340**:17–18.

# 22

# Should ICSI apply to all IVF cycles?

André Van Steirteghem, Anick De Vos, Catherine Staessen, Greta Verheyen and Maryse Bonduelle

**Six years of clinical practice of ICSI** • **Controlled comparison of conventional IVF and ICSI in couples with tubal, idiopathic and borderline male factor infertility** • **Prospective follow-up of pregnancies and children born after ICSI: current results** • **Acknowledgments**

In 1992, our group reported the first pregnancies and births that resulted from replacement of embryos generated by intracytoplasmic sperm injection (ICSI), which involves injection of a single spermatozoon through the zona pellucida directly into the oocyte.[1] It became obvious that ICSI resulted in higher fertilization and cleavage rates than did other assisted fertilization procedures such as partial zona dissection or subzonal insemination.[2]

ICSI has been introduced into clinical practice to treat couples with severe male factor infertility, who cannot be helped by conventional in vitro fertilization (IVF) because they have too few progressively motile spermatozoa with normal morphology.[3–5] The procedure of ICSI is also the technique of choice when epididymal or testicular sperm is obtained surgically from patients with obstructive or non-obstructive azoospermia.[6–10]

This chapter reports on the results of 6 years of ICSI practice (1991–96) at our centre, the preliminary results of controlled studies of ICSI versus IVF in tubal, idiopathic and borderline male factor infertility, and the current results of prospective follow-up of pregnancies and children born after ICSI.

## SIX YEARS OF CLINICAL PRACTICE OF ICSI

### Treatment cycles

Almost 6200 ICSI procedures involving 64 000 metaphase II oocytes were carried out between January 1991 and December 1996.

The ICSI procedure could not be carried out in 185 cycles (2.9%) of 6353 planned ICSI cycles because either there were no cumulus–oocyte complexes or metaphase II oocytes (81 cycles) or there were no spermatozoa available (104 cycles). The latter condition occurred in patients with non-obstructive azoospermia who were scheduled for ICSI with testicular spermatozoa.

ICSI was performed with spermatozoa from the ejaculate in 5391 (87%) cycles where there was no, or only poor, fertilization in conventional IVF cycles or in couples where the man had semen values that were too impaired to be accepted for conventional IVF. Spermatozoa retrieved from the epididymis were used in men with azoospermia caused by congenital or acquired obstruction: freshly collected epididymal spermatozoa were used in 158 cycles (3%) and frozen–thawed epididymal spermatozoa in 116 cycles (2%). ICSI was performed with freshly collected testicular spermatozoa in 503 cycles (8%) from patients with obstructive or non-obstructive spermatozoa.

## Oocytes for ICSI

Controlled ovarial stimulation was usually performed by the association of gonadotrophin-releasing hormone (GnRH) agonists, human menopausal gonadotrophin (hMG) and human chorionic gonadotrophin (hCG). Oocyte retrieval was carried out 36 hours after hCG administration by means of ultrasonically guided transvaginal aspiration.

Our experience is based on a total of 79 731 cumulus–oocyte complexes retrieved during 6353 cycles, which represents a mean of 12.6 complexes per cycle. The cumulus and the corona cells were removed by means of a combination of enzymatic and mechanical procedures. A recent study in our laboratory has indicated that enzymatic denudation is also feasible with only 10 IU hyaluronidase; currently we use this lower concentration in order to avoid the exposure of the oocytes to higher amounts of hyaluronidase.[11] Denuded oocytes are observed under an inverted microscope at a magnification of 200. Observations include assessment of the zona pellucida and the oocyte, and the presence or absence of a germinal vesicle or a first polar body. Of the 79 731 cumulus–oocyte complexes currently studied, 95% contained an oocyte with an intact zona pellucida: 10% contained germinal vesicle stage oocytes, 4% contained metaphase I oocytes that had undergone breakdown of the germinal vesicle but had not yet extruded the first polar body, and 81% contained metaphase II oocytes that had extruded the first polar body. ICSI is only carried out on metaphase II oocytes because they are the only ones that have reached the haploid state and, thus, can be fertilized normally.

## Spermatozoa for ICSI

Before the ICSI cycle, semen assessment is performed according to the recommendations of the World Health Organization except for sperm morphology, which is assessed by strict criteria. Semen values are considered normal if the volume of the ejaculate is at least 2 ml, sperm concentration is at least $20 \times 10^6/\text{ml}$, progressive sperm motility is at least 40% and normal sperm morphology is at least 14%. Analysis of the characteristics of the freshly ejaculated semen used in 5215 ICSI cycles showed that all three semen values were abnormal in 43% of the cycles, two semen values were abnormal in 30% of the cycles, and one semen value was abnormal in 19% of the cycles; normal semen values were observed in 8% of the cycles. Most of the couples with normal semen values had previously undergone conventional IVF treatments without success.

In only 15% of sperm samples, could the swim-up procedure be used to prepare the sperm. The remaining ejaculated sperm samples for ICSI are prepared by centrifugation on a discontinuous gradient initially of Percoll, which has now been replaced by Pure Sperm.

Epididymal sperm are usually recovered from the most proximal part of the caput of the epididymis in a microsurgical procedure. Several epididymal sperm fractions are collected and treated in the same way as ejaculated semen. Whenever possible, some of the freshly recovered epididymal sperm has been frozen for later use in order to avoid surgical procedures in subsequent cycles.

Testicular spermatozoa are isolated from a testicular biopsy, which can be obtained by means of surgical excisional biopsy or fine needle aspiration. Several procedures can be used to recover testicular sperm, including mechanical shredding, sometimes in combination with erythrocyte-lysing buffer or collagenase.[12–14] The second procedure has to be used especially on testicular tissue from patients with non-obstructive azoospermia.

## ICSI procedure

The details of microtool preparation and the actual microinjection procedure have been described earlier in a previous publication.[15] A

**Table 1 Oocyte damage, pronuclear status and embryo cleavage after ICSI**

| | All cycles | Type of sperm | | | |
| --- | --- | --- | --- | --- | --- |
| | | Ejaculated semen | Epididymal | | Testicular |
| | | | Fresh | Frozen–thawed | |
| No. of cycles | 6168 | 5391 | 158 | 116 | 503 |
| No. of injected oocytes | 63 698 | 54 792 | 1850 | 1244 | 5812 |
| Percentage of intact oocytes | 90.3 | 90.3 | 89.6 | 91.7 | 90.1 |
| Percentage of injected oocytes with | | | | | |
| 1 PN | 2.9 | 2.7 | 4.1 | 3.3 | 4.3 |
| 2 PN | 64.8 | 66.1 | 59.4 | 55.9 | 56.3 |
| ⩾3 PN | 3.9 | 3.9 | 5.0 | 5.0 | 3.5 |
| No. of 2 PN oocytes | 41 302 | 36 236 | 1098 | 696 | 3272 |
| Percentage of | | | | | |
| Type A embryos | 65.0 | 6.7 | 7.7 | 3.4 | 5.1 |
| Type B embryos | 56.7 | 58.1 | 48.9 | 44.4 | 47.2 |
| Type C embryos | 16.2 | 15.8 | 14.9 | 18.5 | 20.3 |
| Percentage of transferred or | | | | | |
| frozen embryos | 64.7 | 65.2 | 64.2 | 59.1 | 60.8 |

PN, pronucleus.

single, motile (living), immobilized spermatozoon is aspirated tail first into the injection pipette. The oocyte is fixed with the holding pipette and care is taken that the polar body is situated at the 6 o'clock position. The injection pipette is pushed through the zona pellucida and the oolemma into the cytoplasm at the 3 o'clock position, and the sperm is delivered with the smallest amount of medium.[16] Orienting the oocyte in this way minimizes the risk that the injection pipette will damage the metaphase plate. It is useful to aspirate the cytoplasm gently into the injection pipette before the sperm injection, to be certain that the tip of the pipette has penetrated the oolemma rather than simply indenting it.

**Intactness, pronuclear status and embryo cleavage of injected oocytes** (Table 1)

Oocytes are inspected for damage and pronuclear status 16–18 hours after the ICSI procedure. The number and aspect of polar bodies and pronuclei are recorded. Oocytes are considered to be normally fertilized when two individualized or fragmented polar bodies are present together with two clearly visible pronuclei that contain nucleoli. A mean of 10.3 metaphase II oocytes was injected per cycle. About 10% of the injected oocytes were damaged. The damage rate was similar for the four types of sperm used during the ICSI procedure. The overall normal fertilization rate (oocytes with two pronuclei) was 64.8%, with a variation between 55.9% and 66.1%. The normal fertilization rate for ICSI was higher when ejaculated sperm were used than when other types of sperm were used. Abnormal fertilization occurred as oocytes of one pronucleus in 2.9% of the injected metaphase II oocytes. Abnormal fertilization occurred to a similar extent in the four different groups of spermatozoa. If embryo cleavage occurred from oocytes with one pronucleus to those with three pronuclei, these embryos were never transferred to the patients.

It was very exceptional that none of the injected oocytes fertilized normally. This occurred when: (1) only very few metaphase II oocytes were available for ICSI; (2) only totally immotile spermatozoa could be injected; (3) gross abnormalities were present in the oocytes; (4) round-headed spermatozoa were injected; or (5) all oocytes were damaged in the injection procedure. Most of the patients involved achieved fertilization in a subsequent cycle.[17,18]

Embryo cleavage of normally fertilized oocytes was assessed after 24 hours of further in vitro culture. The cleaving embryos are scored to equality of size of the blastomeres and proportion of anucleate fragments into three categories: (1) excellent, type A embryos with no anucleate fragments; (2) good quality, type B embryos with between 1% and 20% of the volume filled with anucleate fragments; and (3) fair quality, type C embryos with between 21% and 50% of the volume filled with anucleate fragments. Cleaved embryos with less than half of their volume filled with anucleate fragments are eligible for transfer. Supernumerary embryos with less than 20% anucleate fragments are cryopreserved on day 2 or 3 after oocyte retrieval by means of a slow-freezing protocol with dimethylsulphoxide.[13] A higher percentage of good quality embryos was obtained in the group of ejaculated spermatozoa. The percentages of embryos actually transferred or frozen as supernumerary embryos were similar for the four types of spermatozoa.

## Outcome of embryo transfers (Table 2)

Replacement of at least one embryo was possible in 92.6% (5714 of 6168) treatment cycles with ICSI. This could certainly be considered to be a high transfer rate because it represents couples who have had previous fertilization failure in conventional IVF, those for whom the quality of the man's ejaculated sperm is too poor to be included in IVF or men with obstructive or non-obstructive azoospermia. The percentage of transfers was similar for the four groups of sperm used for ICSI and varied from 85.3% to 93%. The overall pregnancy rate with known serum hCG outcome per transfer and per cycle was also similar for the four types of spermatozoa. Particularly high pregnancy rates were observed when elective transfer of two or three embryos was performed.[20]

Delivery rates per transfers with known outcome were calculated for the ICSI treatment cycles performed between 1991 and 1995; they varied from 22.4% to 30.5%.

## CONTROLLED COMPARISON OF CONVENTIONAL IVF AND ICSI IN COUPLES WITH TUBAL, IDIOPATHIC AND BORDERLINE MALE FACTOR INFERTILITY

Should the ICSI procedure be extended to indications other than severe male factor infertility? Are normal fertilization and embryo cleavage better after ICSI than after conventional IVF? Can we avoid unexpected fertilization failures when ICSI is used? If the answers to these questions are positive, the implantation potential of IVF and ICSI embryos should be examined. The ultimate question about safety should then be answered: are there more problems during pregnancy and after delivery when the ICSI procedure has been used instead of conventional IVF?

In a series of ongoing controlled studies we have searched for an answer to these questions in couples with tubal, idiopathic and borderline male factor infertility. Couples who were infertile for the above reasons were included in

**Table 2 Outcome of embryo transfers after ICSI**

| | Type of sperm | | | |
| --- | --- | --- | --- | --- |
| | Ejaculated semen | Epididymal | | Testicular |
| | | Fresh | Frozen–thawed | |
| *1991–1996* | | | | |
| No. of cycles | 5391 | 158 | 116 | 503 |
| No. of transfers | 5011 | 146 | 99 | 458 |
| Percentage of transfers | 93.0 | 92.4 | 85.3 | 91.1 |
| Pregnancy rate per transfer (%)[a] | 36.4 | 44.1 | 33.0 | 33.0 |
| Pregnancy rate per cycle (%)[a] | 33.8 | 40.8 | 27.9 | 30.0 |
| *1991–1995* | | | | |
| No. of transfers with known | | | | |
|    outcome until delivery | 3680 | 131 | 65 | 277 |
| No. of deliveries | 986 | 40 | 19 | 62 |
| Delivery rate per transfer | 26.8 | 30.5 | 29.2 | 22.4 |

[a]With known serum hCG outcome.

these controlled comparisons between conventional IVF and ICSI when at least six cumulus–oocyte complexes were retrieved; half of the cumulus–oocyte complexes were used for conventional IVF and half for the ICSI procedure. Primary endpoints of these studies were fertilization and embryo development (morphology and speed of embryo cleavage after 48 h of in vitro culture).

In 50 infertile couples (caused by tubal infertility in the female partner and normal semen values in the male partner), half of the cumulus–oocyte complexes underwent conventional IVF and the other half the ICSI procedure. A total of 630 cumulus–oocyte complexes were retrieved. As indicated in Table 3, the fertilization rate was higher after ICSI than after IVF. Total fertilization failure after IVF occurred in four patients (20 cumulus–oocyte complexes)

and in only one patient after ICSI (two metaphase II oocytes injected). The total embryo cleavage and distribution of morphological embryo quality were similar in IVF and ICSI. Although the microinjection and insemination of the oocytes were performed at the same time, the embryos used for ICSI were at a more advanced stage of development after 42 h. As the morphologically best embryos were selected for transfer, both sources of embryos were present in most transfers, so preventing evaluation of the implantation potential of IVF or ICSI embryos. A transfer was performed in 49 cycles resulting in 17 pregnancies.[21]

In a similar ongoing controlled comparison of IVF and ICSI involving patients with idiopathic infertility, we have so far recorded similar fertilization rates in 18 treatment cycles with, however, six unexpected complete fertil-

**Table 3  Comparison of conventional IVF and ICSI procedure on sibling oocytes of 50 patients with tubal infertility[a]**

|  | Conventional IVF | ICSI procedure |
|---|---|---|
| No. of cumulus–oocyte complexes | 316 | 314 |
| Normally fertilized oocytes (%) | $56.6 \pm 30.9$[b] | $67.6 \pm 24.6$[b] |
| Cleaved embryos (percentage of fertilized oocytes) | $88.9 \pm 25.4$ | $93.2 \pm 18.3$ |
| Percentage of developmental stages (about 42 h after insemination): |  |  |
| Two-cell embryos | $34.9 \pm 34.1$[c] | $15.8 \pm 23.6$[c] |
| Three-cell embryos | $7.9 \pm 13.2$ | $10.7 \pm 21.2$ |
| Four-cell embryos | $38.7 \pm 28.3$[d] | $60.1 \pm 30.8$[d] |
| Five- to eight-cell embryos | $9.0 \pm 15.1$ | $11.2 \pm 21.8$ |

[a]Results are expressed as mean $\pm$ standard deviation.
[b]$p < 0.05$ paired $t$-test.
[c]$p < 0.0001$ paired $t$-test.
[d]$p < 0.001$ paired $t$-test.

ization failures in conventional IVF.[22] In 16 cycles involving asthenozoospermic semen (<5% type A motility) that had enough progressive motile spermatozoa for IVF, a significantly reduced fertilization rate was observed in conventional IVF (25%) compared with ICSI (66%). Unexpected IVF fertilization failures occurred in seven cycles.[22] Similarly, in 27 teratozoospermic treatment cycles, the fertilization rate was lower in IVF than in ICSI, and in four cycles none of the IVF-treated oocytes were fertilized (G Verheyen, H Tournaye et al, unpublished observations).

These preliminary results need to be confirmed on larger numbers of treatment cycles. Whether ICSI will become the procedure of choice for all couples requiring ART will also depend on the safety aspects of ICSI in comparison to conventional IVF.

## PROSPECTIVE FOLLOW-UP OF PREGNANCIES AND CHILDREN BORN AFTER ICSI: CURRENT RESULTS

When ICSI was introduced in clinical practice there was major concern about its safety: the procedure itself is more invasive and sperm are available that could never have been used in other ART procedures. More concern arose when ICSI was carried out with epididymal or testicular sperm: genomic imprinting may be less complete in these sperm and related anomalies may become manifest only at birth or later in life.

Here we report on 2375 ICSI pregnancies leading to the birth of 1987 children, which were generated in ICSI cycles between April 1991 and September 1997. This follow-up was carried out by the Centre for Medical Genetics in collaboration with the Centre for Reproductive Medicine and has already been partially reported.[22–27]

Initially candidate couples for ICSI procedure were asked to agree to the conditions of the follow-up study which included genetic counselling before pregnancy or at 6–8 weeks of pregnancy, prenatal karyotype analysis and participation in a prospective follow-up study of the resulting children. Prenatal testing was initially strongly recommended; currently couples are informed about the risk factors and left to choose whether or not to have prenatal testing. Pros and cons are discussed in detail: amniocentesis is suggested for singleton pregnancies whereas chorionic villous sampling is proposed for multiple pregnancies. Genetic counselling was attended by 86% of 1513 couples and led to a genetic risk for 557 pregnancies, including increased maternal or paternal age ($n = 415$), chromosomal abnormalities in the parents ($n = 27$), monogenic diseases ($n = 79$, of which 61 were related to cystic fibrosis), multifactorial diseases ($n = 32$) and consanguinity ($n = 7$).

Abnormal fetal karyotypes were found in 28 cases of 1082: 690 amniocenteses (15 of which were abnormal), 392 chorionic villous samplings (13 of which were abnormal) and seven cord blood punctures which were control samples of previous amniocenteses and were all normal. We observed 18, or 1.66%, *de novo* chromosomal aberrations: nine of these, or 0.83%, were sex chromosome aberrations and another nine, or 0.83%, were autosomal aberrations (trisomies and structural aberrations). There is a statistically significant increase in sex chromosomal aberrations compared with data in the literature on a neonatal population. The increase in autosomal aberrations results partly from an increase in trisomies, linked to higher maternal ages. There is also an increase in structural *de novo* aberrations compared with data in the literature. The number of inherited chromosomal aberrations, one of which is unbalanced, are of course higher than in the general population but were predictable for the individual couples, in all but one of whom the father was carrying the structural anomaly.[28]

In a study group of 460 consecutive ICSI singleton pregnancies with amniocentesis and 360 consecutive ICSI singleton pregnancies without amniocentesis, there is no statistical difference in outcome measured in terms of prematurity, low birthweight, very low birthweight or loss of pregnancy. The same findings are observed in 109 consecutive ICSI twin pregnancies with and 174 ICSI twin pregnancies without chorionic villous sampling.[29]

The follow-up study of the expected child was explained further: it consisted of a visit to the geneticist–paediatrician at 2 and 12 months of age, and then once a year. For all pregnancies, written data concerning pregnancy outcome with regard to the babies were obtained from the gynaecologists in charge. Perinatal data, including gestational age, mode of delivery, birthweight, Apgar scores, presence or absence of malformations, and neonatal problems were registered. If any problem was mentioned, detailed information was also requested from the paediatrician in charge. For babies born in our university hospital, a detailed physical examination was done at birth, looking for major and minor malformations and including evaluation of neurological and psychomotor development. For babies born elsewhere, written reports were obtained from gynaecologists as well as from paediatricians, while a detailed morphological examination by a geneticist–paediatrician from our centre was carried out at 2 months whenever possible. Additional investigations were carried out if the anamnestic data or the physical examination suggested them. At follow-up examination at 12 months and 2 years, the physical, neurological and psychomotor examinations were repeated by the same team of geneticists–paediatricians. At about 2 years or more, a Bailey test was performed in order to quantify the psychomotor evolution of the children. Further psychomotor evaluation and social functioning will be evaluated at the age of 4–6 years. If parents did not come spontaneously to the follow-up consultations, they were reminded by telephone to make an appointment. A widely accepted definition of major malformations was used, that is, malformations that generally cause functional impairment or require surgical correction. The remaining malformations were considered to be minor. A minor malformation was distinguished from normal variation by the fact that it occurs in 4% or less of the infants in the same ethnic group. Malformations or anomalies were considered to be synonymous with structural abnormality. The mean birthweight of 1966 liveborn children of at least 20 weeks was 2818 g, the mean length was 47.9 cm and the mean head circumference was 33.5 cm. Prematurity, that is, birth under or at 37 weeks of pregnancy, was observed in 12% of the 1063 singletons, 59% of the 805 twins and 96% of the 98 triplets. Birthweight under 2500 g was observed in 8% of the singletons, 52% of the twins and 85% of the triplets. Very low birthweight under 1500 g was recorded for 2% of the singletons, 5% of the twins and 36% of the triplets. Sex ratio of the males to females was 0.98%.

Major malformations were found in seven interruptions and in four intrauterine deaths, and in a total of 21 stillbirths after 20 weeks of gestation. Major malformations were found in 22 of 1063 (2.1%) singleton children, 22 of 805 (2.7%) twin children and 2 of 98 (2.0%) triplet children. This is 46 of 1966 or 2.3% of all babies born alive. This figure of 2.3% malformation rate is similar to that found in most of the general population national registries and the ART surveys.

These observations should be completed by others and by collaborative efforts such as the ESHRE Task Force on Intracytoplasmic Sperm Injection. In the meantime, before any ICSI treatment is started, couples should be informed on the existing data: the risk of transmitting chromosomal aberrations, the risk of *de novo* sex chromosomal and structural aberrations, and the risk of transmitting fertility problems to the offspring. Patients should also be reassured that there seems to be no higher incidence of major congenital malformations in children born after ICSI.

## ACKNOWLEDGMENTS

We are indebted to many colleagues of the Centres for Medical Genetics and Reproductive Medicine: the clinicians, the clinical embryologists, the scientists, the nurses and laboratory technicians. This work is supported by grants from the Fund for Scientific Research – Flanders (FWO-Vlaanderen), the Brussels Free University Research Council and unconditional educational grant from Organon International.

## REFERENCES

1. Palermo G, Joris H, Devroey P, Van Steirteghem AC. Pregnancies after intracytoplasmic injection of single spermatozoon into an oocyte. *Lancet* 1992;**340**:17–18.

2. Van Steirteghem AC, Liu J, Joris H, et al. Higher success rate by intracytoplasmic sperm injection than by subzonal insemination. Report of a second series of 300 consecutive treatment cycles. *Hum Reprod* 1993;**8**:1055–60.

3. Van Steirteghem AC, Nagy Z, Joris H, et al. High fertilization and implantation rates after intracytoplasmic sperm injection. *Hum Reprod* 1993;**8**:1061–6.

4. Nagy ZP, Liu J, Joris H, et al. The result of intracytoplasmic sperm injection is not related to any of the three basic sperm parameters. *Hum Reprod* 1995;**10**:1123–9.

5. Van Steirteghem A, Nagy P, Joris H, et al. The development of intracytoplasmic sperm injection. *Hum Reprod* 1996;**11**(suppl):59–72.

6. Silber SJ, Nagy ZP, Liu J, et al. Conventional in-vitro fertilization versus intracytoplasmic sperm injection for patients requiring microsurgical sperm aspiration. *Hum Reprod* 1994;**9**:1705–9.

7. Tournaye H, Devroey P, Liu J, et al. Microsurgical epididymal sperm aspiration and intracytoplasmic sperm injection: a new effective approach to infertility as a result of congenital bilateral absence of the vas deferens. *Fertil Steril* 1994;**61**:1045–51.

8. Devroey P, Silber S, Nagy Z, et al. Ongoing pregnancies and birth after intracytoplasmic sperm injection with frozen-thawed epididymal spermatozoa. *Hum Reprod* 1995;**10**:903–6.

9. Devroey P, Liu J, Nagy Z, et al. Pregnancies after testicular sperm extraction and intracytoplasmic sperm injection in non-obstructive azoospermia. *Hum Reprod* 1995;**10**:1457–60.

10. Nagy Z, Liu J, Janssenswillen C, et al. Using ejaculated, fresh, and frozen–thawed epididymal and testicular spermatozoa gives rise to comparable results after intracytoplasmic sperm injection. *Fertil Steril* 1995;**63**:808–15.

11. Van de Velde H, Nagy ZP, Joris H, et al. Effects of different hyaluronidase concentrations and mechanical procedures for cumulus cell removal on the outcome of intracytoplasmic sperm injection. *Hum Reprod* 1997;**12**:2246–50.

12. Verheyen G, De Croo I, Tournaye H, et al. Comparison of four mechanical methods to retrieve spermatozoa from testicular tissue. *Hum Reprod* 1995;**10**:2956–9.

13. Crabbé E, Verheyen G, Tournaye H, Van Steirteghem A. The use of enzymatic procedures to recover testicular germ cells. *Hum Reprod* 1997;**12**:1682–7.

14. Nagy Z, Verheyen G, Tournaye H, et al. An improved treatment procedure or testicular biopsy specimens offers more efficient sperm recovery: case series. *Fertil Steril* 1997;**68**:376–79.

15. Van Steirteghem A, Tournaye H, Van der Elst J, et al. Intracytoplasmic sperm injection three years after the birth of the first ICSI child. *Hum Reprod* 1995;**10**:2527–8.

16. Nagy ZP, Liu J, Joris H, et al. The influence of the site of sperm deposition and mode of oolemma breakage at intracytoplasmic sperm injection on fertilization and embryo development rates. *Hum Reprod* 1995;**10**:3171–7.

17. Liu J, Nagy Z, Joris H, et al. Analysis of 76 total fertilization failure cycles out of 2732 intracytoplasmic sperm injection cycles. *Hum Reprod* 1995;**10**:2630–6.

18. Vandervorst M, Tournaye H, Camus M, et al. Patients with absolutely immotile spermatozoa and intracytoplasmic sperm injection. *Hum Reprod* 1997;**12**:2429–33.

19. Van den Abbeel E, Vitrier S, Camus M, et al. Can further in vitro culture of surviving frozen–thawed multicellular human embryos select viable embryos for transfer? *Assist Reprod Rev* 1997;**7**:202–6.

20. Staessen C, Nagy ZP, Lui J, et al. One year's experience with elective transfer of two good quality embryos in the human in-vitro fertilization and intracytoplasmic sperm injection programmes. *Hum Reprod* 1995;**10**:3305–12.

21. Staessen C, Camus M, De Vos A, Van Steirteghem AC. Conventional IVF versus ICSI in sibling oocytes for non-male indications. *Hum Reprod* 1998;**13**(suppl): in press.

22. Bonduelle M, Desmyttere S, Buysse A, et al. Prospective follow-up study of 55 children born after subzonal insemination and intracytoplasmic sperm injection. *Hum Reprod* 1994;**9**:1765–9.

23. Bonduelle M, Legein J, Derde M-P, et al. Comparative follow-up study of 130 children born after intracytoplasmic sperm injection and 130 children born after in-vitro fertilization. *Hum Reprod* 1995;**10**:3327–31.

24. Bonduelle M, Legein J, Buysse A, et al. Prospective follow-up study of 423 children born after intracytoplasmic sperm injection. *Hum Reprod* 1996;**11**:1558–64.

25. Bonduelle M, Wilikens A, Buysse A, et al. Prospective follow-up study of 877 children born after intracytoplasmic sperm injection (ICSI), with ejaculated epididymal and testicular spermatozoa and after replacement of cryopreserved embryos obtained after ICSI. In: *Genetics and Assisted Human Conception* (Van Steirteghem A, Devroey P, Liebaers I, eds). *Hum Reprod* 1996;**11**, suppl 4:131–59.

26. Bonduelle M, Devroey P, Liebaers I, Van Steirteghem A. Commentary: Major defects are overestimated. *BMJ* 1997;**315**:1265–6. [Commentary Kurinczuk J and Bower C. Birth defects in infants conceived by intracytoplasmic sperm injection: an alternative interpretation. *BMJ* 1997;**315**:1260–6.

27. Bonduelle M, Aytoz A, Van Assche E, et al. Incidence of chromosomal aberrations in children born after assisted reproduction through intracytoplasmic sperm injection. *Hum Reprod* 1998;**13**:781–2.

28. Aytoz A, De Catte L, Bonduelle M, et al. Obstetrical outcome after prenatal diagnosis in intracytoplasmic sperm injection pregnancies. *Hum Reprod* 1998;**13**: in press.

# 23

# In vitro maturation of human oocytes

Anthony J Rutherford, Helen M Picton, Patrick Wynn

**Basic physiology • Practical aspects of human in vitro maturation • Conclusion**

In vitro maturation (IVM) of primordial follicles through to mature graafian follicles, capable of releasing a metaphase II oocyte, would solve many of the difficulties we face in reproductive medicine. One small piece of ovarian cortex, containing an abundant supply of primordial follicles, would provide all the oocytes needed for infertility treatment, whether for returning into the host or for helping others through egg donation. Unfortunately, although feasible in small laboratory animals,[1] the prolonged period of growth necessary for the human oocyte to reach maturity makes this technique impractical in the foreseeable future. At present, the clinical application of IVM of human oocytes extends to immature oocytes from antral stage follicles, removed in the early to midfollicular phase[2] and, to a lesser extent, to immature oocytes retrieved after conventional superovulation. The latter group will contain oocytes that have failed to undergo appropriate nuclear maturation in response to an ovulatory level of human chorionic gonadotrophin (hCG),[3,4] and those in whom hCG was not administered either accidentally[5] or for fear of severe ovarian hyperstimulation.[6]

In theory, IVM is very attractive because it has a number of practical advantages over conventional superovulation. Most IVM protocols are relatively simple, for both the patient and clinician, with fewer consultations, a shorter period of treatment and a significantly reduced drug bill. Both short-term and any potential long-term sequelae of ovarian superovulation (such as the severe ovarian hyperstimulation syndrome and the threat of ovarian neoplasia, respectively) are completely avoided. In addition, the whole process is likely to be cheaper, allowing greater access for patients. Finally, more women may be prepared to donate oocytes, both for research and to help infertile couples, because of the simplicity of the procedure.

Unfortunately, despite excellent results in animals,[7] to date, the pregnancy rate in humans has with, one recent exception,[8] been disappointingly poor.[2,9] This reflects our limited understanding of the physiological events that occur during the process of oocyte development, and the requirements of oocytes once transposed to the laboratory. This chapter briefly reviews the known biology of oocyte maturation, and then presents a practical guide to IVM of human oocytes.

## BASIC PHYSIOLOGY

### Oogenesis

Oogenesis is the developmental process whereby a diploid germ cell is transformed to a haploid cell capable of fertilization. This process not only increases genetic divergence, but provides the oocyte with the means to support the early embryo's nutritional, synthetic and regulatory needs.

## Follicular and oocyte development

In fetal life oogonia stop dividing by mitotic cell division before differentiating into primary oocytes and starting the process of meiosis. They arrest during the first meiotic division at the diplotene (dictyate) stage of prophase and become enclosed by a layer of flattened epithelial cells forming the primordial follicle. Primordial follicles form in the fourth month of gestation,[10] initially in the inner cortex of the developing ovary, and then gradually spreading towards the periphery, with folliculogenesis reaching completion by birth.[10] At this time the ovaries contain between 260 000 and 472 000 primordial follicles. This is a finite supply that slowly dwindles to around a 1000 by the time of the menopause. Primordial follicles are lost through atresia and by entry into the growth phase.[11]

The trigger to initiate follicular growth remains unknown. During the period of growth, which is estimated to be in excess of 90 days, the human oocyte increases from around 35 μm up to 120 μm in diameter.[11] The oocyte develops intimate links with the surrounding granulosa cells through gap junctions, such that the oocyte and granulosa cells act as a functional syncytium.[12] This close association is essential for the development of both oocyte and follicle. The zona pellucida (ZP) starts to form shortly after the resumption of growth, initially as patches of fine filaments that slowly coalesce to form a dense meshwork of interconnected filaments. The ZP contains glycoproteins secreted by the oocyte, important for sperm binding, and later to help prevent polyspermy. The physical continuity between the granulosa cells and oocyte is maintained through long dendritic processes that cross the ZP, and end with the gap junctions on the oocyte (Figure 1). The theca layers start to develop when the follicle has between three and six layers of granulosa cells. Once the theca has formed the follicle is known as a preantral follicle. The granulosa cells proliferate more rapidly as the follicle develops, and there are considerable changes to the intracellular morphology, reflecting their changing function. In humans the follicular antrum forms when the diameter of the follicle has reached about 250 μm. The follicle selected for ovulation comes from a cohort of small, actively growing follicles around 2–5 mm in diameter. In the early follicular phase the healthy follicle will be between 5 mm and 8 mm, increasing by the midfollicular phase to 13 mm, and reaching a maximum diameter when mature of between 18 mm and 27 mm.[11]

The oocyte remains suspended at the dictyate stage through to and beyond puberty, when, with the advent of ovulatory cycles, meiosis is resumed in response to the midcycle luteinizing hormone (LH) surge. To be able to respond appropriately to the LH surge the oocyte needs to have acquired nuclear and cytoplasmic maturation.

## Nuclear maturation

During the period of follicular and oocyte growth, the oocyte acquires both the ability to resume meiosis, and the payload of RNA and proteins required to support complete meiotic maturation, a process known as meiotic competence. Acquisition of meiotic competence appears to take place in two sequential steps: first, from breakdown of the oocyte nucleus (germinal vesicle breakdown, GVBD) to the completion of metaphase I, and second, entry into anaphase, arresting again at metaphase II.

Regardless of the signalling system that initiates GVBD, nuclear maturation of mature oocytes is mediated by dephosphorylation of an active maturation-promoting factor (MPF). This factor consists of a complex of cyclin B and the product of the *cdc2+* gene, a cyclin-dependent protein kinase. The direct action of MPF during GVBD may involve dissolution of the nucleoli, chromosomal condensation and reorganization of the microtubule apparatus to form a functional spindle.[13] Deactivation of MPF is essential for the second step, entry into anaphase I, to take place.

Oocytes from preantral follicles do not have the ability to resume meiosis. In antral oocytes,

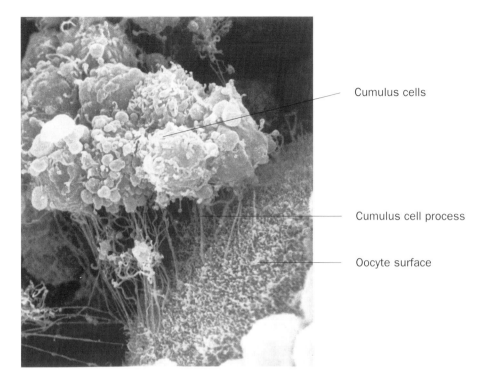

Cumulus cells

Cumulus cell process

Oocyte surface

**Figure 1** Scanning electron micrograph of the oocyte and cumulus oophorus. The zona pellucida (ZP) has been digested revealing the thin cumulus cell processes that penetrate the ZP to form gap junctions and intermediate junctions with the oocyte. (Reprinted from *Human Embryology*, Larsen WJ, ed., 1993, with the permission of Churchill Livingstone).

which are capable of resuming meoisis, meiotic arrest is maintained through inhibitory signals sent via the gap junctions. Although there is probably a degree of species specificity, it would appear that cyclic adenosine 3':5'-monophosphate (cAMP) plays an important role. Reinitiation of meiosis in fully grown oocytes is associated with a fall in intraoocyte cAMP concentration. This appears to be an initial step in the cascade of events, including activation of MPF, which results in oocyte maturation. Once GVBD has started the process is irreversible.

The physiological trigger for resumption of meiosis is provided by the preovulatory surge of LH. These high levels of LH result in a decrease in intracellular cAMP and the attendant loss of gap junctional contacts between the granulosa cells and oocytes which are essential for maintenance of meiotic arrest. In vitro, if antral oocytes are cultured without their cumulus cells they spontaneously resume meiosis.

**Cytoplasmic maturation**

As the oocyte grows there are widespread changes in the infrastructure of the cytoplasm and its organelles. The pattern of protein production changes throughout this growth phase, right through to the second metaphase arrest. Cytoplasmic maturation is essential to prepare the oocyte for fertilization, activation and, then, early preimplantation development before the new embryonic genome is functional. Even though an oocyte may be capable of fertilization, having attained meiotic competence, it may not have achieved the appropriate degree of cytoplasmic maturation necessary to sustain a viable embryo.

It is therefore not surprising that a higher proportion of oocytes recovered from large antral follicles are competent to proceed to form blastocysts compared with those oocytes retrieved from small antral follicles.[14] This is an important consideration which may account in part for the limited clinical success of IVM.

## PRACTICAL ASPECTS OF HUMAN IN VITRO MATURATION

### Background

The initial discovery that mammalian oocytes would undergo in vitro maturation was in 1935, when Pincus and Enzmann[15] demonstrated that oocytes liberated from unstimulated rabbit graafian follicles would undergo meiotic maturation spontaneously in vitro. This showed that the programme of cytoplasmic and nuclear events between the LH surge and subsequent ovulation could take place in culture. In 1965 Edwards et al[16] confirmed and extended these results with a range of mammalian species including the human,[10] and in 1969[17] was able to demonstrate for the first time the fertilization of in vitro matured human oocytes.

The earliest recorded pregnancies after human IVM were in 1983[3] arising from immature oocytes that had failed to respond appropriately to an ovulatory dose of hCG during a conventional in vitro fertilization (IVF) programme. More recently a birth was reported after IVM of immature oocytes obtained in a similar fashion but on this occasion fertilized using intracytoplasmic sperm injection (ICSI).[4] An alternative approach that has proved successful was to collect, and mature in vitro, oocytes from patients in whom hCG was withheld, both unintentionally because of patient forgetfulness[5] and intentionally in a patient at risk of the severe ovarian hyperstimulation syndrome.[6] There are only a handful of published clinical trials that have evaluated the exciting potential of IVM of oocytes from small antral follicles[2,9,18] (Figure 2). Each of these studies has addressed a different aspect of IVM, and all have recorded pregnancies, although the birth rate remains unacceptably low. A review of these studies, and results of our own work, form the basis for the remainder of this chapter. Individual sections cover specific aspects of the IVM technique, from patient selection right through to embryo transfer.

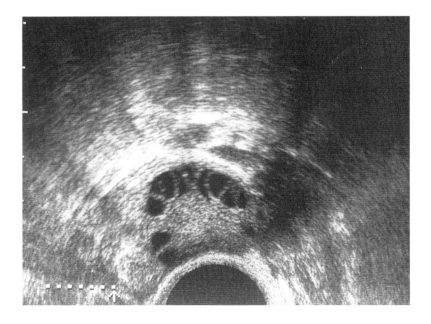

**Figure 2** Transvaginal ultrasonograph of a polycystic ovary. The classic appearance of a 'necklace' of small follicles (2–8 mm) is seen peripherally in the ovary.

## Patient selection

The outcome of any assisted conception treatment cycle is dependent on the quality of the oocytes collected. Three main groups of patients have been used to investigate in vitro maturation of human oocytes. The first group consists of 'rescue' IVM, where women who were undergoing routine superovulated IVF or ICSI, with[3,4] or without[5,6] hCG, and were found to have immature oocytes at collection. The second group consists of those patients who have entered into clinical trials of IVM as part of their fertility treatment. This includes patients with polycystic ovaries (PCO)[9] and, in a more recent study, patients with a range of diagnoses who had all failed at least one cycle of IVF.[2] The third group consists of volunteer patients, some having oophorectomy for gynaecological pathology, such as adenomyosis, endometriosis, uterine fibroids and ectopic pregnancy,[18] and another group of fertile women undergoing a sterilization procedure.[19]

Most of these studies have used oocytes that are potentially suboptimal. All patients in the first two groups suffered from infertility, and many had significant endocrine disturbance, such as raised serum androgens and LH which is commonly seen with the polycystic ovary syndrome (PCOS) and known to be detrimental to oocytes.[20] Others had unresolved infertility after failed conventional IVF, or had oocytes that had failed to respond to a normal ovulatory dose of hCG, despite being given at the appropriate time as judged by follicle size. In addition, in the volunteer group, 18 of the 23 oophorectomy specimens came from patients over the age of 36, with most coming from women aged over 40 years.

In an elegant study, Barnes and colleagues[21] demonstrated that immature oocytes removed from regularly cycling women were found to have a greater developmental capacity, significantly better maturation and fertilization rates, and a trend to higher cleavage rates than those from women with anovular or irregular cycles. Therefore, in an attempt to gain a better understanding of the culture requirements and development capacity of immature human oocytes, we decided to study a group of healthy volunteer patients of proven fertility, age range 23–36 years, in a series of controlled studies.[19]

## Oocyte cumulus priming

One of the major theoretical advantages of IVM is the reduced requirement for ovarian stimulation. However, studies in rhesus monkeys[22] have indicated that mild ovarian stimulation before retrieval markedly improved the proportion of oocytes that were meiotically competent, and that after fertilization would support normal embryonic development. Human evidence is limited, but, in a series of case reports, immature oocytes have been collected after exposure to conventional follicle-stimulating hormone (FSH) stimulation with a follicular phase of relatively normal length. The subsequent maturation rates were generally high and pregnancies were recorded.[3–6] None of the major human trials investigating IVM of oocytes recovered from small antral follicles has used any type of ovarian pre-treatment,[2,9,18] and although it is not appropriate to make a direct comparison, the embryo cleavage rate and the pregnancy rates in these studies have generally been disappointing.

To investigate the potential benefits of FSH priming on human oocyte in vitro maturation, Wynn et al[19] randomly allocated a group of fertile volunteers to receive either mild FSH stimulation or no treatment, before egg retrieval on day 7 of the follicular phase. The stimulation group received a truncated course of recombinant FSH (Gonal F, Serono, Herts, UK) 300 IU on day 2, with additional doses of 150 IU FSH on days 4 and 6 of the menstrual cycle. The results of this study are summarized in Table 1. The mean diameter of the small antral follicles was similar in each group. However, there were significantly more follicles, and hence immature oocytes recovered, in the stimulated group. Although the same proportion of immature oocytes initiated meiosis, a significantly greater percentage of oocytes from pre-treated patients progressed to reach metaphase II. Furthermore, within the FSH-treated group successful oocyte

**Table 1 The effect of FSH pre-treatment in vivo on human oocyte maturation in vitro**

| | Control (n = 9) | FSH treated (n = 17) |
|---|---|---|
| Mean follicle diameter (mm) at collection ± SEM | 8.0 ± 0.5 | 8.9 ± 0.3 |
| Mean number of oocytes collected ± SEM | 5.2 ± 1.3 | 7.5 ± 1.2 |
| Total number of degenerate oocytes after 48 h culture | 8 (17.4) | 6 (5.3) |
| Number of germinal vesicle-stage oocytes after 48 h | 5 (10.9) | 12 (10.5) |
| Number of metaphase I oocytes after 48 h | 13 (28.3) | 15 (13.2) |
| Number of metaphase II oocytes after 48 h | 20 (43.5) | 81 (71.1) |
| Total number of oocytes cultured | 46 | 114 |

From Wynn et al.[19]
Values in parentheses are percentages.
SEM, standard error of the mean.

maturation was positively correlated with follicle size, which is in keeping with findings in other primates[22] and domestic animal species.[14] Interestingly no oocytes capable of maturation were found in follicles less than 5 mm in diameter. Although no attempt was made to fertilize these oocytes and assess embryo development, these findings suggest that FSH priming will be of value in the human setting.

It remains to be elucidated how FSH priming works. Humans and other primates have a much longer follicular phase than other species studied, and it has been postulated that this is to allow time for completion of cytoplasmic maturation.[22] The provision of additional FSH will promote follicular granulosa cell prolifera-

tion, steroid production and, through intercellular signalling, additional oocyte RNA and protein synthesis.

## Oocyte collection

As all experienced in oocyte retrieval will validate, recovering oocytes from 'mature' follicles where hCG has been withheld can be extremely difficult. The classic microscopic appearance of the expanded cumulus–oocyte complex is not found; instead oocytes are surrounded by tightly packed corona and cumulus cells, which can be hard to differentiate from sheets of granulosa cells.[5] It is therefore surprising to find that, with experience, immature oocytes can be recovered relatively easily from antral follicles between 5 mm and 12 mm.[19,21]

Initial attempts at oocyte recovery using a conventional IVF ultrasonographically guided approach were generally unsuccessful.[9] Therefore, Trounson introduced two major changes: first, a new more rigid aspiration needle with a shorter bevel at the tip (Cook, Australia Ltd) and, second, a reduced aspiration pressure of 80 mmHg. These adaptations, combined with experience, led to much higher recovery rates and a reduced need to resort to laparoscopic recovery. Our work indicated that decreasing the aspiration pressure was by far the most significant change. In our preliminary studies we used both the adapted Cook needle and a standard 16-gauge double-lumen needle (DC1S/16G/Clarendon, Casmed, Surrey, UK) with no difference in recovery rates.[19]

Most reports have described the use of a single-lumen needle, under ultrasonographic guidance, with each small follicle aspirated in turn.[9,22] The needle and tubing were then flushed with a warm, pH-buffered, heparinized culture medium to clear the contents. However, using a double-lumen needle, each follicle can be measured, then aspirated and flushed sequentially using known volumes of culture medium, without having to remove the needle. This allows accurate identification of oocytes from follicles of known diameter and volume, which can be correlated with oocyte outcome.

The follicular aspirates are examined using a dissecting microscope to identify the immature cumulus–oocyte complex. To aid detection, embryo filters can be used to remove erythrocytes and other granulosa cell debris.[2,9] In time and with practice, the recovery of immature oocytes from small follicles is no more complex than a routine IVF egg collection for both the clinician and the laboratory.

## Culture media

The mutual interdependence of oocytes and granulosa cells for survival and normal development has important practical implications for strategies aimed at successfully maturing oocytes in vitro. The granulosa–oocyte complex is a metabolically coupled unit. The granulosa cells represent the nutrient and regulatory conduits between the oocyte and its environment, both through their regulation of phosphorylation events within the oocyte, and through the glycolytic activity within the oocyte–cumulus complexes during the resumption of meiosis. Importantly, both the association between granulosa cells and their differentiated status can be profoundly affected by components of the culture environment. Development of a culture medium that supports normal granulosa cell functions is therefore also likely to provide a suitable milieu for oocyte maturation. Although the attainment of oocyte meiotic competence and developmental potential clearly requires inclusion of at least preovulatory levels of FSH and LH, by far the most critical component that can influence the success of IVM is supplementation of the culture medium with serum[2,9,18] or follicular fluid.[18]

Historically, monolayers of granulosa cells cultured in the presence of serum have been used to investigate the effects of hormone treatments on steroidogenesis.[24] Although the inclusion of serum provides a complex mixture of hormones, nutrients, growth and attachment factors (including collagen and fibronectin), which are necessary to support cell proliferation, serum also exerts inhibitory effects on follicular-type functions of granulosa cells. Typically, rat and human granulosa cells cultured in the presence of serum or extracellular matrix proteins[25,26] rapidly proliferate to form flattened, epithelioid monolayers with a dramatically different morphology to that seen in vivo. Furthermore, in the presence of serum or attachment factors, cells spontaneously luteinize and lose the capacity to convert androgens to oestrogens. Aromatase activity and hence oestradiol production by granulosa cells, which are key biochemical markers of the maintenance of follicular phenotype in vitro,[27] are also central to preovulatory follicle selection and oocyte development in vivo.[28,29]

Optimization of the novel serum-free culture system, developed for ovine,[30] bovine[31] and porcine granulosa cells[32,33] to support IVM of human oocytes,[19] offers major advantages over previously published cell culture systems. Using this approach, it is possible to maintain oestradiol production in granulosa cells which are exquisitely sensitive to physiological concentrations of gonadotrophins. Furthermore, controlled luteinization of the cells can be induced by the addition of preovulatory surge levels of gonadotrophins (HM Picton, unpublished data). On the basis of this serum-free culture system, we have used a combination of insulin and the synthetic analogue Long-R3 insulin-like growth factor (IGF), for human IVM[19] with concentrations based on the follicular fluid levels of insulin and IGF-I measured in human antral follicles.[34,35] These additives enhance granulosa cell metabolism and induce, sustain and amplify the actions of FSH and LH on differentiated cell function.

Most importantly using this serum-free approach, cultured granulosa cells form distinct clumps of rounded cells[30–33] which closely resemble the morphology of granulosa cells in vivo.[36] In response to the FSH and insulin[37] in the culture medium, the extensive network of gap junctions between cumulus cells and between cumulus cells and the oocyte is maintained. After exposure to high levels of FSH and LH in vitro, the controlled luteinization of cumulus cells and paracrine signalling breaks these fragile connections and so aids the resumption of nuclear maturation in the oocyte. In contrast, cell proliferation and attachment to the culture surface, caused by inclusion of serum and follicular fluid in the incubation media, may lead to premature disruption of oocyte–cumulus communication and so compromise oocyte maturation potential. The morphological differences of cumulus cells cultured in the presence or absence of serum or follicular fluid, and the associated changes in their actin cytoskeleton,[38] may therefore profoundly affect the success of in vitro maturation systems.

## In vitro maturation and fertilization

In most circumstances, the cumulus–oocyte complex is retrieved 3–7 days before natural ovulation and no attempt is made to mimic the physiological cycle by delaying resumption of meiosis in vitro. The basic assumption is made that the oocyte will have already achieved the necessary cytoplasmic maturation to allow nuclear maturation, fertilization and subsequent normal embryonic development. However, data from human and animal work show that protein synthesis in the oocyte continues throughout the follicular phase until and beyond the time of GVBD.[39,40] These late stages of cytoplasmic maturation may hold the key to explain the poor success in human IVM, but at present there has been no study to define precisely at what stage of follicular development the human oocyte achieves cytoplasmic competence.

Although the functional syncytium found in the intact follicle is lost when the cumulus–oocyte complex is removed at egg collection, the speed at which the gap junctions between cumulus cells and the oocyte are degraded remains unknown. Evidence from human oocytes suggests that this close association continues in culture, because denuded oocytes have reduced developmental potential.[9,19] In all the human studies, oocytes were cultured 'cumulus intact',[2,3,5,6,9,18,19,22,23] with the exception of those stripped for ICSI[4] or to study the time course of maturation.[9,19]

The optimal length of culture for human oocytes to achieve nuclear maturation is impossible to determine from animal data, because there is such a wide species-specific variation, for example, mouse oocytes reach metaphase II by 12–16 hours, and cow oocytes by 24 hours. Culture conditions and methodology will also affect the rate of maturation.[41] In the first paper on human IVM in 1965, Edwards[16] demonstrated that maturation took place over a 40- to 48-hour period. Consequently, many of the later studies adopted a 48-hour culture period (Figure 3),[5,6,19] although others have successfully used a slightly longer fixed culture period of 52–58 hours before attempting fertilization

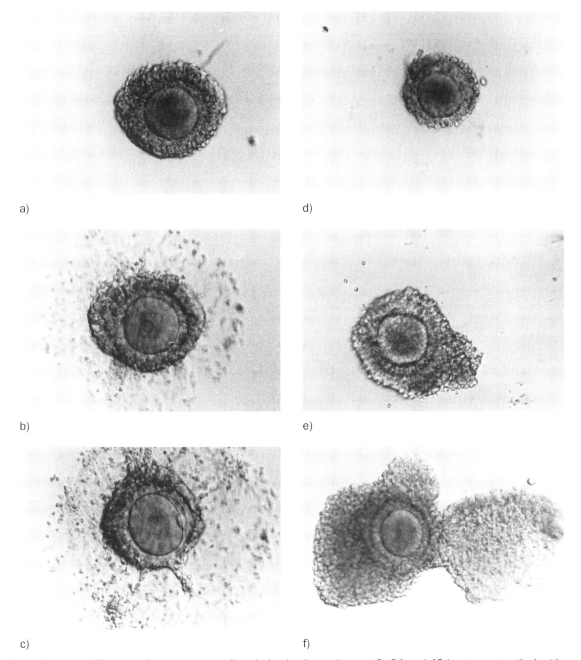

a)

d)

b)

e)

c)

f)

**Figure 3** (a, b, c) The cumulus mass expanding during in vitro culture at 0, 24 and 48 hours, respectively. (d, e, f) The variable cumulus mass seen at collection.

using ICSI.[2] A different approach is to observe the oocytes regularly until the cumulus–granulosa cells have expanded and mucified, or the first polar body is visible, before either insemination or ICSI.[3,4]

A recent detailed examination of the time course of nuclear maturation in human oocytes discovered that, by 28 hours, up to 54% of oocytes had matured to metaphase II; this raises concerns about the potential risks of inseminating oocytes outside the normal fertilization window.[19] However, early insemination, after 29.5–32.5 hours compared with 34.5–35.5 hours in culture, appears to impair the oocytes' capacity to complete maturation and may adversely affect fertilization rates.[9]

In addition to timing, the method of fertilization will affect both the number and quality of embryos produced from in vitro matured human oocytes. Although acceptable fertilization rates have been achieved with conventional insemination,[9,18,21] ICSI minimizes the potential detrimental effects of long-term culture on the ZP.[2] Prolonged culture of the oocyte, in the absence of serum, may cause premature cortical granule release, which leads to hardening of the ZP.[42] This would not only reduce the fertilization potential using conventional insemination, but could also prevent embryo hatching. Zona hardening has been shown to reduce the rate of blastocyst hatching in the rhesus monkey from 77% in serum-based medium to only 25% in serum-free culture.[43] Ultimately it may prove necessary to perform both ICSI and assisted hatching[2,22] for all IVM oocytes and embryos. Alternatively, with adaptations to the culture medium such as the addition of the serum-derived antioxidant fetuin, we might be able to overcome the potential problem of zona hardening.[44]

## Embryo development

Embryos derived from immature oocytes collected after a follicular phase of normal length appear to cleave at a similar rate to oocytes matured in vivo, reaching four to six cells after 42 hours.[4] In contrast, embryos from immature oocytes collected from small antral follicles have a higher rate of arrest at the pronuclear stage, and a significantly lower average cleavage and development rate than in conventional IVF embryos.[21] Furthermore, those embryos from anovulatory patients are even more retarded.[21] Cleavage rates are a good predictor of embryo health and correlate well with the chance of pregnancy.[45,46] This appears to hold true for IVM-derived embryos, because pregnancy is more likely to occur with rapidly dividing embryos.[9]

The failure of slowly dividing embryos may represent an intrinsic abnormality of the original oocyte, or indeed a failure of the culture system.[9] Theoretically both these factors could be implicated. The limited evidence available is reassuring, in that morphologically normal human oocytes matured in vitro have a similar incidence of gross meiotic aberrations (18%)[47] as those oocytes matured in vivo (20%), and apparently lower rates than those seen in oocytes recovered after gonadotrophin stimulation.[48–50] In addition, although morphology alone does not confer normality, the incidence of morphologically abnormal embryos is no greater after IVM than after conventional IVF.[18] Further comparative studies are required, in particular to address the incidence of aneuploidy, and the merits of more complex enriched culture media, specifically designed to encourage development through to the blastocyst.[51]

## Embryo transfer

Healthy viable embryos and a suitable intrauterine environment are both required for successful implantation. Therefore, the timing of embryo development in relation to the physiological stage and degree of development of the endometrium must be considered. Clearly, embryo/endometrial asynchrony does not arise if the developing embryos are either cryopreserved for replacement in a subsequent hormone replacement cycle[5] or used in oocyte donation.[18] In cases of 'rescue IVM' the follicular phase is of normal length and, as patients have received stimulation with FSH, there is sufficient endogenous oestrogen, appropriately supplemented with progesterone after oocyte collection, to ensure a suitable endometrium.[4] However, when oocytes are collected in the midfollicular phase, with no prior ovarian stimulation, evidence suggests that the endometrium is unlikely to have developed sufficiently, despite adding progesterone supplements, to sustain a pregnancy.[19,52] Russell et al[2] successfully overcame this hurdle by introducing midfollicular phase oestradiol supplementation, on cycle days 5–7, in combination with prolonged embryo culture, transferring the embryos on day 3 after fertilization. Interestingly, relatively high-dose oestradiol supplements, given early in the follicular phase starting on day 2 or 3, were found to be detrimental, with poor oocyte maturation rates and a high rate of early cleavage arrest.[2] An alternative strategy is to prolong the period of oocyte and embryo culture, allowing time for endometrial development to occur. This could be achieved by maintaining meiotic arrest in immature oocytes through the addition of cAMP analogues or phosphodiesterase inhibitors.[53] This approach may also provide a bonus by allowing time for the oocyte to undergo the final stages of cytoplasmic maturation in vitro before the resumption of meiosis.

### Pregnancy outcome

There have been too few pregnancies to access the safety of this new technique adequately. So far, concerns about a high rate of aneuploidies in the children born from in vitro matured oocytes has not materialized. All 10 children reported in the literature are described as normal, and many have had their chromosomes analysed. The rate of pregnancy loss appears low with only one biochemical pregnancy.[3]

As these studies are so diverse in their methodology, it would not be valid to collate the results and calculate an overall pregnancy rate. However, the two largest studies in literature[2,9] show a disappointingly low pregnancy rate of 2% and 10%, respectively. More recently, a report from Cha[8] indicates a further 18 pregnancies in two separate studies. The first series of six pregnancies used immature oocytes in an oocyte donation programme. Three of the pregnancies aborted, and there were three live births, two singletons and one twin delivery. The second series consists of patients with PCO undergoing natural cycle immature oocyte collection. Employing a combination of ICSI, prolonged co-culture and assisted hatching they achieved a pregnancy rate similar to that obtained using conventional IVF.[8]

## CONCLUSION

It is too early to be confident that the many problems experienced with IVM have been solved, and that the technique is ready for introduction into routine clinical practice. Nevertheless, if these latest results can be validated through continued research, IVM could revolutionize infertility practice in the twenty-first century.

## REFERENCES

1. Epigg JJ, O'Brien MJ. Development in vitro of mouse oocytes from primordial follicles. *Biol Reprod* 1996;**54:**197–207.
2. Russell JB, Knezevich KM, Fabian KF, Dickson JA. Unstimulated immature oocyte retrieval: early versus midfollicular endometrial priming. *Fertil Steril* 1997;**67:**616–20.
3. Veeck LL, Wortham JWJ, Witmyer J, et al. Maturation and fertilization of morphologically immature human oocytes in a program of in vitro fertilization. *Fertil Steril* 1983;**39:**594–602.
4. Nagy ZP, Cecile J, Liu J, et al. Pregnancy and birth after intracytoplasmic sperm injection of *in vitro* matured germinal vesicle stage oocytes: case report. *Fertil Steril* 1996;**65:**1047–50.
5. Liu J, Katz E, Garcia JE, et al. Successful in vitro maturation of human oocytes not exposed to human chorionic gonadotropin during ovulation induction, resulting in pregnancy. *Fertil Steril* 1997;**67:**566–8.
6. Jaroudi KA, Hollanders JMG, Sieck UV, et al. Pregnancy after transfer of embryos which were generated from in-vitro matured oocytes. *Hum Reprod* 1997;**12:**857–9.

7. Trounson AO, Pushett D, Maclellan LJ, et al. Current status of IVM/IVF and embryo culture in humans and farm animals. *Theriogenology* 1994;**41**:57–66.

8. Cha KY. Oocytes from unstimulated follicles. *Human Oocytes from Physiology to IVF*. Bologna: University of Bologna, 1997: (abstr.) 41.

9. Trounson AO, Wood C, Kausche A. In vitro maturation and fertilization and developmental competence of oocytes recovered from untreated polycystic ovarian patients. *Fertil Steril* 1994;**62**:353–62.

10. Baker TG. A quantitative and cytological study of germ cells in human ovaries. *Proc R Soc Lond [Biol]* 1963;**158**:417–33.

11. Gougeon A. Regulation of ovarian follicular development in primates: facts and hypotheses. *Endocrine Rev* 1996;**17**:121–55.

12. Epigg JJ. The ovary: oogenesis. In: *Scientific Essentials of Reproductive Medicine* (Hillier SG, Kitchener HC, Neilson JP, eds). London: WB Saunders, 1996: 147–59.

13. Dekel N, Galiani D, Sherizly I. Dissociation between the inhibitory and stimulatory action of cAMP on maturation of rat oocytes. *Mol Cell Endocrinol* 1988;**56**:115–21.

14. Pavlok A, Lucas-Hahn A, Niemann H. Fertilisation and developmental competence of bovine oocytes derived from different categories of antral follicles. *Mol Reprod Dev* 1992;**31**:63–7.

15. Pincus G, Enzmann EV. The comparative behaviour of mammalian eggs in vivo and in vitro. *J Exp Med* 1935;**65**:665–75.

16. Edwards RG. Maturation in vitro of human ovarian oocytes. *Lancet* 1965;**ii**:926–9.

17. Edwards RG, Bavister BC, Steptoe PC. Early stages of fertilisation in vitro of Human oocytes matured *in vitro*. *Nature* 1969;**221**:632–5.

18. Cha KY, Koo JJ, Choi DH, et al. Pregnancy after in vitro fertilization of human follicular fluid oocytes collected from nonstimulated cycles, their culture in vitro and their transfer in a donor oocyte program. *Fertil Steril* 1991;**55**:109–18.

19. Wynn P, Picton HM, Krapez JA, et al. FSH pretreatment promotes the number of human oocytes reaching metaphase II by in vitro maturation. *Hum Reprod* 1998; in press.

20. Homburg R, Armar NA, Eshel A, et al. Influence of serum luteinising hormone concentrations on ovulation, conception and early pregnancy loss in polycystic ovary syndrome. *BMJ* 1988;**297**:1024–6.

21. Barnes FL, Kausche A, Tiglias J, et al. Production of embryos from *in vitro* matured primary human oocytes. *Fertil Steril* 1996;**65**:1151–6.

22. Schramm RD, Bavister BD. Follicle-stimulating hormone priming of rhesus monkeys enhances meiotic and developmental competence of oocytes matured *in vitro*. *Biol Reprod* 1994; **51**:904–12.

23. Barnes FL, Crombie A, Gardner DK, et al. Blastocyst development and birth after in-vitro maturation of human primary oocytes, intracytoplasmic sperm injection and assisted hatching. *Hum Reprod* 1995;**10**:3243–7.

24. Erickson GF, Wang C, Hsueh AJW. FSH induction of functional LH receptors in granulosa cells cultured in a chemically defined medium. *Nature* 1979;**279**:336–8.

25. Ham RG, McKeehan WL. Media and growth requirements. *Methods Enzymol* 1979;**58**:44–93.

26. Furman A, Rotmensch S, Dor J, et al. Culture of human granulosa cells from an *in vitro* fertilization program: effects of extracellular matrix on morphology and cyclic adenosine 3',5'-monophosphate production. *Fertil Steril* 1986; **46**:514–17.

27. Amsterdam A, Rotmensch S. Structure–function relationships during granulosa cell differentiation. *Endocrine Rev* 1987;**8**:309–37.

28. Hsueh AJW, Adashi EY, Jones PBC, Welsh TH. Hormonal regulation of the differentiation of cultured ovarian granulosa cells. *Endocrine Rev* 1984;**5**:76–127.

29. Hutz RJ. Disparate effects of estrogens on *in vitro* steroidogenesis by mammalian and avian granulosa cells. *Biol Reprod* 1989;**40**:709–13.

30. Campbell BK, Scaramuzzi RJ, Webb R. Induction and maintenance of oestradiol and immunoreactive inhibin production with FSH by ovine granulosa cells in serum-free media. *J Reprod Fertil* 1996;**106**:7–16.

31. Gutierrez CG, Campbell BK, Webb R. Development of a long term bovine granulosa cell culture system: induction and maintenance of estradiol production response to FSH and morphological characteristics. *Biol Reprod* 1997; **56**:608–16.

32. Picton HM, Campbell BK, Hunter MG. Maintenance of aromatase activity in porcine granulosa cells in serum free culture. *J Reprod Fertil* 1994;**14**:1 (abstract).

33. Picton HM, Campbell BK, Hunter MG. Maintenance of oestradiol production and cytochrome P450 aromatase enzyme messenger ribonucleic acid expression in long-term serum-

free cultures of porcine granulosa cells. *J Reprod Fertil* 1998; in press.

34. Seifer DB, Giudice LC, Dsupin BA, et al. Follicular fluid insulin-like growth factor-I and insulin-like growth factor-II concentrations vary as a function of day 3 serum follicle stimulating hormone. *Hum Reprod* 1995;**10**:804–6.

35. Homburg R, Orvieto R, Bar-Hara I, Ben-Rafael Z. Serum levels of insulin-like growth factor-1, IGF binding protein-1 and insulin and the response to human menopausal gonadotrophins in women with polycystic ovary syndrome. *Hum Reprod* 1996;**11**:716–19.

36. Chang SCS, Anderson W, Lewis JC, et al. The porcine ovarian follicle. II. Electron microscopic study of surface features of granulosa cells at different stages of development. *Biol Reprod* 1997;**16**:349–57.

37. Amsterdam A, May J, Schomberg DW. Synergistic effect of insulin and follicle stimulating hormone on biochemical and morphological differentiation of porcine granulosa cells *in vitro*. *Biol Reprod* 1988;**39**:379–90.

38. Ben-Ze'ev A, Amsterdam A. Regulation of cytoskeletal proteins involved in cell contact formation during differentiation of granulosa cells on extracellular matrix. *Proc Natl Acad Sci USA* 1988;**83**:2894–8.

39. Schultz GA, Gifford DJ, Mahadevan MM, et al. Protein synthetic patterns in immature human oocytes. *Ann NY Acad Sci* 1988;**541**:237–47.

40. Wassarman P. Oogenesis: synthetic events in the developing mammalian egg. In: *Mechanism and Control of Animal Fertilisation* (Hartmann J, ed.). New York: Academic Press, 1983: 1–54.

41. Dekel N, Piontkewitz Y. Induction of maturation of rat oocytes by interruption of communication in the cumulus–oocyte complex. *Bull Assoc Anat* 1991;**75**:51–4.

42. Green DPL. Three-dimensional structure of the zona pellucida. *Rev Reprod* 1997;**2**:147–56.

43. Schramm RD, Bavister BD. Development of in-vitro-fertilized primate embryos into blastocysts in a chemically defined, protein-free culture medium. *Hum Reprod* 1996;**11**:1690–7.

44. Schroeder AC, Schultz RM, Kopf GS, et al. Fetuin inhibits zona pellucida hardening and conversion of ZP2 to ZP2f during spontaneous mouse oocyte maturation in vitro in the absence of serum. *Biol Reprod* 1990;**43**:891–7.

45. Cummings JM, Breen TM, Harrison KL, et al. A formula for scoring human embryo growth rates in in vitro fertilisation: its value in predicting pregnancy and in comparison with visual estimates of embryo quality. *J In Vitro Fertil Embryo Transf* 1986;**3**:284–95.

46. Bolton VN, Hawes SM, Taylor CT, Parsons JH. Development of spare human preimplantation embryos in vitro and analysis of the correlations among gross morphology, cleavage rates and development to the blastocyst. *J In Vitro Fertil Embryo Transf* 1989;**6**:30–5.

47. Racowsky C, Kaufman ML. Nuclear degeneration and meiotic aberrations observed in human oocytes matured in vitro: analysis by light microscopy. *Fertil Steril* 1992;**58**:750–5.

48. Gras L, McBain J, Trounson AO, Kola I. The incidence of chromosomal aneuploidy in stimulated and unstimulated (natural) uninseminated human oocytes. *Hum Reprod* 1992;**7**:1396–401.

49. Munne S, Lee A, Rosenwaks Z, et al. Diagnosis of major chromosomal aneuploidies in human preimplantation embryos. *Hum Reprod* 1993;**8**:2185–91.

50. Delhanty JD, Harper JC, Handyside AH, Winston RM. Multicolour FISH detects frequent chromosomal mosaicisms and chaotic division in normal preimplantation embryos from fertile patients. *Hum Genet* 1997;**99**:755–60.

51. Gardiner DK, Vella P, Lane M, et al. Culture and transfer of human blastocysts increases implantation rates and reduces the need for multiple embryo transfers (abstract O-002). *American Society of Reproductive Medicine Annual Meeting* 1997.

52. Navot D, Anderson TL, Droesch K, et al. Hormonal manipulation of endometrial maturation. *J Clin Endocrinol Metab* 1989;**68**:801–7.

53. Downs SM, Daniel S, Bornslaeger EA, et al. Maintenance of meiotic arrest in mouse oocytes by purines: modulation of cAMP levels and cAMP phosphodiesterase activity. *Gamete Res* 1989;**23**:323–34.

# 24

# Elimination of high-order multiple gestations by blastocyst culture and transfer

David K Gardner, William B Schoolcraft

Frequency of multiple gestations • Clinical problems associated with multiple gestations • Financial problems associated with multiple gestations • Blastocyst culture and transfer to increase implantation rates • Is assisted hatching or zona removal required for blastocyst transfer? • Blastocyst transfer and cryopreservation • Luteal phase support for blastocyst transfer • Endometrial preparation for frozen–thawed blastocyst transfer • Future of blastocyst transfer in the human: towards single embryo transfers • Conclusions

Implantation rates in human in vitro fertilization (IVF) have changed little over the past two decades. Values of between 10% and 20% are routinely reported.[1] Such values are significantly below the 60% implantation rate reported for the transfer of in vivo developed blastocysts.[2] Therefore, to establish and maintain acceptable pregnancy rates, multiple embryos are routinely transferred to patients after IVF. In 1995 in the USA, the average number of embryos transferred to patients of all ages was 4.[3] Unfortunately, although pregnancy rates do increase when up to four embryos are transferred, so does the probability of a multiple gestation. Multiple gestations are now the most common complication of assisted reproduction technology (ART). These pregnancies carry with them great medical, economical, social, ethical, and psychological consequences. Subsequently, IVF units have continued to struggle with the dilemma of maintaining acceptable pregnancy rates while limiting the complication of multiple gestation.

## FREQUENCY OF MULTIPLE GESTATIONS

The 1995 ASRM/SART (American Society for Reproductive Medicine/Society for Assisted Reproductive Technology) annual report revealed a 37% incidence of multiple deliveries with 7% being triplets or higher.[3] As selective embryo reduction was not reported, many of the reported twin pregnancies may have started as higher-order multiples. The increased incidence of maternal and neonatal complications has been well documented.[4,5] Of particular concern is the immediate and long-term neonatal morbidity.[6–8] Despite improved antenatal care for multiple gestations, the perinatal mortality remains up to tenfold higher than that of singleton gestations.[9,10]

## CLINICAL PROBLEMS ASSOCIATED WITH MULTIPLE GESTATIONS

Selective embryo reduction has been proposed as a means of dealing with high-order multiple gestations. Data are conflicting with regard to the increase in perinatal outcome that is achieved with embryo reduction of triplets to twins; however, with four or more fetuses, the improvement in outcome with selective embryo reduction is dramatic.[11] Selective embryo reduction is not without risk, however. Evans et al[12] reported that only 84% of pregnancies reached viability after embryo reduction, and 5% of these had extreme prematurity (25–28 weeks of gestation). However, even after reduction the problems of prematurity are not eliminated, implicating some abnormalities in implantation and placentation.[13–15] Furthermore, there are no prospective studies analyzing the psychological sequelae of selective embryo reduction. Retrospective studies have shown that many couples (32%) are uncomfortable with their decision to reduce.[16]

## FINANCIAL PROBLEMS ASSOCIATED WITH MULTIPLE GESTATIONS

The economic consequences of multiple gestation represent a 'hidden' cost of ART. Goldfarb et al[17] estimated the cost of triplet or greater gestations at $US340 000. The cost of twins has been estimated at $US21 000–39 000. Even this figure does not consider the cost of long-term care for children handicapped as a result of prematurity. In 40% of quadruplet pregnancies, significant developmental delay is present in at least one of the resulting children.[13]

In the USA, insurance coverage typically includes obstetric and neonatal care but excludes ART. Thus, to the patient, the 'economic risk' of a failed IVF cycle is greater than the economic consequences of a multiple gestation. The obvious strategy to limit multiple gestations involves decreasing the number of embryos transferred.[18,19] Indeed, in many countries this policy has been legislated by national governments.

## BLASTOCYST CULTURE AND TRANSFER TO INCREASE IMPLANTATION RATES

The underlying problem culminating in the transfer of numerous embryos, and hence the reason for multiple gestations, is the low implantation rate of cleavage-stage embryos transferred in human IVF. The reason for reported values of 10–20% for embryo implantation rate conceivably results from the premature replacement of the human embryo to the uterus.[1,2,20,21] (see also Chapter 26). The use of sequential serum-free culture media facilitates the routine development of the pronucleate embryo for 4–5 days in culture to the blastocyst stage.[22–24] It is evident that such blastocysts have a higher implantation rate than the cleavage-stage embryo, and therefore the transfer of the human embryo at this later stage of development will facilitate the transfer of fewer embryos, while at the same time maintaining acceptable pregnancy rates.[23] The higher implantation rate of blastocysts developed in culture can be attributed to the transfer of the embryo to the uterus at the appropriate embryonic stage, and by the identification in culture of those embryos with little if any developmental potential.[1,21]

## IS ASSISTED HATCHING OR ZONA REMOVAL REQUIRED FOR BLASTOCYST TRANSFER?

It has been proposed that the removal of the zona pellucida will significantly reduce the energy requirements of the blastocyst, thereby increasing implantation rates. However, this hypothesis may be too simplistic. First, the majority of energy expended by the blastocyst, around 70%, is required to maintain the blastocoel.[25] The embryo does this using basolaterally positioned $Na^+/K^+$ ATPases.[26] Maintenance of the blastocoel, and hence the turgor of the blastocyst, is therefore not a function of the zona. Presumably the blastocoel needs to be fully expanded to facilitate apposition of the trophoectoderm and endometrium. Second, the blastocyst has been shown actively to synthesize a specific enzyme for the degradation of the zona.[27,28] This enzyme will be produced by the blastocyst whether the zona is present or not, and therefore the removal of the zona in the laboratory will not reduce the energy expended by the blastocyst for this function.

Jones et al[24] advocated the use of pronase for complete removal of the zona before transfer of blastocysts developed in sequential culture media. The rationale for this was based on the work of Cohen et al[29] who proposed that hatching was impaired after IVF as a result of hardening of the zona. In contrast, blastocysts do not currently undergo assisted hatching or have their zona removed before transfer at the Colorado Center for Reproductive Medicine.[23] The implantation rate after zona removal with pronase was 23%,[24] whereas the implantation rate for blastocysts transferred with their zona intact was 46%.[23] Although there are several differences between the protocols used for blastocyst culture and transfer between the above two studies, it is evident that blastocysts can implant at high rates when transferred with their zona intact. The question therefore remains whether implantation rates significantly higher than 50% can be obtained by some form of assisted hatching or zona removal.

Should pronase be used to remove the zona, its enzymatic action will be non-specific, and so it will also remove cell surface proteins, glycoproteins, and integrins.[30] This therefore raises the question of whether the blastocyst can replace such cell surface molecules in an appropriate time. It is plausible that the removal of such cell surface molecules may impair embryo apposition and attachment to the endometrium, thereby hindering implantation. An alternative to pronase is trypsin, which does not remove all cell surface glycoproteins or impair the adhesion of cells to fibronectin.[30] Furthermore, the enzyme produced by the trophoectoderm to digest the zona is a trypsin-like protease.[27] So at present it is not clear whether assisted hatching or zona removal is required or even desirable for human blastocyst transfers. However, assisted hatching or complete zona removal may be important for blastocysts conceived after the in vitro maturation of the oocyte, during which time the zona can harden.

## BLASTOCYST TRANSFER AND CRYOPRESERVATION

As blastocysts have an implantation rate of around 50%, one need only transfer two such embryos to the patient to achieve a high pregnancy rate. Indeed, the transfer of more than two blastocysts to a patient can no longer be advocated except under extenuating circumstances. Transfer can successfully be achieved using a Wallace catheter under ultrasonic guidance. Based on an implantation rate of 50%, the theoretical pregnancy rate with two blastocysts transferred is 75%. Of the resultant pregnancies, however, a third will be twins. Therefore, although high-order multiple gestation can be completely eliminated, unless one moves to single blastocyst transfers, multiple births in the form of twins will still be an issue. Present sequential culture media support around 50–60% blastocyst development from the pronuclear stage embryo.[22–24] As only one or two blastocysts are required for transfer, it is essential to have an appropriate freezing system for the cyropreservation of supernumerary blastocysts. Currently, more than 60% of patients having blastocyst transfer at the Colorado Center for Reproductive Medicine have blastocysts for cryopreservation. Historically glycerol has been the cryoprotectant of choice[23,24,31,32] and has resulted in relatively high levels of blastocyst survival and pregnancy after thaw. However, the use of such cryoprotectants as ethylene glycol, which has been used very successfully in the cow, should be considered.[33]

## LUTEAL PHASE SUPPORT FOR BLASTOCYST TRANSFER

The standard luteal support for day 3 embryo transfers at the Colorado Center for Reproductive Medicine involves 50 mg progesterone in oil starting the day after oocyte retrieval. In patients undergoing blastocyst transfer, this replacement dosage is initiated 2 days after oocyte retrieval, that is, one day later. This decision was based on the following:

previous studies have shown that the endometrium of patients undergoing controlled ovarian hyperstimulation is advanced compared with that in natural cycles. This advanced histology is associated with a premature disappearance of endometrial pinopods as assessed by scanning electron microscopy; their presence has been shown to be a marker of the implantation window. Furthermore, elevations in progesterone on the day of administration of human chorionic gonadotropin (hCG) have been associated with a decrease in IVF success, but not in cycles of oocyte donation or in cycles where all embryos were cryopreserved for later transfer.[34] For day 3 transfers in our clinic, we typically utilize assisted hatching, which has been shown to advance the day of implantation by 24 hours. These observations, taken together with the fact that blastocysts grown in culture for 5 days may be developmentally delayed compared with their in vivo counterparts, and the fact that we have not performed assisted hatching on blastocyst stage embryos, led us to a decision to delay progesterone replacement by an additional 24 hours. It was hoped that this would minimize the accelerated endometria seen in hyperstimulation cycles and allow better synchronization between the endometrium and the blastocyst at the time of transfer.

## ENDOMETRIAL PREPARATION FOR FROZEN–THAWED BLASTOCYST TRANSFER

Patients undergoing frozen and thawed blastocyst transfer start taking leuprolide acetate in the midluteal phase of the prior cycle using a subcutaneous dose of 1 mg. After the onset of menses, the dose of leuprolide is decreased to 0.5 mg and estrogen replacement started in the form of a transdermal estrogen patch 0.1 mg daily. After 8 days the dose of estrogen is increased to two patches daily, 2 days later increased further to three patches, and then ultimately to a total of four patches per day. At this time, the estradiol level is checked and transvaginal ultrasonography performed. If the serum estradiol is above 200 pg/ml and the endometrium shows a 9 mm thickness or

greater with a triple pattern, progesterone therapy is started. Progesterone is initiated at an intramuscular dose of 50 mg daily. On day 6 of progesterone administration, frozen and thawed blastocysts are transferred. The blastocysts are thawed late on the afternoon before transfer and allowed to re-expand overnight to confirm viability before transfer. During this time, estrogen patches are continued at a dose of two to four patches per day, depending on estradiol levels. When a pregnancy is confirmed, both estrogen and progesterone administration are continued until the luteal–placental shift is confirmed, signaling the production of endogenous estrogen and progesterone from the placenta. At this time the patient is slowly weaned off her estrogen and progesterone support.

## FUTURE OF BLASTOCYST TRANSFER IN THE HUMAN: TOWARDS SINGLE EMBRYO TRANSFERS

It is evident that new sequential culture media can support the development of viable human blastocysts in culture. That such blastocysts are deemed to be viable is reflected in their high implantation rate. Indeed reported implantation rates using sequential media are equivalent if not higher than those reported using co-culture.[35] As improvements are made to these new serum-free sequential culture media, it should be possible to increase further the percentage of embryos reaching the blastocyst stage in culture. However, it is envisaged that the maximum percentage of blastocyst formation of human embryos conceived through IVF will be around 60–70%, because a significant percentage of oocytes and sperm are not normal. Most such abnormalities are chromosomal. It has been determined that around 25% of oocytes are aneuploid[36] and that this problem is exacerbated with maternal age.[37] Other factors contributing to embryonic attrition include an insufficiency of stored oocyte-coded gene products, and a failure to activate the embryonic genome.[38,39] Although the culture to the blastocyst stage before transfer will eliminate the grossly abnormal embryos, some aneuploids will form blastocysts. It will therefore be important to determine the chromosomal status of those embryos that undergo developmental arrest in culture in order to determine which, if any, aneuploidies and other chromosomal imbalances are incompatible with development during the preimplantation period.

Further to improvements in the culture media used to support blastocyst development (see Chapter 26),[1,21] the ability to identify those blastocysts with the highest developmental potential before transfer should also increase the success of embryo transfer, plausibly leading to single blastocyst transfer. Assessment of embryo metabolism, using the non-invasive approach of ultramicrofluorescence,[40] not only can determine the degree of cellular stress placed on an embryo under different culture conditions,[41] but also can be used to identify those blastocysts with the highest developmental potential.[1,42–45] Most importantly, the non-invasive assessment of blastocyst metabolism can be used prospectively to select the most viable blastocysts before transfer. Using the mouse as the model, individual blastocysts of equivalent morphologies and the same diameter had their glucose consumption and lactate production measured. It was observed that, although the blastocysts had the same appearances, there was a great difference between blastocysts in their metabolic profile, confirming that morphology is a weak criterion on which to base embryo selection.[21,45,46] A hypothesis was set up in which those blastocysts that had a metabolic activity similar to an in vivo developed blastocyst, that is a high rate of glucose consumption but a low level of lactate production, would be the most viable embryos. In contrast, those blastocysts with a low glucose uptake and a high lactate production were deemed to be of low viability. Subsequently individual blastocysts had their metabolism assessed before transfer. The control for this study was transfer of blastocysts based on their morphological appearance alone. Fetal development per blastocyst transferred in the control group was 20%, whereas those blastocysts classified as viable before the transfer had a fetal

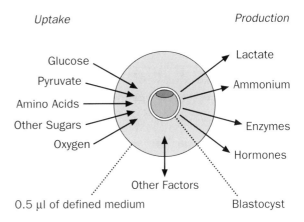

**Figure 1** Non-invasive assessment of blastocyst viability. Blastocysts are incubated individually in a known volume, for example, 0.5 µl, of defined medium. Serial nanoliter samples can then be taken and analyzed for the carbohydrates,[47,48] amino acids,[49] ammonium,[50] oxygen,[51] and enzymes.[52] The concomitant measurement of glucose consumption and lactate production can give an indirect measure of glycolytic activity. The concomitant measurement of amino acid consumption and ammonium production can give an indirect measure of amino acid use. The release of enzymes, such as lactate dehydrogenase, into the surrounding culture medium reflects impairment in membrane integrity, and as such may be useful in assessing freezing damage.

development of 80%. In contrast, blastocysts classified as having low viability had a fetal development of just 6%. Clearly, the measurement of metabolism in human blastocysts is warranted. Figure 1 shows some potential markers of blastocyst viability, all of which can be measured non-invasively. Ultimately, the best indication of viability may come from the simultaneous assessment of several parameters.

## CONCLUSIONS

Multiple gestations are the most common complication of IVF in humans, and represent serious medical, economic, and social problems.

The ability to transfer one or two embryos while still being able to maintain high pregnancy rates is therefore a most attractive proposition. With the development of sequential culture media, routine culture and transfer of human blastocysts have become a reality. Blastocysts developed in such culture systems have a significantly higher implantation rate than cleavage-stage embryos, and therefore fewer blastocysts are required at the time of transfer, thereby eliminating the incidence of high-order multiple gestations. With the concomitant ability to use the non-invasive assessment of metabolism to identify the most viable blastocyst from a given cohort, and to cryopreserve those blastocysts not transferred, the feasibility of performing single blastocyst transfers is increasing.

## REFERENCES

1. Gardner DK, Lane M. Culture and selection of viable human blastocysts: a feasible proposition for human IVF? *Hum Reprod Update* 1997; **3**:367–82.
2. Buster JE, Bustillo M, Rodi IA et al. Biologic and morphologic development of donated human ova by nonsurgical uterine lavage. *Am J Obstet Gynecol* 1985;**153**:211–17.
3. Bustillo M, Zarutskie P. Assisted reproductive technology in the United States and Canada: 1995 results generated from the American Society for Reproductive Medicine/Society for Assisted Reproductive Technology registry. *Fertil Steril* 1998;**69**:389–98.
4. Botting BJ, Davies IM, McFarlane AJ. Recent trends in the incidence of multiple births and associated mortality. *Arch Dis Child* 1987; **62**:941–50.
5. Grutzner-Konnecke H, Grutzner P, Grutzner B et al. High order multiple births: Natural wonder or failure of therapy? *Acta Genet Med Gemellol (Roma)* 1990;**39**:491–5.
6. Elster AD, Bleyl JL, Craven TE. Birth weight standards of triplets under modern obstetrical care in the United States, 1984–1989. *Obstet Gynecol* 1991;**77**:387–93.
7. Kiely JL, Kleinman JC, Kiely M, Triplets and high-order multiple births: time trends and infant mortality. *Am J Dis Child* 1992;**146**:862–8.
8. Lipitz S, Reichman B, Paret G et al. The improving outcome of triplet pregnancies. *Am J Obstet Gynecol* 1989;**161**:1279–84.
9. Lipitz S, Frankel Y, Watts C et al. High order multifetal gestation-management and outcome. *Obstet Gynecol* 1990;**76**:215–18.
10. Neuman RB, Hamer C, Miller MC. Outpatient triplet management: a contemporary review. *Am J Obstet Gynecol* 1989;**161**:547–55.
11. Berkowitz RL, Lynch L, Chitman U et al. Selective reduction of multifetal pregnancies in the first trimester. *N Engl J Med* 1988;**318**:1043–7.
12. Evans MI, Dommergues M, Wapner RJ et al. Efficacy of transabdominal multifetal pregnancy reduction: Collaborative experience among the world's largest centers. *Obstet Gynecol* 1993;**82**:61–6.
13. Evans MI, May M, Drugan A et al. Selective termination: Clinical experience and residual risks. *Am J Obstet Gynecol* 1990;**162**:1568–75.
14. Evans MI, Dommergues M, Timor-Tritsh I et al. Transabdominal versus transcervical and transvaginal multifetal pregnancy reduction: International collaborative experience of more than one thousand cases. *Am J Obstet Gynecol* 1994;**170**:902–9.
15. Cusick W, Gleicher N. Multiple conceptions, implantation, and prematurity. *Assist Reprod Rev* 1995;**5**:246–50.
16. Porreco RP, Harmon RJ, Murrow NS et al. Parental choices in grand multiple gestation: Psychological considerations. *J Maternal–Fetal Med* 1995;**4**:1111–14.
17. Goldfarb JM, Austin C, Lisbona H et al. Cost-effectiveness of in vitro fertilization. *Obstet Gynecol* 1996;**87**:18–21.
18. Nijs M, Geerts L, Van Roosendaal E et al. Prevention of multiple pregnancies in an in vitro fertilization program. *Fertil Steril* 1993;**59**:1245–50.
19. Svendsen TO, Jones D, Butler L, Muasher SJ. The incidence of multiple gestation after in vitro fertilization is dependent on the number of embryos transferred and maternal age. *Fertil Steril* 1996;**65**:561–5.
20. Croxatto HB, Ortiz ME, Diaz S et al. Studies on the duration of egg transport by the human

oviduct. *Am J Obstet Gynecol* 1978;**132**:629–34.

21. Gardner DK, Lane M. Culture of viable human blastocysts in defined sequential serum-free media. *Hum Reprod* 1998;**13**(suppl1):101–12.

22. Gardner DK, Lane M, Kouridakis K, Schoolcraft WB. Complex physiologically based serum-free culture media increase mammalian embryo development. In *In Vitro Fertilization and Assisted Reproduction* (Gomel V, Leung PCK, eds). Bologna; Monduzzi Editore, 1997;87–91.

23. Gardner DK, Vella P, Lane M et al. Culture and transfer of human blastocysts increases implantation rates and reduces the need for multiple embryo transfers. *Fertil Steril* 1998;**69**:84–8.

24. Jones GM, Trounson AO, Gardner DK et al. Evolution of a culture protocol for successful blastocyst development and pregnancy. *Hum Reprod* 1998;**13**:169–77.

25. Benos DJ, Balaban RS. Energy requirements of the developing mammalian blastocyst for active ion transport. *Biol Reprod* 1980;**23**:941–7.

26. Biggers JD, Bell JE, Benos, DJ. Mammalian blastocyst: transport functions in a developing epithelium. *Am J Physiol* 1988;**255**:C419–32.

27. Perona RM, Wassarman PM. Mouse blastocysts hatch in vitro by using a trypsin-like proteinase associated with cells of mural trophectoderm. *Dev Biol* 1986;**114**:42–52.

28. Vu TKH, Liu RW, Haaksma CJ, Tomasek JJ, Howard EW. Identification and cloning of the membrane-associated serine protease, hepsin, from mouse preimplantation embryos. *J Biol Chem* 1997;**272**:31315–20.

29. Cohen J, Elsner C, Kort H et al. Impairment of the hatching process following IVF in the human and improvement by assisted hatching using micromanipulation. *Hum Reprod* 1990;**5**:7–13.

30. Tarone G, Galetto G, Prat M, Comoglio PM. Cell surface molecules and fibronectin-mediated cell adhesion: effect of proteolytic digestion of membrane proteins. *J Cell Biol* 1982;**94**:179–86.

31. Menezo Y, Nicollet B, Herbaut N, Andre D. Freezing cocultured human blastocysts. *Fertil Steril* 1992;**58**:977–80.

32. Kaufmann RA, Menezo Y, Hazout A et al. Cocultured blastocyst cryopreservation: experience of more than 500 transfer cycles. *Fertil Steril* 1995;**64**:1125–9.

33. Lane MW, Ahern TJ, Lewis IM et al. Cryopreservation and direct transfer of in vitro produced bovine embryos; a comparison between vitrification and slow freezing. *Theriogenology* 1998;**49**:170.

34. Silverberg KM, Burns WN, Olive DL et al. Serum progesterone levels predict success of in vitro fertilization/embryo transfer in patients stimulated with leuprolide acetate and human menopausal gonadotropins. *J Clin Endocrinol Metab* 1991;**73**:797–803.

35. Olivennes F, Hazout A, Lelaider C et al. Four indications for embryo transfer at the blastocyst stage. *Human Reprod* 1994;**9**:2367–73.

36. Kola I, Sathanathan AH, Gras L. Chromosomal analysis of preimplantation mammalian embryos. In: *Handbook of In Vitro Fertilization* (Trounson A, Gardner DK, eds) Boca Raton: CRC Press, 1993;173–93.

37. Janny L, Menezo YJ. Maternal age effect on early human embryonic development and blastocyst formation. *Mol Reprod Dev* 1996;**45**:31–7.

38. Braude PR, Bolton VN, Moore S. Human gene expression first occurs between the four- and eight-cell stages of preimplantation development. *Nature* 1988;**332**:459–61.

39. Tesarik J. Developmental failure during the preimplantation period of human embryogenesis. In: *The Biological Basis of Early Human Reproductive Failure* (Van Blerkom J, ed.), New York: Oxford University Press, 1994;327–44.

40. Mroz EA, Lechene C. Fluorescence analysis of picolitre samples. *Anal Biochem* 1980;**102**:90–6.

41. Gardner DK. Changes in requirements and utilization of nutrients during mammalian preimplantation embryo development and their significance in embryo culture. *Theriogenology* 1998;**49**:83–102.

42. Gardner DK, Lesse HJ. Assessment of embryo viability prior to transfer by the non-invasive measurement of glucose uptake. *J Exp Zool* 1987;**242**:103–5.

43. Gardner DK, Leese HJ. Assessment of embryo metabolism and viability. In: *Handbook of In Vitro Fertilization* (Trounson A, Gardner DK, eds) Boca Raton, FL: CRC Press, 1993;195–216.

44. Gardner DK, Pawelczynski M, Trounson A. Nutrient uptake and utilisation can be used to select viable day-7 bovine blastocysts after cryopreservation. *Mol Reprod Dev* 1996;**44**:472–5.

45. Lane M, Gardner DK. Selection of viable mouse blastocysts prior to transfer using a metabolic criterion. *Hum Reprod* 1996;**11**:1975–8.

46. Lane M, Gardner DK. Differential regulation of mouse embryo development and viability by amino acids. *J Reprod Fertil* 1997;**109**:153–64.

47. Leese JH, Barton AM. Pyruvate and glucose uptake by mouse ova and preimplantation

embryos. *J Reprod Fert* 1984;**71**:9–13.

48. Gardner DK, Leese HJ. Non-invasive measurement of nutrient uptake by single cultured preimplantation mouse embryos. *Hum Reprod* 1986;**1**:25–7.

49. Gardner DK, Clarke RN, Lechene CP, Biggers JD. Development of a noninvasive ultramicrofluorometric method for measuring net uptake of glutamine by single preimplantation mouse embryos. *Gamete Res* 1989;**24**:427–38.

50. Gardner DK, Lane M. Amino acids and ammonium regulate mouse embryo development in culture. *Biol Reprod* 1993;**4**:377–85.

51. Houghton FD, Thompson JG, Kennedy CJ, Leese HJ. Oxygen consumption and energy metabolism of the early mouse embryo. *Mol Reprod Devel* 1996;**44**:476–85.

52. Johnson SK, Jordan JE, Dean RG, Page RD. The quantification of bovine embryo viability using a bioluminescent assay for lactate dehydrogenase. *Theriogenology* 1991;**35**:425–33.

# 25

# Cryopreservation of ovarian tissue

Helen M Picton, Roger G Gosden

**The principle of freezing ovarian cells** • **Cryopreservation of oocytes** • **Ovarian tissue cryopreservation**

The first serious attempts to cryopreserve ovarian tissue and restore endocrine function were carried out in rodents in the 1950s.[1–4] At this time, ovarian tissue, which had been frozen in a mixture of glycerol and physiological saline and subsequently autografted onto a subcutaneous site, was shown to restore oestrous activity in ovariectomized rats.[5] Follicle survival rates in these grafts were, however, low. More dramatically, by 1960 the successful isografting of frozen–thawed murine ovaries onto the ovarian bursa had led to the restoration of natural fertility and the birth of healthy pups.[6] Despite this initial success, the technology required to support further progress was not available and the work was largely abandoned. However, with the advent of assisted reproduction technology, extensive research into freezing of spermatozoa[7] and embryos[8,9] in humans and farm species has led to a better theoretical understanding of the principles of cell freezing and significant improvements in the cryoprotective agents available, and in instrumentation and automation to control freezing rates. These advances have generated a resurgence of interest in ovarian cryopreservation.

The potential and application of the ovarian cryobiology in the conservation of female fertility are only now being fully realized (Figure 1) as the survival rates of young people with malignant disease improve[10] and the late effects of chemotherapy and/or radiotherapy on reproductive function become increasingly unacceptable. Frozen banking of ovarian tissues presents an attractive strategy for conserving the fertility of children and young women who are at risk of iatrogenic ovarian failure induced by chemotherapy or abdominal radiation, but who are too young to have either started or completed their families before the start of the treatment. In theory, the only options available to preserve the fertility of these young patients are assisted reproductive techniques which enable collection and storage of mature metaphase II oocytes and, more practically, embryos. Although cryopreservation of metaphase II oocytes has proved unreliable,[11] frozen storage of embryos has occasionally been successfully used before a woman undergoes myeloablative therapy.[12] The requirement for numbers of metaphase II oocytes for in vitro fertilization (IVF) and embryo freezing, however, necessitates ovarian hyperstimulation before oocyte recovery – a procedure that may take several

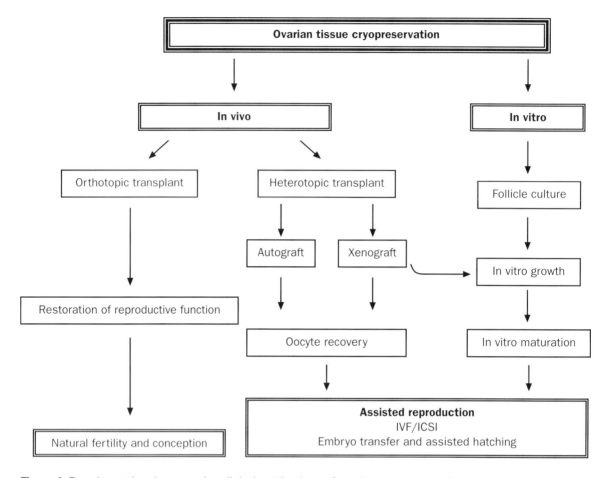

**Figure 1** Experimental and prospective clinical applications of ovarian cryopreservation.

weeks and delay the onset of chemotherapy, so inflicting further hardships on the patient. Although conservation of fertility through the use of existing IVF technologies is sometimes both suitable and acceptable for patients of reproductive age, this approach is clearly inappropriate for prepubertal girls and other patients who may not find frozen embryo banking an acceptable strategy. Ovarian tissue cryopreservation can now be proposed as a more radical and practical alternative treatment for children as well as for adults with or without a male partner. Moreover, it has the potential to restore normal ovarian function and natural fertility which is also attractive to patients and is

less controversial than frozen embryo storage[9,13] or egg donation.

## THE PRINCIPLE OF FREEZING OVARIAN CELLS

Cells undergoing cryopreservation are liable to damage at various stages of cooling and thawing. To minimize freezing injury it is necessary to equilibrate ovarian tissue with cryoprotective agents that are highly water soluble, non-toxic and membrane permeable. Indeed cryoprotectants are essential for the survival of isolated oocytes, follicles or samples of ovarian cortex after freeze-thawing.[14] In the absence of cryo-protectants follicular cells and oocytes are first subjected to cold shock above the freezing point of the solution, and second to a rise in osmolality before the solution freezes,[15,16] and may be irretrievably damaged by the formation of intracellular ice crystals.[17] The colligative properties of cryopreservatives help protect cells against freezing injury by reducing the amount of ice crystal formation at low temperatures which, in turn, decreases external salt concentrations and reduces the likelihood of intracellular freezing. To avoid, or at least reduce, freezing injury cooling rates should be fast enough to minimize exposure of cells to high intracellular concentrations of electrolytes, but slow enough to avoid damaging intracellular ice formation. Finally, the thawing protocol used can profoundly affect oocyte and follicle survival rates. After the thaw cell survival can be improved by: (1) the slow removal of the cryoprotectant; and (2) the inclusion of low concentrations of non-permeable osmolytes, such as sucrose and mannitol, which act as osmotic buffers against swelling during the addition and removal of the protective agents.[18–20] Significantly more pregnancies have been achieved in mice after orthotopic ovarian transplantation when fast (86%) rather than slow (25%) thaw protocols were used.[21]

A major problem of ovarian cryopreservation is achieving adequate permeation of the tissue by the cryoprotectant. This necessitates optimization of protocols for each cell or tissue type because post-thaw survival of ovarian tissue is profoundly affected by both the type of cryoprotectant used[14] and the equilibration time required for cryoprotectant uptake and removal.[20] High rates of solute penetration and high final concentrations of cryoprotectant must be achieved, and preferably at temperatures of 4°C to minimize toxicity.[20] The problems of achieving adequate permeation of tissue fragments can be overcome either by preparation of thin strips of tissue 1 mm or less thick to provide maximal surface area for solute penetration,[14,20] or by dissociation of the tissue into follicles or isolated cells before freezing.[21]

Generally, ovarian cells can be successfully frozen by suspension in an optimal concentration of cryoprotectant and sucrose, by cooling at a rate that allows cellular dehydration but limits the extent of intracellular ice formation, and by avoiding the adverse effects of osmotic stress during thawing. At −196°C ovarian tissues can be stored in liquid nitrogen for as long as required. Using this approach, high post-thaw follicle survival rates have been recorded for human primordial follicles of 84% and 74% for 1.5 mol/l ethylene glycol and dimethyl-sulphoxide (DMSO), respectively, compared with survival rates of only 44% and 10% with 1.5 mol/l propylene glycol and glycerol, respectively.[14] Similar low survival rates were previously recorded for glycerol by Green et al,[5] which was probably the result of osmotic stress by this slowly permeating solute. Our results suggest that the most efficient method for the preservation of human ovarian tissue involves immersion of slices of ovarian cortex that are 1 mm or less thick for 30 min at 4°C in freezing solution containing either 1.5 mol/l ethylene glycol or DMSO with 0.1 mol/l sucrose.[14,20,23]

## CRYOPRESERVATION OF OOCYTES

Oocyte freezing has the potential to be an important adjunct to assisted reproductive technologies. However, the ease and success of cryopreservation programmes for sperm[7] and embryos[9] contrast markedly with the problems associated with freezing mammalian oocytes.[24,25] Despite the first announcements of success by Chen[26] and Van Uem et al,[27] post-thaw survival rates for human oocytes are low[8,19,28] and human oocyte cryopreservation has been slow to be adopted clinically. Several reasons can be offered for the disappointing results. Human oocytes have a short fertile lifespan, are exquisitely sensitive to temperature and the presence of toxic compounds, and have little capacity for repairing damage. Furthermore mature oocytes have reached metaphase II at which stage the cells have a highly organized cytoskeleton, and complex organelles that are enclosed within the zona pellucida. Damage to any of these structures during freezing can potentially reduce post-thaw viability. Freeze storage is, for example, thought to cause premature cortical granule release within the oocyte which results in hardening of the zona pellucida and may profoundly affect fertilization, embryo development and implantation.[24,29] Although hardening of the zona pellucida can be bypassed using micromanipulation techniques and assisted hatching,[11,30] of greater concern is the risk of parthenogenetic activation of the oocyte and increased rates of aneuploidy. Immunocytochemical studies of mouse and human oocytes have demonstrated that both cooling and the cryoprotective solutions themselves can cause depolymerization of the meiotic spindle apparatus[31,32] which may result in non-dysjunction of sister chromatids at fertilization and so increase the risk of aneuploidy after extrusion of the second polar body. Results for human oocytes are, however, inconsistent and thaw survival rates of 60% have been recorded for human oocytes using propanediol and sucrose,[33–35] with no detrimental effects on either fertilization or early embryo development.

To circumvent the obstacles associated with the cryopreservation of metaphase II eggs, an alternative approach is the preservation of fully grown but germinal vesicle (GV) stage oocytes. These immature cells do not possess an organized spindle apparatus and, therefore, represent less of a risk for cooling-induced cytogenetic errors. Although animal data suggest that freezing GV oocytes is feasible,[36] few pregnancies have been achieved after the in vitro maturation of human oocytes[37–39] and none after cryopreservation of immature oocytes which have low post-thaw survival (37%[19] and 43%[35]) and in vitro maturation rates (20%[19] and 27%[35]). At present, and until the efficiency of in vitro maturation of human oocytes improves, cryopreservation of GV oocytes offers little advantage over freeze storage of metaphase II oocytes.

## OVARIAN TISSUE CRYOPRESERVATION

A more attractive alternative strategy to the cryopreservation of oocytes from preovulatory follicles is the possibility of storing oocytes at much earlier stages of follicular development by freezing strips of ovarian cortical tissue. A thin sample of the cortical region of the ovary, obtained by laparoscopy, laparotomy or oophorectomy, can yield large numbers of primordial and primary follicles.[40] This area of a young ovary is packed with hundreds of thousands of quiescent primordial follicles which represents the reserve from which all antral follicles and fertile oocytes will ultimately develop.[41] Furthermore, freeze banking of primordial follicles in situ in slices of the ovarian cortex offers the potential to restore natural fertility by autografting the thawed tissue onto orthotopic or heterotopic sites (see Figure 1). In theory primordial follicles should be better suited to cryopreservation and grafting than secondary follicles because they are smaller, lack a zona pellucida and cortical granules, are relatively metabolically quiescent and undifferentiated and, perhaps most importantly, are by far the most abundant stage present at every age. In addition, primordial follicles are apparently more tolerant to insults, such as immersion in hypotonic cryoprotectant solution and cooling to very low temperatures, than mature oocytes because they are smaller and have more time to repair sublethal damage to organelles and other structures during their prolonged growth phase. Indeed, human,[14,40,42,43] marmoset monkey[44] and mouse[22,45,46] primordial follicles have all successfully survived cryopreservation to liquid nitrogen temperatures.

The in vivo developmental potential of cryopreserved primordial follicles has been assayed by autografting[22] or xenografting cryopreserved tissue under the kidney capsules of immunologically tolerant SCID (severe combined immunodeficiency) mice.[14,44,47] In the human xenograft model both stromal and primordial follicles survived the freeze–thaw and grafting procedures,[14] and follicle growth was initiated and continued up to early antral stages (10–12

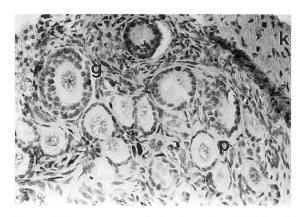

**Figure 2** Human xenograft showing primordial (p) and multilaminar growing (g) human follicles 17 weeks after grafting under the kidney capsule (k) of a SCID mouse. Follicles were stimulated to grow during the last 6 weeks by treatment with recombinant human FSH. Magnification ×400.

layers of granulosa cells) after supplementation with recombinant human follicle-stimulating hormone (FSH)[47] (Figure 2). These data support observations in the marmoset monkey model where large (1–2 mm diameter), oestrogenic, antral follicles developed 21–32 days after transplantation of cryopreserved tissue.[44] The main drawback of the xenograft model is that fertility cannot be tested in vivo. Nevertheless, the primordial follicles and the few growing follicles present in the grafts appeared to be cytologically normal.

After cryopreservation, autografted ovarian tissue has been shown to restore normal reproductive function[46] with the production of live offspring in mice[6,22] and sheep.[23] The restoration of fertility to sheep was reassuring because the ovaries of these animals more closely resemble human ovaries, which are bulkier, more fibrous and with a wider dispersal of primordial follicles than murine ovaries. In the sheep experiments, after freezing and thawing in 1.5 mol/l DMSO, thin slices of cortex were stitched back onto the ovarian pedicle; unfrozen grafts were attached to the contralateral side. Oestrous activity was restored within 3–4 months and, about 9 months after grafting, 11 of the 12 grafts contained follicles. Although few follicles were present in these animals 9 months after grafting, there were no obvious differences between frozen and fresh autografts at this stage, nor was there any evidence that either follicle dynamics or ovarian cycles were abnormal. Indeed, two of the six animals carried pregnancies to full term, one deriving the ovulation from a fresh graft and one from a frozen–thawed graft.[23] In a second group of animals normal ovarian cyclicity was maintained for at least 22 months after ovarian cryopreservation and orthotopic autografting.[48]

Although storage of slices of ovarian cortex is an attractive option, this tissue represents a complex mixture of cells with the potential problem that different cell types will have different cryopreservation optima. Clearly the ability of frozen–thawed ovarian tissue to re-form functional ovaries capable of folliculogenesis, steroidogenesis, ovulation and luteal function suggests that all major ovarian cell types, or their stem cells, were able to survive freezing and thawing. Follicles may, however, be lost at each stage in the procedure. Nevertheless it would appear that, after optimization of the freeze–thaw protocols, most of these losses are not accounted for by cryopreservation[20] but rather some 25–50% of the primordial follicles, depending on species,[14,23,44] will be lost as a result of the grafting itself. This loss probably reflects the effects of acute ischaemia, oxidative stress and reperfusion injury after grafting because revascularization of the graft may take several days.[49] Improved revascularization of the graft through the use of exogenous antioxidants such as vitamin E,[50] together with the relative abundance of endogenous angiogenic growth factors,[51] pituitary gonadotrophins and ovarian steroids,[49,52] may help to reduce ischaemia in the grafted tissue and so improve follicle survival.

Although the available data suggest that it may be possible to store ovarian tissue for patients undergoing sterilizing cancer treatments, the proviso remains that there must be no risk of returning malignant cells with the grafted tissue.[53–55] For a completely safe alternative strategy, it is desirable to grow oocytes to maturity in a culture environment for in vitro fertilization so that embryos, which are free of contamination, can be transferred to the patient. This long-range goal will avoid the risk of transferring disease and also serve to extend the application of ovarian tissue freezing. Although follicle culture technology is still in its infancy in humans,[56,57] its potential has recently been demonstrated in mice with the birth of live young.[58] Encouraging new data from in vitro experiments suggest that we can support antral cavity formation and early antral follicle growth, up to a diameter of at least 1 mm, in follicles from large animal species (H Newton, HM Picton and RG Gosden, unpublished work). Furthermore, progress is being made in the investigation of the conditions required for the successful in vitro maturation of human oocytes.[59] Although the initiation of growth in cultures of isolated human primordial follicles remains elusive, the simpler strategy of primordial follicles culture in situ after cryopreservation of cortical slices may prove more effective.[43,48,60]

These culture techniques may eventually supersede grafting techniques because they are safer for the patient and potentially make more economic use of scarce follicles. Although the original objective of this strategy was to conserve fertility for young women and children (as well as rare and endangered species and transgenic animals), when perfected they will transform assisted reproductive technology and egg donation. These objectives will require a great deal of developmental work to achieve but the benefits of greater safety, convenience and lower costs will surely stimulate continuing efforts.

## REFERENCES

1. Parkes AS, Smith AU. Regeneration of rat ovarian tissue grafted after exposure to low temperatures. *Proc R Soc Lond [Biol]* 1953;**140**:455–67.

2. Deanesley R. Immature rat ovaries grafted after freeze thawing. *J Endocrinol* 1954;**11**:197–200.

3. Parkes AS. Grafting of mouse ovarian tissue after freeze thawing. *J Endocrinol* 1956;**14**:30–1.

4. Parkes AS. Viability of ovarian tissue after freezing. *Proc R Soc Lond [Biol]* 1957;**147**:520–8.

5. Green SH, Smith AU, Zuckerman S. The numbers of oocytes in ovarian autografts after freezing and thawing. *J Endocrinol* 1956;**13**:330–4.

6. Parrot DMV. The fertility of mice with orthotopic ovarian grafts derived from frozen tissue. *J Reprod Fert* 1960;**1**:230–41.

7. Polge C, Smith AU, Parkes AS. Revival of spermatozoa after vitrification and dehydration at low temperatures. *Nature* 1949;**164**:666–7.

8. Trounson AO. Preservation of human eggs and embryos. *Fertil Steril* 1986;**46**:3–11.

9. Trounson AO, Dawson K. Storage and disposal of embryos and gametes. *BMJ* 1996;**313**:1–2.

10. Boring CC. Cancer statistics. *CA* 1994;**44**:7–26.

11. Gook DA, Schiewe MC, Osborn SM, et al. Intracytoplasmic sperm injection and embryo development of human oocytes cryopreserved using 1,2-propanediol. *Hum Reprod* 1995;**10**:2637–41.

12. Atkinson HG, Apperley JF, Dawson K, et al. Successful pregnancy after embryo cryopreservation after BMT for CMI (letter). *Lancet* 1994;**344**:199.

13. Dulioust E, Toyama K, Busmel MC, et al. Long-term effects of embryo freezing in mice. *Proc Natl Acad Sci USA* 1994;**92**:589–93.

14. Newton H, Aubard Y, Rutherford A, et al. Low temperature storage and grafting of human ovarian tissue. *Hum Reprod* 1996;**11**:1487–91.

15. Lovelock JE. The haemolysis of human red blood cells by freezing and thawing. *Biochim Biophys Acta* 1953;**10**:414–26.

16. Meryman HT. Modified model for the mechanism of freezing injury in erythrocytes. *Nature* 1968;**218**:333–6.

17. Mazur P. Kinetics of water loss from cells at subzero temperatures and the likelihood of intracellular freezing. *J Gen Physics* 1963;**47**:347–69.

18. Meryman HT. Cryoprotective agents. *Cryobiology* 1971;**8**:173–83.

19. Mandelbaum J, Junca AM, Planchot M, et al. Cryopreservation of human embryos and oocytes. *Hum Reprod* 1988;**3**:117–19.

20. Newton H, Fisher J, Arnold JPR, et al. Experimental determination of the optimal conditions for cryopreserving human ovarian tissue. *Hum Reprod* 1998; in press.

21. Cox SL, Shaw J, Jenkin G. Transplantation of cryopreserved fetal ovarian tissue to adult recipients in mice. *J Reprod Fertil* 1996;**107**:315–22.

22. Carroll J, Gosden RG. Transplantation of frozen thawed mouse primordial follicles. *Hum Reprod* 1993;**8**:1163–7.

23. Gosden RG, Baird DT, Wade JC, Webb R. Restoration of fertility to oophorectomised sheep by ovarian autografts stored at −196°C. *Hum Reprod* 1994;**9**:597–603.

24. Trounson AO, Kirby C. Problems in the cryopreservation of unfertilized eggs by slow cooling in DMSO. *Fertil Steril* 1989;**52**:778–86.

25. Oktay K, Newton H, Aubard Y, et al. Cryopreservation of immature human oocytes and ovarian tissue – an emerging technology. *Fertil Steril* 1998; in press.

26. Chen C. Pregnancy after human oocyte cryopreservation. *Lancet* 1986;**i**:884–6.

27. Van Uem JFHM, Siebzehnrubl ER, Schuh B, et al. Birth after cryopreservation of unfertilized eggs. *Lancet* 1997;**i**:752–3.

28. Al-Hasani S, Diedrich K, van der Ven H, et al. Cryopreservation of human oocytes. *Hum Reprod* 1987;**2**:695.

29. George MA, Johnson MH. Cytoskeletal organisation and zona sensitivity to digestion by chymotrypsin of frozen-thawed mouse oocytes. *Hum Reprod* 1993;**8**:612–20.

30. Nagy ZP, Loccufier A, Cecile J, et al. Pregnancy and birth after intracytoplasmic sperm injection of *in vitro* matured germinal-vesicle stage oocytes: case report. *Fertil Steril* 1996;**65**:1047–50.

31. Pickering SJ, Braude PR, Johnson MH, et al. Transient cooling to room temperature can cause irreversible disruption of the meiotic spindle in the human oocyte. *Fertil Steril* 1990;**54**:102–8.

32. Vincent C, Johnson MH. Cooling, cryoprotectants and the cytoskeleton of the mammalian oocyte. *Oxf Rev Reprod Biol* 1992;**14**:72–100.

33. Gook DA, Osborn SM, Johnson MH. Cryopreservation of mouse and human oocytes using 1,2-propanediol and the configuration of the meiotic spindle. *Hum Reprod* 1993;**8**:1101–9.

34. Porcu E, Fabbri R, Seracchioli R, et al. Pregnancy after microinjection of a cryopreserved human oocyte. *Hum Reprod* 1997;**12**(1):4.

35. Toth TL, Stavroula GB, Veeck LL, et al. Fertilization and *in vitro* development of cryopreserved human prophase I oocytes. *Fertil Steril* 1994;**61**:891–4.

36. Trounson AO, Pushett D, Maclellan LJ, et al. Current status of IVM/IVF and embryo culture in humans and farm animals. *Theriogenology* 1994;**41**:57–66.

37. Trounson AO, Wood C, Kausche A. *In vitro* maturation and fertilization and developmental competence of oocytes recovered from untreated polycystic ovarian patients. *Fertil Steril* 1994;**62**:353–62.

38. Cha KY, Koo JJ, Choi DH, et al. Pregnancy after *in vitro* fertilization of human follicular fluid oocytes collected from nonstimulated cycles, their culture *in vitro* and their transfer in a donor oocyte program. *Fertil Steril* 1991;**55**:109–18.

39. Russell JB, Knezevich KM, Fabian KF, Dickson JA. Unstimulated immature oocyte retrieval: early versus midfollicular endometrial priming. *Fertil Steril* 1997;**67**:616–20.

40. Oktay K, Nugent D, Newton H, et al. Isolation and characterization of primordial follicles from fresh and cryopreserved human ovarian tissue. *Fertil Steril* 1997;**67**:481–6.

41. Faddy MJ, Gosden RG, Gougeon A, et al. Accelerated disappearance of ovarian follicles in mid-life: implications for forecasting menopause. *Hum Reprod* 1992;**7**:1342–6.

42. Bahadur G, Steele SJ. Ovarian tissue cryopreservation for patients. *Hum Reprod* 1996;**11**:2215–16.

43. Hovatta O, Silye R, Krausz T, et al. Cryopreservation of human ovarian tissue using dimethylsulphoxide and propanediol-sucrose as cryoprotectants. *Hum Reprod* 1996;**11**:1268–72.

44. Candy CJ, Wood MJ, Whittingham DG. Follicular development in cryopreserved marmoset ovarian tissue after transplantation. *Hum Reprod* 1995;**10**:2334–8.

45. Gosden RG. Restitution of fertility in sterilized mice by transferring primordial ovarian follicles. *Hum Reprod* 1990;**5**:499–504.

46. Harp R, Leibach J, Black J, et al. Cryopreservation of murine ovarian tissue. *Cryobiology* 1994;**31**:336–43.

47. Oktay K, Gosden RG. Development of human primordial follicles to antral stages in SCID/*hpg* mice stimulated with follicle stimulating hormone. *Hum Reprod* 1998; in press.

48. Baird DT, Webb R, Campbell B, et al. Autotransplantation of frozen ovarian strips in sheep results in normal oestrous cycles for at least 22 months. *Hum Reprod* 1996;**11**:58 (abstract).

49. Dissen GA, Lara HE, Fahrenbach WH, et al. Immature rat ovaries become revascularized rapidly after autotransplantation and show a gonadotrophin-dependent increase in angio-

genic factor gene expression. *Endocrinology* 1994; **134:**1146–54.

50. Nugent D, Newton H, Gallivan L, Gosden RG. Protective effect of vitamin E on ischaemia–reperfusion injury in ovarian grafts. *J Reprod Fertil* 1998; in press.

51. Koos RD. Potential relevance of angiogenic factors to ovarian physiology. *Semin Reprod Endocrinol* 1989;**7:**29–40.

52. Sato E, Ishibashi, T, Koide SS. Inducement of blood vessel formation by ovarian extracts from mice injected with gonadotrophins. *Experientia* 1982;**38:**1248–9.

53. Shaw JM, Bowles J, Koopman P, et al. Fresh and cryopreserved ovarian tissue samples from donors with lymphoma transmit the cancer to graft recipients. *Hum Reprod* 1996;**8:**1668–73.

54. Gosden RG, Rutherford AJ, Norkolk DR. Ovarian banking for cancer patients: Transmission of malignant cells in ovarian grafts. *Hum Reprod* 1997;**12:**403.

55. Shaw JM, Trounson AO. Oncological implications in the replacement of ovarian tissue. *Hum Reprod* 1997;**12:**403–5.

56. Gosden RG. Prospects for maturing oocytes from small follicles *in vitro*. *Singapore J Obstet Gynaecol* 1996;**27:**66–70.

57. Hartshorne GM. *In vitro* culture of ovarian follicles. *Rev Reprod* 1997;**2:**94–104.

58. Eppig JJ, O'Brien MJ. Development *in vitro* of mouse oocytes from primordial follicles. *Biol Reprod* 1996:**54:**197–207.

59. Wynn P, Krapez J, Picton HM, et al. Randomised study of oocytes matured *in vitro* after collection from unstimulated or mildly stimulated patients. *Hum Reprod* 1997;**12**(abstract book 1):29.

60. Gosden RG. The early stages of follicle development. *Proceedings of the 10th World Congress on In Vitro Fertilization and Assisted Reproduction.* Bologna: Monduzzi, 1997:119–24.

# 26

# Improving embryo culture and enhancing pregnancy rate

David K Gardner

Advantages of blastocyst culture and transfer in human IVF • Lessons learned from the mother
• Changes in embryo physiology and metabolism • Markers of embryo developmental potential
• Types of culture media • Clinical results using blastocyst transfer • Conclusions
• Acknowledgements

The past decade has seen an immense leap forward in our ability to culture the mammalian preimplantation embryo. The term 'mammalian embryo' is used here deliberately, because the improvements have not been restricted to a single species but have been reported for the embryos of the mouse, hamster, goat, sheep, cow, and perhaps most importantly for the human. Interestingly, although significant species differences do exist, and therefore no species can make the perfect model for another, there are some unifying traits between species. Concomitant with an increased ability to culture the zygote throughout the preimplantation period to the blastocyst stage, there has been an increase in our understanding of what regulates embryo viability. Therefore, not only is it possible to obtain an acceptable percentage of blastocyst development in culture, but such blastocysts have a high viability as determined by their ability to go to term after transfer.

In this chapter those findings that have had a direct impact upon the development of novel sequential culture systems for the human embryo conceived through in vitro fertilization (IVF) are discussed. The culmination of this work is that it is now possible to culture the

human embryo to the blastocyst stage at frequencies greater than 50%, but more importantly such resultant blastocysts have an implantation rate of more than 50%. The significance of this is that fewer embryos are required at transfer in order to establish an acceptable pregnancy rate, while at the same time eliminating high-order multiple gestations.

## ADVANTAGES OF BLASTOCYST CULTURE AND TRANSFER IN HUMAN IVF

The significance of improving embryo culture media in human IVF cannot be overstated. Most of the work has concentrated on optimizing the culture conditions from the zygote to the eight-cell stage. This is because, for historical reasons, human embryos are routinely transferred at the four- to eight-cell stage. So why would culturing embryos for a further 2 days to the blastocyst stage be of benefit to human IVF? The answer to this question is twofold: first, in other mammalian species the transfer of cleavage-stage embryos to the uterus results in significantly lower pregnancy rates than the transfer of embryos post-compaction, that is, at the morula or blastocyst stage.[1] The reason for this is that the oviduct and uterus provide different environments for the development of the embryo in vivo;[2] the conditions found in the uterus are not consistent with a high rate of development of the cleavage-stage embryo. As the human embryo resides in the oviduct for up to 80 h after ovulation,[3] that is, up to around the time of compaction, then the replacement of the cleavage-stage embryo in the uterus may compromise development. So by being able to culture the human embryo to the blastocyst stage it is possible to synchronize the stage of development with the uterus. Second, not all gametes and subsequently not all embryos are normal.[4] Therefore, the culture of embryos for 4 days from the pronuclear stage will help to identify those embryos with limited developmental potential.[5,6] It is worth considering that, up to the eight-cell stage, embryo development is under maternal control through proteins and mRNAs synthesized during oocyte maturation. So when assessing the cleavage-stage embryo, one is in effect assessing the quality of the oocyte.[6] In contrast, after the onset of embryonic genome activation at the four- to eight-cell stage,[7] it is possible to assess true embryonic development in culture.

In consideration of the above points, it would appear that the blastocyst has an intrinsically higher developmental potential than the cleavage-stage embryo. This in turn will lead to higher implantation rates. As shown below this indeed appears to be the case. Other advantages of blastocyst culture include: (1) the ability to biopsy the embryo at the four- to eight-cell stage and send the biopsied blastomeres to a separate locale for genetic analysis without the need to cryopreserve the embryo while waiting for results; (2) the ability to biopsy trophectoderm for genetic analysis; this has some important ramifications because trophectoderm is technically non-embryonic; and (3) analysis of physiology past the eight-cell stage should lead to the development of viability assays for the human embryo.[8–11]

## LESSONS LEARNED FROM THE MOTHER

Analysis of oviduct and uterine fluids from naturally cycling patients revealed that there are significant differences in the nutritional milieu to which the embryo is exposed as it develops.[2] The fluid within the oviduct, at the time when the oocyte and early embryo are present, is characterized by relatively high levels of pyruvate and lactate and low levels of glucose. On the other hand, uterine fluid has a relatively high concentration of glucose and lower levels of pyruvate and lactate (Table 1). Such observations are consistent with the carbohydrate requirement of the developing embryo, outlined below. The cumulus cells surrounding the ovulated oocyte and newly formed zygote also contribute to the available nutrient pool. Cumulus cells readily consume glucose and convert it to both lactate and pyruvate, thereby creating an environment rich in carboxylic acids and plausibly devoid of glucose. How long the

**Table 1 Concentration of carbohydrates in the human oviduct and uterus**

|  | Pyruvate (mmol/l) | Lactate (mmol/l) | Glucose (mmol/l) |
|---|---|---|---|
| Oviduct (midcycle) | 0.32 | 10.5 | 0.50 |
| Uterus | 0.10 | 5.87 | 3.15 |

Lactate measured as the biologically active L isoform.[2]

cumulus cells contribute to the nutrient environment within the female tract is uncertain, but at least while the corona cells remain attached to the zona they will alter the environment around the embryo.

## CHANGES IN EMBRYO PHYSIOLOGY AND METABOLISM

The starting stage of preimplantation development, the zygote, and the final stage, the blastocyst, are markedly different in their physiology. Whereas the zygote, and early cleavage-stage embryo, is relatively quiescent and has low levels of oxidation and biosynthesis, the blastocyst is metabolically very active, exhibiting high levels of biosynthesis and consuming relatively large quantities of energy to maintain the blastcoel.[12–15] Such changes in physiology and metabolism are reflected in the changes in nutrient preference and utilization by the embryo. The two most studied groups of nutrients are carbohydrates and amino acids, and hence it is these two groups that are discussed in detail here. However, the role of ions, vitamins, and growth factors should not be overlooked. Studies on the effects of the latter on the regulation of embryo physiology and metabolism should lead to further improvements in IVF and embryo culture.

## Carbohydrates

In contrast to somatic cells, the mammalian cleavage-stage embryo does not appear to utilize glucose to any great extent.[12,16,17] Rather, when present in simple culture media glucose is responsible for the retardation or even developmental arrest of the cleavage-stage embryo from several mammalian species.[18–24] Rather than using glucose as its main energy source, the zygote and subsequent cleavage stages utilize carboxylic and amino acids.[1,12,15,16,25] Premature utilization of glucose by the cleavage-stage embryo is associated with a reduction of oxidative capacity, culminating in reduced embryo development.[15] As a result of its detrimental effect on embryos when present in simple culture media, there is a growing tendency to remove glucose from such media for use in human IVF.[24,26] Although it may be considered physiological to culture the denuded zygote and the first cleavage division in the absence of glucose, the complete removal of glucose from culture media designed to support embryo development beyond the first few cell cycles cannot be considered physiological.

When the cumulus cells have dispersed, the embryo will be exposed to glucose in the female tract, albeit at a low concentration in the oviduct. Therefore, before removing glucose from embryo culture media it is important to consider four things: first, the embryo possesses a specific transporter for glucose, indicating some physiological function for this hexose;[27–30] second, in the presence of suitable regulators of metabolism (such as amino acids and ethylenediaminetetraacetic acid, EDTA) glucose does not impair embryo development;[15,22,31–33] and third, glucose has important cellular functions other than as an energy source. Glucose is a key anabolic precursor and is required for the synthesis of triacylglycerols and phospholipids. It is also a precursor for complex sugars of mucopolysaccharides and glycoproteins. Glucose metabolized by the pentose phosphate pathway (PPP) generates ribose moieties required for nucleic acid synthesis and the NADPH required for the biosynthesis of lipids and other complex molecules.[34,35] NADPH is also required for the reduction of intracellular glutathione, an important antioxidant for the embryo.[13] Consequently, glucose will become increasingly important once the embryonic genome is activated and biosynthetic levels increase. Finally, glucose utilization through glycolysis may well be the only means by which the human and rodent embryos can generate energy during the initial stages of implantation.

Both the human and rodent blastocysts undergo invasive implantation. It has been shown through histological studies in the rat that there is a period of up to 12 h during invasive implantation when there is little, if any, vasculature in the endometrium. The blastocyst will therefore be exposed to a relatively anoxic environment, making glycolysis essential for energy production.[36–38] Should an embryo be cultured in the absence of glucose, it may be forced to use endogenous glucose reserves, in the form of glycogen, which could subsequently compromise implantation. In support of this hypothesis, although blastocysts can be obtained in the absence of glucose in the culture medium,[24,31] resultant blastocysts have significantly impaired implantation and fetal development after transfer compared with blastocysts that developed in the presence of glucose.[31]

## Amino acids

In contrast to the wealth of literature on the role of carbohydrates in embryo development, there is relatively little information on the role of amino acids. Renewed interest in amino acids[1,6,25,39] has led to the proposition that they are among the most important regulators of mammalian preimplantation development, and therefore a key constituent of embryo culture media. Amino acids not only maintain cell function, but are capable of stimulating both development and differentiation of the embryo in vitro, thereby increasing developmental potential after transfer. Furthermore, the inclusion of specific amino acids in embryo culture

media has been shown to alleviate the so-called 'culture blocks' to mammalian embryo development in all species studied to date (hamster,[1,39] mouse,[31] sheep,[40] and cow[41]).

Studies on the mouse embryo initially concentrated on the effects of those amino acids present at high levels in the fluid of the female reproductive tract.[42,43] Interestingly this group of amino acids, with the exception of glutamine, has a striking homology with those present in Eagle's non-essential amino acids,[6,41,44,45] that is, those amino acids not required for the development of somatic cells in culture. This group of amino acids, together with glutamine, was found to stimulate the development of F1 mouse zygotes to the blastocyst stage within 72 h of culture,[45] the time at which the mouse blastocyst is formed in vivo (Table 2). Subsequently, it was shown that these amino acids significantly reduced the duration of the first three cell cycles (Figure 1), resulting in increased rates of development and viability.[46,47] Quite remarkably, the essential group of amino acids (which are present at relatively low levels within the female tract) not only did not confer any benefit to the embryo in culture before the eight-cell stage, but actually negated the beneficial effects of the non-essential amino acids (see all 20 amino acids in Figure 1). Indeed, expo-

---

**Table 2 Effect of amino acids on mouse zygote development after 72 h of culture**

| Media | Stage of development reached (%) | | | | | |
|---|---|---|---|---|---|---|
| | <Morula | Morula | Early blastocyst | Expanded blastocyst | Hatching blastocyst | Total blastocyst |
| mMTF | 0 | 78[a] | 22 | 0 | 0 | 22[a] |
| NEGLN | 6 | 6[ab] | 18 | 36 | 34 | 88[ab] |
| ESS | 8 | 70[b] | 18 | 4 | 0 | 22[b] |

mMTF, modified mouse tubal fluid medium (Gardner and Lane[45]); NEGLN, non-essential amino acids and glutamine; ESS, essential amino acids without glutamine.
Like pairs are significantly different: a, b, $p < 0.01$.
Data from Gardner and Lane.[45]

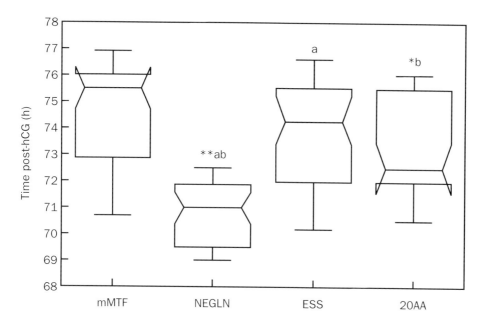

**Figure 1** Effect of amino acids on the timing of the third cleavage division in the mouse. Notches represent the interquartile range, therefore including 50% of the data. Whiskers represent 5% and 95% quartiles.[74] Line across the box represents the mean. NEGLN, mMTF supplemented with Eagle's non-essential amino acids and glutamine; ESS, mMTF supplemented with Eagle's essential amino acids without glutamine; 20AA, mMTF supplemented with all 20 Eagle's amino acids. Significantly different from mMTF: *$p < 0.05$; **$p < 0.01$. Like pairs significantly different: a, $p < 0.01$; b, $p < 0.05$. (From Lane and Gardner[47] with permission.)

sure of the mouse embryo to essential amino acids at the concentration in Eagle's medium before compaction resulted in loss of viability[46] and impaired development to the blastocyst stage in culture.[45,46,48] However, studies on mouse embryos collected from the oviduct/uterine junction at the eight-cell stage, and then placed in culture, showed that the exposure of later stage embryos to the essential group of amino acids was actually stimulatory, specifically increasing the cleavage rate of the inner cell mass (ICM) and subsequent fetal development. Concomitantly, the non-essential amino acids and glutamine were found to stimulate the formation of the blastocoel, increase trophectoderm cell number, and increase hatching rates.[48] Therefore, the highest percentage of blastocyst development and hatching, the highest total cell and ICM number, along with the highest implantation rates and fetal develop-

ment, occurred when mouse zygotes were cultured for the first 48 h in the presence of non-essential amino acids and glutamine, followed by culture for a further 48 h in the presence of all 20 of Eagle's amino acids (that is, both non-essential and essential groups).

One of the more significant observations from these studies was that the implantation rates were equivalent to those of embryos developed in vivo. The importance of a culture system that stimulates ICM proliferation is that ICM development is positively correlated with subsequent fetal development after transfer[48] (see below). The bovine embryo also exhibits a biphasic response to amino acids. Non-essential amino acids and glutamine produce the highest number of eight- to 16-cell embryos after 72 h of culture, with the highest percentage of blastocyst development being obtained after culture in all 20 amino acids for the second 72 h.[49]

Furthermore, in the sheep the culture of zygotes in the presence of amino acids in the culture medium resulted in blastocysts that had an equivalent viability to those developed in vivo.[40] Clearly then, amino acids confer a considerable benefit to the embryo in culture, providing that the toxic effects of their breakdown product ammonium are avoided by renewal of the medium every 48 h.[6,40,41,45,46] It is beyond the scope of this chapter to discuss in detail the various modes of action of amino acids; however, it is evident that they serve not only as biosynthetic precursors, but also as chelators, regulators of carbohydrate metabolism, osmolytes, and buffers of intracellular pH.[6] Amino acids thereby maintain cellular homeostasis and cell function.

## MARKERS OF EMBRYO DEVELOPMENTAL POTENTIAL

To evaluate the merits of new culture media, it is important to understand the significance of the criteria used to assess embryo development in culture. However, no matter which criteria are selected it is paramount that they correlate with subsequent development after transfer, because fetal development is the only true marker of embryo viability. The most commonly reported criteria for assessing embryo development in culture, and therefore the criteria against which new media are assessed, are blastocyst development and hatching. When these criteria were compared with others used to evaluate embryo viability it was evident that blastocyst formation and blastocyst hatching were actually the least sensitive criteria. Instead blastocyst cell number, ICM cell number, ICM outgrowth, and metabolism (measured as glycolysis) were more strongly correlated with fetal development after transfer[48] (Figure 2). Such data therefore question the significance of using blastocyst development and subsequent hatching in vitro as measures for assessing the suitability of a given set of culture conditions.

## TYPES OF CULTURE MEDIA

It is evident that the mammalian embryo is exposed to a changing environment in vivo and that it undergoes changes in its requirements for both carbohydrates and amino acids. However, in spite of this, attempts to optimize embryo culture have focused on the formulation of a single medium to support the entire preimplantation period. Conventionally, the types of culture medium used in human IVF fall into two categories: simple or complex.[25] Those media classified as simple are based upon balanced salt solutions and are routinely supplemented with pyruvate, lactate, and glucose. The protein source is either serum albumin or serum. Examples of such media are HTF[50] and P1.[26] Such media are empirically based and were derived predominantly from the early work on mouse embryo culture performed in the 1960s.[51] In contrast, those media classified as complex, such as Ham's F-10, were designed specifically to support the development of certain somatic cell lines in culture. They are far more complicated than the simple media, containing amino acids, vitamins, and transition metals, and are routinely supplemented with serum.

It is proposed that neither media type is suitable for the culture of the zygote to the blastocyst stage. Rather the formulation of the culture media should change to tailor the changing physiology and metabolism of the embryo as it develops. Simple media cannot adequately support blastocyst development and differentiation. While in complex media the presence of too many components impairs cleavage-stage embryo development, as observed when the essential amino acids are added to the nonessential group (see Figure 1). The use of physiologically based sequential culture media addresses this issue.

### Development of sequential culture media

In light of the dynamics of embryo physiology and the resultant changes in requirements for both carbohydrates and amino acids, two cul-

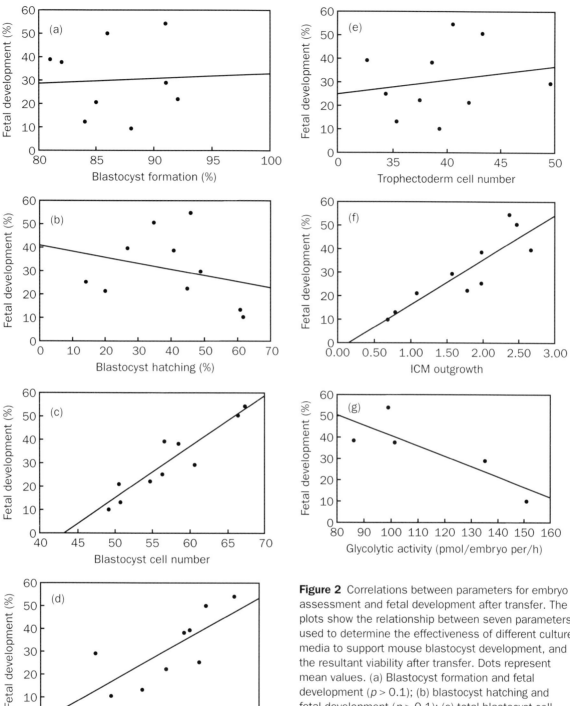

**Figure 2** Correlations between parameters for embryo assessment and fetal development after transfer. The plots show the relationship between seven parameters used to determine the effectiveness of different culture media to support mouse blastocyst development, and the resultant viability after transfer. Dots represent mean values. (a) Blastocyst formation and fetal development ($p > 0.1$); (b) blastocyst hatching and fetal development ($p > 0.1$); (c) total blastocyst cell number and fetal development ($p < 0.01$); (d) inner cell mass cell number and fetal development ($p < 0.05$); (e) trophectoderm cell number and fetal development ($p > 0.1$); (f) inner cell mass outgrowth and fetal development ($p < 0.01$); and (g) glycolytic activity and fetal development ($p < 0.07$). The relationship between glycolysis and viability has been further analysed.[11] (From Lane and Gardner[48] with permission.)

ture media, designated growth 1 and 2 (G1 and G2), were formulated to support the growth of the human pronuclear embryo to the blastocyst stage.[6,41,52] Medium G1 is based on the levels of carbohydrates present in the human oviduct at the time when the cleavage-stage embryo is present. This medium also contains those amino acids that have been shown to stimulate development of the cleavage-stage embryo (that is, the non-essential amino acids and glutamine). The chelator EDTA is also present, not only to sequester any toxic divalent cations present in the system, but also to help minimize glycolytic activity of the embryo, thereby minimizing metabolic perturbations. The mechanisms behind this have been reviewed in detail elsewhere.[6,15,53,54] In contrast, medium G2 is based on the levels of carbohydrates present in the human uterus and contains both non-essential and essential amino acids to facilitate both blastocyst development and differentiation. EDTA is not present in medium G2 because it appears to impair ICM development and function selectively, culminating in a loss of viability.[31,32] The apparent susceptibility of ICM development to EDTA can best be explained from the work of Hewitson and Leese,[55] who demonstrated that the ICM generates its energy exclusively from glycolysis. Therefore anything that specifically inhibits this pathway will inhibit ICM development.

Both media G1 and G2 are supplemented with albumin. Whole serum is not required or desired in embryo culture systems, especially those designed to support blastocyst growth.[6,25,41] The beneficial effects of using sequential media to support mouse embryo development in culture are shown in Figure 3. A most important highlight of this work was the observation that it is possible to generate healthy looking blastocysts in culture, which unfortunately have little if any further developmental potential. This stems from the fact that different components of the culture system affect different aspects of embryo development. So when mouse embryos were cultured in medium G1 for the entire preimplantation period to the blastocyst, although the embryos formed healthy looking blastocysts, most

implantations were lost, that is, they did not have a sufficient ICM to form a viable fetus.[48,54,56] The lack of adequate ICM development stems from the lack of sufficient glucose and the presence of EDTA (both affecting glycolysis) and the omission of essential amino acids. In contrast, those embryos that were switched to medium G2 after 48 h of culture formed blastocysts at the same rate and of equivalent morphologies to those cultured in G1 for the entire period. However, very few implantations were lost as the result of the development of a significant ICM, thereby maintaining a very high pregnancy rate. It is evident that the data represented in Figures 2 and 3 are complementary in that they both demonstrate the weakness of using blastocyst formation and subsequent hatching as indicators of developmental potential after transfer.

This concept, that a well-formed blastocyst does not necessarily equate to a viable blastocyst, is an important one, and one that can perhaps explain why previous attempts to culture the human embryo to the blastocyst stage have resulted in low implantation rates after transfer. For example, Bolton et al,[57] obtained a very respectable 40% blastocyst development from human pronuclear embryos. However, the resultant implantation and pregnancy rate was only 7%. The medium used in their study was Earle's supplemented with pyruvate and 10% maternal serum. Clearly such types of media are not suitable for extended human embryo culture.

## Macromolecules

Irrespective of the type of medium used in IVF, a frequently used supplement is serum. However, the suitability of serum as the protein/fixed nitrogen source for embryos is questionable. Oviduct fluid is not a serum transudate but is formed by the epithelium of the oviduct.[58] In contrast, the pathological clotting of blood forms serum. Furthermore, the composition of serum varies with many factors including patient etiology, day of cycle, state of fasting/diet, so that each patient's embryos are

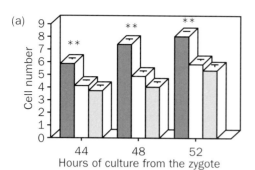

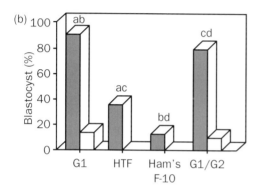

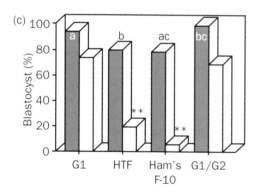

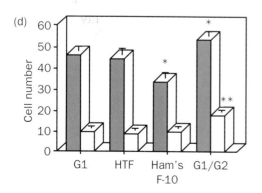

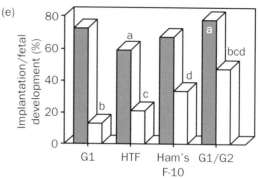

**Figure 3** Effect of sequential culture media on development of F1 (C57BL/6 × CBA/Ca) mouse zygotes in vitro. Zygotes were collected at 20 h post-hCG. All media were supplemented with bovine serum albumin (BSA) 2 mg/ml. All embryos were transferred to fresh medium after 48 h of culture, with the exception of embryos in medium G1, where embryos were transferred to either medium G1 or G2. To compensate for this, twice the number of embryos were originally cultured in medium G1, although only a designated 50% of these embryos were used in statistical analysis of the 44 to 52 h data set.[54,56] (a) Embryo cell number after 44, 48 and 52 h of culture; Values are mean ± SEM; $n = 200$ embryos/medium. Media: G1 (solid bar); HTF (open bar); Ham's F-10 (hatched bar). Significantly different from other media: **, $p < 0.01$. (b) Embryo development after 72 h of culture; $n = 150$ embryos/medium. G1/G2; embryos cultured for 48 h in medium G1 and then transferred to medium G2. Blastocyst (solid bar), hatching blastocysts (as a percentage of total blastocysts; open bar). Like pairs are significantly different: a, c, d, $p < 0.05$; b, $p < 0.01$. (c) Embryo development after 92 h of culture; $n = 150$ embryos/medium. G1/G2; embryos cultured for 48 h in medium G1 and then transferred to medium G2. Blastocyst (solid bar), hatching blastocysts (as a percentage of total blastocysts; open bar). Like pairs are significantly different: a, b, c, $p < 0.05$. Significantly different from medium G1 and G1/G2; **, $p < 0.01$. (d) Cell allocation in the blastocyst after 92 h of culture; $n = 150$ embryos/medium. G1/G2; embryos cultured for 48 h in medium G1 and then transferred to medium G2. Trophoectoderm (solid bars), inner cell mass (open bars). Significantly different from other media: *, $p < 0.05$; **, $p < 0.01$. (e) Viability of cultured blastocysts; $n = $ at least 60 blastocysts transferred per treatment. G1/G2; embryos cultured for 48 h in medium G1 and then transferred to medium G2. Implantation (solid bar), fetal development per implantation (open bar). Like pairs are significantly different: a, d, $p < 0.05$; b, c, $p < 0.01$. (From Gardner and Lane[54] with permission.)

cultured in unique conditions making valid comparisons about embryo development almost impossible.[6,25] In practical terms, it represents extra work in the busy IVF laboratory and also introduces the potential for disease transmission. More importantly, data on the sheep embryo have shown that serum can adversely affect the development of embryos at several levels including: precocious blastcoel formation;[59,60] sequestration of lipid;[40,60] abnormal mitochondrial ultrastructure;[60,61] and perturbations in metabolism.[40] Perhaps, most alarmingly, serum has been associated with the generation of abnormally large lambs.[60] The mechanisms by which serum induces these aberrations have yet to be resolved. However, the role of growth factors in serum in inducing altered patterns of development cannot be overlooked. If serum does perturb embryo development so dramatically, why is it still used in human IVF? The main reason is that embryos are routinely transferred on day 2 or 3 of development, that is, before compaction and possibly before the expression of growth factor receptors. Therefore the many adverse effects of serum observed in the blastocysts of other mammalian species are avoided. Should one wish to move to blastocyst transfers in the human, then the inclusion of serum in the culture system used should be carefully considered. Although serum would seem a rather artificial inclusion in an embryo culture system, it does confer a major advantage in that it is a chelator of potential embryo toxins. It also acts as a pH buffer. As such serum confers a certain degree of protection to the embryo. This has helped perpetuate the inclusion of serum in human embryo culture media.

Fortunately, contrary to popular belief, serum is not required for the successful culture of the mammalian zygote to the fully expanded and hatching blastocyst stage. Rather it can be replaced with an appropriate form of albumin or suitable physiological macromolecule such as the glycosaminoglycan hyaluronate,[62] together with sequential media designed to cater for the changing requirements of the embryo. Hyaluronate is an interesting molecule because not only do its levels increase in the uterus

around the time of implantation,[63] but also the human embryo expresses the receptor for it throughout preimplantation development.[64] Although hyaluronate is a glycosaminoglycan, it is unlike other glycosaminoglycans, such as heparin, in that it possesses no protein moieties and can therefore be considered a polysaccharide. As such, this removes both the problems of variation and contamination, because hyaluronate can be synthesized in a pure form. In a study on CF1 mouse embryo culture and transfer, it was found that hyaluronate 0.5 mg/ml could readily replace serum albumin in the culture medium, but more importantly it significantly increased the implantation rate of resultant blastocysts.[62] Importantly, this increase in implantation rate could be attributed to the presence of hyaluronate in the transfer medium alone.

When embryos were cultured in the appropriate sequential media similar to G1 and G2, there was no evident benefit in vitro to having any macromolecule/protein present. Embryos formed blastocysts at the same rate in medium devoid of any macromolecule, and the blastocysts had equivalent ICM and trophectoderm cells as those embryos cultured with either albumin or hyaluronate. However, when embryos cultured in the absence of any macromolecule were pre-equilibrated in medium with hyaluronate 0.5 mg/ml for just 5 min before transfer in medium with hyaluronate, the resultant implantation rate was equivalent to that obtained for embryo cultured for the entire preimplantation period in the presence of hyaluronate[62] (Figure 4). The beneficial effects of hyaluronate on embryo transfer may be attributed to one or more of its known roles. These include the possible ability to form an antiviral and anti-immunogenic layer around the embryo, an ability to increase angiogenesis, and perhaps, most importantly, an ability to facilitate the rapid diffusion of the contents of the transfer medium (the embryo) with the fluid of the uterus. As uterine fluid is a viscous solution, the transfer of a relatively aqueous solution, such as culture medium with albumin, to the uterine lumen will result in the slow diffusion of the medium and embryo with the luminal contents. In contrast, the transfer of an embryo in a medium containing hyaluronate will facilitate diffusion of the embryo into the luminal environment. Furthermore, hyaluronate may be involved in the initial phases of attachment of the blastocyst to the endometrium. Therefore, investigations into the role of such glycosaminoglycans in human embryo development in culture, and particularly in implantation after transfer, are warranted.

## Significance of incubation conditions

Although the composition of embryo culture media is important, it is essential to consider that media formulations are but one part of the overall culture system, and that in order to optimize embryo development in the laboratory, one has to optimize all aspects of the system.

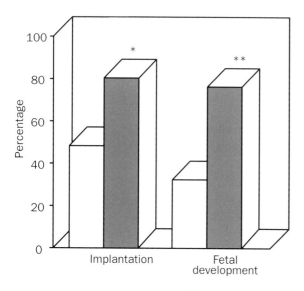

**Figure 4** Effect of hyaluronate when present in the transfer medium on CF1 mouse blastocyst postimplantation development. CF1 mouse zygotes were cultured to the blastocyst stage in the absence of any protein or macromolecule and then transferred to pseudopregnant recipients in the same medium (open bars), or in medium supplemented with 0.5 mg/ml hyaluronate (solid bars). Significantly different from no macromolecule: $*p < 0.05$; $**p < 0.01$.

One aspect of the culture system that has received attention is the effect of incubation volume:embryo ratio on embryo development and viability. It has been shown in several mammalian species that the culture of embryos in reduced volumes of medium and/or in groups significantly increases blastocyst development,[65–67] as well as increasing blastocyst cell number.[66,67,40] More importantly, culturing embryos in reduced volumes increases subsequent viability after transfer.[67] It has been postulated that the benefit of growing embryos in small volumes and groups is the result of the production of specific autocrine/paracrine factor(s) which stimulate an embryo's development or those surrounding embryos in the same microenvironment. Therefore, the culture of embryos in large volumes results in a dilution of the factor so that it becomes ineffectual (Figure 5a,b). This phenomenon is not confined to the mouse, in which several embryos reside in the female tract at one time, but has also been reported for the sheep and cattle, which like the human are monovular.[40,68] Such data have implications for human IVF, especially as there is a tendency to culture human embryos in tubes or four-well plates in relatively large volumes of up to 1 ml culture medium. Recently, it has been demonstrated, in both the mouse and cow, that decreasing the incubation volume:embryo ratio specifically stimulates the development of the ICM. Blastocysts cultured in a reduced incubation volume: embryo ratio had significantly more ICM cells than those cultured in large volumes, whereas the number of trophectoderm cells was unaffected[68,69] (Figure 5c). This would explain the increased viability of embryos cultured in reduced volumes in groups.[67] Possible candidates for such autocrine/paracrine factor(s) include platelet-activating factor and insulin-like growth factors I and II.[70]

## Importance of quality control

For a defined culture system, such as one devoid of serum, to work efficiently it is imperative that adequate quality control procedures

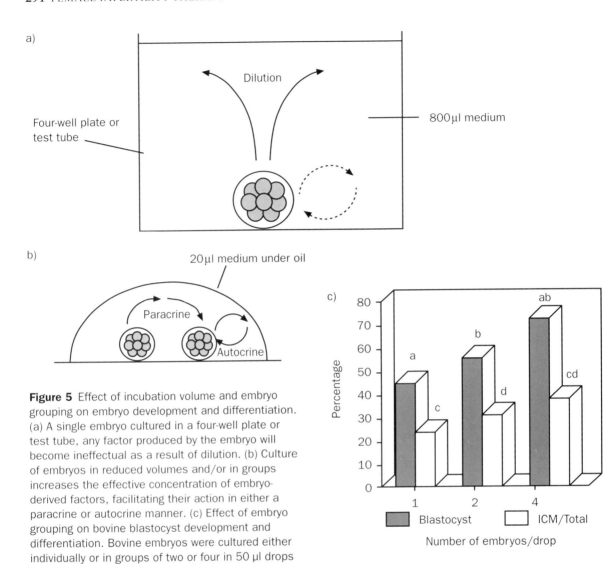

**Figure 5** Effect of incubation volume and embryo grouping on embryo development and differentiation. (a) A single embryo cultured in a four-well plate or test tube, any factor produced by the embryo will become ineffectual as a result of dilution. (b) Culture of embryos in reduced volumes and/or in groups increases the effective concentration of embryo-derived factors, facilitating their action in either a paracrine or autocrine manner. (c) Effect of embryo grouping on bovine blastocyst development and differentiation. Bovine embryos were cultured either individually or in groups of two or four in 50 μl drops of medium.[68] Like pairs are significantly different: $p < 0.05$.

are set in place. Each individual component of the culture media has to be screened using some form of bioassay. Unfortunately there is no guaranteed assay, save for human IVF itself. However, mouse embryos cultured from the pronuclear stage provide a sensitive bioassay, if conditions are set to maximize the sensitivity of the embryos. The presence of serum or albumin in culture media decreases the sensitivity of the bioassay because proteins can mask the toxic effects of certain compounds.[25] Therefore, embryo culture should take place in the absence of any protein, at least from the two-cell stage forward.[25,71] The culture period should be defined and developments quantified at this point only, for example, more than 85% of F1 mouse zygotes should reach the fully expanded blastocyst stage after 96 h of culture. Most embryos will reach the blastocyst stage if the culture period is extended for a further 24 h, but this would make the results of the bioassay meaningless. Ideally blastocyst cell number should be determined, because it is a more sensitive measure of culture conditions. Alternatively, mouse IVF or intracytoplasmic sperm injections (ICSI) could be performed, although the extra time, cost, and logistics may make this impractical for most routine IVF programs.

## CLINICAL RESULTS USING BLASTOCYST TRANSFER

In a pilot trial using frozen–thawed pronucleate human embryos, it was found that the media G1/G2 supported more than 60% blastocyst development after 4 days of culture.[56] In a pilot clinical trial, eight patients underwent routine IVF stimulation and retrieval, but their embryos were cultured for 4 days to the blastocyst stage in the sequential media G1 and G2 before transfer. Pronuclear embryos were cultured for 48 h in medium G1 and then transferred to medium G2 for a further 48 h. In this study 66% of pronuclear embryos cultured in G1 and G2 reached the blastocyst stage. When blastocysts were transferred to the patients an implantation rate of 46% was obtained, culminating in a pregnancy rate of 63% with a mean of 2.7 blastocysts transferred[72] (Figures 6 and 7). In a similar study, but using a simple medium for culture up to the eight-cell stage, it was found that blastocyst culture and transfer resulted in a doubling of implantation rate.[73] In light of the high implantation rate obtained from the transfer of blastocysts, a prospective randomized trial was initiated at the Colorado Center for Reproductive Medicine. After 35 blastocyst transfers, the implantation rate as determined by fetal heart was 53%, with an ongoing clinical pregnancy rate of 71% and a mean of just 2.2 blastocysts transferred. When just two blastocysts are transferred, the implantation rate was 50%, with an ongoing clinical pregnancy rate of 68%. Clearly the use of sequential culture media, be they G1 and G2 or some other combi-

nation that can facilitate normal embryonic development, results in blastocysts with a high developmental potential. The significance of this work is that it is now possible to obtain excellent clinical pregnancy rates with low numbers of blastocysts transferred, thereby eliminating all high-order multiple gestations.

## CONCLUSIONS

Extensive research on the preimplantation embryo of several mammalian species has increased our understanding of embryo physiology, metabolism, and nutrient requirements as development and differentiation proceed. The culmination of this work has been the development of sequential culture media, of which G1 and G2 are examples. The key to the success of such sequential media is that not only do they provide for the changing requirements of the embryo as it develops and differentiates, but they also minimize cellular stress

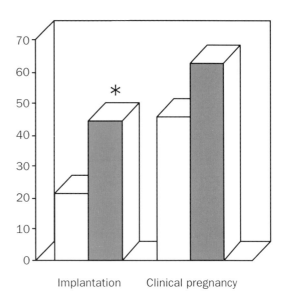

**Figure 6** Effect of day of transfer on implantation and clinical pregnancy rate. Day 3 (open bars), day 5 (solid bars). Significantly different from day 3: *, $p < 0.05$. Significantly fewer embryos were transferred on day 5 (mean of 2.7) than on day 3 (mean of 3.8): $p < 0.01$[72.]

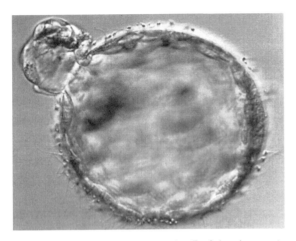

**Figure 7** Human blastocyst on day 5 of development (4 days of culture from the pronuclear stage). The pronuclear embryo was cultured for 48 h in medium G1 and then for 48 h in medium G2. The blastocyst has begun to hatch from the zona pellucida, which has thinned as a result of the action of blastocyst-derived proteases, and by the turgor pressure exerted by the expanding blastcoel cavity.

induced by the very act of culture in vitro.[4,6,15] It is envisaged that, as we increase our understanding of human embryo physiology and metabolism, it should be possible to make further improvements in embryo culture systems. The significance of the transfer medium also cannot be overlooked, specifically the role of glycosaminoglycans such as hyaluronate. Finally, with the application of blastocyst culture systems for the human, the development of new methods of assessing embryo viability before transfer should further increase the overall success of a given IVF cycle.[8–11] The ultimate aim of this work is to be able to perform a single blastocyst transfer while maintaining high pregnancy rates.

## ACKNOWLEDGEMENTS

The author is indebted to Dr William B Schoolcraft and all the staff at the Colorado Center for Reproductive Medicine for their support.

## REFERENCES

1.  Bavister BD. Culture of preimplantation embryos: facts and artifacts. *Hum Reprod Update* 1995;**1**:91–148.
2.  Gardner DK, Lane M, Calderon I, Leeton J. Environment of the preimplantation human embryo in vivo: Metabolite analysis of oviduct and uterine fluids and metabolism of cumulus cells. *Fetil Steril* 1996;**65**:349–53.
3.  Croxatto HB, Ortiz ME, Diaz S, et al. Studies on the duration of egg transport by the human oviduct. *Am J Obstet Gynecol* 1978;**132**:629–34.
4.  Gardner DK, Schoolcraft WB. Human embryo viability: what determines developmental potential and can it be assessed? *J Assist Reprod Genet* 1998; in press.
5.  Dawson KJ, Conaghan J, Ostera GR, et al. Delaying transfer to the third day post-insemination, to select non-arrested embryos, increases development to the fetal heart stage. *Hum Reprod* 1995;**10**:177–82.
6.  Gardner DK, Lane M. Culture and selection of viable blastocysts: a feasible proposition for

human IVF? *Hum Reprod Update* 1997;**3**:367–82.
7.  Braude PR, Bolton VN, Moore S. Human gene expression first occurs between the four- and eight-cell stages of preimplantation development. *Nature* 1988;**332**:459–61.
8.  Gardner DK, Leese HJ. Assessment of embryo viability prior to transfer by the non-invasive measurement of glucose uptake. *J Exp Zool* 1987;**242**:103–5.
9.  Gardner DK, Leese HJ. Assessment of embryo metabolism and viability. In: *Handbook of In Vitro Fertilization* (Trounson A, Gardner DK, eds). Boca Raton, FL: CRC Press, 1993: 195–211.
10. Gardner DK, Pawelczynski M, Trounson A. Nutrient uptake and utilisation can be used to select viable day-7 bovine blastocysts after cryopreservation. *Mol Reprod Dev* 1996;**44**:472–5.
11. Lane M, Gardner DK. Selection of viable mouse blastocysts prior to transfer using a metabolic criterion. *Hum Reprod* 1996;**11**:1975–8.
12. Leese HJ. Metabolism of the preimplantation mammalian embryo. In: *Oxford Reviews of*

*Reproductive Biology* (Milligan SR, ed.), 13. London: Oxford University Press, 1991: 35–72.

13. Rieger D. Relationship between energy metabolism and development of the early embryo. *Theriogenology* 1992;**37**:75–93.

14. Gardner D. Embryo development and culture techniques. In: *Animal Breeding: Technology for the 21st Century* (Clark J, ed.). Reading, Berkshire: Harwood Academic, 1998: 13–46.

15. Gardner DK. Changes in requirements and utilization of nutrients during mammalian preimplantation embryo development and their significance in embryo culture. *Theriogenology* 1998;**49**:83–102.

16. Biggers JD, Whittingham DG, Donahue RP. The pattern of energy metabolism in the mouse oocyte and zygote. *Proc Natl Acad Sci USA* 1967;**58**:560–7.

17. Biggers JD, Gardner DK, Leese HJ. Control of carbohydrate metabolism in preimplantation mammalian embryos. In: *Growth Factors in Mammalian Development* (Rosenblum IY, Heyner S, eds). Boca Raton, FL: CRC Press, 1989: 19–32.

18. Schini SA, Bavister BD. Two-cell block to development of cultured hamster embryos is caused by phosphate and glucose. *Biol Reprod* 1988;**39**:1183–92.

19. Chatot CL, Ziomek CA, Bavister BD, et al. An improved culture medium supports development of random-bred 1-cell mouse embryos in vitro. *J Reprod Fertil* 1989;**86**:679–88.

20. Thompson JG, Simpson AC, Pugh PA, Tervit HR. Requirement for glucose during in vitro culture of sheep preimplantation embryos. *Mol Reprod Dev* 1992;**31**:253–7.

21. Conaghan J, Handyside AH, Winston RML, Leese HJ. Effects of pyruvate and glucose on the development of human preimplantation embryos in vitro. *J Reprod Fertil* 1993;**99**:87–95.

22. Gardner DK, Lane M. The 2-cell block in CF1 mouse embryos is associated with an increase in glycolysis and a decrease in tricarboxylic acid (TCA) cycle activity: alleviation of the 2-cell block is associated with the restoration of in vivo metabolic pathway activities. *Biol Reprod* 1993;**49**(suppl 1):152.

23. Matsuyama K, Miyakoshi H, Fukui Y. Effect of glucose during the in vitro culture in synthetic oviduct fluid medium on in vitro development of bovine oocytes matured and fertilized in vitro. *Theriogenology* 1993;**40**:595–605.

24. Quinn P. Enhanced results in mouse and human embryo culture using a modified human tubal fluid medium lacking glucose and phosphate. *J Assist Reprod Genet* 1995;**12**:97–105.

25. Gardner DK, Lane M. Embryo culture systems. In: *Handbook of In Vitro Fertilization* (Trounson A, Gardner DK, eds). Boca Raton, FL: CRC Press, 1993: 85–114.

26. Pool TB, Atiee SH, Martin JE. Oocyte and embryo culture: Basic concepts and recent advances. In: *Assisted Reproduction: Laboratory considerations* (May JV, ed.). Infertility and Reproductive Medicine Clinics of North America, 1998: in press.

27. Gardner DK, Leese HJ. The role of glucose and pyruvate transport in regulating nutrient utilization by preimplantation mouse embryos. *Development* 1988;**104**:423–9.

28. Hogan A, Heyner S, Charron MJ, et al. Glucose transporter gene expression in early mouse embryos. *Development* 1991;**113**:363–72.

29. Aghayan M, Rao LV, Smith RM, et al. Developmental expression and cellular localization of glucose transporter molecules during mouse preimplantation development. *Development* 1992;**115**:305–12.

30. Dan-Goor M, Sasson S, Davarashvili A, Almagor M. Expression of glucose transporter and glucose uptake in human oocytes and preimplantation embryos. *Hum Reprod* 1997;**12**:2508–10.

31. Gardner DK, Lane M. Alleviation of the '2-cell block' and development to the blastocyst of CF1 mouse embryos: role of amino acids, EDTA and physical parameters. *Hum Reprod* 1996;**11**:2703–12.

32. Gardner DK, Lane MW, Lane M. Bovine blastocyst cell number is increased by culture with EDTA for the first 72 hours of development from the zygote. *Theriogenology* 1997;**47**:278.

33. Lane M, Gardner DK. EDTA stimulates development of cleavage stage mouse embryos by inhibiting the glycolytic enzyme phosophoglycerate kinase. *Biol Reprod* 1997;**57**(suppl 1):193.

34. Reitzer LJ, Wice BM, Kennel D. The pentose cycle: control and essential function in HeLa cell nucleic acid synthesis. *J Biol Chem* 1980;**255**:5616–26.

35. Morgan MJ, Faik P. Carbohydrate metabolism in cultured animal cells. *Biosci Rep* 1981;**1**:669–86.

36. Rogers PAW, Murphy CR, Gannon BJ. Absence of capillaries in the endometrium surrounding the implanting rat blastocyst. *Micron* 1982;**13**:373–4.

37. Rogers PAW, Murphy CR, Gannon BJ. Changes in the spatial organisation of the uterine vascula-

ture during implantation in the rat. *J Reprod Fertil* 1982;**65**:211–14.

38. Rogers PAW, Murphy CR, Rogers AW, Gannon BJ. Capillary patency and permeability in the endometrium surrounding the implanting rat blastocyst. *Int J Microcirc Clin Exp* 1983;**2**:241–9.

39. Bavister BD, McKiernan SH. Regulation of hamster embryo development in vitro by amino acids. In: *Preimplantation Embryo Development* (Bavister BD, ed.). New York: Springer-Verlag, 1993: 57–72.

40. Gardner DK, Lane M, Spitzer A, Batt PA. Enhanced rates of cleavage and development for sheep zygotes cultured to the blastocyst stage in vitro in the absence of serum and somatic cells: amino acids, vitamins and culturing embryos in groups stimulate development. *Biol Reprod* 1994;**50**:390–400.

41. Gardner DK. Mammalian embryo culture in the absence of serum or somatic cell support. *Cell Biol Int* 1994;**18**:1163–79.

42. Miller JGO, Schultz GA. Amino acid content of preimplantation rabbit embryos and fluids of the reproductive tract. *Biol Reprod* 1987;**36**:125–9.

43. Moses DF, Matkovic M, Cabrera Fisher E, Martinez AG. Amino acid contents of sheep oviductal and uterine fluids. *Theriogenology* 1997;**47**:336.

44. Eagle H. Amino acid metabolism in mammalian cell cultures. *Science* 1959;**130**:432–7.

45. Gardner DK, Lane M. Amino acids and ammonium regulate mouse embryo development in culture. *Biol Reprod* 1993;**48**:377–85.

46. Lane M, Gardner DK. Increase in postimplantation development of cultured mouse embryos by amino acids and induction of fetal retardation and exencephaly by ammonium ions. *J Reprod Fertil* 1994;**102**:305–12.

47. Lane M, Gardner DK. Non-essential amino acids and glutamine decrease the time of the first three cleavage divisions and increase compaction of mouse zygotes in vitro. *J Assist Reprod Gen* 1997;**14**:398–403.

48. Lane M, Gardner DK. Differential regulation of mouse embryo development and viability by amino acids. *J Reprod Fertil* 1997;**109**:153–64.

49. Steeves TE, Gardner DK. Temporal effects of amino acids on bovine embryo development in culture. *Biol Reprod* 1997;**57**(suppl):25.

50. Quinn P, Kerin JF, Warnes GM. Improved pregnancy rates in human in vitro fertilization with the use of a medium based on the composition of human tubal fluid. *Fertil Steril* 1985;**44**:493–8.

51. Whittingham DG. Culture of mouse ova. *J Reprod Fertil* 1971;**14**(suppl):7–21.

52. Barnes FL, Crombie A, Gardner DK, et al. Blastocyst development and pregnancy after in vitro maturation of human primary oocytes, intracytoplasmic sperm injection and assisted hatching. *Hum Reprod* 1995;**10**:3243–7.

53. Gardner DK. Embryo metabolism: a marker of embryo development and viability. In: *ART: State of the art* (Rosenwaks Z, Marrs RP, Trounson A, eds). Serono Symposia, USA. New York: Springer-Verlag, 1998: in press.

54. Gardner DK, Lane M. Culture of viable human blastocysts in defined sequential serum-free media. *Hum Reprod* 1998; **Suppl 1:** in press.

55. Hewitson LC, Leese HJ. Energy metabolism of the trophectoderm and inner cell mass of the mouse blastocyst. *J Exp Zool* 1993;**267**:337–43.

56. Gardner DK, Lane M, Kouridakis K, Schoolcraft WB. Complex physiologically based serum-free culture media increase mammalian embryo development. In: *In Vitro Fertilization and Assisted Reproduction* (Gomel V, Leung PCK, eds). Bologna: Monduzzi Editore, 1997: 87–91.

57. Bolton VN, Wren ME, Parsons JH. Pregnancies after in vitro fertilization and transfer of human blastocysts. *Fertil Steril* 1991;**55**:830–2.

58. Leese HJ. Formation and function of oviduct fluid. *J Reprod Fertil* 1998;**82**:843–56.

59. Walker SK, Heard TM, Seamark RF. In vitro culture of sheep embryos without coculture: success and perspectives. *Theriogenology* 1992;**37**:111–26.

60. Thompson JG, Gardner DK, Pugh PA, et al. Lamb birth weight is affected by culture systems utilized during in vitro pre-elongation development of ovine embryos. *Biol Reprod* 1995; **53**:1385–91.

61. Dorland M, Gardner DK, Trouson A. Serum in synthetic oviduct fluid causes mitochondrial degeneration in ovine embryos. *J Reprod Fertil* 1994;**13**:70 (abstract).

62. Gardner DK, Lane M, Rodriguez-Martinez H. Fetal development after transfer is increased by replacing protein with the glycosaminoglycan hyaluronate for embryo culture. *Hum Reprod* 1997;**12**:O-215 (abstract).

63. Zorn TMT, Pinhal MAS, Nader HB, et al. Biosynthesis of glycosaminoglycans in the endometrium during the initial stages of pregnancy of the mouse. *Cell Mol Biol* 1995;**41**:97–106.

64. Campbell S, Swann HR, Aplin JD, et al. CD44 is expressed throughout pre-implantation human embryo development. *Hum Reprod* 1995; **10**:425–30.

65. Wiley LM, Yanami S, Van Muyden D. Effect of potassium concentration, type of protein supplement and embryo density on mouse preimplantation development in vitro. *Fertil Steril* 1986;**45:**111–19.

66. Paria BC, Dey SK. Preimplantation embryo development in vitro: cooperative interactions among embryos and role of growth factors. *Proc Natl Acad Sci USA* 1990;**87:**4756–60.

67. Lane M, Gardner DK. Effect of incubation volume and embryo density on the development and viability of preimplantation mouse embryos in vitro. *Hum Reprod* 1992;**7:**558–62.

68. Ahern T, Gardner DK. Culturing bovine embryos in groups stimulates blastocyst development and cell allocation to the inner cell mass. *Theriogenology* 1998;**49:**194.

69. Gardner DK, Lane MW, Lane M. Development of the inner cell mass in mouse blastocysts is stimulated by reducing the embryo:incubation volume ratio. *Hum Reprod* 1997;**12:**P-132 (abstract).

70. O'Neill C. Evidence for the requirement of autocrine growth factors for the development of mouse preimplantation embryos in vitro. *Biol Reprod* 1997;**56:**229–37.

71. Weiss TJ, Warnes GM, Gardner DK. Mouse embryos and quality control in human IVF. *Reprod Fertil Dev* 1992;**4:**105–7.

72. Gardner DK, Vella P, Lane M, et al. Culture and transfer of human blastocysts increases implantation rates and reduces the need for multiple embryo transfers. *Fertil Steril* 1998;**69:**84–8.

73. Jones GM, Trounson AO, Gardner DK, et al. Evolution of a culture protocol for successful blastocyst development and pregnancy. *Hum Reprod* 1998;**13:**169–77.

74. Kafadar K. Notched box- and whisker plots. *Enc Stat Sci* 1985;**6:**367–70.

# Part VII
# Side Effects of Treatment

# 27

# Ovarian hyperstimulation and the polycystic ovary syndrome

Rina Agrawal, Howard S Jacobs

The ovarian hyperstimulation syndrome is now quite familiar to most people working in reproductive endocrinology and fertility therapy, although it is recommended that those wishing to update their knowledge read the literature about its aetiology[1,2] and its clinical features and management.[3,4] In this chapter we show how the condition is closely linked, both mechanistically and clinically, to the polycystic ovary syndrome.

The cardinal feature that underlies the ovarian hyperstimulation syndrome is an increase in capillary permeability, such that protein-rich fluid escapes from the vascular compartment. The fluid collects in the 'third space', accumulating in the peritoneal cavity but eventually also appearing in the pleural and pericardial spaces. Loss of fluid results in intravascular volume depletion which impairs the circulation, prejudices renal function and causes secondary hyperaldosteronism. Haemoconcentration and the risk of thrombosis result. It is in fact the latter that is the cause of the most severe clinical problems. Usually the condition settles after 10–20 days but, in severe cases, the patient's circulation, hydration and organ function need support, optimally provided in an intensive care unit.

Any theory of aetiology needs to accommodate the clinical observations that, with rare exceptions, the ovarian hyperstimulation syndrome occurs only after therapeutic ovarian stimulation, most particularly after administration of human chorionic gonadotrophin (hCG) and that it is nearly always seen in women with the polycystic ovary syndrome.[5] These observations have suggested that clues to pathogenesis might be found in the process of the ovarian neovascularization that follows rupture of the avascular preovulatory follicle and formation of the highly vascular corpus luteum. For example, Ong et al[6] postulated that release of excessive ovarian renin, known to be involved in ovarian neovascularization, might mediate some of the clinical features of the condition. These workers reported high levels of circulating plasma renin activity in a patient with severe ovarian hyperstimulation at a time when her intravascular volume was normal, as indexed by measurement of central venous pressure, that is, when renally secreted renin would have been expected to be suppressed. The pathophysiological significance of this observation can only be established experimentally, although, as most patients with severe

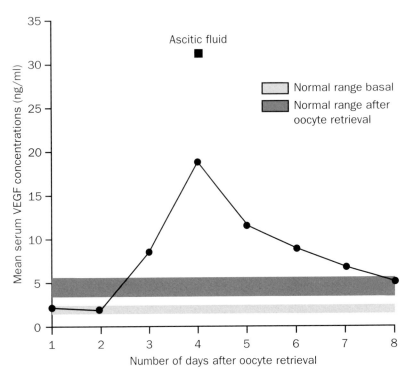

**Figure 1** Serum and ascetic fluid concentrations of VEGF in a woman with severe ovarian hyperstimulation. (From Agrawal et al,[10] with permission.)

ovarian hyperstimulation are pregnant, clinicians have naturally been reluctant to administer peripheral blockers of angiotensin II for fear of their teratogenicity.

Recently attention has shifted to vascular endothelial growth factor (VEGF) as the essential mediator of the ovarian hyperstimulation syndrome. McClure and colleagues,[7] using a laborious bioassay in rabbits which measured vascular permeability in the skin to an injected dye, demonstrated an increase in VEGF bioactivity in ascitic fluid obtained from patients with ovarian hyperstimulation but not in that obtained from women with cirrhosis. The bioactivity could be neutralized by incubation with an antiserum to recombinant VEGF. These results have now been confirmed by others,[8,9] using technically much less demanding immunological methods of measurement. We recently reported one such case[10] in which the time course of development of high levels of VEGF in serum and ascitic fluid can readily be

seen (Figure 1). Further studies from our group (unpublished data) of women undergoing ovarian stimulation for in vitro fertilisation (IVF) have shown that serum VEGF concentrations rise after administration of hCG. The rise is reliably greater in women who develop ovarian hyperstimulation than in those who do not. These studies have allowed us to develop an index which predicts the risk of development of the ovarian hyperstimulation syndrome that is more reliable than measurement of serum oestradiol or counting the total number of follicles detected at the time of hCG administration.

We have previously alluded to the clinical propensity of women with the polycystic ovary syndrome to develop ovarian hyperstimulation. We were not therefore surprised to find that, in our study of VEGF concentrations in women undergoing IVF, all of the highest levels of VEGF were observed in women with polycystic ovaries. We were prompted to measure serum

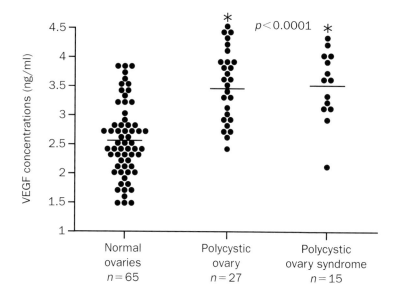

**Figure 2** Serum VEGF concentrations in women with normal ovaries, with polycystic ovaries and those with the polycystic ovary syndrome. (From Agrawal et al,[11] with permission.)

VEGF concentrations before ovarian stimulation in such women. Reference to Figure 2 shows that the concentrations are in fact raised in these women *before* treatment.[11] The results resonate with the immunochemical demonstration by Kamat et al[12] of extensive VEGF staining in the hypercellular theca surrounding a cyst in a polycystic ovary.

The significance of these observations seems to be quite considerable. First, it is of great interest to note that serum VEGF concentrations correlate with ovarian stromal blood flow, as measured by colour Doppler ultrasonography. These changes in blood flow, first demonstrated by Doppler ultrasonography to be raised in the ovarian stroma in women with polycystic ovaries by Zaidi et al[13] and confirmed in this study, may have significance in relation to the characteristically exuberant response to stimulation of the polycystic ovary (see below). Second, the raised levels of VEGF occurred in women with the polycystic ovaries detected by ultrasonography as well as in those with the polycystic ovary syndrome, strongly suggesting that this is a constitutive feature of the polycystic ovary, rather than a result of stimulation by luteinizing hormone (LH) (the usual stimu-

lus to expression of the VEGF gene and, of course, frequently elevated in women with the polycystic ovary syndrome). This observation fits with the observation that the response of the ovary to stimulation by gonadotrophins depends on the ultrasonic appearance of a polycystic pattern rather than on the concentrations of circulating hormones.[14]

There is a striking difference in the ovarian response to gonadotrophic stimulation of women with amenorrhoea and hypogonadotrophic hypogonadism and normal ovaries, compared with women with polycystic ovaries, whether symptomatic (polycystic ovary *syndrome*) or asymptomatic. This is most clearly seen in Figure 3, which is taken from the report of Shoham et al.[14] The results exemplify the notion that the essential feature of the response of the polycystic ovary to gonadotrophic stimulation is loss of the normal intraovarian autoregulatory process that underlies emergence of a single dominant follicle, with suppression of cohort follicles. On ultra- sonography, this persistence of cohort follicles, despite the development of a dominant follicle, can readily be seen in Figure 4. It is of course the failure to maintain a unifollicular response to treatment that

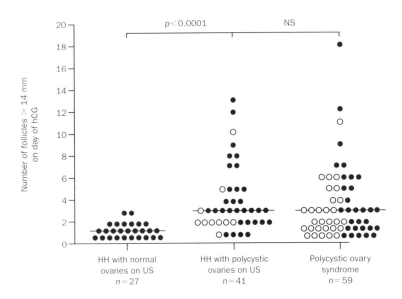

underlies the risks of multiple pregnancy and ovarian hyperstimulation, to which patients with polycystic ovaries are so prone.

The question therefore arises as to what the important factors are that underlie the intra-ovarian autoregulation which results in unifollicular ovulation. Clearly there are endocrine factors to consider, for example, the amount and potency of the gonadotrophin to which the ovary is exposed. Thus, in ovulation-induction therapy there is ample evidence that the risks of multifollicular ovulation, multiple pregnancy and ovarian hyperstimulation are directly related to the dose of gonadotrophin used.[15] Intraovarian paracrine factors are also considered important, particularly the concentration of insulin-like growth factor I, known to augment the granulosa cell response to stimulation by follicle-stimulating hormone (FSH).[16] During development of the dominant follicle, blood is normally diverted to the ovary bearing the dominant follicle and within that ovary there is diversion of blood flow towards the dominant follicle itself. Presumably this change in intra-ovarian blood flow contributes to concentration of FSH in the dominant follicle. Correspondingly, the relative lack of FSH in the non-dominant cohort of follicles presumably contributes to their atresia. We postulate that the widespread distribution of excessive amounts of VEGF in the theca cells of the polycystic ovary (see, for example, Figure 5[12]) prevents this intraovarian redistribution of blood flow, so that non-dominant follicles do not undergo atresia but persist, ready to develop further in response to exposure of the ovary to gonadotrophin stimulation. This would account

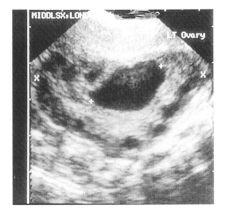

**Figure 4** Ultrasonic image of a polycystic ovary containing a dominant follicle. Note persistence of the cohort follicles. (Image supplied courtesy of Ms Anita Patel.)

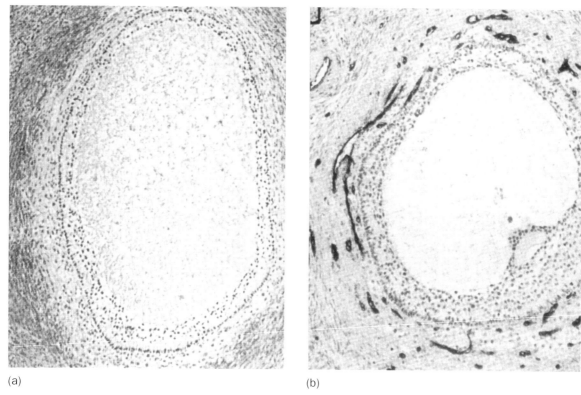

(a)                                                      (b)

**Figure 5** VEGF immunostaining in (a) a section of normal ovary and (b) a section from a polycystic ovary. Note the intense immunostaining in the theca cells surrounding the cyst from the polycystic ovary. (From Kamat et al,[12] with permission.)

for the explosive response of the polycystic ovary in programmes of ovulation induction, with the inevitable increase in the risk of multiple ovulation, pregnancy and ovarian hyperstimulation in women with the polycystic ovary syndrome.[17]

The hypothesis outlined above places an excess of VEGF at centre stage, as a constitutive feature of the polycystic ovary, as underlying

the loss of intraovarian autoregulation and as mediating the major complications of ovarian stimulation. This is no small role for this growth factor to play, but its intimate involvement in the process of (neo)vascularization makes it an attractive candidate for a pivotal place in the pathophysiology of the polycystic ovary syndrome and ovarian hyperresponsiveness.

## REFERENCES

1.  Elchalal U, Schenker JG. The pathophysiology of ovarian hyperstimulation syndrome – views and ideas. *Hum Reprod* 1997;**12**:1129–37.
2.  Rizk B, Aboulghar M, Smitz J, Ron El R. The role of vascular endothelial growth factor and interleukins in the pathogenesis of severe ovarian hyperstimulation syndrome. *Hum Reprod Update* 1997;**3**:255–66.

3. Brinsden PR, Wada I, Tan SL, Balen A, Jacobs HS. Diagnosis, prevention and management of ovarian hyperstimulation syndrome. *B J Obstet Gynaecol* 1995;**102**:767–72.

4. Navot D, Berg RPA, Laufer N. Ovarian hyperstimulation syndrome in novel reproductive technologies: prevention and treatment. *Fertil Steril* 1992;**58**:249–61.

5. MacDougal MJ, Tan SL, Balen AH, Jacobs HS. A controlled study comparing patients with and without polycystic ovaries undergoing in vitro fertilisation. *Hum Reprod* 1993;**8**:233–7.

6. Ong ACM, Eisen V, Rennie DP. The pathogenesis of the ovarian hyperstimulation syndrome (OHSS): a possible role for ovarian renin. *Clin Endocrinol* 1991;**34**:43–9.

7. McClure N, Healy DL, Paw R, et al. Vascular endothelial growth factor as a capillary permeability agent in ovarian hyperstimulation syndrome. *Lancet* 1994;**344**:235–43.

8. Krasnow JS, Berga SL, Guzick DS, Zeleznik AJ, Yeo K-T. Vascular permeability factor and vascular endothelial growth factor in ovarian hyperstimulation syndrome: A preliminary report. *Fertil Steril* 1996;**65**:552–5.

9. Abramov Y, Barak V, Nisman B, Schenker JG. Vascular endothelial growth factor plasma levels correlate to the clinical picture in severe ovarian hyperstimulation syndrome. *Fertil Steril* 1997;**67**(2):261–5.

10. Agrawal R, Chimusoro K, Payne N, Van der Spuy Z, Jacobs HS. Severe ovarian hyperstimulation syndrome: serum and ascitic fluid concentrations of vascular endothelial growth factor. *Curr Opin Obstet Gynaecol* 1997;**9**:141–4.

11. Agrawal R, Sladkevicius P, Engmann L, et al. Serum VEGF concentrations and ovarian stromal blood flow are increased in women with polycystic ovaries. *Hum Reprod* 1998; in press.

12. Kamat BR, Brown LF, Manseau EJ, Senger DR, Dvorak HF. Expression of vascular endothelial growth factor vascular permeability factor by human granulosa and theca lutein cells. Role in corpus luteum development. *Am J Pathol* 1995; **146**:157–65.

13. Zaidi J, Campbell S, Pitroff R, et al. Ovarian stromal blood flow in women with polycystic ovaries – a possible new marker for diagnosis? *Hum Reprod* 1995;**10**:1992–6.

14. Shoham Z, Conway GS, Patel A, Jacobs HS. Polycystic ovaries in patients with hypogonadotropic hypogonadism: similarity of ovarian response to gonadotropin stimulation in patients with polycystic ovarian syndrome. *Fertil Steril* 1992;**58**:37–47.

15. Jacobs HS. Regular dose gonadotrophins in polycystic ovary syndrome: outcome and complications. In: *Ovulation Induction, Update '98* (Filicori M, Flamigni C, eds). New York: The Parthenon Publishing Group, 1998: 41–6.

16. Adashi EY, Resnick CE, D'Ercole AJ. Insulin-like growth factors as intraovarian regulators of granulosa cell growth and function. *Endocrine Rev* 1985;**6**:400–20.

17. Balen AH, Braat DDM, West C, Patel A, Jacobs HS. Cumulative conception and live birth rates after the treatment of anovulatory infertility: safety and efficacy of ovulation induction in 200 patients. *Hum Reprod* 1994;**9**:1563–70.

# 28

# The use of intravenous albumin for prevention of severe ovarian hyperstimulation syndrome

Ariel Weissman, Ami Barash, Zeev Shoham

**Pathophysiology of the OHSS • Human albumin: Physiological properties and proposed mechanism of action • Safety considerations • Clinical experience with intravenous human albumin for prevention of the SOHSS • Conclusion**

The ovarian hyperstimulation syndrome (OHSS) is the most serious complication associated with ovulation induction. Although there had previously been improvements in the monitoring of patients who receive treatment for ovulation induction, at present there is no method that can provide absolute prediction or prevention of the OHSS.[1,2] Some degree of ovarian hyperstimulation occurs in all women who respond to ovulation-induction therapy in assisted reproductive technology (ART) programmes and, in fact, ovulation induction in those cycles has been named 'controlled ovarian hyperstimulation' (COH). In its mild and moderate forms, the OHSS is usually self-limited and requires no active therapy other than observation, and plasma volume and electrolyte replacement. In the severe form of the OHSS, massive ovarian enlargement occurs, accompanied by haemoconcentration and massive transudation of protein-rich fluid in the form of ascites, pleural and pericardial effusion. The full-blown clinical syndrome may be further complicated by renal failure and oliguria, hypovolaemic shock, thromboembolic phenomena, adult respiratory distress syndrome and even death.[1-4] Severe OHSS (SOHSS) is of great clinical significance because 0.5–2% of otherwise healthy young women who participate in ART programmes may develop it[1-4] and experience severe morbidity and even mortality related to this purely iatrogenic condition.

As the key to prevention of the SOHSS is the early identification of patients at risk, there have been many attempts to define this population.[1,2] Navot et al[1] suggested that women with either the hormonal or the morphological signs of polycystic ovarian disease, high serum oestradiol levels before human chorionic gonadotrophin (hCG) administration (>14 685 pmol/l), multiple follicular development (>35), younger age (<35 years) and lean habitus comprise the high-risk group. The risk is further increased if a gonadotrophin-releasing hormone (GnRH) against protocol is used, if hCG is used for luteal support and in the presence of pregnancy. As no single risk factor can reliably predict all cases of the SOHSS, it could be hoped that a combination of features would be more successful.[5-7]

At present, there is no universal agreement on a clear definition for the patient at high risk for development of the SOHSS. Consequently, different investigators have used a wide variety of inclusion criteria in trials on preventive measures for the OHSS. This approach should not necessarily be regarded as negative and, as a matter of fact, it should be considered very reasonable. Assisted reproductive technology programmes may vary in terms of patient characteristics, that is, the prevalence of polycystic ovaries (PCO) or the polycystic ovary syndrome (PCOS), patient's age, etc., the kind and source of fertility drugs, monitoring protocols and techniques, 'aggressiveness' of COH (in terms of starting dosage of gonadotrophins and criteria for hCG administration), luteal support (hCG- or progesterone-based regimens) and hormonal assays. Consequently, there is considerable variability in the reported incidence of the SOHSS, so each programme should establish its own criteria for patients at 'high risk', which may be derived from retrospective analysis of the cases with the SOHSS in that particular programme.

## PATHOPHYSIOLOGY OF THE OHSS

Understanding of the pathophysiology of the OHSS is essential to development of rational prevention strategies. However, the underlying mechanism of the OHSS is currently unknown. Ovarian hyperstimulation is the result of massive follicular luteinization, and it therefore occurs only after hCG administration or, rarely, after an endogenous luteinization hormone (LH) peak. The fact that ovulation (luteinization) is a precondition necessary for the OHSS to occur suggested the involvement of ovarian (luteal) secretions in the pathogenesis of this syndrome, as was shown by Polishuk and Schenker[8] in their classic experimental work in the rabbit. A vasoactive ovarian factor is likely to be involved, and a number of possible endogenous mediators have been suggested. Recent studies seem to indicate the existence of a local ovarian renin–angiotensin system, which may play a major role in the pathogenesis of the OHSS through an effect on angiogenesis and capillary permeability.[9,10] In addition, there is strong evidence to support the role of vascular endothelial growth factor (VEGF) as the capillary permeability agent in the OHSS.[11] Further studies on these substances are awaited with interest.

## HUMAN ALBUMIN: PHYSIOLOGICAL PROPERTIES AND PROPOSED MECHANISM OF ACTION

The exact mechanism by which treatment with human albumin may prevent the development of the SOHSS is still unknown. Albumin is produced by the liver at a rate of approximately 12 g/day.[12,13] It has a low molecular weight (about 69 000), and its average normal half-life is 17–20 days. About 60% of albumin is found in the extravascular spaces, but plasma albumin is still the most abundant circulating protein. Albumin has both osmotic and transport functions: it contributes about 75% of the plasma oncotic pressure, and administration of 50 g human albumin solution will draw more than 800 ml extracellular fluid into the circulation within 15 mins, reducing haemoconcentration and blood viscosity for many hours. This amount of albumin is osmotically equivalent to about 1000 ml (1 l) of normal citrated plasma.[12,13] As a result of these properties, human albumin has already been recognized as a highly effective plasma expander in the treatment of the SOHSS.[1]

It has been suggested that the binding and transport properties of human albumin play the major role in the prevention of the SOHSS.[14–17] As mentioned previously, an hCG-mediated factor secreted by the corpus luteum impedes capillary integrity and leads to the development of the OHSS. This factor could be part of the ovarian renin–angiotensin system or VEGF related, as suggested above, or an as yet undetermined factor. Maybe albumin binds and inactivates this putative factor at a specific and critical time of the cycle and thus helps to prevent the development of the OHSS. The timing of intravenous human albumin administration is, therefore, of major importance. Administration of albumin about 34–36 hours after the injection of hCG, immediately after oocyte retrieval, seems to be reasonable.[14–17] By that time, a sufficient amount of the putative causative factor has been produced, although the clinical signs and symptoms of the OHSS are not yet evident. As different regimens for prophylactic albumin have been suggested, the optimum dosage and timing of administration have yet to be established.

## SAFETY CONSIDERATIONS

Human albumin is non-toxic and considered safe from viral contamination.[12,13] However, the recent concern over bovine spongiform encephalopathy (BSE) and similar diseases in humans, such as Creutzfeldt–Jakob disease (CJD), has led the health authorities in many countries to increase the precautions taken in the collection of human blood and plasma, and in the use of blood-derived products for therapeutic applications. One recent result of these increased precautions has been the withdrawal of several lots of therapeutic human serum albumin (HSA) from use and distribution by the major companies supplying this product in the USA. Until now, the available epidemiological data do not support transmission of CJD via blood transfusion in humans, and transmission by intravenous infusion of whole blood has not been demonstrated in subhuman primates.

Human albumin solutions are convenient to use because no cross-matching is required, and the absence of cellular elements removes the danger of sensitization with repeated infusions. Toxic effects are rare; urticaria, chills and fever may occasionally occur. These reactions are brief and without sequelae. Under circumstances of volume depletion such as in the SOHSS, the oncotic action of administered albumin lasts less than 36 hours, whereas afterwards albumin leaves the intravascular and resides in the interstitium where it can act to draw fluid out of the intravascular space. As the OHSS usually manifests 5–10 days after hCG administration, there is the potential to worsen the fluid derangement in the SOHSS.[18] In addition, albumin should be administered with caution to patients with diminished cardiac reserve because a rapid increase in plasma volume may cause circulatory embarrassment and pulmonary oedema.[12,13] At present, no adverse reactions to the administration of human albumin for prevention of the SOHSS have been reported.

## CLINICAL EXPERIENCE WITH INTRAVENOUS HUMAN ALBUMIN FOR PREVENTION OF THE SOHSS

Asch et al[14,15] were the first to suggest that intravenous human albumin may help to prevent the development of the SOHSS. A proposed mechanism is illustrated in Figure 1. In an uncontrolled study,[15] 50 g human albumin was administered intravenously during and shortly after oocyte retrieval to 36 women considered at high risk ($\geq 28$ oocytes, and serum $> 22\,000$ pmol/l on the day of hCG administration), and in no case had the SOHSS developed. It should be noted, however, that most of the patients (21 of 36) in that uncontrolled study did not undergo embryo transfer, and the overall risk for this group was substantially lower than appreciated.

Prompted by the encouraging results of Asch et al,[14] and our small pilot study,[16] we have conducted a propsective randomized, placebo-controlled study.[17] Our group of patients at highest risk for the SOHSS was defined by reviewing the medical records of the women who had been hospitalized in our department for the condition during the 3 years preceding the study. As it was revealed that all patients had multiple follicular development combined with serum oestradiol concencentration of more than 7000 pmol/l on the day of hCG administration, this concentration was chosen as the cut-off point for inclusion in our study. Thirty-one patients who fulfilled the above criteria were randomized to receive either 50 g human albumin ($n = 16$) or 500 ml 0.9% sodium chloride ($n = 15$). Solutions were infused intravenously at a slow rate over 1 hour immediately after oocyte retrieval. Although no patient developed the SOHSS in the study

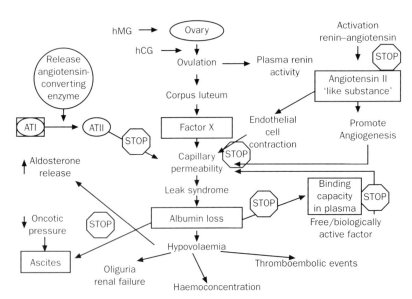

**Figure 1** Proposed mechanisms by which intravenous albumin administration might prevent the development of the severe ovarian hyperstimulation syndrome. ATI, angiotensin I; ATII, angiotensin II; hMG, human menopausal gonadotrophin.

group, there were four such cases in the control group ($p = 0.043$). Three patients in the study group, who had previously experienced the SOHSS after gonadotrophin therapy, did not develop clinically significant OHSS in the present study. There were four pregnancies in the study group and two in the control group. Both pregnant patients in the control group developed the SOHSS.

Shalev et al[19] conducted a randomized controlled trial to evaluate the effectiveness of a single dose of 20 g human serum albumin administered intravenously immediately after oocyte retrieval. The criteria for inclusion in the study were: young age, non-obesity, oestradiol concentration >9200 pmol/l on the day of hCG administration and over 20 follicles of diameter larger than 14 mm observed by transvaginal ultrasonography. There were no cases of the SOHSS in 22 high-risk patients who received intravenous albumin, compared with four cases of the SOHSS in 18 high-risk patients who did not receive ablumin ($p = 0.035$). There were six pregnancies in the study group and two in the control group. When the database was restricted to patients with an oestradiol concentration of more than 15 000 pmol/l on the day

of hCG administration, the results showed that four of six patients in the control group developed the SOHSS, whereas none of the 10 patients in the treatment group did. This was highly significant ($p = 0.00824$).

Isik et al[20] reached the same conclusion in a prospective randomized study comparing two groups of patients undergoing IVF who had oestradiol concentrations of more than 11 010 pmol/l on the day of hCG administration and more than 15 oocytes were retrieved. Patients in the study group received 10 g human albumin as a single intravenous dose just before oocyte retrieval. None of 27 patients developed moderate or severe OHSS in the study group compared with four cases of the moderate OHSS and one case with the SOHSS among the 28 controls ($p < 0.05$).

In addition to the three small-scale, prospective, randomized studies mentioned above, several groups conducted prospective studies comparing patients at high risk for development of the SOHSS who had received intravenous albumin with historical controls. Shahata et al[21] defined their patients with highest risk as those with serum oestradiol of more than 11 000 pmol/l on the day of hCG administration, more than 20 oocytes retrieved and/or more than 30 follicles on ultrasonography, and development of severe symptoms of the OHSS (for example, abdominal pain, nausea, vomiting, increase in weight and girth) before oocyte retrieval. In 41 of 104 treatment cycles, the patients were considered at high risk according to the above criteria, and these patients received 100 ml 20% albumin solution (20 g) at the time of oocyte retrieval. There were no cases of the SOHSS in patients who received albumin, compared with seven cases in 96 cycles (7.3%) completed before the implementation of the albumin protocol ($p < 0.01$).

Using the same approach, Ng et al[22] questioned the efficacy of prophylactic intravenous albumin for prevention of the SOHSS by a cohort study with historical controls. A total of 207 patients, with an oestradiol concentration of more than 10 000 pmol/l and/or more than 15 follicles of over 10 mm in diameter on the day of hCG injection, were reviewed. Of these, 158 women received 500 ml lactated Ringer's solution both before and after egg retrieval, and 49 women received two infusions of 500 ml 5% human albumin (total 50 g) in physiological saline immediately before and repeated immediately after egg retrieval. The SOHSS developed in 2 of 49 patients (4%) who received human albumin and in 10 of 158 women (6.3%) who received physiological saline. This difference was not statistically significant. Whilst six out of ten patients with the SOHSS in the control group conceived, neither of the two patients with the SOHSS in the study group did. Although six of ten patients in the control group had grade 5 OHSS (classification of Golan et al[4]) and five of them were pregnant, neither of the two patients in the study group had grade 5 OHSS (both had grade 4). In conclusion, although there was no significant difference in the occurrence of the SOHSS between the two groups, the authors did note a definite trend towards blunting of the severity of the condition.

Chen et al[23] administered intravenous albumin to 30 patients considered at high risk for the SOHSS (that is, serum oestradiol >13 215 pmol/l on hCG day and/or >20

oocytes retrieved), and compared them with 42 consecutive historical controls. The dosage of albumin was calculated according to the patient's body mass index (BMI), with a mean of 41.5 g (range 30–50 g) being administered. Four (13.3%) of the 30 patients in the treatment group developed the SOHSS, compared with 14 (33.3%) of 42 patients in the control group ($p = 0.047$). Two of 12 patients (16.7%) who had the PCOS developed the SOHSS in the treatment group, compared with 8 of 15 (53.3%) in the control group ($p = 0.057$). None of the 16 patients in the treatment group developed the SOHSS in non-conception cycles, compared with 5 of 23 (21.7%) in the control group ($p = 0.048$). In conception cycles, 4 of 14 patients (28.6%) in the treatment group developed the SOHSS, compared with 9 of 19 (47.4%) in the control group. All patients with the SOHSS in the treatment group carried multiple pregnancies, and all four with multiple pregnancies in the treatment group developed the SOHSS, compared with three of five (60%) in the control group. None of the 10 patients with singleton pregnancies in the treatment group developed the SOHSS, compared with 6 of 14 (42.9%) in the control group ($p = 0.023$). It was therefore concluded that intravenous albumin at the time of egg collection effectively prevents the SOHSS in those high-risk patients who did not conceive or who carried singleton pregnancies, but not in patients with multiple pregnancies.

A recent report of yet another uncontrolled study[24] described the results of administration of human albumin to a group of patients considered at high risk for development of the SOHSS (>25 follicles seen on ultrasonography and >15 oocytes retrieved). Twenty-one patients received 100 ml 20% (20 g) human albumin at the time of oocyte retrieval, and all of them underwent embryo transfer. The clinical pregnancy rate was 38.1%. Only one patient with a twin pregnancy developed grade 3 OHSS (classification of Schenker and Weinstein[25]) and was hospitalized for 3 days during the luteal phase of her IVF cycle, requiring only intravenous fluids.

In a prospective randomized study, Shaker et al[26] compared the efficacy of the administration of intravenous albumin to prevent the SOHSS in patients at risk, with a standard policy of cryopreserving all embryos. The impact of these two treatment approaches on pregnancy rates (PRs) was assessed as well. Twenty-six patients undergoing IVF who were considered to be at high risk of developing the SOHSS (serum oestradiol concentration > 13 000 pmol/l on the day of hCG administration or serum oestradiol > 10 000 pmol/l and > 15 oocytes collected) were randomly allocated to one of the two treatment modalities. In group 1 ($n = 13$) all the generated embryos were cryopreserved, to be transferred subsequently in hormonally manipulated cycles. Patients in group 2 ($n = 13$) received an intravenous infusion of albumin (200 ml 20% albumin [40 g]) on the day of oocyte retrieval and 5 days later. Patients in group 2 had transfers of fresh embryos 2 or 3 days after oocyte retrieval. There were no significant differences in the response to ovarian stimulation between the two groups, but PRs were significantly higher in patients who had all embryos cryopreserved (38.6% vs 0%, $p < 0.05$). No cases of the SOHSS occurred in either group. The authors concluded that both the policy of cryopreserving all generated embryos and the administration of intravenous albumin to be effective in preventing the SOHSS in high-risk patients. No clear explanation could be given for the surprising 0 PR in patients who received intravenous albumin and fresh transfer of embryos. It was speculated that the second dose of albumin, given 5 days after oocyte retrieval, may have bound some putative factors necessary for implantation, thus adversely affecting the PR.

After the initially encouraging reports, several small series and case reports describing patients who developed the SOHSS despite administration of prophylactic albumin appeared in the literature.[27–31] Of special interest were the cases reported by Halme et al[28] and Lewit et al,[30] indicating that the SOHSS may develop even with the combination of two promising preventive measures (intravenous albumin administration and avoidance of embryo transfer). Soon after, it was realized that prophylactic administration of albumin is

not an absolute preventive measure and, eventually, cases of the SOHSS occurred also in the group of Asch when their uncontrolled study was extended to include 169 women at high risk (> 20 oocytes retrieved and/or oestradiol levels on hCG day > 18 350 pmol/l).[32] All the patients who fulfilled the above criteria were treated with 50 g human albumin intravenously during and shortly after oocyte retrieval, but only 108 patients underwent embryo transfer. Five patients (3%) were hospitalized as a result of the SOHSS, whereas 10 (7%) developed the moderate form of the syndrome. However, the overall incidence of the SOHSS was considerably lower than expected for patients at high risk in that particular programme. In a recent uncontrolled study,[33] prophylactic albumin was administered at an intravenous dose of 45 g at the time of oocyte retrieval and immediately after to all patients with serum oestradiol concentrations of more than 15 000 pmol/l at the time of hCG administration, or more than 30 follicles measuring over 14 mm present. Of the 60 patients who received prophylactic albumin, five (8%) developed the SOHSS and eight (13%) developed a moderate form of the syndrome. One patient developed an early form of the SOHSS before embryo transfer, so this transfer was not carried out and the embryos were cryopreserved. Three of the four patients who had embryo transfer conceived (one set of twins and two singletons). Again, the efficacy of human albumin for prevention of the SOHSS was questioned.

## CONCLUSION

Summarizing the studies presented above, one cannot overlook the fact that all three prospective, randomized, controlled trials available to date regarding the use of prophylactic albumin near the time of oocyte retrieval[17,19,20] have shown a significant reduction in the incidence of the SOHSS. If data from all three studies are pooled, despite the differences in inclusion criteria, then the prophylactic effect of albumin becomes highly evident ($p < 0.0011$). Data from prospective studies with historical controls show a similar trend.[21–23] Furthermore, the experience of many of the investigators who had used intravenous albumin as a preventive measure has been that, even if the OHSS has developed, albumin appeared to blunt and ameliorate the severity of the condition. The protective effect of intravenous albumin may be less pronounced in cases where a multiple pregnancy is developing.[23,24,27,31] It has been speculated that the dose of albumin that is currently being administered may be insufficient to counteract the higher amount of hCG and hCG-mediated vasoactive factors produced by multiple pregnancies.[23] Nevertheless, it is difficult to compare and draw firm conclusions from the studies that have been reported to date, because of the marked variability in the inclusion criteria (as discussed above), in the dosage and regimens for albumin administration (doses of 10–50 g albumin have been administered in different regimens), and the fact that several classification systems for the severity of the OHSS are interchangeably used.[1,4,25] Therefore, at present, the use of intravenous albumin as a preventive measure is the subject of ongoing controversy. Further, carefully designed studies are needed in order to establish the ideal timing and optimum dose for prophylactic human albumin administration. Most importantly, a large, randomized, placebo-controlled, clinical trial on a carefully selected and *well*-defined high-risk population is required before prophylactic albumin can be recommended for routine use for the prevention of the SOHSS.

## REFERENCES

1. Navot D, Berg PA, Laufer N. Ovarian hyperstimulation syndrome in novel reproductive technologies: prevention and treatment. *Fertil Steril* 1992;**58**:249–61.
2. Mathur RS, Joles LA, Akande AV, Jenkins JM. The prevention of ovarian hyperstimulation syndrome. *Br J Obstet Gynaecol* 1996;**103**:740–6.
3. Borenstein R, Elhalah U, Lunenfeld B, Schwartz ZS. Severe ovarian hyperstimulation syndrome: a re-evaluated therapeutic approach. *Fertil Steril* 1989;**51**:791–5.
4. Golan A, Ron-El R, Herman A, et al. Ovarian hyperstimulation syndrome: an update review. *Obstet Gynecol Surv* 1989;**44**:430–9.
5. Asch RH, Li HP, Balmaceda JP, et al. Severe ovarian hyperstimulation in assisted reproductive technology: definition of high risk groups. *Hum Reprod* 1991;**6**:1395–9.
6. Morris RS, Paulson RJ, Sauer MV, Lobo RA. Predictive value of serum oestradiol concentrations and oocyte number in severe ovarian hyperstimulation syndrome. *Hum Reprod* 1995;**10**:811–14.
7. Delvigne A, Dubois M, Battheu B, et al. The ovarian hyperstimulation syndrome in vitro fertilization: a Belgian multicentric study. II. Multiple discriminant analysis for risk prediction. *Hum Reprod* 1993;**8**:1361–6.
8. Polishuk WZ, Schenker JG. Ovarian overstimulation syndrome. *Fertil Steril* 1969;**20**:443–50.
9. Navot D, Margalioth EJ, Laufer N, et al. Direct correlation between plasma renin activity and severity of the ovarian hyperstimulation syndrome. *Fertil Steril* 1987;**48**:57–61.
10. Ong AC, Eisen V, Rennie DP. The pathogenesis of the ovarian hyperstimulation syndrome (OHS): a possible role for ovarian renin. *Clin Endocrinol* 1991;**34**:43–9.
11. McClure N, Healy DL, Rogers PAW, et al. Vascular endothelial growth factor as capillary permeability agent in ovarian hyperstimulation syndrome. *Lancet* 1994;**344**:235–6.
12. McClelland DB. Human albumin solutions. *BMJ* 1990;**300**:35–7.
13. Erstad BL. The use of albumin in clinical practice. *Arch Intern Med* 1991;**151**:901–11.
14. Asch RH, Ivery G, Stone SC, Balmaceda JP. Intravenous albumin prevents the development of severe ovarian hyperstimulation in an ART program (Abstract). Presented at the Pacific Coast Fertility Society Annual Meeting, 1992.
15. Asch RH, Ivery G, Goldsman M, et al. The use of intravenous albumin in patients at high risk for severe ovarian hyperstimulation syndrome. *Hum Reprod* 1993;**8**:1015–20.
16. Shoham Z, Borenstein R, Barash A, et al.

Prevention of ovarian hyperstimulation syndrome? [letter]. *Fertil Steril* 1993;**60**:585.

17. Shoham Z, Weissman A, Barash A, et al. Intravenous albumin for the prevention of severe ovarian hyperstimulation syndrome in an in vitro fertilization program: a prospective, randomized, placebo-controlled study. *Fertil Steril* 1994;**62**:137–42.

18. Morris RS, Paulson RJ. Does intravenous albumin prevent ovarian hyperstimulation syndrome? [letter]. *Hum Reprod* 1994;**9**:753–4.

19. Shalev E, Giladi Y, Matilsky M, Ben-Ami M. Decreased incidence of severe ovarian hyperstimulation syndrome in high risk in-vitro fertilization patients receiving intravenous albumin: a prospective study. *Hum Reprod* 1995;**10**:1373–6.

20. Isik AZ, Gokmen O, Zeyneloglu HB, et al. Intravenous albumin prevents moderate-severe ovarian hyperstimulation in in vitro fertilization patients: a prospective randomized and controlled study. *Eur J Obstet Gynecol Reprod Biol* 1996;**70**:179–83.

21. Shahata M, Yang D, Al-Natsha SD, Al-Shawaf T. Intravenous albumin and severe ovarian hyperstimulation (letter). *Hum Reprod* 1994;**9**:2186.

22. Ng E, Leader A, Claman P, et al. Intravenous albumin does not prevent the development of severe ovarian hyperstimulation syndrome in an in-vitro fertilization programme. *Hum Reprod* 1995;**10**:807–10.

23. Chen CD, Wu MY, Yang JH, et al. Intravenous albumin does not prevent the development of severe ovarian hyperstimulation syndrome. *Fertil Steril* 1997;**68**:287–91.

24. Sabatini L, Wilson C, Al Shawaf T, et al. Efficacy of serum albumin to prevent ovarian hyperstimulation syndrome (letter). *Fertil Steril* 1997;**67**:587–8.

25. Schenker JG, Weinstein D. Ovarian hyperstimulation syndrome: a current survey. *Fertil Steril* 1978;**30**:255–68.

26. Shaker AG, Zosmer A, Dean N, et al. Comparison of intravenous albumin and transfer of fresh embryos with cryopreservation of all embryos for subsequent transfer in prevention of ovarian hyperstimulation syndrome. *Fertil Steril* 1996;**65**:992–6.

27. Mukherjee T, Copperman AB, Sandler B, et al. Severe ovarian hyperstimulation despite prophylactic albumin at the time of oocyte retrieval for in vitro fertilization and embryo transfer. *Fertil Steril* 1995;**64**:641–3.

28. Halme J, Toma SK, Talbert LM. A case of severe ovarian hyperstimulation in a healthy oocyte donor. *Fertil Steril* 1995;**64**:857–9.

29. Orvieto R, Dekel A, Dicker D, et al. A severe case of ovarian hyperstimulation syndrome despite the prophylactic administration of intravenous albumin. *Fertil Steril* 1995;**64**:860–2.

30. Lewit N, Kol S, Ronen N, Itskovitz-Eldor J. Does intravenous administration of human albumin prevent severe ovarian hyperstimulation syndrome? *Fertil Steril* 1996;**66**:654–6.

31. Moutus DM, Miller MM, Mahadevan MM. Bilateral internal jugular venous thrombosis complicating severe ovarian hyperstimulation syndrome after prophylactic albumin administration. *Fertil Steril* 1997;**68**:174–6.

32. Goldsman MP, Balmaceda JP, Stone SC, et al. Use of albumin in the prevention of OHSS (Abstract). Presented at the Pacific Coast Fertility Society Annual Meeting, 1995.

33. Ndukwe G, Thornton S, Fishel S, et al. Severe ovarian hyperstimulation syndrome: is it really preventable by prophylactic intravenous albumin? *Fertil Steril* 1997;**68**:851–4.

# 29

# How to avoid multiple pregnancy

Per Olof Janson, Lars Hamberger

**Problems involved in multiple pregnancy** • **New strategies for treatment of infertility** • **Embryo reduction**
• **Summary and conclusions**

Ever since the introduction of gonadotrophin treatment at the start of the 1960s, multiple pregnancy has been an almost inevitable complication in many instances. The public reaction has been, on the whole, positive, not only to twins but also to higher-order multiple births, illustrated recently by the enthusiasm about the heptacepts born after gonadotrophin treatment and intrauterine insemination (IUI).

On the other hand, the professional reaction, predominantly of paediatricians, has been very negative, pointing to the fact that even twins constitute a perinatal problem of a much higher magnitude than singletons. The aim of gynaecologists responsible for treatment of various types of infertility should therefore be clear: avoid multiple pregnancy under almost all circumstances. In this chapter we try to divide the problem into particular subgroups and point to solutions that may have a specific 'Scandinavian flavour' because Scandinavia has the lowest multiple pregnancy rate in the world, at least based on international statistics from treatment with in vitro fertilization (IVF).

## PROBLEMS INVOLVED IN MULTIPLE PREGNANCY

Multiple pregnancy is partly a natural phenomenon and partly an iatrogenic one, as a result of ovulation induction with or without various procedures of assisted reproduction. In spontaneously occurring pregnancies, twins are the most common type with an average incidence of one in 85 deliveries. Triplet and quadruplet pregnancies are very uncommon, each occurring in one in 85 deliveries.[1,2] Higher orders of pregnancy are extremely rare. In twin pregnancies small differences between races have been shown (Asians 0.64%; white Europeans 1.13%; Africans 1.43%), caused predominantly by differences in the incidence of dizygotic twinning. In recent years an increase in the incidence of spontaneous twinning of up to 2–3% has been reported in the USA.[3] This could result partly from delayed child birth.

### Maternal and fetal complications

Twin gestations are justifiably regarded as risk pregnancies with complications affecting both mother and fetus. It has been difficult to obtain reliable figures on complications as a result of the lack of controlled studies comparing twins with singleton pregnancies. However, large American studies[1] involving 1253 twin pregnancies and 5119 controls, and those of Gardner et al[2] including 33 873 deliveries with 432 sets of twins, have presented valuable information on the prevalence of some of the complications.

The frequency of spontaneous abortion is estimated to be two to three times higher in multiple gestations than in singletons. About 30% of all twin pregnancies appear, however, to be spontaneously converted to singletons. The incidence of prematurity (delivery before the end of 37 weeks of gestation) has been reported to be three times more common among twins compared with singletons. Of the deliveries presented from the data set by Gardner et al,[2] 54% of the twins were pre-term compared with 9.6% among singletons. The reason for the high prematurity among twin pregnancies is believed to be increased uterine distension resulting in premature labour. Other complications, such as hyperemesis, hypertension in pregnancy/pre-eclampsia, bleeding resulting from placental abruption, anaemia, pyelonephritis and symptoms of increased pressure exerted by the uterus, also occur more frequently in twins than in singletons. However, it has to be pointed out that, although there are significant differences in complications between twin and singleton pregnancies, the rate of each of the complications other than prematurity amounts to less than 10%.

## Neonatal complications

Among neonatal complications the most common are low birthweight, caused by prematurity and probably also by placental dysfunction, and congenital malformations which are three to four times more common than in singletons. Finally, the perinatal mortality is five to six times higher among twins. This results for several reasons, such as prematurity, intrauterine growth retardation and increased risks during delivery (placental abruption, placenta praevia,

umbilical cord compression). Gardner et al[3] reported that 9.6% of all fetal deaths and 15.4% of all neonatal deaths occurred in twin pregnancies.

## Multiple pregnancies of higher order

In triplet and higher-order multiple pregnancies, the pattern of complications is the same as for twin pregnancies, with the important proviso that the complications tend to be very serious. Papiernik[4] has indicated that the mean gestational length for twin pregnancy is, on average, 37 weeks, and those of triplet and quadruplet pregnancies 33 and 31 weeks, respectively. Among women with quadruplets, every other pregnancy is complicated by pre-eclampsia.[5] In an analysis of 71 quadruplet pregnancies, Collins and Bleyl[6] reported 98% prematurity, 35% first trimester haemorrhages, 25% hypertension in pregnancy/pre-eclampsia, 25% anaemia, 14% cervical incompetence and 14% urinary tract infections.

Data from England and Wales show that, between 1980 and 1993, the higher-order maternity rate more than doubled and that, compared with singletons, neonatal morbidity was more than 20 times higher in triplets and higher-order births.[7]

## Cerebral palsy and multiple pregnancy

Pharoah and Cooke[8] reported, from a study carried out in the UK, a crude prevalence of cerebral palsy of 2.3 per 1000 infant survivors in singletons, 12.6 per 1000 in twins and 44.8 per 1000 in triplets. Similar figures, with a six times higher cerebral palsy rate in twins than in singletons, has been reported from New York by Laplaza et al.[9] From California, Grether et al[10] reported that twin pregnancies produced a child with cerebral palsy 12 times more often than in singleton pregnancies. From Western Australia, Petterson et al[11] reported a prevalence figure of cerebral palsy eight times higher for twins than for singletons, whereas in the same study cerebral palsy occurred 47 times more often in triplets than in singletons. According to recent literature, there are at least three independent risk factors for cerebral palsy in multiple gestations, namely lower gestational age, lower birthweight distribution and a higher risk among infants of normal birthweight.[8,12]

### Iatrogenic multiple pregnancy

The iatrogenic form of multiple pregnancy occurs after ovulation induction with clomiphene citrate, pulsatile gonadotrophin-releasing hormone (GnRH) agonists and gonadotrophins, with reported incidence figures of 5–10%, 7–10% and 16–40% respectively.[13] The most common result is twinning, but the greatest relative increase is constituted by triplet and quadruplet pregnancies. The number of multiple births increased steadily in the Western World during the 1980s, partly because of the 'ageing' of the female population at the time of reproduction, and partly and quantitatively more important as a consequence of assisted reproduction technologies (ART). For example, from 1982, after the introduction of in vitro fertilization (IVF), to 1988, the number of twin births increased by 18% and triplets and higher-order births by 58%, compared with only a 7% increase in total US births.[14] ART has affected the rate of multiple births in two ways: first, the procedures themselves have a direct influence on the incidence of multiple pregnancy and, second, the number of couples undergoing infertility treatment has increased dramatically.

Interestingly, the rate of monozygotic pairs, a phenomenon previously thought to be a biological constant, has been shown to be significantly increased in women undergoing ovulation induction and in women undergoing IVF with or without micromanipulation.[15–17] The reason for this is still a matter of speculation, but the fact that there is an increase in monozygotic splitting clearly indicates that hormonal induction of ovulation, and handling of the oocyte and the early embryo, both have an action on the embryo before implantation.

The first successful human IVF pregnancy followed retrieval of a single oocyte in a spontaneous menstrual cycle.[18] Subsequent attempts to utilize the natural cycle on a large scale have shown disappointingly low pregnancy rates with this approach, with delivery rates per retrieval of only 6%.[19] The low cost-effectiveness of unstimulated IVF can, however, vary between different centres and may become a future alternative for selected groups of patients, also avoiding the ethical dilemma of how to use or preserve spare embryos.[20] On the other hand, comparison with stimulated cycles must take into consideration the potential for cryopreserving excess embryos in stimulated cycles for future transfer(s) without superovulation. It is well known that the pregnancy rate in IVF rises with the number of embryos transferred, but it is also obvious that the rate of multiple births rises with an increased number of embryos transferred.

## NEW STRATEGIES FOR TREATMENT OF INFERTILITY

Currently, treatment options for mild-to-moderate female mechanical infertility are endoscopic microsurgical procedures or IVF. With a careful preselection of cases suitable for operative procedures, results equal or in excess of those obtained with IVF have been achieved.[21,22] Microsurgery also has the advantage of not being associated with an increased multiple pregnancy rate (Figure 1).

In cases with patent tubes and in those with mild male subfertility, IUI has been an attractive treatment option in many programmes. As the results from natural cycles are inferior to those from gonadotrophin-stimulated cycles, this has become the treatment of choice. Also cases with so-called unexplained infertility are frequently treated with IUI in stimulated cycles. In our opinion, it is, however, doubtful if this widely adopted treatment is optimal and in the patient's best interest. Even if strict rules are applied, that is, not allowing more than two follicles larger than 18 mm in diameter to occur at the time of ovulation induction, there is obviously the risk that ultrasonography may not

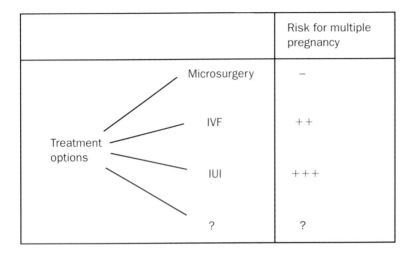

| | Risk for multiple pregnancy |
|---|---|
| Microsurgery | – |
| IVF | + + |
| IUI | + + + |
| ? | ? |

**Figure 1** Relative risks for multiple pregnancy when comparing different options for treatment of infertility.

reveal all follicles or that smaller follicles will ovulate at a slightly later stage. Further, and especially in couples with unexplained infertility, if pregnancy fails to occur, little knowledge is gained concerning the cause of the infertility.

For these reasons we recommend that IVF be used after one (possibly two) failure with IUI. In our own setting, all couples are informed in advance that a scheduled IUI treatment may be acutely converted into an IVF treatment, in case more than two preovulatory follicles are visible on the ultrasound screen at the time for ovulation induction. In a series of such acutely 'switched' patients in our IVF unit, a clinical pregnancy was established in 46% of the cases, although the overall pregnancy rate for IUI was only 26% per treatment cycle.[23]

It is thus obvious that IVF has come to replace both microsurgery and IUI because in a majority of infertile couples, it is more effective and also possible to use for a wider spectrum of indications. Therefore, investigation of couples with long-standing infertility can be simplified, because the exact cause of the infertility is frequently of less importance and not decisive for the type of treatment. The crucial question is whether or not a couple can be regarded as optimal for treatment with IVF. Ultrasonographically guided evaluation of the uterine cavity and fallopian tubes seems sufficient in most cases, possibly combined with measurements of a few endocrine parameters such as serum follicle-stimulating hormone (FSH), prolactin and luteal phase progesterone. For the man, one sperm analysis seems to be sufficient in order to decide if conventional IVF or intracytoplasmic sperm injection (ICSI) should be used. With this new insight about which method is preferable comes the responsibility for carrying it through as safely as possible. Avoidance of multiple pregnancy is, in this connection, of first priority.

The introduction of controlled ovarian hyperstimulation (COH) with gonadotrophins, later combined with down-regulation using GnRH agonists, has resulted in a dramatic increase in multiple pregnancy rates. In the latest World Statistics Report on IVF pregnancy outcome, the USA has a 36% multiple pregnancy rate and a triplet pregnancy rate of 6%.[24] It can be asked who should be held responsible for these high rates of multiple pregnancies. The answer is simple: large IVF centres with high impact factors and high multiple pregnancy rates. IVF teams all over the world now make attempts to achieve a balance between a satisfactory pregnancy rate and an acceptable rate of multiple pregnancy in deciding the number of embryos to transfer. In so doing, they have to consider several factors contributing to the patient's or the physician's *perception* of what is satisfactory or acceptable, including biological, psychological, ethical and financial considerations. Often as a result of the fact that these factors are not quantifiable, they do not readily fit into a risk–benefit analysis. Should, for instance, a high-order multiple gestation that does not even result in a single live baby be considered 'a success' and can it ever be regarded as 'acceptable'?

Risk versus benefit of multiple oocyte/embryo transfer has been the subject of a great deal of debate. Already, in 1987, the Voluntary Licensing Authority of the UK introduced voluntary guidelines, limiting the number of embryo transfers during ART procedures to 'three or exceptionally four', in response to concerns about higher-order multiple births. As a result of a continuing steep rise of multiple births in Britain, and the strain placed on the provincial neonatal services, a rigorous enforcement of licensing authority guidelines has been urged.[25] In Scandinavia, voluntary guidelines have been issued[26] recommending replacement of a maximum of two embryos per cycle.

From the recently published World Report on IVF,[24] based on 34 000 deliveries and almost 50 000 children, it is obvious that different countries have, apart from their replacement policy, very different results. The world average is 15% for conventional IVF and ICSI. Belgium and Sweden report 25% whereas the figures for the Netherlands and Australia are somewhat lower, with 20% and 15% respectively. The USA reports an average of 27%, which is most probably the result of their 'liberal' policy regarding the number of embryos transferred (Table 1).

According to the World Report,[24] twin pregnancies occur at every fourth delivery with fairly similar figures from different countries. However, the incidence figures of triplets with a mean value of 4% differs considerably between countries. For example, Sweden reported 0.9%, whereas the UK and the USA reported 5% and 6%, respectively. Quadruplets or higher-order pregnancies average 0.2% of

**Table 1 Different embryo transfer policies**

- Replace only one to two embryos
- Replace three to five embryos but inform the patient about embryo reduction
- Replace three to seven embryos and let the paediatricians take care of the problems

deliveries. Even though triplets and higher-order pregnancies have become increasingly more rare, especially in the countries that have adopted a restrictive transfer policy with only one or two embryos per treatment cycle, the incidence of twins is relatively high and should be a matter of further concern and research.

To achieve an acceptable pregnancy rate per cycle even if only one or two embryos are replaced, a better selection of optimal embryos must be made. Milder gonadotrophin stimulation might be one way to avoid immature oocytes, or oocytes of suboptimal quality, being included. Another possibility is to monitor fertilization and embryo development more intensely. In our programme, the embryos are checked at both 18 and 25 hours after fertilization, in order to trace those embryos that cleave most rapidly. By the development of more optimal media for embryo culture, human embryos can be grown for 5–6 days before transfer without using co-culture systems.[27] Replacement of one expanded blastocyst at a time, in combination with an optimal blastocyst freezing protocol, is one endeavour and we are planning to include an increasing number of couples in this type of treatment in our own programme. Assisted hatching before replacement has been discussed intensely in recent years and both mechanical and instrumental techniques have been described. The introduction of assisted hatching with the use of laser might be an attractive alternative for the future.[17]

## EMBRYO REDUCTION

In 1978, Åberg and co-workers[28] described what they called 'selective termination in a case of a foetus with multiple malformations'. Almost a decade later Dumaz and Oury[29] introduced the expression 'multi-fetal pregnancy reduction' where apparently normal fetuses were terminated in order to increase the chances of the remainder surviving and developing. In connection with IVF, selective embryo reduction has been used to overcome some of the risks associated particularly with multiple pregnancies of higher order. Various techniques of termination have been described but currently there seems to be a general agreement that: week 7–8 from the last menstrual period is an optimal time; the paracervical vaginal route is preferable; and ultrasound-guided aspiration of the embryo is better than injections of agents such as KCl to arrest heart activity. If a termination is performed at an earlier stage, certain spontaneous reductions may be missed and, if performed later, technical difficulties will increase and the weight gain of a remaining fetus(es) is smaller or completely lost.

## SUMMARY AND CONCLUSIONS

Multiple pregnancies are risk pregnancies, particularly triplets and higher-order gestations. As ovulation induction and ART procedures are responsible for the steady increase in multiple births in the Western World, a number of strategies have to be applied to prevent this complication. Restrictive embryo transfer policies limiting the number of embryos transferred to two, or at the most three, have reduced higher-order pregnancies to almost acceptable, low levels whereas higher-order multiple births are still significant problems in ovulation induction in anovulatory women or in COH in ovulating women. Also, in ART the rate of twins is still very high. In spite of the fact that a twin pregnancy after ART procedures is presently regarded as acceptable or even desirable or satisfactory, the high rate of prematurity with inherent complications in twins should, in our opinion, encourage the development of strategies to minimize further multiple pregnancies. A crude way of compensating for the therapeutic mishap of term triplets and higher-order gestations is embryo reduction. Embryo reduction is a valuable tool for the management of exceptional cases, mostly related to ovulation induction or superovulation therapy, and in the future should not be a necessary procedure in the management of ART pregnancies.

The novel strategies for avoiding multiple pregnancies in infertility treatment involves the proper selection of candidates for non-ART procedures, such as tubal and ovarian microsurgery, and an evaluation of the indications for COH with or without IUI, using prospective, randomized trials. An option in cases of COH with multifollicular development is to convert to IVF. In ovulation inductions and IVF methodology one might apply milder gonadotrophin-stimulating regimens, according to the low-dose scheme suggested by, for example, Franks.[30]

In IVF cycles an improved monitoring of fertilization and embryo development, together with the use of new media allowing prolonged embryo cultures, may also contribute to the development of *one*-embryo transfer regimens. Likewise, the replacement of *one* expanded blastocyst may, in conjunction with an optimal freezing programme, be instrumental in reducing the number of multiple pregnancies. In this context, we believe that stimulated cycles will also, in the future, be superior to spontaneous cycle IVF, as a result of the possibility of freezing excess embryos for use in subsequent cycles. Further, the natural cycle cannot generally be recommended for IVF because large treatment groups (female cycle irregularities, male factor infertility) are excluded.

Finally, further development of the technique of assisted hatching and results from basic research on biochemical markers for oocyte and embryo quality will help to minimize the number of multiple births. In cases of pregnancy, we will always have to accept some degree of monozygotic twinning in spite of the transfer of only one embryo. Such twins will never, in our opinion, be subject to embryo reduction, which would do more harm than good.

Until these slightly futuristic strategies have been fully evaluated, we will reluctantly have to accept the replacement of two embryos as a temporary policy.

## ACKNOWLEDGEMENT

We thank Sabine Geiser for expert secretarial assistance. We acknowledge grants from the Swedish Medical Research Council (2873).

## REFERENCES

1. Spellacy WN, Handler A, Ferre CD. A case-control study of 1253 twin pregnancies from a 1982–1987 perinatal base. *Obstet Gynecol* 1990; **75**:168.
2. Gardner MO, Goldenberg RL, Chuer S, Tucker JM, Nelson KG, Copper RL. The ongoing and outcome of preterm twin pregnancies. *Obstet Gynecol* 1995;**85**:53–7.
3. Luke B. The changing pattern of multiple births in the United States: maternal and infant characteristics, 1993 and 1990. *Obstet Gynecol* 1994;**84**:101–6.
4. Papiernik E. The very tiny baby, multiple births and other questions about preterm delivery. *Curr Opin Obstet Gynecol* 1991;**3**:4.
5. Petrikovski BM, Vihtzileos AM. Management and outcome of multiple pregnancy of high fetal order: literature review. *Obstet Gynecol Surv* 1989;**44**:578.
6. Collins MS, Bleyl JA. Seventy-one quadruplet pregnancies: management and outcome. *Am J Obstet Gynecol* 1990;**162**:1384.
7. Doyle P. The outcome of multiple pregnancy. *Hum Reprod* 1993;**11**:110–17.
8. Pharoah POD, Cooke T. Cerebral palsy and multiple births. *Arch Dis Child* 1996;**75**:F174–7.
9. Laplaza FJ, Root L, Tassanawipas A, Cervera P. Cerebral palsy in twins. *J Med Child Neurol* 1992;**34**:1053–63.
10. Grether J, Nelson KB, Cummins S. Twinning and cerebral palsy. Experience in four northern California counties, births 1983 through 1985. *Pediatrics* 1993;**92**:854–8.
11. Petterson B, Nelson KB, Watson L, Stanley F. Twins, triplets and cerebral palsy in births in Western Australia in the 1980's. *BMJ* 1993; **307**:1239–43.
12. Williams K, Hennessy E, Alberman E. Cerebral palsy: effects of twinning birth weight and gestational age. *Arch Dis Child* 1996;**75**:F178–82.
13. Speroff L, Glass RH, Kase NG. *Clinical Gynecologic Endocrinology and Infertility*, 5th edn. Baltimore, MA: Williams & Wilkins, 1994: 897–930.
14. Hecht BR. The impact of assisted reproductive technology on the incidence of multiple gestation. In: *Multiple Pregnancy* (Keith LG, Papiernik E, Keith DM, Luke B, eds). London: Parthenon, 1995:175–90.
15. Derom C, Vlietinck R, Van den Berghe H, Tiery M. Increased monozygotic twinning rate after ovulation induction. *Lancet* 1987;**i**:1236–8.
16. Edwards RG, Mettler L, Walters DE. Identical twins and in vitro fertilization. *J In Vitro Fertil* 1986;**3**:114.
17. Cohen J, Alikani M, Trowbridge J, Rosenwaks Z. Implantation enhancement of selective assisted hatching using zona drilling of human embryos with poor prognosis. *Hum Reprod* 1992;**7**:685.
18. Steptoe PC, Edwards RG. Birth after reimplantation of a human embryo. *Lancet* 1978;**ii**:366.
19. Paulson RJ, Sauer MV, Frances MM, et al. In vitro fertilization in unstimulated cycles. The University of South California experiences. *Fertil Steril* 1992;**57**:290.
20. Zayed F, Lenton EA, Cooke ID. Natural cycle in vitro-fertilization in couples with unexplained infertility: impact of various factors on outcome. *Hum Reprod* 1997; **12**:2402–7.
21. Dubuisson JB, Chapron C, Nos S, Morice P, Aubrist FX, Gamier P. Sterilization reversal: fertility results. *Hum Reprod* 1998;**10**:1145–51.
22. Edén B, Bryman I, Strandell A, Thorburn J. Laparoscopic surgery for infertility – a last effective alternative to IVF. *Proc Ann Mtg Swed Med Assoc* (Abstract) 1995:289.
23. Bergh C, Bryman I, Nilsson L, Janson PO. Results of gonadotrophic stimulation with the option to convert cycles to in vitro fertilization in cases of multi follicular development. *Acta Obstet Gynecol Scand* 1998;**77**:68–73.
24. World Report on IVF. *J Assist Reprod Genet* 1997;**5**:250–65.
25. Levene MI, Wild J, Steer P. Higher multiple births and the modern management of infertility in Britain. *Br J Obstet Gynacol* 1992;**99**:607.

26. Yding-Andersen S, Hovatta O, Hreinsson J, Hazekamp J, Nygren KG. Clinical and laboratory guidelines for assisted reproductive technologies in the Nordic countries. *J Assist Reprod Genet* 1997;**5**:250–65.

27. Gardner DK, Vella P, Lane M, Wagley L, Schlenker T, Schoolcraft WB. Culture and transfer of human blastocysts increases implantation rates and reduces the need for multiple embryo transfers. American Society for Reproductive Medicine 1997 abstracts of the Scientific Oral and Poster Sessions, Oct 18–22, 1997.

28. Åberg A, Miterian F, Cantz M, et al. Cardiac puncture of fetus with Hurler's disease avoiding abortion of unaffected co-twin. *Lancet* 1978; **ii**:990–1.

29. Dumaz Y, Oury JF. Method for first trimester selective abortion in multiple pregnancy. *Gynecol Obstet* 1986;**15**:50–3.

30. Hamilton-Fairly D, Kiddy D, Watson H, Sagle M, Franks S. Low-dose gonadotrophin therapy for induction of ovulation in 100 women with polycystic ovary syndrome. *Hum Reprod* 1991; **6**:1095–9.

# 30

# What are the cancer risks?

Liat Lerner-Geva, Bruno Lunenfeld

**Ovarian cancer** • **Breast cancer** • **Endometrial cancer** • **Melanoma** • **Conclusion**

Infertility is one of the most prevalent conditions affecting many women. More than 15% of couples will require treatment during their reproductive years.[1] Infertility by itself was found to be a risk factor for cancer,[2] and, according to its aetiology, a risk factor for other conditions such as cardiovascular disease. Many adverse effects related to infertility treatments have been reported,[3,4] including short-term effects – multiple pregnancies[5–7] and the hyperstimulation syndrome[8–10] – and recently long-term effects such as genital tract cancer. This last effect, namely the possible development of cancer in reproductive organs in infertile women and, in particular, after treatment with ovulation-inducing drugs, is the subject of this chapter.

## OVARIAN CANCER

Ovarian cancer represents the sixth most common female cancer and is the most fatal gynaecological malignancy with 5-year survival rate of about 40%.[11,12]

The incidence of ovarian cancer varies widely among countries ranging from 15 new cases of ovarian cancer per 100 000 women-years in Europe and North America to two new cases per 100 000 women-years in Japan.[13] It is predicted that one of every 70 newborn females will eventually have ovarian cancer.[14]

A number of identifiable factors have been associated with increased risk of ovarian cancer including: environmental,[15–17] hormonal[18,19] and genetic,[20–22] most recently, the presence of *BRCA-1* and *BRCA-2* gene mutations.[23]

Parity and oral contraceptive use have well-documented protective effects in ovarian cancer.[24–29] In addition, tubal ligation and hysterectomy (without bilateral oophorectomy) have been associated with a decreased risk for ovarian cancer.[30] The rationale for these protective effects is unclear and possibly involves decreased ovulation after these procedures or blockage of ovarian carcinogens.

An inability to conceive has been suggested as a risk factor for ovarian cancer independent of nulliparity.[19,31–38] Nulliparous women who have tried but failed to conceive have a higher rate of ovarian cancer than those who have not planned to become pregnant. A 20% rise in cancer risk with every additional 5 years of unprotected intercourse was calculated.[35]

Fathala in 1971[39] was the first to suggest the relationship between ovarian cancer and 'incessant ovulation'. With each ovulation the ovarian epithelium was thought to incur minor trauma. The cumulative effect of repetitive surface injury was hypothesized to contribute to the development of ovarian neoplasms. Zajicak[40] postulated that epithelial inclusion cysts of the ovarian surface epithelium, which occur in association with ovulation, may be the source of such neoplasms. In 1979, Casagrande et al[41] advocated a relationship between ovarian cancer risk and 'ovulatory age'. This is based on the theory that the number of ovulatory cycles between menarche and menopause is directly proportional to a woman's risk of ovarian cancer. Periods of anovulation caused by pregnancy or oral contraceptive use are considered 'protected time' and are subtracted from the menarche to menopause time interval to yield a woman's 'ovulatory age'. As ovarian tissue is responsive to gonadotrophins, a hypergonadotrophic state has also been implicated as a contributing factor to the development of ovarian cancer.[42–44]

In 1983, Cramer and Welch[45] proposed a model for the pathogenesis of ovarian cystadenocarcinoma. The model consisted of two stages: entrapment of the ovarian epithelium within the ovarian stroma resulting in inclusion cysts and stimulation of the entrapped epithelium by oestrogens and gonadotrophins resulting in proliferation and malignant transformation.

It has been well established that the frequency of ovarian germ cell tumours is increased in patients with gonadal dysgenesis.[46,47] In these patients, gametes are absent resulting in continuously elevated levels of pituitary gonadotrophins. The occurrence of a few reported cases of ovarian cystadenocarcinomas in patients with gonadal dysgenesis has been suggested to support the role of gonadotrophins in the aetiology of epithelial ovarian cancer. On the other hand, if elevated gonadotrophin levels increase cancer risk, an increased cancer incidence after the menopause would have been expected. This trend has not been demonstrated, because the incidence of

ovarian cancer tends to level off after the menopause.[48] In addition, the reported incidence of ovarian cancer among patients with early menopause is not always increased, possibly because the longer duration of elevated gonadotrophins in these patients is offset by a decrease in ovulatory cycles.[25,49]

The concern that there may be a causative relationship between ovulation-inducing drugs and ovarian cancer was first raised by a number of case reports[50–58] (Table 1). Eleven additional cases of epithelial ovarian malignancies have been reported by Kaufman et al.[59] A series of articles, published by Whittemore et al[60–62] and Harris et al[63] in 1992, led to renewed interest in the potentially carcinogenic effects of infertility and ovulation-inducing drugs used to treat infertility.

In 1987, Ron et al[64] published one of the earliest studies concerning treatment for infertility and ovarian cancer. The study cohort consisted of 2632 Israeli women treated for infertility between 1964 and 1974. Among women with non-hormonal infertility, there was a suggestion of non-significant increased risk of ovarian cancer (SIR = 3.2; 95% confidence interval, 95% CI = 0.3–32.9). The authors found no association between the exposure to ovulation-inducing drugs and ovarian cancer, although the many different hormones that were used during the course of therapy made it impossible to distinguish between independent treatment effects. Shu et al[65] observed, in a case-control study of 229 cases of ovarian cancer, that women who had used 'hormone to help become pregnant' had an increased but insignificant risk for developing ovarian cancer (odds ratio, OR = 2.1; 95% CI = 0.2–22.7).

In 1992, Whittemore et al[60–62] and Harris et al[63] and the Collaborative Ovarian Cancer Group reported the findings of meta-analysis of 12 case-control studies of ovarian cancer. In three of these studies information was available on the use of 'fertility drugs'. This report found that infertile women using fertility drugs had about three times the risk for invasive epithelial ovarian cancer as women without a history of infertility (OR = 2.8; 95% CI = 1.3–6.1). Even greater risk was observed among nulliparous

| Table 1 Published case reports of ovarian cancer associated with ovulation induction | | | | |
|---|---|---|---|---|
| Author | Year | Age (years) | Histology | Ovulation induction regimen |
| Bamford and Steele[50] | 1982 | 32 | Endometrioid | hMG 11 cycles |
| Atlas and Menczer[51] | 1982 | 26 | Serous LMP | Clomiphene citrate |
| Ben-Hur et al[52] | 1986 | 27 | Serous LMP | Clomiphene citrate |
| | 1986 | 22 | Serous | Clomiphene citrate 3 cycles |
| Kulkarni and McGarry[53] | 1989 | 34 | Serous | Clomiphene citrate 3 cycles, cyclofenil |
| Dietl[54] | 1991 | 34 | Serous | Clomiphene citrate '1 year', hMG one cycle |
| Goldberg and Runowicz[55] | 1992 | 28 | Serous LMP | hMG 2 cycles |
| Balasch and Barri[56] | 1993 | 35 | Serous LMP | Clomiphene citrate 6 cycles |
| Karlan et al[57] | 1994 | 39 | Serous | Clomiphene citrate 5 cycles |
| Salle et al[58] | 1997 | Unk | Serous LMP | Clomiphene citrate 6 cycles |
| | 1997 | 29 | Mucinous LMP | Clomiphene citrate 6 cycles |

LMP, low malignant potential; Unk, Unknown.

infertile women using fertility drugs compared with nulligravid controls (OR = 2.7; 95% CI = 2.3–315.6). In contrast, infertile women who did not use fertility drugs were found to have no increased risk (OR = 0.9; 95% CI = 0.66–1.3).

This report received a great deal of criticism mainly with regard to methodological issues.[66–68] The major disadvantages included selection bias, wide confidence intervals and lack of information regarding the aetiology of infertility, and the specific medication used. In addition, no attempt was made to control for confounders such as infertility itself or family history of ovarian cancer. The main concern, however, was the temporal incompatibility between treatment for infertility and the licensing of modern fertility drugs in relation to the study period.[67,69] Clomiphene citrate was registered in 1967, and human menopausal gonadotrophin (hMG) was registered in 1969; thus those subjects in the Whittemore report who were treated for infertility during the late 1950s and early 1960s were exposed to pituitary irradiation[70] (which, according to RS Finkler, was a universally accepted procedure), pregnant mare serum gonadotrophins[71] and diethylstilboestrol,[72] none of which is used currently.[67]

Rossing et al[73] examined the risk of ovarian cancer among a cohort of 3837 women evaluated for infertility between 1974 and 1985. Eleven cases of ovarian cancer were observed and compared with 135 randomly selected infertile controls, matched for age and time of enrollment. Nine ovarian cancer patients were exposed to clomiphene, five of whom had used clomiphene for 12 or more monthly cycles. The analysis revealed that prolonged use of clomiphene was associated with a statistically significant increased risk for ovarian cancer (OR = 11.1; 95% CI = 1.5–82.3). By contrast, women exposed to fewer cycles of clomiphene or to other infertility treatments, such as hMG or human chorionic gonadotrophin (hCG), did not demonstrate a significant association with ovarian cancer development.

The strength of this study lies in the selection of the infertile cohort for both study and control patients and that data were abstracted from medical files, thus avoiding recall bias. However, a wide variety of tumours was considered to be 'ovarian cancer' (four invasive, five borderline and two granulosa cell tumours), whereas it is not clear whether these tumours can be biologically grouped together.[74] In addition, the association between cancer diagnosis and clomiphene might be the result of detection bias, because women on repeated clomiphene cycles will be exposed to more examinations by ultrasonography. Another concern is that infertile women using clomiphene for one to eleven cycles had demonstrated no increased risk for ovarian cancer (relative risk, RR = 0.8; 95% Cl = 0.1–5.7). If the relationship between clomiphene use and ovarian cancer was truly causal, a more evident dose–response relationship would have been expected.[44,69,75]

Preliminary results of an ongoing case–control study in Italy[76] revealed no increased risk of ovarian cancer associated with exposure to fertility drugs (OR = 0.73; 95% Cl = 0.16–3.30). This study included only two of 195 cases and 15 of 1339 controls which ever used fertility drugs during a period when clomiphene was used relatively rarely.

Shushan et al,[77] in another case–control study, interviewed 200 living women with histologically confirmed diagnosis of ovarian cancer and 408 controls who lived in the same areas based on the local telephone area codes. The risk for ovarian cancer was found to be increased in the subgroup of women with borderline tumours who had used any fertility drugs (OR = 3.52; 95% Cl = 1.23–10.09) and particularly in those who used hMG (OR = 9.38; 95% Cl = 1.66–52.08). No excess risk was observed in women exposed to clomiphene or to a combination of clomiphene and hMG, thus contradicting previous reports. Only patients who were alive during the study period were interviewed, thus implying that the result may be relevant only to the less severe cases of ovarian cancer. This also supports the large proportion of borderline malignancies included as cases.

Recently, Mosgaard et al[78] published the results of a case-control study based on the nationwide and public registries in Denmark. Included in the analysis were 684 cases of ovarian cancer that were diagnosed during the period 1989–94 and 1721 age-matched population controls. Among parous as well as nulliparous women, treatment with fertility drugs did not increase the risk for ovarian cancer compared with non-treated infertile women (OR = 0.8; 95% Cl = 0.4–2.0 and OR = 0.6; 95% Cl = 0.2–1.3, respectively).

Modan et al[79] updated the cohort analysis of Ron et al[64] with an additional 10 years of follow-up, reaching more than 50 000 womenyears. The cohort consisted of 2496 infertile Israeli women who were followed for cancer development through 1991. Twelve cases of ovarian cancer were observed compared with the 7.2 that would be expected in the population matched for age and ethnic origin (SIR = 1.6; 95% Cl = 0.8–2.9). Sensitivity analysis revealed that nulliparity by itself might explain these findings.

The most prominent excess risk for ovarian cancer was evident in the subgroup of women with mechanical or male-related infertility and normal ovulatory cycles (SIR = 2.7; 95% Cl = 1.0–6.0). The risk for ovarian cancer was similar among patients treated with any ovulation-induced agent compared with untreated patients (SIR 1.7 vs 1.6). Patients treated with clomiphene only revealed a borderline significant excess risk of ovarian cancer (SIR = 2.7; 95% Cl = 0.97–5.8), although the data are based on a small number of cases.

The possible link between ovulation-inducing drugs and ovarian cancer might not necessarily be a causal one, but rather the enhancement or stimulation of an already existing lesion. Bandera et al[80] described a case of a nulliparous patient diagnosed and treated for ovarian cancer before the start of ovulation-induction treatments for infertility. Shortly after ovulation induction she suffered tumour recurrence. Additional case reports by Karlan et al[57] revealed two patients diagnosed with ovarian cancer, one during infertility evaluation and one shortly after the start of treatment.

Recently, another two cases of ovarian cancer

in infertile women were published by Salle et al.[58] One case described a woman who had an ovarian cyst before treatment which enlarged under induction of ovulation. In the second case, during the first ultrasonography at the start of the cycle an ovarian cyst was discovered, and proved to be malignant before the start of treatment. The report concluded that the presence of an ovarian cyst, or any other ovarian pathology, before treatment should be closely observed.

All of these cases were observed in women with limited exposure to ovulation induction, thus implying that the treatment was merely coincidental to their pre-existing ovarian tumour, which could be more clinically evident during the treatment, or may even be the cause of the infertility.[69]

In vitro fertilization (IVF) procedures include not only ovarian hyperstimulation but also repeated minor trauma for ovum pick-up. Multiple case reports showed ovarian cancer among women treated with IVF, mostly during or shortly after a small number of treatment cycles[55,81–84] (Table 2). Venn et al[85] examined the incidence of breast and ovarian cancer in a cohort of 10 358 women referred to IVF treatment between 1978 and 1982. The 'exposed' group of 5564 women had had ovarian stimulation to induce multiple folliculogenesis,

whereas the 'unexposed' group of 4794 women had been referred for IVF but were untreated or had had 'natural cycle' treatment without ovarian stimulation. They observed no excess risk for ovarian cancer in the treated compared with the untreated group (RR = 1.45, 95% Cl = 0.28–7.55). Women with unexplained infertility, independent of IVF exposure, had significantly increased risk for ovarian cancer compared with women with known causes of infertility (RR = 19.19; 95% Cl = 2.23–165.0). J Dor, L Lerner-Geva, J Rabinovici, A Chetrit, B Lunenfeld, S Mashiach and B Modan (unpublished data) assessed the incidence of cancer among all 1254 women who participated in an IVF treatment programme between 1981 and 1992 and compared them with the general population matched for sex, age and ethnic origin. Not even a single case of ovarian cancer was observed.

Close medical surveillance and repeated ultrasonographic examination may explain the incidental diagnosis of ovarian cancer during treatment with IVF. Large cohort studies have still failed to prove an assocation between ovulation induction in IVF and ovarian cancer development. The relatively short follow-up available since the introduction of IVF[86] allows only limited conclusions to be drawn.

| Table 2 Published case reports of ovarian cancer associated with IVF | | | | |
|---|---|---|---|---|
| **Author** | **Year** | **Age (years)** | **Histology** | **Number of IVF cycles** |
| Carter and Joyce[81] | 1987 | 25 | Serous | 3 |
| Goldberg and Runowicz[55] | 1992 | 32 | Serous LMP | 2 |
| | 1992 | 25 | Serous LMP | 3 |
| Nijman et al[82] | 1992 | 38 | Serous LMP | 2 |
| Lopes and Mensier[83] | 1993 | 37 | Serous LMP | 5 |
| Grimbizis et al[84] | 1995 | 32 | Serous LMP | 1 |

LMP, low malignant potential.

## BREAST CANCER

Breast cancer is the leading cancer in women, with an incidence of 80 new cases per 100 000 population per year.[11] The risk for breast cancer has been associated with family history and genetic mutations of the *BRCA* genes,[87] higher socio- economic status, nulliparity and late age at first pregnancy.[88,89] The use of oral contraceptives (especially in breast cancer diagnosed in young women) and the use of hormonal replacement therapy as risk factors for breast cancer remain controversial.[90–92]

Cowan et al[93] examined breast cancer incidence in infertile women, treated between 1945 and 1965. They identified 17 cases of breast cancer and concluded that 'progesterone deficiency' infertility may be associated with increased risk of premenopausal breast cancer. Another study[94] of a cohort of infertile women revealed 12 cases of breast cancer compared with the 8.25 expected, but the excess was limited to postmenopausal women. Ron et al[64] followed a cohort of 2632 infertile women and observed 15 cases of breast cancer compared with the 14.14 expected. No association between specific subgroups of infertility and breast cancer risk was noted. Other studies also failed to observe excess risk of breast cancer among infertile women.[95,96]

Ovulation induction could possibly be associated with breast cancer risk. High progesterone levels produced during the simultaneous ovulation of multiple follicles, combined with higher oestrogen levels during the follicular phase of ovulation-induction cycles, may expose infertile women to an environment that could have the potential for the development of breast cancer.[4] However, one commonly used ovulation-inducing agent, clomiphene citrate, is structurally similar to tamoxifen and, like tamoxifen, has been reported to exert antiproliferative effects on human breast cancer cells.[97]

Laing et al[98] published a case report of nulliparous woman with infiltrating ductal breast cancer which was diagnosed shortly after two failed IVF cycles. Bilateral breast cancer associated with clomiphene exposure was published even earlier.[99] Another case report[100] described a patient with family history of breast cancer who developed an early onset breast cancer after four cycles of IVF.

Brzezinski et al[101] examined 950 patients treated with ovulation induction and observed 16 cases of breast cancer. The excess risk was crudely calculated to be 2.2 times the national average rate for breast cancer (with no confidence intervals given). On the contrary, Rossing et al[102] found no excess risk for breast cancer among a large cohort of infertile women when compared with population rates. Moreover, treatment with clomiphene citrate appeared to reduce the risk relative to patients who did not use this drug (SIR = 0.5; 95% CI = 0.2–1.2). Braga et al[103] again observed no excess risk for breast cancer among women who reported receiving infertility treatments compared with those who did not (OR = 1.08; 95% CI = 0.8–1.5).

Modan et al[79] currently updated the analysis previously published by Ron et al,[64] revealing 59 breast cancer cases versus the 46.6 expected (SIR = 1.3; 95% CI = 0.96–1.6) more than 21 years after infertility treatments. A non-significant excess risk was confined to women with 'progesterone deficiency' infertility and infertility of unknown cause (SIR = 1.4; 95% CI = 0.9–2.1 and SIR = 1.5; 95% CI = 0.9–2.3, respectively). Most cases of breast cancer (*n* = 34) were observed among women who were not treated with ovulation induction (SIR = 1.4; 95% CI = 1.0–2.0).

The incidence of breast cancer among women exposed to IVF was assessed by Venn et al.[85] No excess risk for breast cancer was observed in the entire cohort of infertile women (SIR = 0.89; 95% CI = 0.55–1.46), as well as among subgroups of infertile women. J Dor, L Lerner-Geva, J Rubinovici, A Chetrit, B Lunenfeld, S Mashiach and B Modan (unpublished data) examined cancer incidence among 1254 women treated with IVF between 1981 and 1992. Six cases of breast cancer were observed compared with the 3.43 expected (SIR = 1.75; 95% CI = 0.64–3.81), most of them shortly after the IVF treatments. Women of Asian–African origin had the most profound risk for breast cancer (SIR = 4.65; 95% CI = 0.93–13.48), especially when they failed to conceive after IVF (SIR = 6.52; 95% CI = 1.31–19.06). However, the unique multiparity tradition among this specific ethnic group may be a strong protective factor, which does not benefit infertile women.[104,105]

According to the reviewed literature, no excess risk for breast cancer can be attributed to ovulation induction. On the contrary, some agents, such as clomiphene citrate, could be considered protective because of their similarity to tamoxifen. Again, diagnosis of breast cancer during or shortly after infertility treatment should warrant close medical surveillance before and during such treatments.

## ENDOMETRIAL CANCER

Excluding breast cancer, endometrial cancer is the most frequently occurring cancer of the reproductive tract among women.[11,106] Case series and epidemiological studies have identified an association between infertility and endometrial cancer.[107–109]

Escobedo et al[110] investigated the association between specific subgroups of infertility and endometrial cancer. Compared with women who had no infertility problem, women with diagnosed infertility had an increased risk for endometrial cancer (OR = 1.7; 95% Cl = 1.1–2.6). The risk was more profound among women who reported infertility resulting from ovarian factors (OR = 4.2; 95% Cl = 1.7–10.4). In addition, there is no doubt that the risk for endometrial cancer in all women, whether or not infertile, increases considerably when unopposed oestrogen is administered.[91,111,112] A three- to five-fold increased risk is observed after exposure to unopposed oestrogen for more than 5 years, and the risk continues to rise the longer the oestrogen is used.[113]

Ron et al[64] observed five cases of endometrial cancer compared with the 1.05 expected (SIR = 4.8; 95% Cl = 1.7–10.6) among a cohort of infertile women. Four of these cases were diagnosed in women with hormonal infertility (anovulatory cycles, amenorrhoea, oligomenorrhoea or irregular periods) (SIR = 8.0; 95% Cl = 2.5–19.3). A current update on this cohort[79] observed 21 cases of endometrial cancer compared with the 4.3 expected, thus revealing a

similar excess risk (SIR = 4.8; 95% Cl = 3.0–7.4). Confounding by nulliparity, obesity and oral contraceptive use or hysterectomy could not explain this increased risk ratio, which was limited to women with the hormonal status of unopposed oestrogen (SIR = 9.4; 95% Cl = 5.0–16.0). The risk for endometrial cancer was not found to be significantly different among women treated with ovulation induction versus untreated women (SIR = 6.8; 95% Cl = 3.6–11.5 and SIR = 3.3; 95% Cl = 1.4–6.6, respectively).

The study by Venn et al,[85] who investigated cancer incidence among IVF-treated women, also observed an excess risk of endometrial cancer among women who were not exposed to treatment (SIR = 3.48; 95% Cl = 1.12–10.8). The risk was even greater for women with unexplained infertility (SIR = 6.34; 95% Cl = 1.06–38.0).

Endometrial cancer presents with higher incidence rates among infertile women in general, and those with unopposed oestrogen status in particular. The excess risk remains the same even after long periods of follow-up and does not seem to be related to ovulation induction. Nevertheless, special attention should be made during follow-up for the early detection of this malignancy.

## MELANOMA

Increased risk for melanoma associated with infertility characteristics, such as late age at first birth and nulliparity, has been observed in some case-control studies, but not in others.[114–118] A cohort study by Brinton et al[96] observed an increased risk for melanoma among a subgroup of infertile women with progesterone deficiency compared with other types of infertility. Ron et al[64] observed a non-significant twofold increase in the risk for melanoma, which was limited to women with hormonal infertility. This risk was abolished in a recent update[79] that observed eight melanoma cases compared with the 7.0 expected (SIR = 1.1).

Kuppens et al[119] were the first to report a case of multiple primary melanomas after almost 2 years of treatment with clomiphene citrate in a woman with familial dysplastic naevus syndrome. Rossing et al[120] observed 12 cases of melanoma among a cohort of infertile women; this was greater than expected but not significant (SIR = 1.8; 95% CI = 0.9–3.1). Women with ovulatory problems and women who have received more than 12 cycles of clomiphene citrate were at increased risk (SIR = 2.4; 95% CI = 0.9–5.1 and SIR = 2.2; 95% CI = 0.5–10.2).

All of these reports analyse small numbers of melanoma cases, giving rise to difficulties in assessment of the possible association with infertility or infertility treatments. In addition, women who seek treatment for infertility may differ from the general population with respect to access and use of health care services, and these differences may lead to earlier diagnosis of melanoma. This possibility is emphasized by the results reported by Ron et al[64] who observed an increase risk for melanoma which disappeared with a longer follow-up period.[79]

## CONCLUSION

Although the risk of cancer of all sites combined does not appear to be increased among infertile women, an elevated risk of endometrial cancer, particularly among women with infertility of hormonal origin, has been observed repeatedly. Cancer of the ovary has also been associated with a history of infertility, but the results are less consistent. Whether there is an association between the risk of breast cancer and infertility is not clear at this time.

According to the literature published to date, and our long-term results,[79,121] no excess risk for cancer development could be attributed to ovulation-inducing drugs by themselves. When adding assisted reproductive techniques to ovulation induction, it seems that similar conclusions might be drawn. However, the short follow-up allows only limited conclusions to be drawn, until the women reach their peak incidence years.

Taking into consideration the short latency periods that were observed between ovulation induction and cancer diagnosis, it seems justified to recommend that, before ovulation induction, any ovarian pathology should be excluded. Moreover, clinical examination of the breast is also warranted.

Infertile women with unopposed oestrogen status should be considered a high-risk group for endometrial cancer, independent of ovulation-induction treatments. They should be followed closely during their reproductive life and after its cessation.

## REFERENCES

1. Mosher WD, Pratt WF. Fecundity and infertility in the United States: incidence and trends. *Fertil Steril* 1991;**56**:192–8.
2. Friedlaner M, de Souza P, Segelov E. Risk factors, epidemiology, screening and prognostic factors in female genital cancer. *Curr Opin Oncol* 1992;**4**:913–22.
3. Johannes CB, Caro JJ, Hartz SC, Marrs R. Adverse effects of ovulatory stimulants: A review. *Assist Reprod Rev* 1993;**3**:68–74.
4. Schenker JG, Ezra Y. Complications of assisted reproductive techniques. *Fertil Steril* 1994;**61**:411–22.
5. Schenker JG, Laufer N, Weinstein D, Yarkoni S.

Quintuplet pregnancies. *Eur J Obstet Gynecol Reprod Biol* 1980;**10**:257–68.
6. Hack M, Brish M, Serr D, et al. Outcome of pregnancy after induced ovulation. Follow-up of pregnancies and children born after clomiphene therapy. *JAMA* 1973;**220**:1329–33.
7. Oelsner G, Menashe Y, Tur-Kaspa I, et al. The role of gonatropins in the etiology of ectopic pregnancy. *Fertil Steril* 1989;**52**:514–16.
8. Bider D, Menashe Y, Oelsner D, et al. Ovarian hyperstimulation syndrome due to exogenous gonadotropin administration. *Acta Obstet Gynecol Scand* 1989;**68**:511–14.
9. Schenker J, Weinstein D. Ovarian hyperstimula-

tion syndrome: A current survey. *Fertil Steril* 1978;**30:**255–61.

10. Navot D, Relou A, Birkenfeld A, et al. Risk factors and prognostic variables in the ovarian hyperstimulation syndrome. *Am J Obstet Gynecol* 1988;**159:**210–15.

11. Parkin DM, Muir CS, Whelan SL, et al. *Cancer Incidence in Five Continents*, Vol. VI. Lyon: IARC Scientific Publications, no. 120, 1992.

12. Heintz AP, Hacker NF, Lagasse LD. Epidemiology and etiology of ovarian cancer: A review. *Obstet Gynecol* 1985;**66:**127–35.

13. Parazzini F, Franceschi S, La Vecchia C, Fasoli M. The epidemiology of ovarian cancer. *Gynecol Oncol* 1991;**43:**9–23.

14. Greene M, Clark J, Blayney D. The epidemiology of ovarian cancer. *Semin Oncol* 1984; **11:**209–26.

15. Mori M, Harabuchi I, Miyake H, et al. Reproductive, genetic, and dietary risk factors for ovarian cancer. *Am J Epidemiol* 1988; **128:**771–7.

16. West RO. Epidemiologic study of malignancies of the ovaries. *Cancer* 1966;**19:**1001–7.

17. Cramer DW, Welch WR, Scully RE, Wojciechowski CA. Ovarian cancer and talc: A case-control study. *Cancer* 1982;**50:**372–6.

18. McGowan L, Norris HJ, Hartge P, et al. Risk factors in ovarian cancer. *Eur J Gynaecol Oncol* 1988;**9:**195–9.

19. Joly DJ, Lilienfeld AM, Diamond EL, Bross ID. An epidemiologic study of the relationship of reproductive experience to cancer of the ovary. *Am J Epidemiol* 1974;**99:**190–209.

20. Lynch HT. Genetic risk in ovarian cancer. *Gynecol Oncol* 1992;**46:**1–3.

21. Schildkraut JM, Thompson WD. Familial ovarian cancer: population based case-control study. *Am J Epidemiol* 1988;**128:**456–66.

22. Lynch HT, Watson P, Lynch JF, et al. Hereditary ovarian cancer. Heterogeneity in age at onset. *Cancer* 1998;**71:**(suppl):573–81.

23. Easton DF, Bishop DT, Ford D, et al. Genetic linkage analysis in familial breast and ovarian cancer: results from 214 families. *Am J Hum Genet* 1993;**52:**678–701.

24. Demopoulos RI, Seltzer V, Dubin N, Gutman E. The association of parity and marital status with the development of ovarian carcinoma: clinical implications. *Obstet Gynecol* 1979;**54:**150–5.

25. Risch HA, Weiss NS, Lyon JL, et al. Events of reproductive life and the incidence of epi-

thelial ovarian cancer. *Am J Epidemiol* 1983;**117:**128–39.

26. Wu ML, Whittemore AS, Paffenbarger RJ, et al. Personal and environmental characteristics related to epithelial ovarian cancer. I. Reproductive and menstrual events and oral contraceptive use. *Am J Epidemiol* 1988;**128:**1216–27.

27. Gwinn ML, Lee NC, Rhodes PH, et al. Pregnancy, breast feeding, and oral contraceptives and the risk of epithelial ovarian cancer. *J Clin Epidemiol* 1990;**43:**559–68.

28. The Cancer and Steroid Hormone Study of the Centers for Disease Control and the National Institute of Child Health and Human Development. The reduction in risk of ovarian cancer associated with oral-contraceptive use. *N Engl J Med* 1987;**316:**650–5.

29. Rosenberg L, Shapiro S, Slone D, et al. Epithelial ovarian cancer and combination oral contraceptives. *JAMA* 1982;**247:**3210–12.

30. Booth M, Beral V, Smith P. Risk factors for ovarian cancer: a case-control study. *Br J Cancer* 1989;**60:**592–8.

31. Weiss NS. Measuring the separate effects of low parity and its antecedents on the incidence of ovarian cancer. *Am J Epidemiol* 1988; **128:**451–5.

32. Hartge P, Schiffman MH, Hoover R, et al. A case-control study of epithelial ovarian cancer. *Am J Obstet Gynecol* 1989;**161:**10–16.

33. Parazzini F, La Vecchia C, Negri E, Gentile A. Menstrual factors and the risk of epithelial ovarian cancer. *J Clin Epidemiol* 1989;**42:**443–8.

34. Nasca PC, Greenwald P, Chorost S, et al. An epidemiologic case-control study of ovarian cancer and reproductive factors. *Am J Epidemiol* 1984;**119:**705–13.

35. Whittemore AS, Wu ML, Paffenbarger RJ, et al. Epithelial ovarian cancer and the ability to conceive. *Cancer Res* 1989;**49:**4047–52.

36. Harlow BL, Weiss NS, Roth GJ, et al. Case-control study of borderline tumors: reproductive history and exposure to exogenous female hormones. *Cancer Res* 1988;**48:**5849–52.

37. Kvale G, Heuch I, Nilssen S, Beral V. Reproductive factors and risk of ovarian cancer: a prospective study. *Int J Cancer* 1988;**42:**246–51.

38. Franceschi S, La Vecchia C, Helmrich SP, et al. Risk factors for epithelial ovarian cancer in Italy. *Am J Epidemiol* 1982;**115:**714–19.

39. Fathalla MF. Incessant ovulation – a factor in ovarian neoplasia? *Lancet* 1971;**ii:**163.

40. Zajicek J. Prevention of ovarian cystomas by

inhibition of ovulation: a new concept. *J Reprod Med* 1978;**2**:114.

41. Casagrande JT, Louie EW, Pike MC, et al. 'Incessant ovulation' and ovarian cancer. *Lancet* 1979;**ii**:170–3.

42. Stadel BV. The etiology and prevention of ovarian cancer. *Am J Obstet Gynecol* 1975;**123**:772.

43. Daly MB. The epidemiology of ovarian cancer. *Hematol Oncol Clinics North Am* 1992;**6**:729–38.

44. Bristow RE, Karlan BY. Ovulation induction, infertility and ovarian cancer risk. *Fertil Steril* 1996;**66**:499–507.

45. Cramer DW, Welch WR. Determinants of ovarian cancer risk. II. Inferences regarding pathogenesis. *J Natl Cancer Instit* 1983;**71**:717–21.

46. Goldberg NB, Scully AL. Gonadal malignance in gonadal dysgenesis: Papillary pseudo-mucinous cystadenocarcinoma in a patient with Turner's syndrome. *J. Clin Endocrinol Metab* 1967;**27**:341–7.

47. Miller DS, Teng N, Ballon S. Epithelial ovarian carcinoma in patient with intersex disorders: The role of pituitary gonadotropins in ovarian tumorigenesis. *Gynecol Oncol* 1986;**24**:229–308.

48. Mohle J, Whittemore A, Pike M, et al. Gonadotropins and ovarian cancer risk. *J Natl Cancer Instit* 1985;**75**:178–9.

49. Stein DE, Santoro N. Infertility, gonadotrophins and ovarian cancer. *Infertil Manag* 1997;**8**:289–303.

50. Bamford PN, Steele SJ. Uterine and ovarian carcinoma in a patient receiving gonadotrophin therapy. Case report. *Br J Obstet Gynaecol* 1982;**89**:962–4.

51. Atlas M, Menczer J. Massive hyperstimulation and borderline carcinoma of the ovary. A possible association. *Acta Obstet Gynaecol Scand* 1982;**61**:261–3.

52. Ben-Hur H, Dgani R, Lancet M, et al. Ovarian carcinoma masquerading as ovarian hyperstimulation syndrome. *Acta Obstet Gynaecol Scand* 1986;**65**:813–14.

53. Kulkarni R, McGarry JM. Follicular stimulation and ovarian cancer. *BMJ* 1989;**229**:740.

54. Dietl J. Ovulation and ovarian cancer. *Lancet* 1991;**338**:445.

55. Goldberg GL, Runowicz CD. Ovarian carcinoma of low malignant potential, infertility, and induction of ovulation – is there a link? *Am J Obstet Gynecol* 1992;**166**:853–4.

56. Balasch J, Barri PN. Follicular stimulation and ovarian cancer? *Hum Reprod* 1993;**8**:990–6.

57. Karlan BY, Marrs R, Lagasse LD. Advanced-stage ovarian carcinoma presenting during infertility evaluation. *Am J Obstet Gynecol* 1994;**171**:1377–8.

58. Salle B, de Saint Hilaire P, Devouassoux M, et al. Another two cases of ovarian tumours in women who had undergone multiple ovulation induction cycles. *Hum Reprod* 1997;**12**:1732–5.

59. Kaufman SC, Spirtas R, Alexander NJ. Do fertility drugs cause ovarian tumors? *J Women's Hlth* 1995;**4**:247–59.

60. Whittemore AS, Harris R, Itnyre J, Halpern J. Characteristics relating to ovarian cancer risk: collaborative analysis of 12 US case-control studies. I. Methods. Collaborative Ovarian Cancer Group. *Am J Epidemiol* 1992;**136**:1175–83.

61. Whittemore AS, Harris R, Itnyre J. Characteristics relating to ovarian cancer risk: collaborative analysis of 12 US case-control studies. II. Invasive epithelial ovarian cancers in white women. Collaborative Ovarian Cancer Group. *Am J Epidemiol* 1992;**136**:1184–203.

62. Whittemore AS, Harris R, Itnyre J. Characteristics relating to ovarian cancer risk: collaborative analysis of 12 US case-control studies. IV. The pathogenesis of epithelial ovarian cancer. Collaborative Ovarian Cancer Group. *Am J Epidemiol* 1992;**136**:1212–20.

63. Harris R, Whittemore AS, Itnyre J. Characteristics relating to ovarian cancer risk: collaborative analysis of 12 US case-control studies. III. Epithelial tumors of low malignant potential in white women. Collaborative Ovarian Cancer Group. *Am J Epidemiol* 1992;**136**:1204–11.

64. Ron E, Lunenfeld B, Menczer J, et al. Cancer incidence in a cohort of infertile women. *Am J Epidemiol* 1987;**125**:780–90.

65. Shu XO, Brinton LA, Gao YT, Yuan JM. Population-based case-control study of ovarian cancer in Shanghai. *Cancer Res* 1989;**49**:3670–4.

66. Spirtas R, Kaufman SC, Alexander NJ. Fertility drugs and ovarian cancer: red alert or red herring? *Fertil Steril* 1993;**59**:291–3.

67. Cohen J, Forman R, Harlap S, et al. IFFS experts group report on the Whittemore study related to the risk of ovarian cancer associated with the use of fertility agents. *Hum Reprod* 1993;**8**:996–9.

68. Walters DE. Ovarian cancer and pregnancy: comment on a paper by Whittemore et al. *Fertil Steril* 1994;**61**:239–42.

69. Shoham Z. Epidemiology, etiology and fertility drugs in ovarian epithelial carcinoma: Where are we today? *Fertil Steril* 1994;**62**:433–48.

70. Finkler RS. Evaluation of hormonal and radiation therapy in 190 cases of functional sterility and secondary amenorrhea. *J Obstet Gynecol* 1949;**58**:559–64.

71. Ryberg E. Gonadotropic hormones in gynecologic therapy. *Ugesk Laeger* 1939;**101**:375–82.

72. Swyer GI. Induction of ovulation in the human – older and newer approaches. *Proc R Soc Med* 1963;**56**:39–46.

73. Rossing MA, Daling JR, Weiss NS, et al. Ovarian tumors in a cohort of infertile women. *N Engl J Med* 1994;**331**:771–6.

74. Willemsen W, Kruitwagen R, Bastiaans B, et al. Ovarian stimulation and granulosa-cell tumors. *Lancet* 1993;**341**:986–8.

75. Del Priore G, Robischon K, Phipps WR. Risk of ovarian cancer after treatment for infertility. *N Engl J Med* 1995;**332**:1300.

76. Franceschi S, La Vecchia C, Negri E, et al. Fertility drugs and the risk of epithelial ovarian cancer in Italy. *Hum Reprod* 1994;**9**:1673–5.

77. Shushan A, Paltiel O, Ischovich J, et al. Human menopausal gonadotrophin and the risk of epithelial ovarian cancer. *Fertil Steril* 1996;**65**:13–18.

78. Mosgaard BJ, Lidegaard O, Kjaer SK, et al. Infertility, fertility drugs and invasive ovarian cancer: a case-control study. *Fertil Steril* 1997;**67**:1005–12.

79. Modan B, Ron E, Lerner-Geva L, et al. Cancer incidence in a cohort of infertile women. *Am J Epidemiol* 1998; in press.

80. Bandera CA, Cramer DA, Friedman AJ, Sheets EE. Fertility therapy in the setting of a history of invasive epithelial ovarian cancer. *Gynecol Oncol* 1995;**58**:116–18.

81. Carter ME, Joyce DN. Ovarian carcinoma in a patient hyperstimulated by gonadotrophin therapy for in vitro fertilization: a case report. *J In Vitro Fert Embryo Transf* 1987;**4**:126–8.

82. Nijman HW, Burger CW, Baak JPA, et al. Borderline malignancy of the ovary and controlled hyperstimulation. A report of 2 cases. *Eur J Cancer* 1992;**28**:1971–3.

83. Lopes P, Mensier A. Ovarian cancer and assisted reproductive technique. *Eur J Obstet Gynecol Reprod Biol* 1993;**51**:171–3.

84. Grimbizis G, Tarlatzis BC, Bontis J, et al. Two cases of ovarian tumors in women who had undergone multiple ovarian stimulation attempts. *Hum Reprod* 1995;**10**:520–3.

85. Venn A, Watson L, Lumley J, et al. Breast and ovarian cancer incidence after infertility and in-vitro fertilization. *Lancet* 1995;**346**:995–1000.

86. Edwards RG, Steptoe PC, Purdy JM. Establishing full-term human pregnancies using cleaving embryos grown in vitro. *Br J Obstet Gynaecol* 1980;**87**:737–68.

87. Couch FJ, DeShano ML, Blackwood A, et al. BRCA1 mutations in women attending clinics that evaluate the risk of breast cancer. *N Engl J Med* 1997;**336**:1409–15.

88. Westhoff C. Infertility and breast cancer. *Gynecol Oncol* 1996;**60**:1–2.

89. Gross J, Modan B, Bertini B, Spira D. Relationship between steroid secretion patterns and breast cancer incidence in Israeli women of various origin. *J Natl Cancer Instit* 1977;**59**:7–11.

90. Harlap S. Oral contraceptives and breast cancer. *J Reprod Med* 1991;**36**:374–95.

91. Wren B. Hormonal therapy and genital tract cancer. *Curr Opin Obstet Gynecol* 1996;**8**:38–41.

92. La Vecchia C, Negri E, Francesch S, et al. Oral contraceptives and breast cancer: a cooperative Italian study. *Int J Cancer* 1995;**60**:163–7.

93. Cowan LD, Gordis L, Tonascia J, Jones GS. Breast cancer incidence in women with history of progesterone deficiency. *Am J Epidemiol* 1981;**114**:209–17.

94. Coulam C, Annegers J, Kranz J. Chronic anovulation syndrome and associated neoplasia. *Obstet Gynecol* 1983;**61**:403–7.

95. Gammon M, Thompson WD. Infertility and breast cancer: A population-based case-control study. *Am J Epidemiol* 1990;**132**:708–16.

96. Brinton LA, Melton LJ, Malkasian GD, et al. Cancer risk after evaluation for infertility. *Am J Epidemiol* 1989;**129**:712–22.

97. Sutherland RL, Watts CKW, Hall RE, Ruenitz PC. Mechanisms of growth inhibition by non-steroidal anti-estrogens in human breast cancer cells. *J Steroid Biochem* 1987;**27**:891–7.

98. Laing RW, Glaser MG, Barret GSA. A case of breast carcinoma in association with in-vitro fertilization. *J R Soc Med* 1989;**82**:503.

99. Bolton PM. Bilateral breast cancer associated with clomiphene. *Lancet* 1977;**ii**:1952.

100. Albour L, Narod S, Glendon G, et al. In-vitro fertilization and family history of breast cancer. *Lancet* 1994;**344**:610–11.

101. Brzezinski A, Peretz T, Mor-Yosef S, Schenker JG. Ovarian stimulation and breast cancer: Is there a link? *Gynecol Oncol* 1994;**52**:292–5.

102. Rossing MA, Daling JR, Weiss MS, et al. Risk of breast cancer in a cohort of infertile women. *Gynecol Oncol* 1996;**60**:3–7.

103. Braga C, Negri E, La Vecchia C, et al. Fertility treatment and risk of breast cancer. *Hum Reprod* 1996;**11**:300–3.

104. Modan B. Role of ethnic background in cancer development. *Isr J Med Sci* 1974;**10**:1112–16.

105. Modan B. Role of migrant studies in understanding the etiology of cancer. *Am J Epidemiol* 1980;**112**:289–95.

106. Ludwig H. Women and cancer. *Int J Gynecol Obstet* 1994;**46**:195–202.

107. Kelsey JL, LiVolsi VA, Holford TR, et al. A case-control study of cancer of the endometrium. *Am J Epidemiol* 1982;**116**:333–42.

108. Vessey MP, Painter R. Endometrial and ovarian cancer and oral contraceptives – finding in a large cohort study. *Br J Cancer* 1995;**71**:1340–2.

109. Levi F, Franceschi S, Negri E, La Vecchia C. Dietary factors and the risk for endometrial cancer. *Cancer* 1993;**71**:3575–81.

110. Escobedo LG, Lee NC, Peterson HB, et al. Infertility-associated endometrial cancer risk may be limited to specific subgroups of infertile women. *Obstet Gynecol* 1991;**77**:124–8.

111. Smith DC, Prentice R, Thompson DL, Herrman WL. Association of exogenous estrogens and endometrial cancer. *N Engl J Med* 1975;**293**:1164–8.

112. Mack TM, Pike MC, Henderson BE, et al. Estrogens and endometrial cancer in retirement community. *N Engl J Med* 1976;**294**:1262–7.

113. Antunes CMF, Stolley PD, Rosenstein NB, et al. Endometrial cancer and estrogen use. *N Engl J Med* 1979;**300**:9–13.

114. Zanetti R, Franceschi S, Rosso S, et al. Cutaneous malignant melanoma in females: the role of hormonal and reproductive factors. *Int J Epidemiol* 1990;**19**:522–6.

115. Holly EA, Weiss NS, Liff JM. Cutaneous melanoma in relation to exogenous hormones and reproductive factors. *J Natl Cancer Instit* 1983;**70**:827–31.

116. Holman CDJ, Armstrong BK, Heenan PJ. Cutaneous malignant melanoma in women: exogenous sex hormones and reproductive factors. *Br J Cancer* 1984;**50**:673–80.

117. Gallaghar RP, Elwood JM, Hill GB, et al. Reproductive factors, oral contraceptive use and risk of malignant melanoma: Western Canada Melanoma Study. *Br J Cancer* 1985;**52**:901–7.

118. Osterlind A, Tucker MA, Stone BJ, Jensen OM. The Danish case-control study of cutaneous malignant melanoma. III. Hormonal and reproductive factors in women. *Int J Cancer* 1988;**42**:821–4.

119. Kuppens E, Bergman W, Welvaart K, et al. Multiple primary melanomas in a patient with familial-type DNS during clomiphene-induced pregnancy. *Melanoma Res* 1992;**2**:71–4.

120. Rossing MA, Daling JR, Weiss NS, et al. Risk of cutaneous melanoma in a cohort of infertile women. *Melanoma Res* 1995;**5**:123–7.

121. Ron E, Lunenfeld B. A review of infertility and its treatment in the etiology of female reproductive and other cancers. *J Women's Hlth* 1995;**4**:1–12.

# 31

# Benign ovarian teratomas (dermoid cysts): changing trends in management and impact on fertility

Benjamin Caspi, Asnat Groutz

**Clinical presentation and complications** • **Diagnosis** • **Fertility** • **Management**

Benign ovarian teratomas (dermoid cysts) are the most common type of ovarian germ cell tumours, accounting for about 25% and 50% of all ovarian neoplasms and benign ovarian tumours, respectively. The incidence of dermoid cysts is unknown. Westhoff et al,[1] in their population-based, case–control study, reported an annual incidence of 8.9 per 100 000 women. These tumours occur more frequently during the second and third decades of life, but have been reported to occur during childhood and after the menopause. In patients under 30 years of age, the growths account for 70% of benign ovarian tumours,[2] and are bilateral in 15% of affected patients. They are often composed of tissues of ectodermal, mesodermal and endodermal origin, although the ectodermal component is the most prominent. The typical cyst is filled with sebaceous material, degenerated squamous cells and hair. Other mature tissues, such as teeth or bones, may also be present.[3] Most of these tumours have a normal 46XX karyotype,[4] but mosaicism has been found in some.[5] It is generally accepted that dermoid cysts are of germ cell origin because of their histological, cytogenetic and biochemical features.

However, the precise histogenesis of these tumours remains controversial.[6,7]

The development of the dermoid is probably associated with an attempt of the germ cells to complete meiosis and to form a zygote within the ovary without the stimulus of fertilization.[8] Abnormalities at various stages in the meiotic process could result in cells from which a diploid tumour could arise. The trigger for these precocious divisions is unknown. Several investigators have suggested that ovarian teratomas may be caused by a failure of meiosis I,[7,8] whereas others suggested that they arise from a single germ cell after the first meiotic division with failure of meiosis II,[9–11] or from an endoreduplication of a mature ovum.[7] Some immature teratomas may also arise from fusion of two ova.[12] The entity of familial ovarian dermoids exists, and is probably associated with genetic factors. To date, 12 familial cases comprising 33 women have been described in the literature.[13]

## CLINICAL PRESENTATION AND COMPLICATIONS

Most patients with a dermoid cyst are asymptomatic. The tumour is typically an incidental finding during physical examination, imaging of the pelvis or surgery. In a recently published series of dermoid cysts, 90.7% of the cases were found incidentally during ultrasonography.[14] Radiological examination of the abdomen may demonstrate calcifications and, in some instances, even teeth, and transvaginal ultrasonography may facilitate an accurate diagnosis. Large dermoid cysts could cause vague symptoms of pelvic pressure, abdominal pain, or compression of the bladder or bowel.

Complications associated with dermoid cysts include torsion, rupture, fistula formation, infection, haemolytic anaemia and malignant transformation.[15–18] Torsion is the most common complication, occurring in up to 16% of cases;[15,16] it is found more frequently in dermoids of intermediate size, the small and the extremely large ones being less likely to be affected.[16,18] Comerci et al[19] reported a relatively low rate of torsion (3.4%) in a series of 517 women with dermoid cysts. In another series of 360 women with dermoid cysts, who were referred to our centre over the last decade, 220 were operated on for various indications. Among these, only six patients underwent surgery because of torsion; none had a cyst smaller than 6 cm (unpublished data). These data suggest that the risk of torsion is lower than previously estimated, and is most probably very low in dermoid cysts smaller than 6 cm. If the torsion is not too severe, only venous drainage may be affected. The resulting congestion could lead to haemorrhage, usually within the cyst itself. The congestion could also induce an inflammatory reaction in the cyst wall, leading to adhesions to neighbouring viscera.[16]

Rupture of a dermoid cyst is a rare complication, occurring in only 0.7–1.3% of cases.[15,16,20] Possible explanations for rupture include: partial torsion of the tumour, resulting in circulatory compromise and subsequent tumour wall necrosis; infection; malignant transformation; and mechanical factors.[21] Intraperitoneal rupture may cause an acute abdominal crisis as a result of chemical irritation of the peritoneum.[22] Recently, Coccia et al[23] reported a case of acute abdomen after dermoid cyst rupture during transvaginal ultrasonographically guided retrieval of oocytes. A slow leakage of the tumour contents after rupture could cause an extensive granulomatous peritoneal reaction, which cannot always be distinguished macroscopically from tuberculosis or carcinomatosis.[15,22] Adhesions of the tumour to adjacent organs and an inflammatory reaction may result in a fistula and drainage into various organs. Several reports documented spontaneous rupture of dermoid cysts into the urinary bladder, small bowel, rectum, sigmoid colon and vagina.[20,21]

Although pregnancy is believed to be associated with increased risk of dermoid complications, no such evidence could be found in the published data. Caruso et al[18] reported on 31 pregnancies among 295 patients with dermoid cysts. The rate of torsion during pregnancy was 6.5%, compared with 9.3% in non-pregnant patients. Likewise, no evidence was found concerning the possible increased incidence of infection, rupture or malignant transformation of dermoid cysts during pregnancy. Data collected from an expectant management programme of dermoid cysts,[14] conducted at the Kaplan Medical Centre, Israel, confirm these results. Forty-nine women with ultrasonographically diagnosed dermoid cysts smaller than 6 cm were followed up prospectively during pregnancy and delivery. The tumour growth rate was similar to that of the expected growth rate in non-pregnant women. Furthermore, none of the women developed any dermoid-related complications during pregnancy or delivery.[14]

### Growth rate

Caspi et al[14] prospectively evaluated the growth rate of ultrasonographically diagnosed small (< 6 cm) dermoid cysts in premenopausal and postmenopausal women. The growth rate in the premenopausal women was $1.77 \pm 3.86 \, mm/$ year. In the postmenopausal group, the growth rate was practically zero. The difference in the growth rate between the two groups was statistically significant. This difference may be attributed to oestrogen and progesterone deprivation in postmenopausal women. It has been suggested that ovarian dermoid cysts increase in size after puberty because of the hormonally induced growth of the sebaceous glands contained in these tumours.[24]

## Malignant transformation

Malignant transformation of a dermoid cyst is a rare event, occurring in 1–2% of all cases.[25,26] Some investigators are sceptical about this low percentage.[18,27] Caruso et al,[18] in a 20-year retrospective review of 305 consecutive ovarian teratomas, found the incidence of malignant teratomas to be 2.95%. Chadha and Schaberg[27] recommended that any thick area in the wall of a dermoid cyst be selected and sectioned for histology, to avoid inaccurate diagnosis. Any of the tissues present in a dermoid cyst may undergo malignant transformation, and subsequently a wide variety of malignancies have been reported. Squamous cell carcinoma is the most common (75%) malignancy encountered, followed by adenocarcinoma and carcinoids.[27–30]

The frequency of malignant transformation is related to age. Dermoid cysts with malignant transformation are rarely found in young women. Over 75% of the patients are aged over 40 years, the average age being 50.[27–29] The frequency of malignant transformation is most probably also related to the size of the tumour. Caruso et al[18] found the average size of the malignant lesions to be about threefold larger than the average benign cystic teratoma.

Malignant cystic teratomas are rarely recognized preoperatively because of the similarity of clinical symptoms to those of uncomplicated mature cystic teratomas. Kimura et al[31] evaluated the efficacy of a squamous cell carcinoma-associated antigen, TA-4, as a tumour marker for diagnosis and monitoring of patients with squamous cell carcinoma arising in mature cystic teratoma. Five of the six cases studied showed an elevated level of TA-4 in the sera obtained preoperatively. No elevated TA-4 level was detected in the sera of 28 patients with benign dermoids. Moreover, serial determinations of the serum TA-4 level showed a good correlation between the clinical course and the serum TA-4 level. Thus, measurement of TA-4 in the sera of women who have been clinically diagnosed as having a dermoid cyst may be a useful aid for diagnosing and monitoring patients with malignant transformation.

## DIAGNOSIS

Until recently, diagnosis of ovarian dermoid cysts was made at laparoscopy or laparotomy undertaken because of an adnexal mass. With the use of high-resolution ultrasonic equipment and the experience gained by ultrasonographers, diagnosis of a dermoid cyst is now possible before surgery. The typical sonographic signs of a benign ovarian cystic teratoma include a dermoid plug,[32] 'tip of an iceberg',[33] fat–fluid level,[34] cysts with a pearl-grey appearance[35] and dermoid mesh.[36] Recently, Caspi et al[37] suggested a new, simple classification of the pathognomonic echo patterns of ovarian cystic teratoma. The characteristic echo patterns were classified into three major groups (I–III), with a subclassification of the first group into further three subgroups (Ia, Ib and Ic):

*Ia* – an echogenic mass in which the borders of the tumour are clearly visible (Figure 1).
*Ib* – an echogenic mass in which most of the tumour is visible, except its distal border (Figure 2).
*Ic* – an echogenic mass in which only the border of the tumour proximal to the transducer is seen, producing a 'tip of an iceberg' effect (Figure 3).
*II* – the presence of echogenic particles in a hypoechoic medium, creating a 'mesh-like' appearance within the tumour (Figure 4).

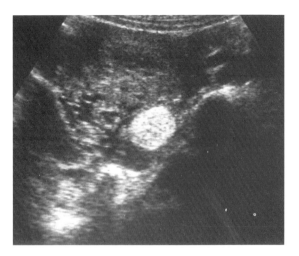

**Figure 1** An echogenic mass in which the borders of the tumour are clearly visible (classification Ia). (With permission from reference 37.)

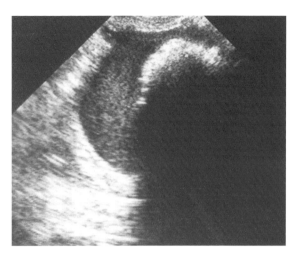

**Figure 3** An echogenic mass in which only the border of the tumour proximal to the transducer is seen, producing a 'tip of an iceberg' effect (classification Ic). (With permission from reference 37.)

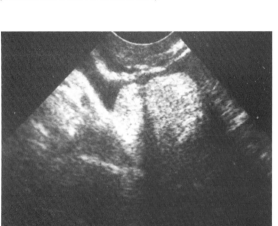

**Figure 2** An echogenic mass in which most of the tumour is visible, except its distal border (classification Ib). (With permission from reference 37.)

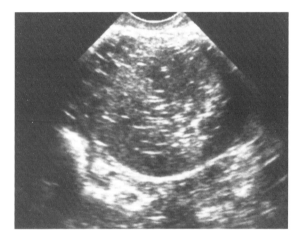

**Figure 4** The presence of echogenic particles in a hypoechoic medium, creating a 'mesh-like' appearance with the tumour (classification II). (With permission from reference 37.)

*III* – a cyst with a fat–fluid level (Figure 5).

Schematic representation of this classification is shown in Figure 6.

The appearance of an acoustic shadow, when present together with one of these typical echo patterns, should further strengthen the ultrasonographic diagnosis of dermoid cysts. In a prospective study of 118 echogenic adnexal masses with postoperative histological confirmation, this classification facilitated the correct diagnosis in 115 cases (accuracy rate, 97.45%). This high rate of accuracy in ultrasonographic diagnosis of dermoid cysts was also confirmed in two studies.[38,39]

Doppler flow characteristics of dermoid cysts

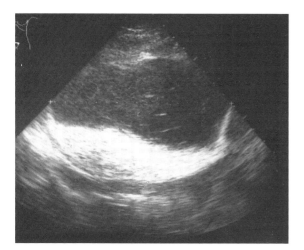

**Figure 5** A cyst with a fat–fluid level (classification III). (With permission from reference 37.)

were evaluated by Zalel et al.[40] In 74 dermoid cysts, when blood flow patterns were detected (detection rate, 24.3%), they were obtained only from the ovarian tissue surrounding the dermoid cavity, with a mean resistance index (RI) of $0.6 \pm 0.1$. In four cases, which proved postoperatively to be the stroma of the ovary, blood flow was detected not only from the cyst capsule, but also from the centrally positioned solid area, with a mean RI of $0.565 \pm 0.08$. Therefore, when apparently vascularized solid

tissue is detected in the central part of an ultrasonographically suspected dermoid, it is highly likely to be the stroma of the ovary.

## FERTILITY

Data about possible associations between ovarian dermoid cysts and female fertility are scarce. Westhoff et al[1] compared 120 women with pathologically confirmed dermoid cysts with 119 age-matched controls. Patients with dermoid cysts reported slightly later menarche. By 14 years of age, 44% of the patients, compared with only 31% of controls, did not have regular cycles ($p = 0.04$). Furthermore, patients with dermoids were less likely to report regular 27- to 31-day cycles. Although both groups (patients and controls) began sexual activity at similar ages and used oral contraceptives for similar durations, there were significantly fewer pregnancies ($p = 0.0004$) and children ($p = 0.003$) in the dermoid group. The difference in number of pregnancies persisted after adjusting for age at marriage. Infertile patients in the dermoid group reported a longer time to achieving pregnancy, compared with infertile controls (an average of 60 months versus 49 months, respectively). The authors suggested that both the infertility and the irregular menses reported by their study population may

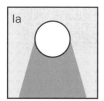
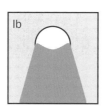
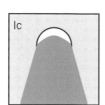
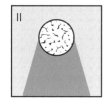
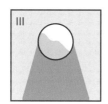

**Figure 6**
I, An echogenic mass of varying density and shadowing:
a, all the borders are visible;
b, the distal border is not visible;
c, only the proximal border is visible ('tip of the iceberg')
II, Echogenic thin bond-like echoes ('dermoid mesh')
III, Fat/fluid level
(With permission from reference 37.)

have reflected some underlying hormonal abnormality, which also led to growth of the tumour. Alternatively, the preclinical tumour may have caused some local ovarian dysfunction many years before diagnosis.

Caspi et al[14] reported the follow-up results of five patients who conceived after ovulation induction with the dermoid cysts in situ. All tumours were less than 6 cm in diameter. The patients were followed up conservatively by serial ultrasonographic examinations during ovulation induction and pregnancy. Two of these women received therapy for ovulation induction with gonadotrophin, and three conceived after in vitro fertilization–embryo transfer (IVF/ET). Ovulation was induced by treatment with gonadotrophin-releasing hormone agonists and gonadotrophin. In all five patients, the size of the dermoid cysts remained stable during treatment. In the three patients who were treated with IVF/ET, the dermoid cysts were not punctured during the procedure. All the pregnancies were uneventful and resulted in healthy infants.

## MANAGEMENT

### Surgery

Cystectomy with conservation of the remaining ovarian tissue has become the standard of care in the management of dermoid tumours in women of reproductive age. Laparoscopic cystectomy for removal of dermoid cysts has been used increasingly as a result of the enhanced diagnostic accuracy of current radiological modalities and the decrease in morbidity and hospital stay associated with laparoscopy. Three laparoscopy techniques can be used when treating dermoid cysts:[41] intraperitoneal cystectomy, transparietal cystectomy and ovariectomy. Intraperitoneal cystectomy is the optimum treatment in women of reproductive age. Radical treatment is indicated under two circumstances: difficulty with conservative treatment and in patients over 40 years. Transparietal cystectomy is best reserved for specific voluminous dermoid cysts. The laparoscopic technique reduces

hospitalization and recovery time;[41–43] however, it is associated with a higher incidence of leakage of the cyst contents.[43] Intraoperative spillage of cyst contents may cause postoperative chemical peritonitis, chronic granulomatous peritonitis, adhesion formation and subsequent impairment in fertility.[15,16,22] Spillage of a malignant dermoid cyst may lead to malignant dissemination.[18,44,45]

Intraoperative spillage and related complications may be reduced by use of a large suction probe or endoscopic bag, and liberal irrigation of the peritoneal cavity until the irrigation fluid is devoid of any hair or sebum. Further studies are required to establish strict indications and contraindications for the laparoscopic management of ovarian dermoid cysts.

### Expectant management

The incidence of adhesion formation after ovarian dermoid cystectomy is still not known. However, spillage of dermoid material during the operation may increase the severity of the adhesions, potentially resulting in impaired fertility. Fiedler et al[46] investigated in a rabbit model whether peritoneal exposure to dermoid cyst material produces inflammation and adhesions above control levels, and whether saline lavage reduces the degree of peritoneal reaction. Dermoid material was found to produce a significant peritonitis. Results of the clinical evaluation demonstrated that saline lavage brought inflammation and adhesion formation close to control levels. From observations of rabbits receiving instillation of dermoid with or without lavage, using histological criteria, lavage tended to decrease inflammation and adhesion formation; however, it failed to bring the level of inflammation and adhesion formation down to that found in the control groups. This finding raises the concern that inflammation and adhesions that are not clinically apparent, but are detectable with histological evaluation, may have some effect on human fertility. Therefore, women with small dermoid cysts who would like to become pregnant may benefit from postponing surgical intervention.

In 1985 we initiated a programme of expectant management for selected patients at our centre, postponing surgery until the completion of family planning.[14] The programme consisted of strict ultrasonographic follow-up. Exclusion criteria included a mean cyst diameter of over 6 cm, proximity to menopause, an annual cyst growth rate of more than 2 cm and persistent abdominal pain. The mean growth rate of dermoid cysts in premenopausal women was found to be 1.8 mm/year. No evidence of torsion or malignancy was found in any of our study patients. The primary considerations should relate to the safety of our expectant management programme. The potential risk of missing a malignant tumour is disturbing, but this did not occur in our study. In two series made up of 48 women who had dermoid cysts with malignant transformation, the mean size of the tumours was 17 cm.[27,29] In a recent clinicopathological study of 517 women with mature cystic teratoma,[19] the mean cyst diameter was 6.4 cm. In that study, low rates of malignant transformation (0.17%) and torsion (3.4%) were found. Furthermore, all the published series have rarely shown malignant tumours measuring less than 6 cm. This supports the possibility that malignant transformation is associated with large tumours. In view of these findings, and provided the tumour growth rate is less than 2 cm/year, we suggest that, in premenopausal women with dermoid cysts of smaller than 6 cm in diameter, conservative follow-up would be safe. As an additional safety measure, serum CA-125 concentrations should also be measured. By postponing surgical intervention in young women who have not completed their family planning, we may avoid possible impairment of fertility.

## REFERENCES

1. Westhoff C, Pike M, Vessey M. Benign ovarian teratomas: a population-based case-control study. *Br J Cancer* 1988;**58**:93–8.
2. Koonings PP, Campbell K, Mishell DR, Grimes DA. Relative frequency of primary ovarian neoplasms: a 10-year review. *Obstet Gynecol* 1989; **74**:921–6.
3. Baker TR. Ovarian germ cell tumors. In: *Handbook of Gynecologic Oncology* (Piver MS, ed.). Boston, MA: Little, Brown & Co., 1996: 41.
4. Corfman PA, Richart RM. Chromosome number and morphology of benign ovarian cystic teratomas. *N Engl J Med* 1964;**271**:1241–4.
5. Patil SR, Kaiser-McCaw B, Hecht F, et al. Human benign ovarian teratomas: chromosomal and electrophoretic enzyme studies. *Birth Defects* 1978;**14**:297–301.
6. Mutter GL. Teratoma genetics and stem cells: a review. *Obstet Gynecol Surv* 1987;**42**:661–70.
7. Surti U, Hoffner L, Chakravarti A, Ferrell RE. Genetics and biology of human ovarian teratomas. I. Cytogenetic analysis and mechanism of origin. *Am J Hum Genet* 1990;**47**:635–43.
8. Parrington JM, West LF, Povey S. The origin of ovarian teratomas. *J Med Genet* 1984;**21**:4–12.
9. Dahl N, Gustavson KH, Rune C, et al. Benign ovarian teratomas – An analysis of their cellular origin. *Cancer Genet Cytogenet* 1990;**46**:115–23.
10. Linder D, Power J. Further evidence for potmeiotic origin of teratomas in the human female. *Ann Hum Genet* 1970;**34**:21–30.
11. Linder D, Kaiser McCaw B, Hecht F. Parthenogenetic origin of benign ovarian teratomas. *N Engl J Med* 1975;**292**:63–6.
12. Hoffner L, Shen-Schwarz S, Deka R, et al. Genetics and biology of human ovarian teratomas: III. Cytogenetics and origins of malignant ovarian germ cell tumors. *Cancer Genet Cytogenet* 1992;**62**:58–65.
13. Kim R, Bohm-Velez M. Familial ovarian dermoids. *J Ultrasound Med* 1994;**13**:225–8.
14. Caspi B, Appelman Z, Rabinerson D, et al. The growth pattern of ovarian dermoid cysts: a prospective study in premenopausal and postmenopausal women. *Fertil Steril* 1997;**68**:501–5.
15. Peterson WF, Prevost EC, Edmunds FT, et al. Benign cystic teratomas of the ovary: a clinicostatistical study of 1,007 cases with a review of the literature. *Am J Obstet Gynecol* 1955; **70**:368–82.
16. Pantoja E, Noy MA, Axtmayer RW, et al. Ovarian dermoids and their complications: comprehensive historical review. *Obstet Gynecol Surv* 1975;**30**:1–20.
17. Pantoja E, Rodriguez-Ibanez I, Axtmayer RW, Noy MA, Pelegrina I. Complications of dermoid

tumors of the ovary. *Obstet Gynecol* 1975; **45**:89–94.

18. Caruso PA, Marsh MR, Minkowitz S, Karten G. An intense clinicopathologic study of 305 teratomas of the ovary. *Cancer* 1971;**27**:343–8.

19. Comerci JT, Licciardi F, Bergh PA, et al. Mature cystic teratoma: a clinicopathological evaluation of 517 cases and review of the literature. *Obstet Gynecol* 1994;**84**:22–8.

20. Stern JL, Buscema J, Rosenshein NB, Woodruff JD. Spontaneous rupture of benign cystic teratomas. *Obstet Gynecol* 1981;**57**:363–6.

21. Shiels WE, Dueno F, Hernandez E. Ovarian dermoid cyst complicated by an entero-ovarian fistula. *Radiology* 1986;**160**:443–4.

22. Abitol MM, Pomerance W, Mackles A. Spontaneous peritoneal rupture of benign cystic teratomas: review of the literature and report of two cases. *Obstet Gynecol* 1959;**13**:198–203.

23. Coccia ME, Becattini C, Bracco GL, Scarselli G. Acute abdomen following dermoid cyst rupture during transvaginal ultrasonographically guided retrieval of oocytes. *Hum Reprod* 1996;**11**:1897–9.

24. Blackwell WJ, Dockerty MB, Masson JC, Mussey RD. Dermoid cysts of the ovary: their clinical and pathologic significance. *Am J Obstet Gynecol* 1946;**51**:151–72.

25. Scully RE. Tumors of the ovary and maldeveloped gonads. In: *Atlas of Tumor Pathology* (Hartmann WH, ed.), Second series, 16th fascicle. Washington, DC: Armed Forces Institute of Pathology, 1979: 246–86.

26. Kelly RR, Scully RE. Cancer developing in dermoid cysts of the ovary. A report of eight cases including a carcinoid and a leiomyosarcoma. *Cancer* 1961;**14**:989–1000.

27. Chadha S, Schaberg A. Malignant transformation in benign cystic teratomas: dermoids of the ovary. *Eur J Obstet Gynecol Reprod Biol* 1988;**29**:329–38.

28. Climie ARW, Heath LP. Malignant degeneration of benign cystic teratomas of the ovary. *Cancer* 1968;**22**:824–32.

29. Stamp GWH, McConnell EM. Malignancy arising in cystic teratomas. A report of 24 cases. *Br J Obstet Gynaecol* 1983;**90**:671–5.

30. Krumerman MS, Chung A. Squamous carcinoma arising in benign cystic teratoma of the ovary. *Cancer* 1977;**39**:1237–42.

31. Kimura T, Inoue M, Miyake A, et al. The use of serum TA-4 in monitoring patients with malignant transformation of ovarian mature cystic teratoma. *Cancer* 1989;**64**:480–3.

32. Quinn SF, Erickson S, Black WC. Cystic ovarian teratomas: the sonographic appearance of the dermoid plug. *Radiology* 1985;**155**:477–8.

33. Guttman PH. In search of the elusive benign cystic ovarian teratoma: application of the ultrasound 'tip of the iceberg' sign. *J Clin Ultrasound* 1977;**5**:403–6.

34. Owre A, Pedersen JF. Characteristic fat–fluid level at ultrasonography of ovarian dermoid cyst. *Acta Radiol* 1991;**32**:317–19.

35. De Meglio A, Di Meglio G, Esposito A, et al. Echo patterns of ovarian dermoid tumor. *Eur J Gynaecol Oncol* 1988;**9**:242–5.

36. Malde HM, Kedar RP, Chadha D, Sandeep N. Dermoid mesh: a sonographic sign of ovarian teratoma. *Am J Roentgenol* 1992;**159**:1349–50.

37. Caspi B, Appelman Z, Rabinerson D, et al. Pathognomonic echo patterns of benign cystic teratomas of the ovary: classification, incidence and accuracy rate of sonographic diagnosis. *Ultrasound Obstet Gynecol* 1996;**7**:275–9.

38. Bronshtein M, Yoffe N, Brandes JM. Hair as a sonographic marker of ovarian teratomas: improved identification using transvaginal sonography and simulation model. *J Clin Ultrasound* 1992;**19**:351–5.

39. Ekici E, Soysal M, Kara S, et al. The efficiency of ultrasonography in the diagnosis of dermoid cysts. *Z Gynäkol* 1996;**118**:136–41.

40. Zalel Y, Caspi B, Tepper R. Doppler flow characteristics of dermoid cysts: unique appearance of struma ovarii. *J Ultrasound Med* 1997;**16**:355–8.

41. Chapron C, Dubuisson JB, Samouh N, et al. Treatment of ovarian dermoid cysts: place and modalities of operative laparoscopy. *Surg Endosc* 1994;**8**:1092–5.

42. Nezhat C, Winer WK, Nezhat F. Laparoscopic removal of dermoid cysts. *Obstet Gynecol* 1989;**73**:278–80.

43. Lin P, Falcone T, Tulandi T. Excision of ovarian dermoid cyst by laparoscopy and by laparotomy. *Am J Obstet Gynecol* 1995;**173**:769–71.

44. Peterson WF. Malignant degeneration of benign cystic teratomas of the ovary: a collective review of the literature. *Obstet Gynecol Surv* 1957; **12**:793–830.

45. Genadry R, Parmley T, Woodruff JD. Secondary malignancies in benign cystic teratomas. *Gynecol Oncol* 1979;**8**:246–51.

46. Fiedler EP, Guzick DS, Guido R, et al. Adhesion formation from release of dermoid content in the peritoneal cavity and effect of copious lavage: a prospective, randomized, blinded, controlled study in a rabbit model. *Fertil Steril* 1996;**65**:852–9.

# Part VIII
# Endometriosis

# 32

# Endometriosis: pathophysiological and diagnostic considerations

Ivo Brosens

**The history of the identification of endometriosis  •  Appearances of endometriosis  •  Pathophysiological considerations  •  Diagnosis**

In an attempt to describe the current concept of endometriosis, we first follow the path of discoveries that led to the identification of endometriosis; subsequently we discuss aspects of pathophysiology and criteria on which the diagnosis and modern management are based. Unfortunately, in the absence of an understanding of the disease, much of our knowledge is derived not from deductive evidence but from observational concepts. However, the maxim *'ars medica tota in observationibus'* ('the skill of medicine lies completely in the observation') still holds true for the quality of data collection on which scientific evidence is based.

## THE HISTORY OF THE IDENTIFICATION OF ENDOMETRIOSIS

The discovery of what is currently defined as endometriosis can be described in three phases.[1] Exactly 100 years ago Iwanoff claimed that he had already published a paper in Russian on adenomyoma. It was, however, the work of TS Cullen[2] that made scientists recognize that adenomyomas contained heterotopic uterine epithelium, stroma and glands. Cullen collected adenomyomas of the body of the uterus, uterine horn, the round, utero-ovarian and uterosacral ligaments, and the posterior fornix of the vagina. He stressed that adenomyoma 'consists of a matrix of non-striped muscle and fibrous tissue, (and) ... scattered throughout this matrix isolated glands or groups of glands sometimes lying in direct contact with the muscle but usually in a characteristic stroma. The glands resemble in every particular those found in the mucosa lining the body of the uterus.' Cullen's view on the nature of glands in adenomyomas remained controversial. The first gynaecologist to describe a second type of endometrial-like tissue outside the uterus was Russel in 1899. He described a haemorrhagic ovarian cyst enveloped in adhesions on the posterior face of the broad ligament' and was 'astonished to find areas which were exact prototype of the uterine glands and interglandular connective tissue'.[1] It is remarkable that it took more than 20 years to recognize the endometrial origin of the haemorrhagic ovarian cyst. In 1921 Sampson[3] observed, when he operated, that in women who were menstruating the heterotopic endometrial-like tissue also showed menstrual shedding, a specific feature of endometrial tissue. He also described the third type of endometriosis when he observed menstrual bleeding in small peritoneal implants. The disease was subsequently called endometriosis and was defined histologically by the presence of glands and stroma outside the uterine cavity. Smooth muscle cell hyperplasia, as originally described in the nodules, was no longer included in the definition.

With the advent of laparoscopy, peritoneal endometriosis became the most common type of endometriosis observed in patients with infertility and chronic pelvic pain. The dark pigmented lesions became the classic criteria for the visual diagnosis of endometriosis. Subtle, so-called atypical lesions were rediscovered at laparoscopy. Endometriosis in all its appearances was found in up to 18% of asymptomatic fertile women.[4] In addition, microscopic lesions observed at scanning electron microscopy were also described, although it was not clear what exactly they represented in the evolution of peritoneal endometriosis.[5] It should be noted that Sampson's definition of endometriosis was based on the presence of endometrial-like tissue with evidence of menstrual shedding. Direct or indirect evidence of cyclic bleeding provides the functional evidence for the diagnosis of endometriosis.

## APPEARANCES OF ENDOMETRIOSIS

### Peritoneal endometriosis

Peritoneal endometriosis has many different appearances such as non-haemorrhagic, glandular excrescences, serous and haemorrhagic blebs, and puckered, pigmented and fibrotic lesions. Tridimensional studies using scanning electron microscopy have shown that early peritoneal lesions are mesothelial vesicles formed by secretions with small polyps emerging from underlying glandular structures.[5,6] These polypoidal lesions are highly vascularized and show hormone-dependent bleeding (red lesions). The so-called typical, puckered, pigmented lesions (black lesions) are characterized by the presence of a variable amount of fibrosis, a moderately vascularized stroma, glands with intraluminal debris and haemosiderin-laden macrophages. Lesions with extensive fibrosis (white lesions) have minimal stroma, poor vascularization and some glandular debris.

It is now generally accepted that black and white peritoneal lesions represent an evolution from the red, active lesions,[7] in which chronic, recurrent bleeding and inflammatory reaction (black lesion) ultimately lead to fibrosis and healing (white lesion).[8] Demographic data lend support to this conjecture. The petechial implant is the only type present in 20% of adolescents with endometriosis, whereas black and white fibrotic lesions apparently dominate at later ages.[9] Oligomenorrhoea is most frequently associated with vesicular lesions.[10]

Active superficial endometriosis is associated with adhesion formation. Fibrin deposits and non-connecting, filmy adhesions are masked by the positive intraperitoneal pressure, and are frequently noticed on the ovary and ovarian fossa in patients with mild endometriosis, when they are explored under fluid.[11]

### Ovarian endometrioma

The structure of the ovarian endometrial cyst when studied in situ is most instructive for understanding the complex appearance of endometriosis. Sampson,[3] studying hysterectomy and bilateral salpingoophorectomy specimens with the endometrioma in situ, always found the endometrioma to be adherent to the surrounding tissue. At the site of adhesions the cyst showed a stigma which he originally called the 'site of perforation'. Hughesdon[12] demonstrated, on serial sections of ovaries with the endometrioma in situ, that in 93% of cases the wall of the cyst was formed by ovarian cortex as demonstrated by the presence of primordial follicles. The 'site of perforation' changed into the 'site of inversion'. It is interesting to note that Sampson[13] accepted this possibility of invagination when he presented his theory of menstrual regurgitation and implantation. The adhesions were no longer considered as the sequelae of perforation but could be the cause of cyst formation. The location of the endometrioma on the side of the ovary opposing the posterior wall of the broad ligament, the presence of adenomyotic lesions at the site of stigma and surrounding adhesions all suggest an extraovarian origin. Apparently, a pseudo-cyst is formed by invagination of ovarian cortex and colonized by a superficial, endometrial-like mucosa. There is no evidence that 'ectopic endometrium ate its way into the ovary like insects are eating into an apple'.[12]

Our observations, based on endoscopic in situ inspection of the endometrioma and selective biopsies, support the view that endometrial-like tissue is colonizing the invaginated cortex.[14] In young girls the endometrial-like tissue consists of a highly vascularized endometrial-like mucosa, loosely attached to the wall and covering the white cortex patchily. At the site of invagination chronic haemorrhage is most prominent. In older women the wall of endometrioma is yellow, brown or black, and pigmented or fibrotic. At the site of inversion the vascularization is replaced by fibrosis and organized blood clots. The vessels of the mucosal lining (free implants) in the endometrioma show cyclic changes that correspond fully to the vascular changes in the upper functional layer of eutopic endometrium, including menstrual flow.[15]

Three lesions are frequently associated with the ovarian endometrioma. First, ovarian endometriomas larger than 2 cm are associated with adhesions in 86–100%.[3,16] Small endometriomas are less frequently adherent, but laparoscopy may underestimate ovarian adhesions in endometriosis. In addition, interconnecting filmy adhesions in the ovarian fossa are easily destroyed at laparoscopy by manipulation to expose it. Second, at or near the site of invagination, typical foci of endometriosis with glands and stroma (enclosed implants) are found. On hysterectomy specimens with endometriomas in situ, Sampson[3] found adenomyotic implants at the site of adhesions in 93%. The presence of nodular endometriosis, rather than the cyst, may explain why the endometrioma is frequently associated with chronic pelvic pain.[17] Failure to recognize the nodular endometriosis at surgery may lead to incomplete surgery and recurrence of cyst formation and pelvic pain. It is also important to note that ovarian endometriomas can develop after hysterectomy and bilateral salpingo-oophorectomy

in women receiving unopposed oestrogen or sequential oestrogen–progestogen therapy.[18] Third, large endometriomas, when multilocular, are frequently combined with luteal cysts and in 8% a communicating luteal cyst is found.[16] Some of the communicating luteal cysts also show early colonization by endometrial surface epithelium at the site of communication.[3,16]

## Rectovaginal endometriosis

Rectovaginal endometriosis is described as a deep, nodular lesion found in the posterior fornix. The lesion is usually more prominent on vaginal examination than at laparoscopy. Similar solid lesions can be found in other fibromuscular pelvic structures such as the uterosacral and utero-ovarian ligaments and vesicouterine fold. The nodule consists largely of fibromuscular tissue and rather scanty stromal tissue surrounding the glandular tissue. Nodules in the posterior fornix have the histological appearance of adenomyosis more frequently than at other sites.[19] In contrast with the free, mucosal implant, the nodular lesions are less hormone responsive and the vessels show congestion, but not vascular necrosis and bleeding at menstruation.[15] Deep nodular endometriosis is also focally associated with microendometriomas that are 500–2000 mm in diameter,[20] and at some sites, particularly in the loose tissue underlying the vaginal epithelium and rectal and vesical mucosa, the endometriomas are more obvious.

## PATHOPHYSIOLOGICAL CONSIDERATIONS

With current knowledge, endometriosis can be distinguished as three major entities, namely peritoneal, ovarian and rectovaginal endometriosis. Whether they represent different pathogenic entities or are simply the appearance of the same endometriotic tissue in different topographical environment remains to be elucidated. Severe, progressive endometriosis includes the haemorrhagic, endometrial cyst usually found at the site of the ovary and the solid, fibromuscular nodule in the posterior fornix and pelvic supporting structures.

They cystic type is lined focally, partially or completely by an endometrial-like mucosa, although glandular structures are frequently lacking. The mucosal vessels respond to ovarian steroids as those in the upper functional layer of the uterus do by cyclic bleeding.[15] Menstruation-dated ectopic endometrium was found in a much higher proportion of the cycles of women with ovarian implants than in other sites.[21] Recent histochemical studies[22–25] have shown that in the eutopic endometrium the matrix metalloprotease-1 expression is restricted, in space, to stromal foci of the functionalis layer and, in time, to the premenstrual period of the cycle. In endometriosis metalloprotease-1 RNA is expressed focally in red, peritoneal and ovarian endometriomas, but without restriction to the perimenstrual period. Foci of expression are closely related to matrix breakdown, with absence of progesterone receptors in adjacent epithelial cells.[26]

The nodular type is composed of fibromuscular tissue with glands and sometimes with scanty stroma. The lesion is also typically infiltrated by lymphoid aggregates containing T1 lymphocytes. In eutopic endometrium the lymphoid aggregates are confined to the endometrial–myometrial junction zone and consist mainly of activated CD3-positive T cells.[27] Recently, it has become clear that these cells play an important role in polarizing the endometrium. Both the phenotypical responsiveness to sex steroids and the endometrial proliferation are maximal in the functional layer and gradually decrease towards the basal layer. The low proliferative and secretory activity in the basal layer is associated with a marked increase in expression of human leukocyte class II antigen (HLA-DR) by glandular epithelium in this layer. Tabibzadeh and coworkers[27] demonstrated in vitro that interferon-γ (IFNγ) released by activated T cells can induce a high HLA-DR expression in endometrial-epithelial cells and dramatically inhibit their proliferative activity. The mechanism of surrounding smooth muscle hyperplasia in a nodular lesion is not known. Growing evidence suggests that, in the uterus, ovarian hormone action on smooth muscle cells may be mediated through cytokines and uterotonines locally released by the basal endometrial layer and endometrial T lymphocytes.[26] The most typical adenomyotic lesion is found at the posterior fornix of the vagina. As the posterior fornix is derived from the paramesonephric tract, although at a higher level than the anterior fornix,[29] it is not surprising to see the development of adenomyotic lesions that are similar, if not identical, to uterine adenomyosis. If this view is correct, rectovaginal endometriosis is not endometriosis of the rectovaginal septum but rather cervicovaginal adenomyosis. This would explain the consistent involvement of the vaginal but not the rectal wall in the lesion.

## DIAGNOSIS

The visualization of endometriosis is related to the current or past hormone responsiveness of the ovarian implant. Menstrual shedding is one of the functional manifestations of endometrial tissue, and therefore direct or indirect evidence of hormone-dependent bleeding is a solid basis for the diagnosis of active endometriosis.

### Rectovaginal examination early during the menses

For many years it has been recommended to look for endometriosis via vaginal and, particularly, rectovaginal examination early in the menses, when ovarian implants are larger and more tender. This recommendation has been made to detect endometriosis in patients at risk for obstructive uropathy which, although uncommon, may occur insidiously at laparoscopy in patients with minimal endometriosis.[30]

### Laparoscopy

The gold standard for diagnosis of pelvic endometriosis is laparoscopy. Visual inspection by laparoscopy has increased the awareness of the multiple, subtle and typical appearances of peritoneal endometriosis. However, there is the risk that the clinical significance of endometriosis is overestimated if whatever looks like endometriosis at laparoscopy, or represents some endometrial-like tissue at histopathology, is considered to be evidence of disease. The visual concept of endometriosis has several pitfalls, making endometriosis an illusive disease to diagnose.

## Peritoneal endometriosis

Peritoneal endometriosis in humans was shown to have a variable and changing appearance[31] which is probably related to the irregular, hormone-dependent menstrual shedding.[21] Remodelling makes peritoneal implants appear and disappear on the peritoneal surface. Failure to recognize the relationship between the hormone status and the visibility of the ovarian implants has for many years led to a visual illusion when the efficacy of hormone treatment in endometriosis was evaluated at laparoscopy. Second-look laparoscopy, as recommended by the Food and Drug Administration and other drug regulatory agencies, was performed at the end of therapy and compared with laparoscopy before treatment. The peritoneum will appear dry and clean, masking the subperitoneal implants at the end of a 6-month period of ovarian-suppressive therapy using any medication provided amenorrhoea has been induced. Evers[32] has shown that, as soon as menstruation has resumed, the 'beneficial' effect will have disappeared. As menstruation-suppressive therapy appears to be more successful after 6 months than after 2 or 3 months of therapy, it is assumed that the optimal duration of medical therapy is 6 months. At the microscopic level, however, there is no evidence that prolonged use of medication results in increased regression of the implant.[33] In clinical practice, relief of pelvic pain is achieved by 2 or 3 months once amenorrhoea has been established. Second-look laparoscopy at the end of therapy should not therefore be inflicted on women to assess the efficacy of ovarian-suppressive therapies because the effect is predictable. It should be taken into account that cycle irregularity, use of oral contraceptives and pregnancy may affect or change the visibility. It is interesting to note that, in a series of 91 women with the polycystic ovary syndrome, all with follicle-stimulating hormone (FSH) values within the normal range of the follicular phase, pelvic endometriosis was observed at laparoscopy in women with regular menses or oligomenorrhoea but not in those with amenorrhoea for more than 3 months.[10]

## Progressive endometriosis

Progression of endometriosis is usually evaluated by the increase in the score of the American Fertility Society (r-AFS) classification system.[34] The numerical score for the different appearances of endometriosis and adhesions is arbitrarily chosen and the concept that an increase in the r-AFS score represents progression of the disease has never been validated. Progression at laparoscopy largely depends on the presence and extent of adhesions and cyst formation. The technique of laparoscopy is not ideal for accurate investigation of adhesion formation. Access from the umbilicus requires manipulations to expose the tubo-ovarian structures, resulting in destruction of filmy adhesions in the ovarian fossa before their visualization; the intra-abdominal pressure of $CO_2$–pneumoperitoneum masks the non-connecting filmy adhesions. Fifty per cent more free-floating adhesions are seen in patients with endometriosis when explored under fluid (unpublished data).

The increase in the r-AFS score is frequently seen as evidence of progressive, invasive endometriosis in recurrent disease after conservative surgery. The increase is, however, likely to reflect postoperative adhesive disease as much as any progression of endometriosis. Ovarian haemorrhagic cysts after conservative surgery are present in more than 50% of lutein cysts. The more surgery there is, the more adhesive disease with recurrent pain and cyst formation occurs. The ultimate hysterectomy and bilateral oophorectomy in such patients is not evidence of progressive endometriosis but of surgical failure. It is no surprise that there is a high interobserver variation in the diagnosis of extensive endometriosis, reflecting difficulties in evaluating depth and extension at laparoscopy and interpretation of visual findings. Unfortunately, clinical and research studies continue to use the r-AFS classification indiscriminately to assess the severity and to monitor the evolution of the disease.

## Biopsy

Biopsies are essential for the detection of malignancies or atypias. Atypical peritoneal lesions, especially if they do not have the characteristics of haemorrhagic, red or fibrotic or black lesions, should be biopsied because they can be confused with other, possibly malignant lesions of the peritoneum. Ovarian and posterior fornix lesions should always be biopsied because they are the most frequent sites for malignancy in endometriosis. The histological diagnosis of endometriosis depends on the selection of biopsy site and the criteria used for the histopathological diagnosis. For peritoneal endometriosis, the reported incidence of a positive biopsy for the pigmented black lesions varies from 72% to 100%, for the red lesions from 65% to 100% and for the white lesions from 22% to 91%. For random ovarian endometriomas biopsies reveal endometrial-like tissue in less than 50% and large resected specimens show no endometriosis in one-third of cases. In the absence of endometrial tissue the diagnosis of endometriosis is based on the presence of haemosiderin-laden macrophages in fibroreactive tissue. Selecting the red areas at cystoscopy for biopsy increases the rate of positive biopsies to 83%.[14] In addition, biopsies should be taken not only from the wall of the cyst but also from the site of dense adhesions. For deep lesions it is unfortunate that there are no criteria for evaluating the presence of smooth muscle hyperplasia and lymphocyte aggregates. Deep lesions as diagnosed at laparoscopy and excision cover a range of lesions from purely fibrotic to adenomyotic. Further criteria are required to define so-called deep lesions by histopathological criteria in order to avoid the present visual confusion.

## Imaging techniques

### Ultrasonography

Ultrasonography is accepted as the initial modality of choice in the detection of ovarian endometriomas. Endometriomas present different ultrasonographic patterns, for example, purely cystic, cystic with few septations or minimal debris, complex combinations of cystic and solid elements, and largely solid. The sensitivity, specificity and accuracy of ultrasonographic diagnosis are reportedly 84%, 90% and 88%, respectively. As a result of the non-specific nature of ultrasonography, the mass has to be differentiated from other ovarian cysts and occasionally from a cystadenoma or tubo-ovarian abscess. The technique is, however, useful in the identification of the presence and location of endometriomas and may also be helpful in following the size of a cystic structure in response to therapy. The diagnostic accuracy can be improved by colour Doppler ultrasonography. The vascular pattern is typically focal and located in the caudal pole of the cyst. Low impedance–high diastolic flow is seen when there is a haemorrhage during menstruation. Aspiration of the cyst under ultrasonography can reveal the chocolate-coloured contents, although similar chocolate-coloured haemorrhagic contents may be found in some follicle haematomas, lutein cysts or even in cystadenomas.

### Magnetic resonance imaging

Ultrasonography continues to be the initial modality of choice for evaluating adnexal masses, although magnetic resonance imaging (MRI) is increasingly used for problem solving when further characterization is needed. MRI has a higher accuracy than ultrasonography and appears to be the most accurate method of differentiating an endometrioma from other gynaecological masses. The haemorrhagic cyst can be accurately distinguished from non-haemorrhagic cysts by MRI. The blood element of a chronic stage haematoma exhibits a hyperintense signal on both T1- and T2-weighted images, and the thick viscous content is likely to explain the shading of the fluid's signal intensity. The signal intensity typical of acute haematomas (intermediate intensity on T1-weighted masses) and subacute haematomas (hyperintensity with a distinct central area of hypointensity on T1-weighted images) allows the differentiation from chronic bleeding in the endometrial cyst. Using the fat saturation technique, endometriomas bigger than 4 mm can be reliably detected. The overall diagnostic sensitivity, specificity and accuracy for MRI diagnosis of endometrial cysts are reportedly 90%, 98% and 96%, respectively. Given the 96% accuracy, MRI is an acceptable diagnostic test on which clinical decisions can be based. The technique is non-invasive, more cost-effective than laparoscopy, and can be performed repeatedly.

Recently, we described the medical management of obstructive uropathy secondary to endometriosis based on MRI.[35] MRI was used to detect the haemorrhagic lesion obstructing the ureter and to monitor the lesion during hormone therapy. The resorption of the lesion and clearance of the obstruction during progestogen therapy indicated that the obstruction was caused by compression and not by fibrotic stricture. As the patient was reaching the menopause, she preferred to continue progestogen therapy rather than undergo surgery.

## Laboratory analysis

### Serum markers
CA-125 has been the first and most frequently used marker. Several studies have shown varying specificity and sensitivity rates with different cut-off points. The CA-125 markers, as well as markers for inflammatory conditions such as C-reactive protein, are elevated in patients with advanced endometriosis, mainly during the first days of the menstrual cycle.

### Cyst aspiration
Cytological examination for diagnosis has been abandoned. Biochemical assay of the aspirate has been proposed to differentiate between endometrioma and functional ovarian cyst. It should be noted that large endometriomas are frequently combined or even have a communication with a luteal cyst.

## Therapeutic trial

A case can be made for the use of a therapeutic trial to diagnose endometriosis or adenomyosis in patients with chronic pelvic pain. It is well established that chronic pelvic pain caused by endometriosis or adenomyosis improves as soon as menstruation is suppressed. After 2 or 3 months of menstruation-suppressive therapy, no further significant improvement of pain occurs. A 3-month menstruation-suppressive medical therapy can therefore be a useful, additional tool in the differential diagnosis of chronic pelvic pain.

## REFERENCES

1. Benagiano G, Brosens I. The history of endometriosis: identifying the disease. *Hum Reprod* 1991;**6**:963–7.
2. Cullen TS. The distribution of adenomyoma containing uterine mucosa. *Arch Surg* 1920; **1**:215–83.
3. Sampson JA. Perforating hemorrhagic (chocolate) cysts of the ovary. *Arch Surg* 1921;**3**:245–323.
4. Moen MH. Endometriosis in women at interval sterilization. *Acta Obstet Gynaecol Scand* 1987; **66**:451–4.
5. Vasquez G, Cornillie F, Brosens IA. Peritoneal endometriosis: scanning electron microscopy and histology of minimal pelvic endometriosis lesion. *Fertil Steril* 1984;**42**:696–703.
6. Donnez J, Nisolle M, Casanas-Roux F. Three-dimensional architectures of peritoneal endometriosis. *Fertil Steril* 1992;**57**:980–3.
7. Vernon MW, Beard SJ, Graves K. Classification of endometriotic implants by morphologic appearance and capacity to synthesize prostaglandin F. *Fertil Steril* 1986;**46**:801–6.

8. Nisolle M, Casanas-Roux F, Anaf V, et al. Morphometric study of the stromal vascularization in peritoneal endometriosis. *Fertil Steril* 1993;**59**:681–4.

9. Redwine DB. Age-related evolution in color appearance of endometriosis. *Fertil Steril* 1987; **48**:1062–3.

10. Singh KB, Patel YC, Wortsman J. Coexistence of polycystic ovary syndrome and pelvic endometriosis. *Obstet Gynecol* 1989;**74**:650–2.

11. Gordts S, Campo R, Rombauts L, Brosens I. Transvaginal hydrolaparoscopy as an outpatient procedure for infertility investigation. *Hum Reprod* 1998;**13**:99–103.

12. Hughesdon PE. The structure of the endometrial cysts of the ovary. *J Obstet Gynaecol Br Emp* 1957;**44**:481–7.

13. Sampson JA. Peritoneal endometriosis due to the menstrual dissemination of endometrial tissue into the peritoneal cavity. *Am J Obstet Gynecol* 1927;**14**:422–69.

14. Brosens IA, Puttemans PJ, Deprest J. The endoscopic localization of endometrial implants in the ovarian chocolate cyst. *Fertil Steril* 1994; **61**:1034–8.

15. Nieminen U. Studies on the vascular pattern of ectopic endometrium with special reference to cyclic changes. *Acta Obstet Gynaecol Scand* 1962; **41**:1–81.

16. Nezhat F, Nezhat C, Allan C, et al. Clinical and histologic classification of endometriomas. *J Reprod Med* 1992;**37**:771–6.

17. Fedele L, Bianchi S, Bocciolone L, et al. Pain symptoms associated with endometriosis. *Obstet Gynecol* 1992;**79**:767–9.

18. Brosens I. Endometriosis – A disease because it is characterized by bleeding. *Am J Obstet Gynecol* 1997;**176**:264–7.

19. Brosens IA. New principles in the management of endometriosis. *Acta Obstet Gynaecol Scand Suppl* 1994;**159**:18–21.

20. Cornillie FJ, Oosterlynck D, Lauwereyns JM, et al. Deeply infiltrating pelvic endometriosis: histology and clinical significance. *Fertil Steril* 1990;**53**:978–83.

21. Metzger DA, Olive DL, Haney AF. Limited hormonal responsiveness of ectopic endometrium: histologic correlation with intrauterine endometrium. *Hum Pathol* 1988;**19**:1417–24.

22. Rodgers WH, Matrisian LM, Giudice LC, et al. Patterns of matrix metalloproteinase expression in cycling endometrium imply differential functions and regulation by steroid hormones. *Am Soc Clin Invest* 1994;**94**:946–53.

23. Hampton AL, Salamonsen LA. Expression of messenger ribonucleic acid encoding matrix metalloproteinases and their tissue inhibitors is related to menstruation. *J Endocrinol* 1994; **141**:R1–3.

24. Kokorine I, Marbaix E, Henriet P, et al. Focal cellular origin and regulation of interstitial collagenase (matrix metalloproteinase-1) are related to menstrual breakdown in the human endometrium. *J Cell Sci* 1996;**109**:2151–60.

25. Marbaix E, Kokorine I, Moulin P, et al. Menstrual breakdown of human endometrium can be mimicked *in vitro* and is selectively and reversibly blocked by inhibitors of matrix metalloproteinases. *Proc Natl Acad Sci USA* 1996;**93**:9120–5.

26. Kokorine I, Nisolle M, Donnez J, et al. Expression of interstitial collagenase (matrix metalloproteinase-1) is related to the activity of human endometriotic lesions. *Fertil Steril* 1997;**68**:246–51.

27. Tabibzadeh S, Sun XZ, Kong QF, et al. Induction of a polarized micro-environment by human T cells and interferon-gamma in three-dimensional spheroid cultures of human endometrial epithelial cells. *Hum Reprod* 1993;**8**:182–93.

28. Brosens JJ, Barker FG, de Souza NM. Myometrial zonal differentiation and uterine junctional zone hyperplasia in the non-gravid uterus. *Hum Reprod* 1997; in press.

29. O'Rahilly R. Prenatal human development. In: *Biology of the Uterus*, 2nd edn (Wynn RM, ed.). New York: Plenum Press, 1997: 53.

30. Kane C, Drouin P. Obstructive uropathy associated with endometriosis. *Am J Obstet Gynecol* 1985;**151**:207–11.

31. Wiegerinck MAHM, Van Dop PA, Brosens IA. The staging of peritoneal endometriosis by the type of active lesion in addition to the revised American Fertility Society Classification. *Fertil Steril* 1993;**60**:461–4.

32. Evers J. The second look laparoscopy for the evaluation of the results of controlled trials in endometriosis-associated infertility. *Fertil Steril* 1987;**47**:502–4.

33. Brosens IA, Verleyen A, Cornillie F. The morphologic effect of short-term medical therapy of endometriosis. *Am J Obstet Gynecol* 1987; **157**:1215–21.

34. American Fertility Society. Revised classification of endometriosis. *Fertil Steril* 1985;**43**:351–2.

35. Deprest J, Marchal G, Brosens I. Obstructive uropathy secondary to endometriosis. *N Engl J Med* 1997;**337**:1174–5.

# 33

# Endometriosis and infertility: pathogenesis and work-up

Stephen K Smith

Epidemiology • The angiogenic hypothesis for endometriosis • Endometriosis and infertility
• Work-up • Conclusion

## EPIDEMIOLOGY

Endometriosis is the diagnosis of endometrium implanted at ectopic sites. The cause of endometriosis is unknown, and furthermore it is not clear whether it is a cause or a consequence of infertility. Of the many hypotheses proposed for this disease, retrograde menstruation is currently the favourite. The reasons for this are severalfold. Young girls with occlusive congenital lesions of the lower genital tract, giving rise to haematocolpos and haematometra, frequently have endometriosis.[1,2] Endometriosis is more common in older women who choose to restrict their family[3] and it is assumed that this is because they have more periods resulting in cumulatively greater endometrial deposits in the peritoneal cavity. Women who are long-term users of the intrauterine contraceptive device (IUCD) have a three times greater chance of getting the disease than women not using the coil.

Multiple pregnancies[4] and long-term use of the oral contraceptive pill are protective to endometriosis.[5,6] In the former case, reduction of menstruation by the pregnancy and lactational amenorrhoea reduce the volume of endometrial soiling, whereas, in the latter, oral contraceptive use reduces menstrual blood loss by about 50%,[7] also reducing the volume of menstrual detritus. Asian women are eight times more likely to develop endometriosis than white women[6] and their average menstrual loss is 50 ml compared with 30 ml.

The cellular basis for the retrograde menstruation hypothesis is reviewed by Haney.[8] Viable endometrium is present in menstrual effluent, can be maintained in culture, and endometrial cells and tissue are found in the peritoneal cavity at menstruation. This tissue is also viable as judged by subsequent in vitro culture.

Yet all of these facets are associative and none provides conclusive evidence for retrograde menstruation as the cause of endometriosis.

## THE ANGIOGENIC HYPOTHESIS FOR ENDOMETRIOSIS

Recently a new hypothesis for the induction of endometriosis has arisen which tries to bring together the more obvious clinical observations. The starting point for this view was with the acceptance that retrograde menstruation is needed for the induction of endometriosis in most cases. If all women deposit endometrium into the uterine cavity at menstruation, why do some women go on to have the syndrome complex of endometriosis? The explanation starts with the observation that many women, especially younger women[9] with endometriosis, complain of dysmenorrhoea.[10] An apparently unconnected observation then continues the story. Peritoneal fluid of women with endometriosis has an increased angiogenic activity compared with that in women who do not have the disease.[11] Endometriotic nodules are characterized by intense angiogenic activity. Endometrium is a rich source of growth factors which promote angiogenesis including the fibroblast growth factors, FGF1 and FGF2, and the vascular endothelial growth factor (VEGF)[12–14] Furthermore, these agents are expressed in endometriotic nodules. Peritoneal fluid of women with endometriosis has increased levels of VEGF in the proliferative phase of the cycle.[15]

So, how can increased uterine contractions cause endometriosis? Dysmenorrhoea is associated with increased plasma levels of vasopressin.[16,17] Vasopressin induces uterine contractions,[17] but it also increases contractility of the uterine resistance arteries.[18] In addition, other peptides including oxytocin, endothelin and noradrenaline contribute to this action on blood levels. The consequence is a large reduction in blood flow in the uterus and particularly to the endometrium during uterine contractions.[19] In addition to this gross effect on endometrial blood flow, it has been known for over 50 years that intense contraction of the spiral arterioles leads to menstrual shedding.[20]

Hypoxia is a critical activator of genes, especially for VEGF.[21,22] Hypoxia induces expression of the hypoxia-inducible factor α which dimerizes with the aryl hydrocarbon receptor nuclear translocator (ARNT). This complex binds to the hypoxic response element in the 3'-enhancer region of the VEGF gene which promotes mRNA stability. Hybridization for VEGF in the endometrium is intense and greatest in the glands at menstruation.[23] Recent studies have confirmed that the epithelial cells of the endometrium are, cell for cell, ten times more capable of inducing VEGF expression than stromal cells.[24] However, both glandular and stromal cells respond to hypoxia by stabilizing VEGF messages which results in increased translation for the VEGF protein.[24] Thus the greater hypoxia in the uteri of women with severe dysmenorrhoea results in increased production of VEGF, facilitating angiogenesis at the implantation site of the desquamated endometrium. This process is enhanced because activated macrophages in the peritoneal cavity produce large amounts of VEGF. Indeed supernatant collected from peritoneal fluid macrophages that have been taken from women with the disease has significantly greater angiogenic activity than that obtained from cells from women without the disease. This increased activity is blocked by antibodies to VEGF.[15]

It is not known why women have severe dysmenorrhoea. This explanation for the association between endometriosis and dysmenorrhoea is simple and is not dependent on changes in the immune system, or on the induction of autoantibodies to endometrium; all of these have proved difficult to establish. However, it does provide exciting new treatment options based on anti-angiogenic strategies.

## ENDOMETRIOSIS AND INFERTILITY

In view of the possibility that endometriosis is in some way associated with increased menstruation, it would not be surprising to find it in women who have failed to achieve a pregnancy. This might simply be a consequence of the infertility. However, endometriosis is rare in women presenting for sterilization,[6] although it is found in about 30% of women receiving laparoscopy for infertility.[25,26] However, there seems to be a poor or at the most a small correlation between the severity of the disease and infertility.[27]

The pathophysiology of endometriosis-associated infertility is therefore difficult to determine. Women with mild or moderate disease are assumed to have unexplained infertility. Several hypotheses have been suggested.

## Ovarian cycle

Subtle changes in the hypothalamopituitary–ovarian axis have been proposed as possible causes of infertility associated with endometriosis. These range from subtle changes in the luteinizing hormone (LH) surge,[28,29] raised plasma prolactin concentrations,[30,32] the luteinized unruptured follicle syndrome,[33] to defective corpus luteal function.[28,32] None of these has been confirmed and the consensus view is that they are not causes of infertility in women with endometriosis.[34,35]

## Peritoneal fluid

Peritoneal fluid of women with endometriosis contains activated macrophages and a wide range of cytokines and growth factors including inferon-γ (IFNγ), the interleukins IL-1, IL-6 and IL-8, colony-stimulating factor 1 (CSF-1), monocyte chemotactic protein (MCP-1), which are all associated with inflammation; the peritoneal fluid of endometriotic women is toxic to mice embryos (for a review see Hurst and Rock[36]). Alternatively, the inflammatory response may alter tubal motility, interfering with fertilization. Finally, if endometriosis arises because of abnormal endometrium, this may alter implantation when the embryo eventually arrives in the endometrial cavity. The evidence for these views is not strong. Fertility after removal of the peritoneal fluid is slightly increased in the following cycle. This could be an effect that is toxic to an embryo or a tubal motility effect. A disturbance of implantation seems less likely because success rates for patients with endometriosis is the same as for women without the disease.

More severe stages of endometriosis are classified based on the degree of distortion of the pelvic anatomy. This does not take into account the depth of invasion or the severity of the associated pain. However, tubal occlusion would be expected.

## Endometriosis and assisted reproduction

Several possibilities remain to explain the apparent increased incidence of infertility with endometriosis. It may reflect abnormal oocytes, the development of defective embryos or failed implantation. In effect all of these questions can be answered by studying the impact of assisted reproduction of fertility rates in women with the disease. Many such studies have now been completed. Several show that there are no differences in gamete intrafallopian transfer (GIFT) success rates between women with and those without the disease.[37–40] However, several other studies suggest that a difference does exist. Wardle et al[41] showed reduced pregnancies per oocyte transferred and per couple as did Khan et al,[42] when comparing women with endometriosis and those with unexplained infertility. Yovich et al[37] found an even poorer success rate in women with more severe disease. This finding is confirmed by observations in baboons in which the spontaneous pregnancy rates are reduced in animals with more severe disease.[43] Arici et al[44] studied 89 cycles of IVF in women with endometriosis compared with 147 cycles in patients with tubal disease and 48 cycles in women with endometriosis. The pregnancy rate per transfer was reduced in the endometriosis patients, being 14.8%, 25.7% and 23.3%, respectively. Similarly, Pellicer et al[45] compared 96 cycles in women with tubal disease with 96 cycles of IVF in women with endometriosis. Pregnancy rates were significantly reduced when calculated as pregnancies per cycle, per transfer and per embryo replaced. In addition these authors found a reduced pregnancy rate in an ovum donation programme when the oocytes were retrieved from women with endometriosis. Finally, they found poorer in vitro development of blastocysts in women with endometriosis. These findings point to subtle changes in patients with endometriosis but are less than conclusive.

## WORK-UP

### History

The classic history of women with endometriosis consists of three specific types of pain: dysmenorrhoea, dyspareunia and abdominal pain during the menstrual cycle. The correlation between dysmenorrhoea and endometriosis is most persistent and interesting.

Prostaglandins (PGs) are increased in women with dysmenorrhoea. Endometrial production of $PGF_{2\alpha}$ is increased[46] and $PGF_{2\alpha}$ and $PGE_2$ levels are raised in the menstrual blood of women with dysmenorrhoea.[47] Prostaglandin production is increased in women with endometriosis and dysmenorrhoea.[48] Increased uterine contractions may be expected to deposit more endometrium into the peritoneal cavity. In addition, endometriotic patients may have altered peristaltic movements in which the motility of the myometrium results in peristaltic activity towards the peritoneal cavity instead of towards the cervix.[49]

### Examination

Making the diagnosis of endometriosis is not possible on the basis of the physical examination. However, several features are of importance. First, uterosacral nodularity associated with pain is more common in women with endometriosis although the numbers are low – 7.5%.[50] Retroversion is also slightly more common in women with endometriosis. Interestingly, in this study of 174 women with endometriosis the clinical findings on vaginal examination did not correlate with the revised AFS (American Fertility Society) score.

In more severe disease, endometriomas can be palpated and are often fixed. The uterus is usually retroverted and fixed.

### Special investigations

The only way to diagnose endometriosis is to perform a laparoscopy. Although in the past insufficient women underwent this essential diagnostic procedure, the increased awareness of the disease has produced a difficult dilemma for clinicians. Many patients are given a presumptive diagnosis which is the worst of all worlds. Endometriosis is a chronic debilitating disease with important consequences for infertility. Clinicians must be sure of their diagnosis before burdening women with this disease and must not pass it off as a throw-away diagnosis.

### Peritoneal endometriosis

Examination of the peritoneal cavity by an experienced clinician will in almost all cases find endometrial deposits. Indeed this is universal at the time of menstruation. The presence of endometrial deposits must be associated with the symptoms of the disease syndrome. The findings at laparoscopy have been described extensively. The peritoneal deposits may be clear, red, blue, brown or white. This reflects the age of the deposit. At first, lesions look like and are fresh endometrium. As they become encapsulated they may bleed and the darkening feature reflects fresh blood and subsequently haemosiderin[51,52] identifies three lesions. The nodular lesion contains inactive glandular epithelium but there is fibrosis and pigmentation. The vesicular lesion is a small lesion of less than 5 mm which contains endometrial tissue in 95% of cases. It demonstrates increased vascularization and angiogenesis in the peritoneum surrounding the lesion. The stroma is well vascularized. Finally, the papular lesion is also small but contains whitish or yellow lesions, which are cystic glandular and stromal structures situated in the subperitoneal tissue. This lesion also has extensive vascularization in the peritoneum overlying the implant.

Most deposits are situated on the uterosacral ligaments. This is explained by the presence of endometrial deposits sitting on the peritoneal fluid. Varying degrees of invasion can be seen and may be very deep and extensive, but they are not usually visible at laparoscopy. As the lesion progresses fibrosis ensues with the development of blood vessels and the deposition of adhesions. This may cause close dense apposition between structures in the peritoneal cavity. Large and small bowel are often involved in more extensive disease. In addition to the lesions themselves and the associated fibrosis, peritoneal pockets can form which probably reflect organizing adhesions across peritoneal surfaces.

*Ovarian endometriosis*
The ovary is a common site for endometriosis and may present either with superficial lesions or the more classic endometrioma or endometriotic cyst. Superficial lesions consist of small deposits of endometrium arising probably in the same way that peritoneal endometriosis does. These lesions may often be found in the periovarian fossa and this area must be inspected at laparoscopy. Adhesions also form in this area. The chocolate ovarian cyst is not actually a cyst. The lining of these lesions is the outside of the ovary, not the inside.[53] It is not known how they form. The finding of loss of heterozygosity in endometriotic lesions close to endometrioid and clear cell ovarian malignancies[54] suggests that the lesions are superficial in all cases. Within the cyst bleeding points can be identified which are histologically like eutopic endometrium.

*Extrapelvic endometriosis*
Endometrium has been identified in almost every organ in the body (for a review see Markham[55]). The most frequently seen in the clinic is that involving the bowel, which may arise in about 5% of cases.[56–58] The clinical symptoms are of rectal bleeding at menstruation. This is clearly a difficult diagnosis. Occasionally obstruction may arise giving rise to abdominal pain and distension.

Endometriosis may present at any location in the urinary tract with the bladder being the most frequent site followed by the lower ureter and the kidney.[59,60] Cyclical haematuria associated with dysuria, frequency and urgency may reflect involvement of the lower urinary tract.[61]

Haematuria associated with loin pain reflects disease in the upper renal tract. Occasionally ureteric endometriosis can occlude the ureter with loss of the kidney.[60,62]

Occasionally the lung may be involved when the presentation is of haemoptysis and pleuritic pain at menstruation.[63]

**Blood test**

CA-125 is a cell surface antigen expressed by derivatives of coelomic epithelium, peritoneum and the cervix.[36] It is elevated in the peritoneal fluid of women with moderate and severe disease and is raised in the serum of such patients.[64,65] However, it is not specific to endometriosis and may be raised with pelvic infection; it is therefore a poor screening test for endometriosis. Its use comes in monitoring disease progression. There are currently no other blood markers for the disease.

**Imaging**

Transvaginal ultrasonography is not effective in identifying peritoneal endometriosis. However, it is effective in identifying endometriotic cysts in the ovary. It is not possible to determine the nature of the cyst on ultrasonography although some centres are needling the lesion to obtain chocolate fluid which can result in a diagnosis. This is still a questionable practice for diagnosis but may be used when previously identified endometriotic cysts need to be deflated before oocyte retrieval.

Magnetic resonance imaging provides the latest attempt at a non-invasive diagnosis for endometriosis. However, if the lesions are less than 2 cm they are difficult to identify.

**CONCLUSION**

Endometriosis is a common disease. It is more common in women with infertility. Beyond this the relationship between endometriosis and infertility become less clear. The consensus view is that severe cases of endometriosis with occlusion or severe entrapment of the fallopian tubes do cause infertility. It is likely that moderate endometriosis is in some way causative of the infertility. Mild endometriosis is probably not a cause of infertility but is found more frequently in women who have chosen to delay child bearing. The aetiology of endometriosis remains a goal for research in reproductive medicine. The latest techniques of familial genetics with gene and protein arrays are likely to identify the elusive nature of this debilitating disease.

## REFERENCES

1. Huffman W. Endometriosis in young teenage girls. *Pediatr Ann* 1981;**10**:44.
2. Olive DL, Henderson DY. Endometriosis and mullerian anomalies. *Obstet Gynecol* 1987;**69**:412.
3. Cramer DW, Wilson E, Stillman R. The relation of endometriosis characteristics, smoking and exercise. *JAMA* 1986;**255**:1904.
4. Parazzini F, Ferraroni M, Fedele L, Bocciolone L, Rubessa S, Riccardi A. Pelvic endometriosis: reproductive and menstrual risk factors at different stages in Lombardy, northern Italy. *J Epidemiol Commun Health* 1995;**49**:61–4.
5. Buttram VC. Cyclic use of combination oral contraceptions and the severity of endometriosis. *Fertil Steril* 1979;**31**:347.
6. Sangi-Haghpeykar H, Poindexter AN. Epidemiology of endometriosis among parous women. *Obstet Gynecol* 1995;**85**:983–92.
7. Nilsson L, Rybo G. Treatment of menorrhagia. *Am J Obstet Gynecol* 1971;**110**:713–20.
8. Haney AF. The pathogenesis and aetiology of endometriosis. In: *Modern Approaches to Endometriosis* (Thomas E, Rock J, eds). Amsterdam: Kluwer Academic Publishers, 1991; 3–19.
9. Punnonen RH, Nikkanen VP. Endometriosis in young women. *Infertility* 1980;**3**:1–10.
10. Mahmood TA, Templeton AA, Thomson L, Fraser C. Menstrual symptoms in women with pelvic endometriosis. *Br J Obstet Gynaecol* 1991;**98**:558–63.
11. Oosterlynck DJ, Meuleman C, Sobis H, Vandeputte M, Koninckx PR. Angiogenic activity of peritoneal fluid from women with endometriosis. *Fertil Steril* 1993;**59**:778–82.
12. Ferriani RA, Charnock-Jones DS, Prentice A, Thomas EJ, Smith SK. Immunohistochemical localization of acidic and basic fibroblast growth factor in normal human endometrium and endometriosis and the detection of their mRNA by polymerase chain reaction. *Hum Reprod* 1993;**8**:11–16.
13. Charnock-Jones DS, Sharkey AM, Rajput-Williams J, et al. Identification and localization of alternately spliced mRNAs for vascular endothelial growth factor in human uterus and steroid regulation in endometrial carcinoma cell lines. *Biol Reprod* 1993;**48**:1120–8.
14. Sangha RK, Xiao Feng L, Shams M, Ahmed A. Fibroblast growth factor receptor-1 is a critical component for endometrial remodeling: Localization and expression of basic fibroblast growth factor and FGF-R1 in human endometrium during the menstrual cycle and decreased FGF-R1 expression in menorrhagia. *Lab Invest* 1997;**77**:389–402.
15. McLaren J, Prentice A, Charnock-Jones DS, Smith SK. Vascular endothelial growth factor (VEGF) concentrations are elevated in peritoneal fluid of women with endometriosis. *Hum Reprod* 1996;**11**:220–3.
16. Akerlund M, Stromberg P, Forsling M-L. Primary dysmenorrhoea and vasosuppression. *Br Obstet Gynaecol* 1979;**86**:484–7.
17. Ekstrom P, Akerlund M, Forsling M, Kindahl H, Laudanski T, Mrugacz G. Stimulation of vasopressin release in women with primary dysmenorrhoea and after oral contraceptive treatment – effect on uterine contractility. *Br J Obstet Gynaecol* 1992;**99**:680–4.
18. Ekstrom P, Alm P, Akerlund M. Differences in vasomotor responses between main stem and smaller branches of the human artery. *Acta Obstet Gynaecol Scand* 1991;**70**:429–33.
19. Akerlund M, Andersson K-E. Vasosuppression response and terbutaline inhibition of the uterus. *Obstet Gynecol* 1976;**47**:484–7.
20. Markee JE. Morphological basis for menstrual bleeding. *Bull NY Acad Med* 1948;**18**:159.
21. Ikeda E, Achen MG, Breier G, Risau W. Hypoxia-induced transcriptional activation and increased mRNA stability of vascular endothelial growth factor in C6 glioma cells. *J Biol Chem* 1995;**270**:19761–6.
22. Levy AP, Levy NS, Goldberg MA. Post-tran-

scriptional regulation of vascular endothelial growth factor by hypoxia. *J Biol Chem* 1995;**271**:2746–53.

23. Charnock-Jones DS, Sharkey AM, Boocock CA, et al. Vascular endothelial growth factor receptor localization and activation in human trophoblast and choriocarcinoma cells. *Biol Reprod* 1994;**51**:524–30.

24. Sharkey AM, Charnock-Jones DS, Day K, et al. Vascular endothelial growth factor expression in human endometrium is regulated by hypoxia and steroids *in vitro* and *in vivo*. *J Clin Endocrinol Metab* 1998; in press.

25. Petersohn EP, Behrman SJ. Laparoscopy of the infertile patient. *Obstet Gynecol* 1970;**30**:363–7.

26. Goldenberg RL, Magendantz HG. Laparoscopy and the infertility investigation. *Obstet Gynecol* 1976;**47**:410–14.

27. Guzick DS, Silliman NP, Adamson GD, et al. Prediction of pregnancy in infertile women based on the American Society for Reproductive Medicine's revised classification of endometriosis. *Fertil Steril* 1997;**67**:822–9.

28. Cheeseman KL, Ben-Nun I, Chatterton RT, Cohen MR. The relationship of luteinizing hormone, pregnadiol-3-glucuronide and estriol-16-glucuronide in the urine of infertile women with endometriosis. *Fertil Steril* 1982;**38**:542–8.

29. Cahill DJ, Wardle PG, Maile LA, Harlow CR, Hull MGR. Pituitary–ovarian dysfunction as a cause for endometriosis-associated and unexplained infertility. *Hum Reprod* 1995;**10**:3142–6.

30. Hirschowitz JS, Soler NG, Worstman J. The galactorrhea–endometriosis syndrome. *Lancet* 1978;**i**:896–8.

31. Machida T, Taga M, Minaguchi H. Prolactin secretion in endometriotic patients. *Eur J Obstet Gynaecol Reprod Biol* 1997;**72**:89–92.

32. Hargrove JT, Abraham GE. Abnormal luteal function in endometriosis. *Fertil Steril* 1980; **34**:302.

33. Brosens IA, Koninckx PR, Corvelyn PA. A study of plasma progesterone, oestradiol-17-beta, prolactin and LH levels and of the luteal phase appearance of the ovaries in patients with endometriosis and infertility. *Br J Obstet Gynaecol* 1978;**85**:246–50.

34. Thomas EJ. Endometriosis and infertility. In: *Modern Approaches to Endometriosis* (Thomas E, Rock J, eds). Amsterdam: Kluwer Academic Publishers, 1991:113–28.

35. Matorras R, Rodriguez F, Pijoan JI, et al. Are there any clinical signs and symptoms that are related to endometriosis in infertile women? *Am J Obstet Gynecol* 1996;**174**:620–3.

36. Hurst BS, Rock JA. The peritoneal environment in endometriosis. In: *Modern Approaches to Endometriosis* (Thomas E, Rock J, eds). Amsterdam: Kluwer Academic Publishers, 1991: 79–96.

37. Yovich JL, Matson PL, Blackledge DG, Turner SR, Yovich JM, Edrisinghe WR. The treatment of normospermic infertility by gamete intrafallopian transfer (GIFT). *Br J Obstet Gynaecol* 1988;**95**:316–19.

38. Wong PC, Ng SC, Hamilton MP, Anandakumar C, Wong YC, Ratnam SS. Eighty consecutive cases of gamete intra-fallopian transfer. *Hum Reprod* 1988;**3**:231–3.

39. Borerro C, Ord T, Balmaceda JP, Rojas FJ, Asch RH. The GIFT experience: an evaluation of the outcome of 115 cases. *Hum Reprod* 1988;**3**:227–30.

40. Braeckmans P, Devroey P, Camus M, et al. Gamete intra-fallopian transfer: evaluation of 100 consecutive attempts. *Hum Reprod* 1987; **2**:201–5.

41. Wardle PG, McLaughlin EA, McDermott A, Mitchell JD, Ray BD, Hull MGR. Endometriosis and ovulatory disorder: Reduced fertilisation in vitro compared with tubal and unexplained infertility. *Lancet* 1985;**ii**(8449):236–9.

42. Khan I, Camus M, Staessen C, Wisanto A, Devroey P, Van Steirteghem AC. Success rate in gamete intrafallopian transfer using low and high concentrations of washed spermatozoa. *Fertil Steril* 1988;**50**:922–7.

43. D'Hooghe TM, Bambra CS, Raeymaekers BM, Riday AM, Suleman MA, Koninckx PR. The cycle pregnancy rate is normal in baboons with stage I endometriosis but decreased in primates with stage II and stage III–IV disease. *Fertil Steril* 1996;**66**:809–13.

44. Arici A, Duleba A, Oral E, Olive DL, Bukulmez O, Jones EE. The effect of endometriosis on implantation: Results from the Yale University *in vitro* fertilization and embryo transfer program. *Fertil Steril* 1996;**65**:603–7.

45. Pellicer A, Oliveira N, Ruiz A, Remohi J, Simon C. Exploring the mechanism(s) of endometriosis-related infertility: An analysis of embryo development and implantation in assisted reproduction. *Hum Reprod* 1995;**10**(suppl 2):91–7.

46. Lundstrom V, Green K. Endogenous levels of prostaglandin $F_{2\alpha}$ and its main metabolites in plasma and endometrium of normal and dysmenorrheic women. *Am J Obstet Gynecol* 1978;**130**:640–6.

47. Lumsden MA, Kelly RW, Baird DT. Primary dysmenorrhoea: the importance of both prostaglandins $E_2$ and $F_{2\alpha}$. *Br J Obstet Gynaecol* 1983;**90**:1135–40.

48. Koike H, Egawa H, Ohtsuka T, Yamaguchi M, Ikenoue T, Mori N. Correlation between dysmenorrheic severity and prostaglandin production in women with endometriosis. *Prostaglandins Leukotrienes Essential Fatty Acids* 1992;**46**:133–7.

49. Leyendecker G, Kunz G, Wildt L, Beil D, Deininger H. Uterine hyperperistalsis and dysperistalsis as dysfunctions of the mechanism of rapid sperm transport in patients with endometriosis and infertility. *Hum Reprod* 1996;**11**:1542–51.

50. Mattoras R, Rodriguez F, Perez C, Pijoan JI, Neyro JL, Rodriguez-Escudero FJ. Infertile women with and without endometriosis: A case control study of luteal phase and other infertility conditions. *Acta Obstet Gynaecol Scand* 1996; **75**:826–31.

51. Redwine DB. The distribution of endometriosis in the pelvis by age groups and fertility. *Fertil Steril* 1987;**47**:173–5.

52. Brosens IA. The endometriotic implant. In: *Modern Approaches to Endometriosis* (Thomas E, Rock J, eds). Amsterdam: Kluwer Academic Publishers, 1991:21–31.

53. Hughesdon PE. The structure of the endometrial cyst of the ovary. *J Obstet Gynaecol Br Emp* 1957;**64**:481–7.

54. Jiang X, Hitchcock A, Bryan EJ, et al. Microsatellite analysis of endometriosis reveals loss of heterozygosity at candidate ovarian tumor suppressor gene loci. *Cancer Res* 1996;**56**:3534–9.

55. Markham SM. Extrapelvic endometriosis. In: *Modern Approaches to Endometriosis* (Thomas E, Rock J, eds). Amsterdam: Kluwer Academic Publishers, 1991:151–82.

56. Masson JC. Present conception of endometriosis and its treatment. *Trans West Surg Assoc* 1945;**53**:35.

57. Weed JC, Ray JE. Endometriosis of the bowel. *Obstet Gynecol* 1987;**69**:727.

58. Williams TJ. Endometriosis. In: *TeLinde's Operative Gynecology*, 6th edn (Mattingly RF, Thompson JD, eds). Philadelphia: JB Lippincott, 1985:257.

59. Koszczuk JC, Fogliette M, Perez JF, Dono FV, Thomas RJ. Urinary tract endometriosis. *J Am Osteopathol Assoc* 1989;**89**:83.

60. Kerr SW. Endometriosis involving the urinary tract. *Clin Obstet Gynecol* 1966;**9**:331.

61. Yates-Bell AJ, Molland EA, Pryor JP. Endometriosis of the ureter. *Br J Urology* 1972;**40**:58–67.

62. Stanley KE, Utz DC, Dockerty MD. Clinically significant endometriosis of the urinary tract. *Surg Gynecol Obstet* 1965;**120**:491.

63. Lancaster JM, Prentice A, Smith SK. Successful medical treatment of sub-diaphragmatic endometriosis. *J Obstet Gynaecol Br Emp* 1995; **15**:206–9.

64. Williams RS, Rao CV, Yussman MA. Interference in the measurement of CA-125 in peritoneal fluid. *Fertil Steril* 1988;**49**:547.

65. Moretuzzo RW, Lauro SD, Jenison E, Chen SL, Reindollar RH, McDonagh PG. Serum and peritoneal lavage fluid CA-125 levels in endometriosis. *Fertil Steril* 1988;**50**:430.

# 34

# Genetic factors in endometriosis

Stephen Kennedy

**Familial clustering in humans and rhesus monkeys** • **Increased prevalence in first-degree relatives** • **OXEGENE (Oxford Endometriosis Gene) Study** • **Candidate gene analysis** • **Miscellaneous associations** • **Acknowledgments**

The aetiology of endometriosis is unknown but there is increasing evidence to suggest that the disease has a genetic basis. This does not imply that the condition is transmitted as a mendelian trait. Endometriosis is more likely to be a complex trait, that is, a condition like diabetes, hypertension or asthma, without a clear mendelian pattern of inheritance. In such complex traits, multiple gene loci conferring susceptibility to the condition interact with each other and the environment to produce the phenotype.

The evidence that genetic susceptibility has a role in endometriosis is that: (1) there is familial clustering in humans[1] and rhesus monkeys;[2] (2) concordance has been reported in monozygotic twins;[3,4] (3) the age at onset of pain symptoms is very similar in non-twin concordant sisters;[5] (4) the prevalence of the disease is six to nine times greater in the first-degree relatives of affected women compared with the general population;[6–8] and (5) certain genetic polymorphisms may be more prevalent in affected women than in controls.[9–12]

This chapter reviews the current literature on the genetics of endometriosis using the databases EMBASE (January 1980 to December 1997) and MEDLINE (January 1966 to December 1997) and the search terms endometriosis and genetic. The chapter also describes the OXEGENE study which aims, using genetic linkage analysis, to identify susceptibility loci involved in the development of endometriosis.

## FAMILIAL CLUSTERING IN HUMANS AND RHESUS MONKEYS

The impression that endometriosis has a genetic basis has been gained largely from case reports, for example, catamenial pneumothorax in sisters,[13] and poorly controlled studies of larger groups of affected women[14,15] documenting an apparent tendency for familial clustering. Adding to this anecdotal evidence, the Oxford Group recently described the clinical characteristics of 100 families containing 230 women with surgically confirmed endometriosis.[1] The families were recruited for linkage analysis by placing advertisements in the newsletters of endometriosis self-help groups in the UK, Ireland, the USA, Canada, Australia and New Zealand. They consisted of 19 mother–daughter pairs, one set of cousins and 56 sister pairs; there were also five families with three affected sisters, one family with five affected sisters, and 18 families with more than three affected members in more than one generation. Seventy-nine women (34%) had revised American Fertility Society (r-AFS)[16] stage I–II disease and 151 (66%) had r-AFS stage III–IV disease.

These studies all suffer from ascertainment bias, but defining the familial tendency more thoroughly in whole populations is difficult because surgery is required to establish the diagnosis. Segregation analysis to determine the mode of inheritance is not possible because of the difficulties inherent in determining who is and who is not affected. However, a clearer understanding of the inheritability of the disease may emerge from studying spontaneous endometriosis in rhesus monkey (*Macaca mulatta*) colonies.

The clinical features, appearance at surgery and histological characteristics of the disease in the rhesus monkey mimic those in humans.[17] Large colonies therefore represent a unique opportunity to study the epidemiology and inheritability of the disease. The Oxford Group is collaborating with two Regional Primate Research Centers in the USA: one at the University of California, Davis, and the other at the University of Wisconsin, Madison, both of which house large colonies of rhesus monkeys.

At the California Regional Primate Research Center (CRPRC), we have identified 121 (8.3%) affected rhesus monkeys among the autopsy records of the 1459 female animals that died, aged 4 years or more, in the colony between 1982 and 1996 (manuscript in preparation). We are trying to determine the familial tendency in these affected animals by analysing the entire colony records of over 9000 females from 1965 to 1997, but it is proving difficult to construct a large pedigree at CRPRC because paternity cannot be determined for all the animals. At the Wisconsin Regional Primate Research Center (WRPRC), however, the animals are bred under different conditions and paternity can almost always be determined. In addition, it appears that the animals at WRPRC have been exposed to a number of experimental procedures, such as hysterotomy and oestradiol implants, which appear to be risk factors for endometriosis and which may have led to a higher prevalence in this colony than at CRPRC.[2]

Hadfield et al examined the autopsy records of the 399 female rhesus monkeys that died in the WRPRC colony between 1980 and 1995 and reported a prevalence rate of 20% (81 of 399) in animals aged 4 years or older at death and 29% (81 of 284) in animals aged 10 years or older at death.[2] The majority (78%) had the equivalent of r-AFS stage III–IV disease. In this colony, age also appeared to be a significant risk factor for the development of endometriosis: the mean age at death was significantly greater in the affected group compared with those animals without disease (Figure 1).

To investigate other risk factors, 62 affected animals were matched, by age at death and date of death, with an equal number of controls without disease. Of the affected animals, 26 (42%) were related to one animal or more within the affected group but only 13 (21%) of the matched controls were related to one animal or more within the matched control group. The related animals (affected and unaffected) were in a number of family groups which could be amalgamated in the lowest generations to produce an extended, multi-generational pedigree of over 1600 animals. To increase the informativeness of the pedigree for segregation analysis, magnetic resonance imaging (MRI) scans have been performed on the 116 monkeys aged 10 years or older that are the living descendants of the dead, affected animals. These images are currently being analysed.

## INCREASED PREVALENCE IN FIRST-DEGREE RELATIVES

The strongest evidence in favour of a genetic basis for endometriosis is provided by three studies showing that the prevalence of the disease is higher in the first-degree relatives of affected women than in controls, who are taken to be representative of the general population. Simpson et al[6] noted a sevenfold higher risk among the first-degree relatives of American patients compared with their husbands' first-degree relatives. Coxhead and Thomas[7] found a sixfold increased risk among the first-degree relatives of English patients compared with those of unaffected case controls. Moen and Magnus[8] reported a sevenfold increase in risk for endometriosis and/or adenomyosis among

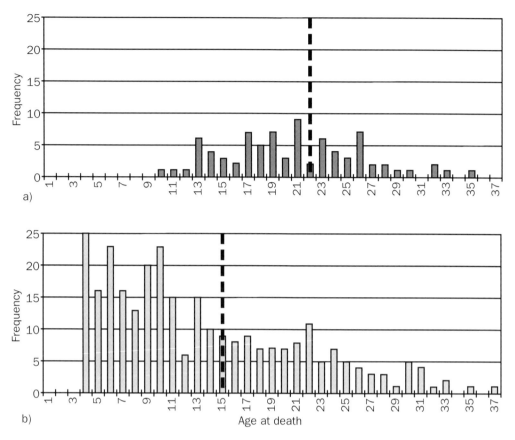

**Figure 1** Age at death in rhesus monkeys (a) with and (b) without endometriosis at autopsy. (a) Mean 20.7 (10–35) years; $n = 81$; (b) Mean 13.4 (4–37) years; $n = 318$.

the first-degree relatives of Norwegian patients compared with those of case controls; among the women with endometriosis, severe disease was significantly more common in those with an affected relative ($p < 0.01$). These data are summarized in Table 1.

The reported figures of 0.6–1.6% disease prevalence in the controls are compatible with the best estimates of disease prevalence in the general population, namely 0.5–2.5%.[18,19] The higher reported prevalence in the first-degree relatives of affected women suggests that $\lambda_R$ (the recurrence risk for the relative of an affected individual divided by the risk for the general population) is 6–9 which is similar to complex traits such as inflammatory bowel disease.

Further evidence for a genetic basis to endometriosis, based upon analyses of sisters, is provided by the case reports documenting concordance in monozygotic twins[3,4] and by the finding that concordant non-twin sisters tend to develop pain symptoms at the same age.[5]

## OXEGENE (OXFORD ENDOMETRIOSIS GENE) STUDY

### Linkage analysis

The development of large-scale, automated screening of the genome using fluorescent-labelled dinucleotide tandem repeat (micro-

**Table 1 Disease prevalence in the first-degree relatives of affected women**

| Authors | Controls | Sisters | Mothers | Sisters or mothers |
|---|---|---|---|---|
| Simpson et al[6] | First-degree relatives of patients' husbands | 9/153 (5.8%) vs 1/104 (1%) | 10/123 (8.1%) vs 1/107 (0.9%) | – |
| Coxhead and Thomas[7] | First-degree relatives of women with a normal pelvis | – | – | 6/64 (9.4%) vs 2/128 (1.6%) |
| Moen and Magnus[8]* | First-degree relatives of women with a normal pelvis | 25/523 (4.8%) vs 1/169 (0.6%) | 20/515 (3.9%) vs 1/149 (0.7%) | – |

* Disease defined as endometriosis and/or adenomyosis.

satellite) markers in linkage studies has already led to the identification of susceptibility loci in complex traits such as type 1 diabetes[20] and asthma.[21] A similar approach is planned to identify susceptibility loci in endometriosis.

We aim to establish linkage using affected sib-pair analysis which involves studying affected sibs to determine how often marker alleles are shared identical by descent (inherited from a common parent). Allele sharing at a chromosomal region that is not consistent with random mendelian segregation (occurring more frequently than expected by chance) is indicative of linkage.

The main advantages of this non-parametric statistical approach are that: (1) only affected women and their parents are genotyped; (2) no assumptions are made about the mode of inheritance; and (3) families as small as two sister-pairs can be recruited. There is therefore no need to find large pedigrees with both affected and unaffected members which would obviously be difficult to achieve in endometriosis given the need to perform laparoscopy to establish the diagnosis.

## Disease phenotype

In any linkage study it is vital to use a reliable definition of phenotype, that is, to have a clear definition of who is affected. For the purpose of determining linkage, we are using a restricted phenotypic definition of surgically confirmed r-AFS stage III–IV disease because: (1) severe phenotypic types usually display the highest $\lambda_R$ ratios (the power to detect linkage being related to the size of this ratio); (2) there is often histological confirmation if disease of this severity is present; and (3) minimal endometriosis may not be a disease state.[22] Any woman whose diagnosis cannot be confirmed by scrutinizing the surgical records provided by her gynaecologist is excluded from the study.

## Family collection

DNA from sisters with surgically confirmed r-AFS stage III–IV disease and their parents are being collected to perform a genome-wide screen. Families are being recruited: (1) through advertisements placed in the newsletters of national endometriosis self-help groups, such as the Endometriosis Association in the USA; (2) with the collaboration of leading research centres throughout the world; (3) in Oxford alone, by screening the sisters of women with stage III–IV disease using MRI scanning and confirming disease status in those with a positive scan;[23] and (4) via the OXEGENE web-site.

## OXEGENE web-site

The address is http://www.medicine.ox.ac.uk/ ndog/oxegene/oxegene.htm. We have demonstrated that the World Wide Web provides a rapid and cost-effective means of recruiting families for genetic linkage analysis.[24] Visitors are invited to participate in the research by e-mailing us directly or by completing an electronic form, asking for simple personal details and information outlining which family members are affected by endometriosis. The OXE-GENE web site was accessed by 10 445 people between March and December 1997 and we had 203 responses from women with a family history of endometriosis who were willing to participate in the study.

## Current status

Through the endometriosis self-help groups and the web-site, the Oxford Group have contacted 668 families containing 1003 affected women from Argentina (1), Australia (35), Bermuda (1), Canada (29), Chile (1), Germany (3), the Netherlands (1), Hong Kong (1), Ireland (11), Israel (1), Italy (3), Mexico (2), New Zealand (16), Philippines (1), Slovenia (1), Sweden (1), the UK (419) and the USA (476). These families contain 60 sister-pairs with stage III–IV disease. The collaborators have identified another 168 sister-pairs with stage III–IV disease. Additional collaborators are joining the OXEGENE Study all the time as we continue to collect as many sister-pairs as possible.

## CANDIDATE GENE ANALYSIS

The use of linkage analysis alone is often insufficient to localize susceptibility genes in complex traits because of the limited resolution of the method for fine mapping. As a complementary approach, candidate genes need to be investigated in association studies by comparing the frequency of marker alleles in affected cases and normal controls. Differences in frequency arise if the marker is causally implicated in the disease or if it is in linkage disequilibrium with a susceptibility locus, that is, haplotype combinations of alleles at different loci occur more frequently than would be expected from random association. Examples of association reported in complex traits include apolipoprotein E in Alzheimer's disease[25] and angiotensin-converting enzyme (ACE) polymorphisms in hypertension.[26]

There are no obvious candidate genes to investigate in endometriosis but two genetic associations have already been reported which warrant further investigation in larger samples. The first is a polymorphism in galactose-1-phosphate uridyl transferase (GALT) in a North American sample;[9] GALT is an enzyme involved in galactose metabolism. The second is a null mutation in glutathione *S*-transferase M1 (GSTM1) reported in French[10] and Slavic samples;[11] GSTM1 is an enzyme involved in the detoxification of dioxin, an environmental pollutant.

## Galactose-1-phosphate uridyl transferase

The GALT enzyme catalyses the formation of uridyl diphosphate (UDP)-galactose and glucose 1-phosphate from galactose 1-phosphate and UDP-glucose. Some polymorphisms without enzyme activity cause galactosaemia, a recessive condition with a 1:50 000 incidence; other variants have reduced enzyme activity without clinical manifestations. The most common polymorphism is Q188R (an $A_{1470}$ to $G_{1470}$ transition in exon 6 substituting arginine[188] for glutamine[188]). Q188R homozygotes have galactosaemia and Q188R heterozygotes have 15% enzyme activity. The second most common polymorphism is N314D (an $A_{2744}$ to $G_{2744}$ transition in exon 10 substituting aspartate[314] for asparagine[314]). N314D homozygotes have 50% and heterozygotes 75% activity.

The N314D variant has been associated with ovarian cancer,[27] early menopause[28] and müllerian anomalies, in particular Mayer–Rokitansky–Kuster–Hauser syndrome.[29] Cramer et al[29] investigated the prevalence of the variant in endometriosis given the known association between the disease and müllerian anomalies (which can also be familial[30–32]). They reported that 30% (10 of 33) of women with endometriosis (r-AFS I–IV) carried at least one N314D allele compared with 14% (15 of 111) of controls (premenopausal women from the general population excluding those with a past history of endometriosis, hysterectomy or bilateral oophorectomy).[9] Six of the 11 (55%) women with III–IV disease carried at least one N314D allele.

Reduced GALT activity associated with N314D may be an aetiological factor in endometriosis but it is more likely that this polymorphism is in linkage disequilibrium with a disease susceptibility locus. The GALT gene locus (9p21) is in a region where loss of heterozygosity in endometriotic tissue has been reported.[33]

## Glutathione *S*-transferase M1

Enzymes belonging to the glutathione *S*-transferase (GSTM1) family are involved in the two-stage detoxification of 2,3,7,8-tetrachlorodibenzo-*p*-dioxin (dioxin). This is an environmental pollutant produced by the combustion and manufacture of chlorinated carbon products such as PVC. Dioxin is a carcinogen and teratogen in rodents and a null mutation in one of the GST enzymes, GSTM1, is associated with environmentally induced lung[34] and bladder cancers[35] in humans caused by the lack of enzyme activity. Dioxin has numerous effects on the reproductive health of humans as well and it

may be a risk factor for endometriosis. Rhesus monkeys given 5–25 parts per trillion in their food over 4 years were at increased risk of developing the disease compared with unexposed controls.[36] There is also some evidence that dioxin levels may be higher in women with endometriosis compared with controls[37] and the incidence of endometriosis is high in Belgium, a country with one of the worst dioxin pollution records in the world.[38]

GSTM1 homozygotes for the mutation (a 10-kilobase-pair or kb deletion at 1p13) were more common in a group of French women with endometriosis: 86% (43 of 50) of affected (r-AFS stages I–IV) women had the null mutation compared with 46% (33 of 72) of controls (women undergoing termination of pregnancy).[10] If only women with stage III–IV disease were included then over 90% had the mutation. In a Slavic sample, recruited in northwestern Russia, 81% (34 of 42) of women with endometriosis (disease severity not specified) had the null mutation compared with 39% (26 of 67) of healthy male and female controls.[11]

## MISCELLANEOUS ASSOCIATIONS

A number of associations and molecular changes have been reported in the literature which add weight to the theory that endometriosis has a genetic basis and may prove useful in identifying candidate genes. For example, familial clustering occurs in adenomyosis which may be a similar disease to endometriosis[39] and a karyotypic abnormality, del(7) (q21.2–q31.2), previously only described in uterine leiomyomas, has been found in cultured adenomyotic cells.[40]

Spitsyn et al[12] have reported associations with certain ABO blood types and polymorphisms in pseudocholinesterase, C3 complement component, transferrin and phosphoglucomutase (PGM1).[12] In particular, rare alleles at the esterase D locus were more common in Russian women with endometriosis than in healthy controls.

Associations have also been reported with

red hair,[41] dysplastic naevi,[42] atopy[43] and poly-cystic ovaries;[44] there is no known association between endometriosis and HLA type.[45–47] Lastly, susceptibility for the disease may vary between ethnic groups as higher prevalence rates have been reported in Japanese[48] and Asian women[49,50] than in white European women, and endometriosis is rarely found in ultra-Orthodox Jews.[51]

## Conclusions

There is increasing evidence to suggest that endometriosis is inherited as a complex trait, like diabetes, hypertension or asthma. This implies that there are environmental factors, such as dioxin, that interact with multiple genetic susceptibility loci to produce the pheno-type. The OXEGENE study, an international collaborative project, seeks to identify the sus-ceptibility loci using linkage analysis; the aim then is to use positional cloning techniques to identify genes that predispose women to the disease. Analysis of the biochemical function of the gene products will lead to a better under-standing of the pathophysiology and aetiology of endometriosis. New therapies may be designed based on knowledge of the gene func-tion and disease-associated genetic markers may be used to identify women at high risk of developing the disease.

## ACKNOWLEDGMENTS

The OXEGENE Collaborative group is com-prised of members of the Oxford Endometriosis Group (David Barlow, Ruth Hadfield, Stephen Kennedy, Sanjiv Manek, Helen Mardon and Satoshi Nakago) and the following 52 centres around the world: David Adamson, Palo Alto; Leila Adamyan, Moscow; Robert Albee, Atlanta; Kulenthran Arumugam, Kuala Lumpur; Ronald Batt, Buffalo; Agneta Bergqvist, Huddinge; Michel Canis, Clermont-Ferrand; Ming Yang Chang, Taiwan; Paul Claman, Ottawa; Chan Clement, Singapore; Fabian Correa, Bogota; Pier Crosignani/Paolo Vercellini, Milan; E Darai, Paris; Mike Diamond, Detroit; Paul Dmowski, Chicago; Geoffrey Driscoll, Sydney; Keith Edmonds and Gillian Rose, London; Roger Fay, Sydney; Cindy Farquhar, Auckland; Sylvia Fernandez-Shaw, Madrid; Ian Fraser, Sydney; Linda Giudice, Stanford; Mark Hamilton, Aberdeen; David Heeley, Melbourne; Thomas Hilgers, Omaha; Minaguchi Hiroshi, Yokohama; Masumi Inui, Japan; Philippe Koninckx, Leuven; Sr T Lillian, Bangalore; Salvador Livas, Mexico; Paul van der Linden, The Netherlands; FH Loh, Singapore; Edward Loong, Hong Kong; Peter Maher, Melbourne; Mamta Deenadayal, Secunderbad; Dan Martin, Memphis; Suneeta Mittal, New Delhi; Mette Moen, Trondheim; Hugh O'Connor, Dublin; Colm O'Herlihy and Mary Wingfield, Dublin; David Olive, Yale; Engin Oral, Istanbul; Matt Peterson, Salt Lake City; David Redwine, Bend; Bob Schenken, San Antonio; Robert Shaw, Cardiff; Martin Sillem, Heidelberg; Zephne van der Spuy, Cape Town; Lawrence Tang and Alice Wong, Hong Kong; Gurgan Timur, Ankara; Mike Vernon, Lexington; Kuwabara Yoshinori and Naoki Mituhashi, Tokyo. Research in the rhesus macaque is being con-ducted with the collaboration of the Wisconsin Regional Primate Research Center, University of Wisconsin, Madison (Joe Kemnitz, Leslie Knapp, Joan Scheffler and Hideo Uno) and the California Regional Primate Research Center, University of California, Davis (Andrew Hendrickx, Anne Ketchum and Jenny Short) and the Harlow Primate Laboratory, Department of Psychology, University of Wisconsin, Madison (Chris Coe). There are additional collaborations with groups at the Universities of Reykjavik (Reynir Geirsson – prevalence and familial tendency in Iceland), Oxford (John Bell – genotyping; Pat Yudkin – statistics; Stephen Golding – MRI studies) and Pittsburgh (Daniel Weeks – biostatistics). I thank the National Endometriosis Society of Great Britain, the American Endometriosis Association and Mary-Lou Ballweg, in particular, for their invaluable help. Family collection, the human MRI studies and Ruth Hadfield have been supported by an MRC-ROPA grant. The WRPRC is supported by grant P51 RR00167 from the National Institutes of Health.

## REFERENCES

1. Kennedy SH, Mardon HJ, Barlow DH. Familial endometriosis. *J Assist Reprod Genet* 1995;**12**:32–4.
2. Hadfield RM, Yudkin PL, Coe CL, et al. Risk factors for endometriosis in the rhesus monkey (Macaca mulatta): A case-control study. *Hum Reprod Update* 1997;**3**:109–15.
3. Moen MH. Endometriosis in monozygotic twins. *Acta Obstet Gynaecol Scand* 1994;**73**:59–62.
4. Hadfield RM, Mardon HJ, Barlow DH, Kennedy SH. Endometriosis in monozygotic twins. *Fertil Steril* 1997;**68**:941–2.
5. Kennedy SH, Hadfield RM, Mardon HJ, Barlow DH. Age of onset of pain symptoms in non-twin sisters concordant for endometriosis. *Hum Reprod* 1996;**11**:403–5.
6. Simpson JL, Elias S, Malinak LR, Buttram VCJ. Heritable aspects of endometriosis. I. Genetic studies. *Am J Obstet Gynecol* 1980;**137**:327–31.
7. Coxhead D, Thomas EJ. Familial inheritance of endometriosis in a British population. A case control study. *J Obstet Gynecol* 1993;**13**:42–4.
8. Moen MH, Magnus P. The familial risk of endometriosis. *Acta Obstet Gynaecol Scand* 1993;**72**:560–4.
9. Cramer DW, Hornstein MD, Ng WG, Barbieri RL. Endometriosis associated with the N314D mutation of galactose-1-phosphate uridyl transferase (GALT). *Mol Hum Reprod* 1996;**2**:149–52.
10. Baranova H, Bothorishvilli R, Canis M, et al. Glutathione S-transferase M1 gene polymorphism and susceptibility to endometriosis in a French population. *Mol Hum Reprod* 1997;**3**:775–80.
11. Baranov VS, Ivaschenko T, Bakay B, et al. Proportion of the GSTM1 0/0 genotype in some Slavic populations and its correlation with cystic fibrosis and some multifactorial diseases. *Hum Genet* 1996;**97**:516–20.
12. Spitsyn VA, Andreeva EN, Adamian LV, Agapova RK, Sandoval P. Genetic aspects of endometriosis: features of the distribution of polymorphic gene frequencies. *Genetika* 1996;**32**:1693–9.
13. Hinson JM Jr, Brigham KL, Daniell J. Catamenial pneumothorax in sisters. *Chest* 1981;**80**:634–5.
14. Ranney B. Endometriosis. IV. Hereditary tendency. *Obstet Gynecol* 1971;**37**:734–7.
15. Lamb K, Hoffmann RG, Nichols TR. Family trait analysis: a case-control study of 43 women with endometriosis and their best friends. *Am J Obstet Gynecol* 1986;**154**:596–601.
16. American Fertility Society. Revised classification of endometriosis: 1985. *Fertil Steril* 1985;**43**:351–2.
17. MacKenzie WF, Casey HW. Animal model of human disease. Endometriosis. Animal model: endometriosis in rhesus monkeys. *Am J Pathol* 1975;**80**:341–4.
18. Haupt BJ. Utilization of short-stay hospitals: annual summary for the United States, 1980. *Vital Health Stat 13* 1982;**13**(64):1–60.
19. Houston DE, Noller KL, Melton LJ III, Selwyn BJ, Hardy RJ. Incidence of pelvic endometriosis in Rochester, Minnesota, 1970–1979. *Am J Epidemiol* 1987;**125**:959–69.
20. Davies JL, Kawaguchi Y, Bennett ST, et al. A genome-wide search for human type 1 diabetes susceptibility genes. *Nature* 1994;**371**:130–6.
21. A genome-wide search for asthma susceptibility loci in ethnically diverse populations. The Collaborative Study on the Genetics of Asthma (CSGA). *Nat Genet* 1997;**15**:389–92.
22. Koninckx PR. Is mild endometriosis a condition occurring intermittently in all women? *Hum Reprod* 1994;**9**:2202–5.
23. Kennedy SH, Hadfield RM, Barlow DH, Weeks DE, Laird E, Golding S. Use of MRI in genetic studies of endometriosis. *Am J Med Genet* 1997;**71**:371–2.
24. Suchard MA, Hadfield RM, Elliott T, Kennedy SH. Beyond providing information: the Internet as a research tool in reproductive medicine. *Hum Reprod* WWW site. 1997, Issue 5.
25. Poirier J, Davignon J, Bouthillier D, Kogan S, Bertrand P, Gauthier S. Apolipoprotein E polymorphism and Alzheimer's disease. *Lancet* 1993;**342**:697–9.
26. Soubrier F, Cambien F. The angiotensin I-converting enzyme gene polymorphism: implication in hypertension and myocardial infarction. *Curr Opin Nephrol Hypertens* 1994;**3**:25–9.

27. Cramer DW, Muto MG, Reichardt JK, et al. Characteristics of women with a family history of ovarian cancer. I. Galactose consumption and metabolism. *Cancer* 1994;**74**:1309–17.

28. Cramer DW, Xu H, Harlow BL. Family history as a predictor of early menopause. *Fertil Steril* 1995;**64**:740–5.

29. Cramer DW, Goldstein DP, Fraer C, Reichardt JK. Vaginal agenesis (Mayer–Rokitansky–Kuster–Hauser syndrome) associated with the N314D mutation of galactose-1-phosphate uridyl transferase (GALT). *Mol Hum Reprod* 1996;**2**:145–8.

30. Elias S, Simpson JL, Carson SA, Malinak LR, Buttram-VC J. Genetics studies in incomplete mullerian fusion. *Obstet Gynecol* 1984;**63**:276–9.

31. Ergun A, Pabuccu R, Atay V, Kucuk T, Duru NK, Gungor S. Three sisters with septate uteri: another reference to bidirectional theory. *Hum Reprod* 1997;**12**:140–2.

32. Verp MS, Simpson JL, Elias S, Carson SA, Sarto GE, Feingold M. Heritable aspects of uterine anomalies. I. Three familial aggregates with Müllerian fusion anomalies. *Fertil Steril* 1983; **40**:80–5.

33. Jiang X, Hitchcock A, Bryan EJ, et al. Microsatellite analysis of endometriosis reveals loss of heterozygosity at candidate ovarian tumor suppressor gene loci. *Cancer Res* 1996;**56**:3534–9.

34. Seidegard J, Pero RW, Markowitz MM, Roush G, Miller DG, Beattie EJ. Isoenzyme(s) of glutathione transferase (class Mu) as a marker for the susceptibility to lung cancer: a follow up study. *Carcinogenesis* 1990;**11**:33–6.

35. Kempkes M, Golka K, Reich S, Reckwitz T, Bolt HM. Glutathione *S*-transferase GSTM1 and GSTT1 null genotypes as potential risk factors for urothelial cancer of the bladder. *Arch Toxicol* 1996;**71**:123–6.

36. Rier SE, Martin DC, Bowman RE, Dmowski WP, Becker JL. Endometriosis in rhesus monkeys (*Macaca mulatta*) following chronic exposure to 2,3,7,8-tetrachlorodibenzo-p-dioxin. *Fundam Appl Toxicol* 1993;**21**:433–41.

37. Mayani A, Barel S, Soback S, Almagor M. Dioxin concentrations in women with endometriosis. *Hum Reprod* 1997;**12**:373–5.

38. Koninckx PR, Braet P, Kennedy SH, Barlow DH. Dioxin pollution and endometriosis in Belgium. *Hum Reprod* 1994;**9**:1001–2.

39. Arnold LL, Ascher SM, Simon JA. Familial adenomyosis: a case report. *Fertil Steril* 1994; **61**:1165–7.

40. Pandis N, Karaiskos C, Bardi G, et al. Chromosome analysis of uterine adenomyosis. Detection of the leiomyoma-associated del(7q) in three cases. *Cancer Genet Cytogenet* 1995;**80**:118–20.

41. Woodworth SH, Singh M, Yussman MA, Sanfilippo JS, Cook CL, Lincoln SR. A prospective study on the association between red hair color and endometriosis in infertile patients. *Fertil Steril* 1995;**64**:651–2.

42. Hornstein MD, Thomas PP, Sober AJ, Wyshak G, Albright NL, Frisch RE. Association between endometriosis, dysplastic naevi and history of melanoma in women of reproductive age. *Hum Reprod* 1997;**12**:143–5.

43. Nichols TR, Lamb K, Arkins JA. The association of atopic diseases with endometriosis. *Ann Allergy* 1987;**59**:360–3.

44. Brincat M, Galea R, Buhagiar A. Polycystic ovaries and endometriosis: a possible connection. *Br J Obstet Gynaecol* 1994;**101**:346–8.

45. Moen M, Bratlie A, Moen T. Distribution of HLA-antigens among patients with endometriosis. *Acta Obstet Gynaecol Scand Suppl* 1984; **123**:25–7.

46. Simpson JL, Malinak LR, Elias S, Carson SA, Radvany RA. HLA associations in endometriosis. *Am J Obstet Gynecol* 1984;**148**:395–7.

47. Steele RW, Dmowski WP, Marmer DJ. Immunologic aspects of human endometriosis. *Am J Reprod Immunol* 1984;**6**:33–6.

48. Miyazawa K. Incidence of endometriosis among Japanese women. *Obstet Gynecol* 1976;**48**:407–9.

49. Sangi Haghpeykar H, Poindexter AN. Epidemiology of endometriosis among parous women. *Obstet Gynecol* 1995;**85**:983–92.

50. Arumugam K, Templeton AA. Endometriosis and race. *Aust NZ J Obstet Gynaecol* 1992; **32**:164–5.

51. Bocker J, Tadmor OP, Gal M, Diamant YZ. The prevalence of adenomyosis and endometriosis in an ultrareligious Jewish population. *Asia Oceania J Obstet Gynaecol* 1994;**20**:125–9.

# 35

# Principles of management of endometriosis: surgical treatment

Philippe R Koninckx, David Barlow

**History of surgical techniques** • **Minimal and mild endometriosis** • **Cystic ovarian endometriosis** • **Deep endometriosis** • **Discussion and conclusions** • **Acknowledgements**

Our understanding of endometriosis has changed dramatically over the last decade. Introduced clinically at the beginning of this century, as ovarian 'chocolate cysts'[1] and as adenomyosis externa,[2–4] it was defined as endometrial glands and stroma outside the uterus. According to this definition, black puckered lesions in the pelvis were soon recognized as endometriosis, making it a frequently observed disease. When, in the 1980s, non-pigmented endometriotic lesions were also described,[5–8] the prevalence of the disease increased from 5–20% to over 60–80% of women with infertility and/or pelvic pain.[9–18] Simultaneously with the increasing awareness of the prevalence of endometriosis, our concepts of aetiology, pathophysiology, natural history and therapy have evolved. Endometriosis has been considered for decades to be the result of the implantation of retrograde menstruated endometrial cells,[19] or metaplasia[20,21] induced by this menstrual debris or lymphatic spread.[22,23] It has been shown that retrograde menstruation occurs in almost all women;[24,25] this fluid contains viable cells[26] which can implant in the peritoneum.[27] Progression to cystic ovarian endometriosis and/or deep infiltrating endometriosis was assumed to be the natural course of the disease.[28] In recent years this concept of implantation and progression has been challenged by a new concept that considers superficial endometriosis to be a physiological condition occurring intermittently in all women, retaining only deep and cystic ovarian endometriosis as a true disease.[29,30]

Treatment of endometriosis consisted of surgical destruction or medical inactivation. As recurrences were considered to be frequent, surgery was often radical. In the last decade, especially since the introduction of endoscopic surgery, concepts such as debulking of deep endometriosis and focal therapy of cystic endometriosis have questioned the concept that surgery should be radical, that endometriotic disease is always progressive, and that recurrence rates are high. Hormone replacement therapy given to women with endometriosis has, moreover, questioned our concepts about medical therapy and peritoneal fluid.[31]

To evaluate critically surgery for endometriosis first we discuss the differences in surgical techniques and subsequently evaluate indications and results of treatment.

## HISTORY OF SURGICAL TECHNIQUES

To interpret the literature describing the results of surgery for endometriosis, a clear understanding of the evolution and limitations of the various techniques is necessary. Up to the end of the 1970s, minimal and mild endometriosis was destroyed endoscopically by heat application (endothermia) and by unipolar or bipolar coagulation. Treatment of more severe endometriotic disease was mostly radical by hysterectomy, often leaving some rectovaginal endometriosis, whereas in younger women adnexectomies, rather than cystectomies and anterior resections of the rectum, were performed. The literature of this period focuses on infertility and mild endometriosis, and is biased by the fact that deep endometriosis – unless very severe and extensive – was not recognized. All series of this period are thus 'contaminated' by some 5–20% of undiagnosed and thus untreated deep endometriosis. In the late 1970s and the early 1980s, microsurgery was promoted, emphasizing careful destruction of superficial endometriosis by bipolar coagulation or resection and removal of cystic ovarian endometriosis, followed by reconstruction of the ovary. The underdiagnosing of deep endometriosis continued to be a problem.

From 1986 to 1987 onwards, the concept of minimal endometriosis and/or non-pigmented endometriosis was introduced.[32] This has caused an important shift in the reported incidence of endometriosis, which depends on recognition and awareness. This increasing recognition of endometriosis has resulted in a progressive shift of women, who would previously have been classified as 'normal', to women classified as having minimal endometriosis. This is important in the interpretation of data of that time, such as results of surgery, because the reported groups of 'normal' women thus contain variable numbers of (unrecognized and untreated) women with minimal endometriosis. Simultaneously, the severity of the disease in groups of women with minimal and mild disease progressively decreases, through dilution by those women with minimal disease. The bias of non-

recognition of the majority of deep endometriotic disease still existed.

The increasing use of endoscopic surgery for the treatment of cystic ovarian endometriosis was paralleled by a diversification of techniques with possibly different results. The removal of the cyst wall by stripping followed by suturing or gluing of the ovary is technically similar to microsurgery. Vaporization of the cyst wall is poorly defined, ranging from focal treatment to superficial vaporization to deeper vaporization. Besides these differences in techniques used, the various studies are biased by the fact that the technique varies with the volume of the endometriotic cyst, but not always to the same extent. In addition combined endoscopic and microsurgical techniques have been proposed.[33]

In the 1990s, deep endometriosis has been recognized increasingly during laparoscopic surgery,[18,34] or by clinical examination during menstruation.[35] 'Resection of deep endometriosis' comprises techniques ranging from complete resection to debulking and resection–reanastomosis of the rectum, a difference that is rarely stated clearly in the literature. With the recent trend to recognize and to treat deep endometriosis this 'enthusiasm' is already producing and will continue to produce a progressive shift of the severity of the reported series of deep endometriosis, which will include increasing numbers of women with less severe deep endometriosis previously diagnosed as mild disease. To interpret correctly data in the literature it is thus important to consider: (1) the awareness of minimal endometriosis, which is important to judge the 'contamination' of the normal group with minimal endometriosis together with the overall severity of endometriosis in the group with minimal endometriosis; (2) the awareness of deep endometriosis which will determine the incidence of 'unrecognized' deep endometriosis in the minimal–mild groups; whereas (3) only depth of penetration and volume will permit evaluation of the 'enthusiasm' of the surgeon to include small spots infiltrating 4–5–6 mm; and (4) the size of cystic ovarian endometriosis, the presence of adhesions, the pathological confirmation of the disease and the technique used, in comparing reported series on cystic ovarian endometriosis.

## MINIMAL AND MILD ENDOMETRIOSIS

### Methods of destruction

Ideally these endometriosis lesions are vaporized or excised with a high-power $CO_2$ laser. We consider this to be the method of choice because this treatment rapidly removes all the endometriosis and only the endometriosis, leaving a minimal amount of necrotic tissue. The choice between vaporization and excision depends on the size of the endometriotic lesion, larger lesions being excised more rapidly. This method takes full advantage of the characteristics of a $CO_2$ laser as a bloodless and precise cutting instrument, with a thermal damage to the surrounding tissue of 100 μm or less. It requires, however, a high power $CO_2$ laser, which is expensive, and a high flow insufflator of more than 20 l/min,[36] to evacuate smoke and prevent blooming and to maintain a high-power density necessary for a minimal thermal damage, at least with a conventional $CO_2$ laser.

Alternative methods of destruction are bipolar coagulation, endothermia and sharp excision. The former two methods are less adequate than laser vaporization/excision for typical lesions, because depth of infiltration is difficult to assess by inspection and palpation only. Moreover, the amount of necrotic tissue left behind could increase the number of postoperative adhesions. Sharp excision is theoretically equivalent to $CO_2$ laser excision. In our hands, however, this method makes it more difficult to find the exact borders between the lesion and the healthy tissue, a process that is more visual than tactile. Sharp dissection, moreover, balances extensive prophylactic coagulation – which results in tissue damage and difficult planes of cleavage – and no prophylactic coagulation which is always associated with capillary bleeding and poor visualization.

### Is destruction necessary?

If minimal and possibly mild endometriosis is considered a natural condition occurring intermittently in all women,[29–30] it would be logical to postulate that treatment is not necessary because it is not a disease, it will disappear spontaneously and can reappear later at another site.

From a surgical point of view, however, this is an academic discussion. Indeed the vaporization of minimal endometriosis, that is, a few subtle lesions, is so easily performed in a few seconds and generally without risks, that it might be unwise to leave the possibility that some of these lesions would be or become more invasive or aggressive. For slightly larger typical lesions, excision is mandatory to ascertain the depth of infiltration.

### Is destruction useful?

It is uncertain whether it is useful to treat endometriosis to prevent progression; although most minimal lesions will disappear spontaneously at some stage, it remains extremely likely that at least some of these lesions may have the potential to develop into a more aggressive disease and will eventually do so. To demonstrate this in randomized controlled trials can be argued to be clinically irrelevant because destruction is so easy, and scientifically it might be impossible to achieve. With a 60% prevalence of minimal–mild endometriosis and a progression to severe disease in some 10% after 5 years, it would moreover require a randomized trial of hundreds of patients over many years, which is unrealistic.

Whether it is useful as a treatment of pain is unknown. Indeed, we favour the hypothesis that subtle and typical endometriosis is rarely painful, except when associated with deeper disease and possibly when larger areas are involved. This view relates to the concept of the activation of spare nociceptors[37,38] with inflammation and the observation that these lesions are specifically painful when stimulated.[39] This discussion, however, is more academic than clinically irrelevant.

That it is useful as an infertility treatment has become increasingly clear. During the late 1970s an association was shown between endometriosis, luteal phase insufficiency, unexplained infertility and the luteinized unruptured follicle syndrome (LUF).[40–42] To understand why this association has been questioned later, it might be important to realize the shift that had taken place in the groups of women reported because of the recognition of subtle non-pigmented lesions.[43–46] Studies in the baboon confirmed experimentally that endometriosis was associated with the LUF syndrome, the LUF syndrome was recurrent and the LUF syndrome, diagnosed by inspection of the ovaries, correlated with the absence of ovulation.[47] Recently, it was shown in humans that treatment improved fertility.[48] It should be realized that these observations do not contradict the concept of a natural condition being present intermittently in all women, because subfertility, for example, an LUF syndrome, might be present predominantly in those months that the lesions are present. If, in women with infertility, subtle endometriotic lesions are more frequently encountered, this might reduce the overall monthly fecundity rate, for example, through an LUF syndrome. Again this discussion could be academic because surgical destruction can be done so easily and rapidly.

In conclusion, treatment of minimal and subtle endometriosis can be considered both unnecessary and impossible if it is a recurrent natural condition. The surgical reality of a simple, rapid and harmless destruction, however, favours destruction during laparoscopy, because some of these lesions could have more aggressive behaviour in the long run, it can be very difficult or impossible to evaluate with certainty the depth of infiltration without excision, and finally fertility is enhanced in the months after destruction. This argument is based on the assumption that there are facilities for the rapid deployment of the laser or that, if more destructive technology is used, the surgeon is able to appreciate situations where the position of a lesion may make it unsuitable for destruction.

## CYSTIC OVARIAN ENDOMETRIOSIS

### Pitfalls of diagnosis

The treatment of cystic ovarian endometriosis remains hampered by misdiagnosing of a cystic corpus luteum as a cystic ovarian endometrioma. This problem has not been addressed specifically in the literature. Even if only women with pathologically confirmed cystic endometriosis were considered, these data do not permit a judgement of the extent to which cystic corpora lutea had been operated on. A clinical history of the persistence of a cyst is unreliable for diagnosing cystic ovarian endometriosis.

Over the years we have operated on several women, with a 'chocolate cyst' on ultrasonography persisting for more than 4 months, even during treatment with a luteinizing hormone-releasing hormone (LHRH) agonist or oral contraceptive. We are fully aware that this clinical observation does not allow any conclusion about frequency, but it is consistent with the observation that ovarian cysts can develop during ovarian down-regulation.[49] Imaging, such as ultrasonography and computed tomography, has a sensitivity of 70–80% and a specificity of 90–95%.[50–54] This is a valuable method of diagnosis that helps clinical management. It will not, however, prevent errors of judgement during surgery. Ovarian flow measurement does not seem to improve specificity or sensitivity substantially.[50]

CA-125 in chocolate fluid has been reported to have a sensitivity and a specificity of almost 100%.[55,56] Unfortunately, a rapid test, for example, a stick assay, is not available to make the diagnosis during surgery. Our clinical rule of thumb is that, as cystic ovarian endometriosis is so strongly associated with adhesions,[18] a 'chocolate cyst' without adhesions has a high probability of being a cystic corpus luteum, whereas the presence of severe adhesions especially in the fossa ovarica enhances the suspicion of endometriosis. This, together with the inspection of the inside of the cyst by ovarioscopy[57] or by inspection with the laparoscope,[58] will help to make a correct judgement in most women. Those with a flattened appearance and red or red and brown mottled ridges generally were endometriosis and those with a dark uniform base, an intracavitary clot or a yellowish rim generally were corpus lutea or albicans.

In conclusion, however, awareness of the problem, preoperative imaging and CA-125 assays, and preoperative scrutiny did not prevent misdiagnoses in over 10% of women.

## Physiopathology

The physiopathology of cystic endometriosis is not entirely understood. It is attractive to consider that much, if not most, of the cystic ovarian endometriosis originates from invagination of superficial implants.[59] Particularly when the ovary becomes adherent to the pelvic wall by endometriotic implants, it seems logical that a 'pseudocyst' is formed by the accumulation of old blood and debris, thus stretching the ovarian capsule over this cyst.[60,61] This phenomenon of invagination and stretching of the ovarian capsule can explain why the inside of the cyst wall is not always entirely covered by endometriosis, but is instead localized as focal endometriotic spots. It thus seems logical to postulate that only these endometriotic spots should be destroyed, and that removing the cyst wall is equivalent to removing the ovarian surface. This mechanism of invagination and stretching of the ovarian capsule does not preclude some cysts having a different origin and a lining covered by endometriosis. A careful histology of the cyst wall moreover reveals that endometriotic glands can be present in the so-called cyst wall up to a depth of at least 5–6 mm.

## Surgical pragmatism of size

From a surgical point of view, the size of the ovarian cyst is most important. For smaller cysts ($< 5\,cm$) the cyst wall can generally be stripped easily from the ovary. This process seems to follow a natural plane of cleavage, confirmed indirectly by the fact that it is associated with little bleeding. For cysts larger than 5 cm in diameter, the discussion of whether the cyst wall should be removed or destroyed, or whether a focal treatment will be sufficient, is purely academic. Indeed, in those women with a large cyst, the remaining ovarian rim will be so thin that resection becomes either technically impossible or practically unrealistic because minimal ovarian tissue will be left. Also the extensive vaporization of these very large areas is unrealistic.

## Methods of treatment

Aspiration and rinsing of cystic ovarian endometriosis have been attempted but the recurrence rate is high.[62–64] Ultrasonically guided aspiration will result in 'chocolate in the pelvis' the next day (unpublished data), which could increase adhesion formation,[65] although we have shown that chocolate fluid does not induce adhesions when injected intraperitoneally in mice.[66]

For smaller cysts, that is, less than 5 cm in diameter, the method of stripping the cyst from the ovary, as initially described by the Clermont Ferrand group, seems most attractive.[67–69] It is rapid and technically relatively easy. It is also a complete treatment when invading glands are present. Closure of the ovary by Tissucol (Immuno, Vienna, Austria) when necessary results in a 'normal ovary' after surgery with no denuded areas. The cyst wall could be vaporized. Some report excellent results,[59] but we stopped using this method because it was too difficult to judge the correct depth of vaporization. Destruction that is too superficial will result in an incomplete treatment, whereas destruction that is too deep often causes bleeding. The cyst wall could be destroyed by unipolar or semi-bipolar coagulation. Although attractive, the reported series are too small to compare this technique with vaporization. The third option besides wall excision and wall destruction is focal treatment.[70] We feel that this is less indicated because it is difficult in most women to judge which areas are not involved, making focal treatment generally equivalent to vaporization of the wall.

For larger cysts, the pragmatism of size in practice excludes excision and/or vaporization. The method of making a large window in the cyst wall, followed by rinsing and focal treatment, is attractive and promising. It remains unclear, however, whether during this surgery it is important to do a full adhesiolysis, if necessary, or whether the surgery should be kept to a strict minimum, that is, marsupialization to reduce the surgical trauma and possibly adhesion formation. It is also unclear whether medical therapy is helpful postoperatively. This is logical because it will prevent development of a corpus luteum and a hypo-oestrogenic milieu could reduce adhesion formation. It also remains unclear whether second-look surgery should always be performed. The number of 'large' endometriomas are insufficient in most centres to perform randomized trials, whereas the rapid technical evolution of endoscopic surgery has made a large randomized trial impossible in practice.

We favour keeping surgery to a minimum during the first laparoscopy making it a 5–10 minute procedure that vaporizes superficially all visible endometriotic spots, then giving LHRH agonists for 3 months, followed by ultrasonography. If a cyst still persists, a second laparoscopy will generally find a small one. If no cyst is found, and if there are no complaints of pain or infertility, a second intervention is no longer necessary. This concept has the indirect advantage that the first operation can always be scheduled as a day case, without bowel preparation, whereas the need for bowel preparation in the second intervention will be known in advance.

## Results

The results of endoscopic and microsurgical treatment are comparable,[71] ranging between a 60% and 80% cure of pain, a cumulative pregnancy rate of 60–70% after 6 months to 1 year, and a recurrence rate of some 20%.[72–76] It remains unclear whether preoperative or postoperative medical treatment or ovarian downregulation affects the results of surgery significantly.[77]

## Conclusion

Cystic ovarian endometriosis has to be treated, because this condition is associated with pain and infertility, and carries the risk of spontaneous rupture; surgery is the only real treatment, because medical treatment can only inactivate endometriosis and reduce the size of the cyst.[78] As a result of technical and practical surgical considerations, we favour excision of smaller cysts by stripping, followed by closure of the remaining flaps if necessary. For larger cysts, we propose a minimal first intervention, consisting of marsupialization, rinsing and focal treatment, followed by LHRH agonists for 3 months and a second intervention when a cyst persists.

## DEEP ENDOMETRIOSIS

### Diagnosis, types and prevalence

Endometriosis can infiltrate the surrounding tissues resulting in an important sclerotic and inflammatory reaction, which clinically translates into nodularity, bowel stenosis and ureteral obstruction. The most severe forms, such as rectovaginal endometriosis and endometriosis invading the rectum or the sigmoid, have been known since the early 1900s. These conditions, however, are relatively rare with an estimated prevalence of less than 1%. This estimation is derived from the observation in Leuven of some 10–20% deep endometriosis in 1988–91,[79] a period during which endoscopic surgery was not yet well developed, and in which deep endometriosis was not yet a well-known entity. Referralls were thus only those for infertility and pain, and not those for deep endometriosis. Assuming that laparoscopies for infertility are performed in some 10–15% of the population, and taking into account that Leuven is a tertiary referral centre, the prevalence of deep endometriosis can be estimated to be between 1% (the prevalence is 10% in younger age groups with infertility which can be estimated at 15% of the population; in a tertiary centre the prevalence is probably slightly overestimated) and 3% (prevalence of 20% of the older age group with infertility). Taking into account the observation that, using menstrual clinical examination, deep endometriosis is more frequent, prevalences of between 3% and 10% seem a fair estimate.

The endoscopic excision of endometriosis has revealed that endometriosis invading deeper than 5–6 mm is associated with pain and infertility. Three subtypes were described.[80]

Type I is characterized by a large pelvic area of typical and sometimes some subtle endometriotic lesions surrounded by white sclerotic tissue. Only during excision does it become obvious that the endometriotic lesion infiltrates deeper than 5 mm. Typically the endometriotic area becomes progressively smaller as it grows deeper; the lesion is thus cone shaped.

Type II lesions are characterized by retraction of the bowel. Clinically they are recognized by the obvious bowel retraction around a small typical lesion. In some women, however, no endometriosis can be seen through the laparoscope, and the bowel retraction is the only clinical sign. Diagnosis is generally not too difficult because, during laparoscopy, the retraction under which an induration is felt is obvious. In some women, however, the retraction is hardly seen and the induration can be hardly felt. Only during excision does the endometriotic nodule become apparent, emphasizing the need for a preoperative diagnosis and training in recognition of these lesions.

Type III lesions are spherical endometriotic nodules in the rectovaginal septum. In their most typical manifestation these lesions are felt as painful nodularities in the rectovaginal septum. At laparoscopy they generally present as a small typical lesion, and in some women a careful vaginal examination reveals some dark blue cysts (3–4 mm) in the fornix posterior. Type III lesions are the most severe lesions, and they often spread laterally up and around the uterine artery, sometimes causing sclerosis around the ureter. The spread along the uterine artery can be so obvious that this can be considered as an indirect argument for the hypothesis that

deep endometriosis has escaped from the inhibitory influence of peritoneal fluid and is mainly under peripheral circulation control. Although being prominent in most women, these lesions are very often missed as will be discussed later. Sclerosing endometriosis, invading the sigmoid, is similar to rectal endometriosis, but is situated 10 cm above the rectovaginal septum. This is another form of deep endometriosis, which is fortunately a rare condition and which we could classify as type IV.

Diagnosis of deep endometriosis should be made before surgery. A retrospective analysis showed that using a routine clinical examination only 50% of the larger lesions are diagnosed. A menstrual clinical examination is the most powerful tool actually available for diagnosing deep endometriosis types I, II and III. By clinical examination during menstruation, painful nodularities are found in some 30% of women with pain or infertility. In the absence of cystic ovarian endometriosis, these nodularities were present in most of the women and were caused by deep endometriosis. The concentrations of CA-125 are increased in women with deep endometriosis and in those with cystic ovarian endometriosis and were proposed as a screening tool. Although specifically increased during menstruation, the variability does not improve the diagnostic accuracy.[81] A late follicular sample has a sensitivity of some 70–90% of endometriotic disease with a specificity of around 95%.[82] Ultrasonography and magnetic resonance imaging (MRI)[83] can be used to diagnose deep endometriosis, but their sensitivity is low especially for the smaller lesions. For type IV lesions a contrast enema and/or rectoscopy is necessary. Although hard data are not available, we presume that this diagnosis is easily missed, making prevalences higher than actually believed.

In conclusion, the most powerful tool to diagnose deep endometriosis is a menstrual clinical examination, whereas a routine clinical examination will reveal mainly the very large lesions. A CA-125 assay is a useful screening aid for deep endometriosis, and it might prove useful as a screening method for type IV lesions which, although severe, are easily missed and cannot be diagnosed by clinical examination. The final diagnosis is the estimation of the depth of infiltration during excisional surgery. The prevalence of the disease increases with age and is estimated at 1–10% in the general population and at 10–30% in women with pain and/or infertility. A menstrual clinical examination will increase these figures by diagnosing deep endometriosis in women with pain, which is insufficient to perform a laparoscopy.

## Surgical treatment

Surgery for deep endometriosis can be difficult and dangerous. Therefore a preoperative contrast enema and intravenous pyelography should be considered, whereas surgery itself requires a full bowel preparation in order to allow any kind of bowel surgery. This may require the collaboration of a colorectal surgeon, depending on the experience and training of the gynaecologist. If gross distortion of the ureter is present, preoperative ureter stents are recommended. The surgical excision of deep endometriosis itself relies upon a combination of perfect visual inspection and tactile information.

For types I, II and III, one of the authors (PK) prefers to use a $CO_2$ laser (80 watts, Sharplan; Tel Aviv, Israel) together with a high-flow insufflator (Thermoflator, Storz AG; Tüttlingen, Germany). Guided by visual inspection together with tactile information about the softness of the tissue, the peritoneum is incised below the lesion at the border between the normal and soft tissue and the harder endometriosis, glowing yellowish under the $CO_2$ laser beam. First the lateral edges of the nodule are dissected to free the nodule, if necessary, from the ureter, the uterine artery and the spinosacral ligament. This is technically the most difficult part of the surgery. Subsequently, the posterior part of the nodule is dissected thus freeing the rectum. We feel that it is important, during this dissection, that the nodule remains attached to the uterus and cervix or vagina,

thus elevating the nodule, whereas the rectum progressively falls down by gravity. This dissection is continued as far as possible, at least until the rectum is completely liberated from the rectovaginal septum. Only after completion of the dissection of the posterior part, is the anterior side of the nodule dissected from the cervix and the vagina. In some 20% of women, part of the vaginal fornix has to be removed because of endometriotic invasion, whereas we estimate that, in some 20% of women, the rectum has to be opened to permit a complete resection.[84] In the Leuven series, it is noteworthy that resection of the rectum has not been necessary in any of these women.

A careful description of the excisional technique is mandatory to understand the pros and cons of the reported techniques. The advantages of the technique as described are the perfect visualization and the angle of access. Using $CO_2$ laser excision through the operating laparoscope, excisional surgery is performed with great magnification: excision can be performed with the laparoscope close in because the laparoscope carries the 'knife'; excision also has to be performed close in because the focal length of the $CO_2$ laser lens is some 2 cm from the laparoscope. A third advantage is that the direction of access of the rectovaginal septum, and especially the posterior side of the node, is easier through the laparoscope than through a secondary port. Obviously, this technique requires a high-flow insufflator[85] to maintain a clear picture throughout the excision, and to permit continuous use of the laser, without interruption.

Three other techniques are used for the resection of deep endometriosis: sharp dissection together with electrosurgery through the laparoscope; sharp dissection together with electrosurgery through the secondary ports; and a partial rectum resection followed by reanastomosis, usually with a circular stapler. It is obvious that each surgeon performs best using the techniques he or she is most familiar with, and that few endoscopic surgeons are familiar with all techniques. Most, indeed, have developed the technique that they started with generally for historical reasons. This should not, however, prevent discussion of the relative advantages of the different approaches, as evaluated by expert surgeons performing surgical procedures, often arranged on the basis of friendship. Sharp dissection, together with electrosurgery through the laparoscope as developed by David Redwine,[86–90] is technically almost identical to the $CO_2$ laser excision, that is, it permits a very posterior approach, working close in with great magnification in a bloodless operating field. The disadvantage is that this technique is physically demanding although less suited for video-endoscopic surgery, thus reducing the possibility of help from an assistant. This technique, however, probably combines the advantage of an improved depth of vision (as not using a video screen) with enhanced tactile information (as with sharp dissection). Sharp dissection together with electrosurgery through the secondary ports is the most widely used technique[68,91–100] for several reasons: it is derived from the other endoscopic procedures, it does not require a $CO_2$ laser and, possibly even more important, a high-flow insufflator was not available during its development. As the angle of access is much sharper, surgeons using this technique generally start dissection at the anterior site of the nodule, thus freeing nodule and rectum from the rectovaginal septum.

Subsequently the rectum is dissected from the nodule which has become freely mobile. Most of these procedures aim at debulking the endometriosis, rather than performing a complete resection. The word 'debulking' is chosen when the surgeon prefers not opening the rectum, even if the resection is less complete. It is difficult to estimate whether this 'debulking' attitude is a consequence of the technique used, or of the philosophy often dictated by local and medicolegal considerations. The experience of one of the authors (PK) was that resection of endometriosis using this technique is much more difficult than using the $CO_2$ laser approach, and that the best method to avoid bowel lesions was by avoiding traction and using only gravity. These same considerations could explain why some authors – probably in order to perform a complete resection and to

avoid recurrences – perform a partial resection and anastomosis in women with larger nodules. Currently, it is not known whether those performing a complete resection are overtreating their patients, or whether those aiming at debulking the lesion are undertreating the endometriosis.

Type IV endometriosis requires a resection and subsequent reanastomosis. PK attempted to carry out conservative surgery in three of these women, but was unsuccessful: the angle of access was too difficult, a third secondary port was necessary to stabilize the sigmoid and the procedures took more than 2 hours.

## Complications, treatment and prevention[101–103]

When part of the rectum wall has to be removed, or when the rectum is accidentally opened, the pelvis is rinsed with a 1% Hibitane (chlorhexidine) solution and the wall is sutured endoscopically with two layers of 3/0 Vicryl (Ethicon, Cincinnati, USA). A defect in the posterior vaginal fornix is sutured either vaginally or endoscopically. Care is taken to suture these defects so that they are water tight. PK prefers to suture these defects laparoscopically, for reasons of sterility: during laparoscopic suturing a continuous flow of $CO_2$ from the abdominal cavity to the vagina prevents contamination.

Surgical excision of deep endometriosis is thus difficult surgery because it often necessitates dissection far laterally around the ureter and uterine artery. Also the excision from the bowel wall is difficult, because in 10% of women part of the bowel wall will have to be resected. In 20% of women, especially those with rectovaginal endometriosis, that is, type III lesions, excision has to be performed up to and including the posterior vaginal fornix. It is important that neither resection of part of the bowel wall nor resection of the vaginal fornix should be considered as complications of surgery, because the postoperative follow-up has been uneventful in a series of over 300 women (series of PK).

Complications of surgery ($n = 225$) have been the trans-section of the uterine artery in two women necessitating clipping, a ureter lesion in one woman and a late bowel perforation in six women. A ureteric lesion is a serious complication, and therefore we advocate a pre-operative intravenous urogram, a careful dissection of the ureter from its landmarks at the pelvic brim and liberal preventive stenting if necessary. This is judged even more important, because it became evident that a ureter that is only half cut can rather easily be sutured endoscopically over a double J.[104] A late bowel perforation is an even more serious complication which has occurred in six women: two with a type II lesion (1989 and 1991) and one with a type III lesion (1992) were readmitted after a week with progressively increasing symptoms of peritonitis; one (1992) with a type I lesion and a history of pouch anastomosis for colitis ulcerosa was observed for 1 week with atypical symptoms which later proved to be a rectum perforation; and two (1994) with a type II lesion had acute pelvic pain, 12 hours after surgery and 2 days after surgery respectively. Although symptoms of peritonitis were minimal, an immediate laparoscopy revealed a bowel perforation in both.

It is important to realize that bowel perforations can occur during the early postoperative days, thus necessitating a low-fibre diet and eventually hospitalization. A perforation generally occurs during straining, with acute pelvic pain as the only symptom. Disturbingly, this pain disappears over the subsequent hours with slight peritoneal irritation as the only symptom. A liberal use of early second-look laparoscopies is advocated in these women before symptoms of peritonitis develop. In five women one of the authors (PK) did indeed recently demonstrate that even a bowel perforation can safely be sutured endoscopically thus avoiding a colostomy.

Prevention of a late perforation is even more important. Since January 1996, liberal prophylactic suturing of the rectum has been used whenever a suspicion of a lesion to the muscularis existed. Since then this complication has disappeared.

## Medical treatment

Medical therapy before surgery has been discussed for many years and surgeons have claimed that deep lesions were less vascularized after medical therapy. Recently, it was demonstrated that pre-treatment for 3 months with an LHRH agonist could shrink deep lesions.[84] Indeed, in this series triptorelin (Decapeptyl) 3.75 mg/month had been given specifically to women with the most severe disease, especially deep lesions. Analysis of data showed that women pre-treated with this LHRH agonist had a higher rAFS (revised American Fertility Society) score at surgery than those without treatment, confirming the selection bias. Similarly, pre-treated women had more and larger areas of cystic ovarian endometriosis, also pointing to the selection bias. As expected, women with pre-treatment had a smaller pelvic area of endometriosis. Pre-treated women had, however, a smaller volume of deep endometriosis notwithstanding the fact that, as a result of the selection bias, they almost certainly had a much higher volume before treatment. For this reason we advocate pre-treating women with severe deep endometriosis medically for 3 months with a gonadotrophin-releasing hormone (GnRH) agonist. We have the impression that danazol might be equally effective but the series was too small to prove this statistically. Other medical therapies have not been used frequently enough to be evaluated.

Medical treatment after excision of deep endometriosis has not been evaluated properly. If excision has been performed completely, medical treatment is probably not necessary. Medical therapy should, however, be considered instead of repeat or more radical surgery for recurring symptoms or failures of excision.

Medical treatment alone has not been addressed specifically in any study because of the lack of a clear-cut diagnosis of deep endometriosis without excision. Medical treatment using danazol, GnRH agonists or gestrinone does not cure endometriosis.[105–109] They all inactivate the endometriotic lesions which reappear rapidly after treatment has been stopped.[110] None of these therapies has an important beneficial effect on subsequent fertility.[111] They all improve pelvic pain and the effect persists often for many months after therapy has been stopped.[112] As deep endometriosis is strongly associated with pelvic pain, and as cystic ovarian endometriosis does not respond well to medical therapy, it is suggested that the observations and conclusions concerning severe pelvic pain are probably related to deep endometriosis.

## Results

Nehzat[97] reported 25 pregnancies in 67 women after excision of deep endometriosis. We (PK) evaluated cumulative pregnancy rates (CPR) in a consecutive series of 900 women with primary or secondary infertility without severe tubal damage and with a severely subfertile husband. Cumulative pregnancy rates were slightly lower in advanced stages of endometriosis according to the revised AFS classification, being 62% and 44% in classes I and IV, respectively. When, however, the duration of infertility was taken into account – which was the strongest predictor of subsequent conception – the differences in CPR between classes I and IV disappeared suggesting that the differences found between mild and severe endometriosis were mainly a consequence of differences in duration of infertility and possibly in age of the women.[113,114]

The only single group with a significantly higher CPR after surgery consisted of women with deep endometriosis. Using Cox's multivariate regression analysis, the following model was established: pregnancy was predicted most strongly by a shorter duration of infertility and by the surgical treatment of cystic ovarian endometriosis and/or deep endometriosis. From these results it can be concluded that aggressive and complete excision of deep endometriosis can be advocated, with subsequent spontaneous pregnancy rates of up to 60% within 1 year. These results can be considered excellent taking into account the severity of disease and the large denuded area in the

pelvis after excision of deep endometriosis. It remains unclear whether those women who did not conceive after 1 year should be oriented towards IVF or to second-look laparoscopy. Medical treatment alone, as can be derived from indirect evidence, is probably not the treatment of choice for deep endometriosis and infertility. As has been pointed out, medical pre-treatment seems to be useful to facilitate surgery as has been suggested for cystic ovarian endometriosis.[115] Both surgical and medical treatment were reported to be highly successful in treating pelvic pain. Candiani reported absence of dyspareunia and dysmenorrhoea in six and four out of ten after 40 months.[96] Nezhat reported moderate to complete pain relief in 162 women out of 175 but in some two or more interventions had been necessary.[97]

Preliminary analysis of our results in 250 women, in whom deep endometriosis has been excised with a $CO_2$ laser, showed a cure rate of pelvic pain in 70% with a recurrence rate of less than 5% over a follow-up period of up to 5 years. These data should be interpreted carefully, because the completeness of excision has steadily increased. The results of recent years strongly suggest an almost complete cure rate without recurrences; this, however, could be an overoptimistic clinical impression which will have to be proved by careful analysis of the data. In addition, medical treatment of pelvic pain is highly efficient, and the effect of treatment often persists after treatment has been stopped.[112]

## DISCUSSION AND CONCLUSIONS

We advocate (Fig. 1) a first-line approach to the diagnosis and treatment of endometriosis, which relies on a menstrual clinical examination, ultrasonography and eventually an assay of CA-125. After these examinations, four groups of women can be considered. When the clinical examination during menstruation does not reveal any nodularities, no ovarian cysts are found at ultrasonography and the CA-125 concentration is normal, women with infertility and/or pain are scheduled for a day-case diagnostic laparoscopy. If an endometrioma is

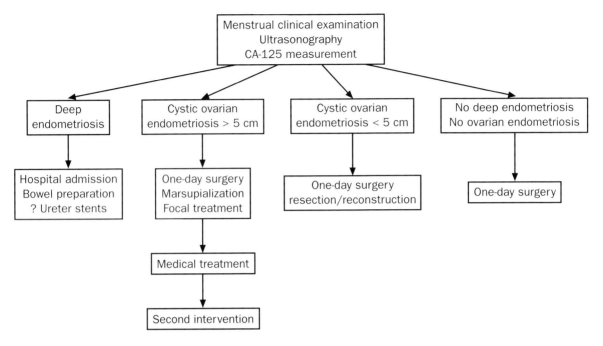

**Figure 1** Treatment of endometriosis.

found, larger than 5 cm in diameter, these women are also scheduled as a day case for an initial procedure during which the cyst is opened, rinsed and focally treated. Postoperatively these women are treated for 3 months with a GnRH analogue, and eventually scheduled for a second intervention. If a small endometrioma is found on ultrasonography, these women are also scheduled for a day case procedure. They are advised that the probability that a bowel preparation would be necessary cannot be excluded, but is probably less than 5%. If a deep endometriotic nodule is found, the necessity of a preoperative medical treatment, and of a preoperative contrast enema and intravenous urography should be considered. These women always receive a bowel

preparation and are admitted to the hospital for at least 48 hours.

This approach has the advantage that the preoperative clinical examination together with ultrasonography are used to decide whether the patient will be admitted to the hospital or treated in the day-case clinic, and whether a bowel preparation will be given. From our experience over the last few years, the accuracy of this procedure is close to 100% because unexpected deep endometriosis and unnecessary bowel treatments have virtually disappeared from the department.

Surgery remains the cornerstone of the treatment of endometriosis. Medical treatment seems to be indicated, both pre- and postoperatively as discussed, for women with recurrent pelvic endometriosis and pain, or when adequate surgery is not available or too dangerous.

## ACKNOWLEDGEMENTS

Dr Stephen Kennedy, Nuffield Department of Obstetrics and Gynaecology, Oxford, UK, is thanked for reviewing this manuscript. We thank our co-workers and our co-authors of the articles, of which data have been reviewed. Stefan Lempereur MD, Ipsen NV, Belgium and Freddy Cornillie PhD, Director, Centocor Europe, are thanked for their support and cooperation. This work was supported partially by the NFWO research grant No. 9-002090. This manuscript was typed by Mrs Diane Wolput.

## REFERENCES

1. Sampson JA. Peritoneal endometriosis due to the menstrual dissemination of endometrial tissue into the peritoneal cavity. *Am J Obstet Gynecol* 1927;**14**:422–69.
2. Cullen TS. Adenoma-myoma uteri diffusum benignum. *Johns Hopkins Hosp Bull* 1896;**6**:133–7.
3. Cullen TS. Adeno-myoma of the round ligament. *Johns Hopkins Hosp Bull* 1896;**7**:112–14.
4. Cullen TS. The distribution of adenomyomata containing uterine mucosa. *Am J Obstet Gynecol* 1919;**80**:130–8.
5. Jansen RPS, Russel P. Nonpigmented endometriosis: Clinical, laparoscopic, and pathologic definition. *Am J Obstet Gynecol* 1986;**155**:1154–9.
6. Stripling MC, Martin DC, Chatman DL, Vander Zwaag R, Poston WM. Subtle appearance of pelvic endometriosis. *Fertil Steril* 1988;**49**:427–31.
7. Stripling MC, Martin DC, Poston WM. Does endometriosis have a typical appearance? *J Reprod Med Obstet Gynecol* 1988;**33**:879–84.
8. Martin DC, Hubert GD, Van der Zwaag R, El Zeky FA. Laparoscopic appearances of peritoneal endometriosis. *Fertil Steril* 1989;**51**:63–7.
9. Mahmood TA, Templeton A. Prevalence and genesis of endometriosis. *Hum Reprod* 1991;**6**:544–9.
10. Rawson JMR. Prevalence of endometriosis in asymptomatic women. *J Reprod Med Obstet Gynecol* 1991;**36**:513–15.
11. Wheeler JM. Epidemiology of endometriosis-associated infertility. *J Reprod Med* 1989;**34**:41–6.
12. Houston DE, Noller KL, Melton LJ, Selwyn BJ, Hardy RJ. Incidence of pelvic endometriosis in Rochester, Minnesota, 1970–1979. *Am J Epidemiol* 1987;**125**:959–69.
13. Moen, MH. Endometriosis in women at interval sterilization. *Acta Obstet Gynaecol Scand* 1987; **66**:451–4.
14. Hull MGR, Glazener CMA, Kelly NJ et al. Population study of causes, treatment, and outcome of infertility. *BMJ* 1985;**291**:1693–7.
15. Strathy JH, Molgaard CA, Coulam CB, Melton LJIII. Endometriosis and infertility: A laparoscopic study of endometriosis among fertile and infertile women. *Fertil Steril* 1985;**44**:83–8.
16. Nikanen V, Punnonen R. External endometriosis in 801 operated patients. *Acta Obstet Gynaecol Scand* 1984;**63**:699–701.
17. Bitzer J, Korber HR. Laparoscopy findings in infertile women. *Geburts Frauenheilkd* 1983; **43**:294–8.
18. Koninckx PR, Meuleman C, Demeyere S, Lesaffre E, Cornillie FJ. Suggestive evidence that pelvic endometriosis is a progressive disease, whereas deeply infiltrating endometriosis is associated with pelvic pain. *Fertil Steril* 1991;**55**:759–65.
19. Sampson JA. Peritoneal endometriosis due to the menstrual dissemination of endometrial tissue into the peritoneal cavity. *Am J Obstet Gynecol* 1927;**14**:422–69.
20. El Mahgoub S, Yaseen S. A positive proof for the theory of coelomic metaplasia. *Am J Obstet Gynecol* 1980;**137**:137–40.
21. Suginami H. A reappraisal of the coelomic metaplasia theory by reviewing endometriosis occurring in unusual sites and instances. *Am J Obstet Gynecol* 1991;**165**:214–18.
22. Moore JG, Binstock MA, Growdon WA. The clinical implications of retroperitoneal endometriosis. *Am J Obstet Gynecol* 1988; **158**:1291–8.
23. Ueki M. Histologic study of endometriosis and

examination of lymphatic drainage in and from the uterus. *Am J Obstet Gynecol* 1991;**165:**201–9.

24. Koninckx PR, Ide P, Vandenbroueke W, Brosens IA. New aspects of the pathophysiology of endometriosis and associated infertility. *J Reprod Med* 1980;**24:**257–60.

25. Halme J, Hammond MG, Hulka JF, et al. Retrograde menstruation in healthy women and in patients with endometriosis. *Obstet Gynecol* 1984;**64:**151–4.

26. Kruitwagen RF. Menstruation as the pelvic aggressor. *Baillière's Clin Obstet Gynaecol* 1993; **7:**687–700.

27. van der Linden PJQ, de Goeij AFPM, Dunselman GAJ, Erkens HWH, Evers JLH. Amniotic membrane as an in vitro model for endometrium – extracellular matrix interactions. *Gynecol Obstet Invest* 1998;**45:**7–11.

28. Redwine DB, Koninckx PR, D'Hooghe T, Oosterlynck D. Endometriosis: Will the real natural history please stand up? *Fertil Steril* 1991;**56:**590–1.

29. Koninckx PR. Is mild endometriosis a condition occurring intermittently in all women? *Hum Reprod* 1994;**9:**2202–5.

30. Vercellini P, Bocciolone L, Crosignani PG. Is mild endometriosis always a disease? *Hum Reprod* 1992;**7:**627–9.

31. Koninckx PR, Kennedy, SH, Barlow DH. Endometrium and endometriosis: the role of peritoneal fluid. *Hum Reprod* 1998; in press.

32. Jansen RP, Russell P. Nonpigmented endometriosis: clinical, laparoscopic, and pathologic definition. *Am J Obstet Gynecol* 1986;**155:**1154–9.

33. Goldenberg M, Oelsner G, Bider D, Admon D, Rabinowich O, Mashiach S. A new approach to ovarian cystectomy – a combined laparoscopic and extra-abdominal microsurgical technique. *Gynecol Obstet Invest* 1994;**37:**196–8.

34. Cornillie FJ, Oosterlynck D, Lauweryns JM, Koninckx PR. Deeply infiltrating pelvic endometriosis: histology and clinical significance. *Fertil Steril* 1990;**53:**978–83.

35. Koninckx PR, Meuleman C, Oosterlynck D, Cornillie FJ. Diagnosis of deep endometriosis by clinical examination during menstruation and plasma CA-125 concentration. *Fertil Steril* 1996;**65:**280–7.

36. Koninckx PR, Vandermeersch E. The persufflator: an insufflation device for laparoscopy and especially for $CO_2$-laser-endoscopic surgery. *Human Reprod* 1991;**6:**1288–90.

37. Cervero, F. Visceral pain: mechanisms of peripheral and central sensitization. *Ann Med* 1995;**27:**235–9.

38. Cervero F, Janig W. Visceral nociceptors: a new world order? *Trends Neurosci* 1992;**15:**374–8.

39. Koninckx PR, Renaer M. Pain sensitivity of and pain radiation from the internal female genital organs. *Hum Reprod* 1997;**12:**1785–8.

40. Brosens IA, Koninckx PR, Corveleyn PA. A study of plasma progesterone, oestradiol-17β, prolactin and LH levels, and of the luteal phase appearance of the ovaries in patients with endometriosis and infertility. *B J Obstet Gynaecol* 1978;**85:**246–50.

41. Koninckx PR, Brosens IA. Clinical significance of the luteinized unruptured follicle syndrome as a cause of infertility. *Eur J Obstet Gynecol Reprod Biol* 1982;**13:**355–68.

42. Koninckx PR, Brosens IA. Endometriosis: new aspects of the pathophysiology. *Proc FIGO Tokyo*, Excerpta Medica, 1977.

43. Schenken RS, Werlin LB, Williams RF, Prihoda TJ, Hodgen GD. Histologic and hormonal documentation of the luteinized unruptured follicle syndrome. *Am J Obstet Gynecol* 1986;**154:**839–47.

44. Haines, CJ. Luteinized unruptured follicle syndrome. *Clin Reprod Fertil* 1987;**5:**321–32.

45. Scheenjes E, te Velde ER, Kremer J. Inspection of the ovaries and steroids in serum and peritoneal fluid at various time intervals after ovulation in fertile women: implications for the luteinized unruptured follicle syndrome. *Fertil Steril* 1990;**54:**38–41.

46. Mio Y, Toda T, Harada T, Terakawa N. Luteinized unruptured follicle in the early stages of endometriosis as a cause of unexplained infertility. *Am J Obstet Gynecol* 1992;**167:**271–3.

47. D'Hooghe TM, Bambra CS, Raeymaekers BM, Koninckx PR. Increased incidence and recurrence of recent corpus luteum without ovulation stigma (luteinized unruptured follicle syndrome?) in baboons with endometriosis. *J Soc Gynecol Invest* 1996;**3:**140–4.

48. Marcoux S, Maheux R, Berube S, and the Canadian collaborative group on endometriosis. Laparoscopic Surgery in infertile women with minimal and mild endometriosis. *N Engl J Med* 1997;**337:**217–22.

49. Jenkins JM, Anthony FW, Wood P, Rushen D, Masson GM, Thomas E. The development of functional ovarian cysts during pituitary down-regulation. *Hum Reprod* 1993;**8:**1623–7.

50. Alcazar JL, Laparte C, Jurado M, Lopez-Garcia

G. The role of transvaginal ultrasonography combined with color velocity imaging and pulsed Doppler in the diagnosis of endometrioma. *Fertil Steril* 1997;**67**:487–91.

51. Mais V, Guerriero S, Ajossa S, Angiolucci M, Paoletti AM, Melis GB. The efficiency of transvaginal ultrasonography in the diagnosis of endometrioma. *Fertil Steril* 1993;**60**:776–80.

52. Outwater EK, Dunton CJ. Imaging of the ovary and adnexa: Clinical issues and applications of MR imaging. *Radiology* 1995;**194**:1–18.

53. Guerriero S, Ajossa S, Paoletti AM, Mais V, Angiolucci M, Melis GB. Tumor markers and transvaginal ultrasonography in the diagnosis of endometrioma. *Obstet Gynecol* 1996;**88**:403–7.

54. Guerriero S, Mais V, Ajossa S, Paoletti AM, Angiolucci M, Melis GB. Transvaginal ultrasonography combined with CA-125 plasma levels in the diagnosis of endometrioma. *Fertil Steril* 1996;**65**:293–8.

55. Koninckx PR, Muyldermans M, Moerman P, Meuleman C, Deprest J, Cornillie F. CA 125 concentrations in ovarian 'chocolate' cyst fluid can differentiate an endometriotic cyst from a cystic corpus luteum. *Hum Reprod* 1992;**7**:1314–17.

56. Koninckx PR. CA 125 in the management of endometriosis. *Eur J Obstet Gynecol Reprod Biol* 1993;**49**:109–13.

57. Brosens IA, Puttemans PJ, Deprest J. The endoscopic localization of endometrial implants in the ovarian chocolate cyst. *Fertil Steril* 1994;**61**:1034–8.

58. Martin DC, Demos Berry J. Histology of chocolate cysts. *J Gynecol Surg* 1990;**6**:43–6.

59. Donnez J, Nisolle M, Gillet N, Smets M, Bassil S, Casanas Roux F. Large ovarian endometriomas. *Hum Reprod* 1996;**11**:641–6.

60. Hughesdon PE. Benign endometrioid tumours of the ovary and the müllerian concept of ovarian epithelial tumours. *Histopathology* 1984;**8**:977–90.

61. Brosens I, Puttemans P, Deprest J. Appearances of endometriosis. *Baillières Clin Obstet Gynaecol* 1993;**7**:741–57.

62. Vercellini P, Vendola N, Bocciolone L, Colombo A, Rognoni MT, Bolis G. Laparoscopic aspiration of ovarian endometriomas. Effect with postoperative gonadotropin releasing hormone agonist treatment. *J Reprod Med* 1992;**37**:577–80.

63. Giorlandino C, Taramanni C, Muzii L, Santillo E, Nanni C, Vizzone A. Ultrasound-guided aspiration of ovarian endometriotic cysts. *Int J Gynaecol Obstet* 1993;**43**:41–4.

64. Aboulghar MA, Mansour RT, Serour GI, Rizk B. Ultrasonic transvaginal aspiration of endometriotic cysts: an optional line of treatment in selected cases of endometriosis. *Hum Reprod* 1991;**6**:1408–10.

65. Muzii L, Marana R, Caruana P, Catalano GF, Mancuso S. Laparoscopic findings after transvaginal ultrasound-guided aspiration of ovarian endometriomas. *Hum Reprod* 1995;**10**:2902–3.

66. Kennedy SH, Cederholm-Williams SA, Barlow DH. The effect of injecting endometriotic 'chocolate' cyst fluid into the peritoneal cavity of mice. *Hum Reprod* 1992;**7**:1329.

67. Bruhat MA, Mage, G, Chapron C, Pouly JL, Canis M, Wattiez A. Present day endoscopic surgery in gynecology. *Eur J Obstet Gynecol Reprod Biol* 1991;**41**:4–13.

68. Bruhat MA, Mage G, Pouly JL, Canis M, Wattiez A, Chapron C. Advances in pelviscopic surgery. *Ann NY Acad Sci* 1991;**626**:367–71.

69. Bruhat MA, Wattiez A, Mage G, Pouly JL, Canis M. $CO_2$ laser laparoscopy. *Baillière's Clin Obstet Gynaecol* 1989;**3**:487–97.

70. Brosens IA, Van Ballaer P, Puttemans P, Deprest J. Reconstruction of the ovary containing large endometriomas by an extraovarian endosurgical technique. *Fertil Steril* 1996;**66**:517–21.

71. Crosignani PG, Vercellini P. Conservative surgery for severe endometriosis: should laparotomy be abandoned definitively? *Hum Reprod* 1995;**10**:2412–18.

72. Adamson GD, Pasta DJ. Surgical treatment of endometriosis-associated infertility: Meta-analysis compared with survival analysis. *Am J Obstet Gynecol* 1994;**171**:1488–505.

73. Brosens IA. New principles in the management of endometriosis. *Acta Obstet Gynaecol Scand Suppl* 1994;**159**:18–21.

74. Wood C. Endoscopy in the management of endometriosis. *Baillière's Clin Obstet Gynaecol* 1994;**8**:735–57.

75. Canis M, Mage G, Wattiez A, Chapron C, Pouly JL, Bassil S. Second-look laparoscopy after laparoscopic cystectomy of large ovarian endometriomas. *Fertil Steril* 1992;**58**:617–19.

76. Fayez JA, Vogel MF. Comparison of different treatment methods of endometriomas by laparoscopy. *Obstet Gynecol* 1991;**78**:660–5.

77. Muzii L, Marana R, Caruana P, Mancuso S. The

impact of preoperative gonadotropin-releasing hormone agonist treatment on laparoscopic excision of ovarian endometriotic cysts. *Fertil Steril* 1996;**65**:1235–7.

78. Chang SP, Ng HT. A randomized comparative study of the effect of leuprorelin acetate depot and danazol in the treatment of endometriosis. *Chung Hua I Hsuch Tsa Chih Taipei* 1996; **57**:431–7.

79. Koninckx PR, Meuleman C, Demeyere S, Lesaffre E, Cornillie FJ. Suggestive evidence that pelvic endometriosis is a progressive disease, whereas deeply infiltrating endometriosis is associated with pelvic pain. *Fertil Steril* 1991;**55**:759–65.

80. Koninckx PR, Martin DC. Deep endometriosis: A consequence of infiltration or retraction or possibly adenomyosis externa? *Fertil Steril* 1992;**58**:924–8.

81. Hompes PG, Koninckx PR, Kennedy SH, van Kamp GF, Verstraeten RA, Cornillie F. Serum CA-125 concentrations during midfollicular phase, a clinically useful and reproducible marker in diagnosis of advanced endometriosis. *Clin Chem* 1996;**42**:1871–4.

82. Koninckx PR, Meuleman C, Oosterlynck D, Cornillie FJ. Diagnosis of deep endometriosis by clinical examination during menstruation and plasma CA-125 concentration. *Fertil Steril* 1996;**65**:280–7.

83. Deprest J, Marchal G, Koninckx PR. MRI in the diagnosis of deeply infiltrating endometriosis. Abstract AAGL 22nd annual meeting 1993.

84. Koninckx PR, Timmermans B, Meulemann C, Pennickx F. Complications of $CO_2$ laser endoscopic excision of deep endometriosis. *Hum Reprod* 1996;**11**:2263–8.

85. Koninckx PR, Vandermeersch E. The persufflator: an insufflation device for laparoscopy and especially for $CO_2$-laser-endoscopic surgery. *Hum Reprod* 1991;**6**:1288–90.

86. Redwine DB. Conservative laparoscopic excision of endometriosis by sharp dissection: Life table analysis of reoperation and persistent or recurrent disease. *Fertil Steril* 1991; **56**:628–34.

87. Redwine DB. Laparoscopic en bloc resection for treatment of the obliterated cul-de-sac in endometriosis. *J Reprod Med* 1992;**37**:695–8.

88. Sharpe DR, Redwine DB. Laparoscopic segmental resection of the sigmoid and rectosigmoid colon for endometriosis. *Surg Laparoscopy Endosc* 1992;**2**:120–4.

89. Redwine DB, Koning M, Sharpe DR. Laparoscopically assisted transvaginal segmental resection of the rectosigmoid colon for endometriosis. *Fertil Steril* 1996;**65**:193–7.

90. Redwine DB. Severe intestinal (GI) endometriosis (E) and pelvic mapping. *Fertil Steril* 1997; ASRM abstr, S22–S22.

91. Donnez J, Nisolle M, Gillerot S, Smets M, Bassil S, Casanas-Roux F. Rectovaginal septum adenomyotic nodules: a series of 500 cases. *B J Obstet Gynaecol* 1997;**104**:1014–18.

92. Crosignani PG, De Cecco L, Gastaldi A et al. Leuprolide in a 3-monthly versus a monthly depot formulation for the treatment of symptomatic endometriosis: A pilot study. *Hum Reprod* 1996;**11**:2732–5.

93. Vercellini P, Trespidi L, De Giorgi O, Cortesi I, Parazzini F, Crosignani PG. Endometriosis and pelvic pain: relation to disease stage and localization. *Fertil Steril* 1996;**65**:299–304.

94. Donnez J, Nisolle M, Casanas–Roux F, Bassil S, Anaf V. Rectovaginal septum, endometriosis or adenomyosis: Laparoscopic management in a series of 231 patients. *Hum Reprod* 1995; **10**:630–5.

95. Martin DC. Pain and infertility – a rationale for different treatment approaches. *Br J Obstet Gynaecol* 1995;**102**(suppl 12):2–3.

96. Candiani GB, Vercellini P, Fedele L, Roviaro G, Rebuffat C, Trespidi L. Conservative surgical treatment of rectovaginal septum endometriosis. *J Gynecol Surg* 1992;**8**:177–82.

97. Nezhat C, Nezhat F, Pennington E. Laparoscopic treatment of infiltrative rectosigmoid colon and rectovaginal septum endometriosis by the technique of videolaparoscopy and the $CO_2$ laser. *Br J Obstet Gynaecol* 1992;**99**:664–7.

98. Reich H, McGlynn F, Salvat J. Laparoscopic treatment of cul-de-sac obliteration secondary to retrocervical deep fibrotic endometriosis. *J Reprod Med Obstet Gynecol* 1991;**36**:516–22.

99. Ripps BA, Martin DC. Focal pelvic tenderness, pelvic pain and dysmenorrhea in endometriosis. *J Reprod Med* 1991;**36**:470–2.

100. Martin DC. Laparoscopic and vaginal colpotomy for the excision of infiltrating cul-de-sac endometriosis. *J Reprod Med* 1988;**33**:806–8.

101. Koninckx PR, Timmermans B, Meuleman C, Pennickx F. Complications of $CO_2$-laser endoscopic excision of deep endometriosis. *Hum Reprod* 1996;**11**:2263–8.

102. Van Rompaey B, Deprest JA, Koninckx PR. Enterocele as a consequence of laparoscopic

resection of deeply infiltrating endometriosis. *J Am Assoc Gynecol Laparosc* 1996;**4:**73–5.

103. Tate JJT, Kwok S, Dawson JW, Lau WY, Li AKC. Prospective comparison of laparoscopic and conventional anterior resection. *Br J Surg* 1993;**80:**1396–8.

104. Neven P, Vandeursen H, Baert L, Koninckx PR. Ureteric injury at laparoscopic surgery: The endoscopic management. Case review. *Gynaecol Endoscop* 1993;**2:**45–6.

105. Shaw RW. Endometriosis: current evaluation of management and rationale for medical therapy. In: *The Current Status of Endometriosis* (Brosens IA, Donnez J, eds) New York: Parthenon Publishing, 1993;371–83.

106. Fedele L, Bianchi S, Bocciolone L, Dinola G, Franchi D. Buserelin acetate in the treatment of pelvic pain associated with minimal and mild endometriosis – a controlled study. *Fertil Steril* 1993;**59:**516–21.

107. Fedele L, Arcaini L, Bianchi S, Baglioni A, Vercellini P. Comparison of cyproterone acetate and danazol in the treatment of pelvic pain associated with endometriosis. *Obstet Gynecol* 1989;**73:**1000–4.

108. Fedele L, Bianchi S, Arcaini L, Vercellini P, Candiani GB. Buserelin versus danazol in the treatment of endometriosis-associated infertility. *Am J Obstet Gynecol* 1989;**161:**871–6.

109. Redwine DB, Elstein M, Shaw R, Barlow DH, Kellerman LA. Nafarelin versus danazol versus surgery. *Fertil Steril* 1992;**58:**455–6.

110. Evers JLH. The second-look laparoscopy for evaluation of the result of medical treatment of endometriosis should not be performed during ovarian suppression. *Fertil Steril* 1987;**47:**502–4.

111. Hughes, EG, Fedorkow DM, Collins JA. A quantitative overview of controlled trials in endometriosis-associated infertility. *Fertil Steril* 1993;**59:**963–70.

112. Shaw RW. Nafarelin in the treatment of pelvic pain caused by endometriosis. *Am J Obstet Gynecol* 1990;**162:**574–6.

113. Koninckx PR, Stukkens K, Meuleman C. Cumulative pregnancy rates following $CO_2$-laser-endoscopic surgery for deeply infiltrating endometriosis. *FIGO Proceedings*, Singapore, 1991.

114. Koninckx PR, Deprest J, Janssen G, Oosterlynck D, Meuleman C. Cumulative pregnancy rates following $CO_2$-laser endoscopic excision of deeply infiltrating endometriosis. *Fertil Steril* 1993; AFS abstr.

115. Buttram VC. Rationale for combined medical and surgical treatment of endometriosis. In: *The Current Status of Endometriosis* (Brosens IA, Donnez J, eds) New York: Parthenon Publishing, 1993;32–406.

# Part IX
# Implantation

# 36

# The implantation process: lessons from ART

Carlos Simón, Carlos Moreno, Antonio Pellicer

**Basic aspects of human implantation** • **Current strategies to improve implantation in patients undergoing ART** • **Future strategies to improve implantation in patients undergoing ART**

Since the introduction of in vitro fertilization (IVF) (20 years ago), there has been substantial improvement in ovulation induction, oocyte retrieval, fertilization capability and embryonic development. However, the endpoint, which is to improve implantation and pregnancy rates after transferring three to four embryos, remains below physiological expectations. It has been estimated that clinical implantation in the human is efficient in no more than 30% of cases[1] considering that only one embryo is present in natural cycles, which gives us a 30% implantation rate. The responsibility for this low implantation efficiency has to be shared between the embryo (30% of blastocysts are morphologically abnormal at the time of implantation in vivo[2]), and a defective embryonic–endometrial dialogue (30% of early pregnancy losses occur before the expected time of menstruation).[3]

This implantation efficiency seems to be very poor when compared with other animal species, but is still unachievable using assisted reproduction technologies (ART). Implantation ability deteriorates in ovum donation programmes (18% implantation rate) in which hormone replacement therapy (HRT) is used to prepare the endometrium, and this is even worse during controlled ovarian hyperstimulation (COH) used for IVF, wherein the implantation rate is not more than 12% of embryos,[4] resulting in 50% and 30% pregnancy rate per transfer respectively.[4] We know from basic studies that the success of embryonic implantation relies upon a perfect dialogue between good quality embryos and a receptive endometrium. The main reason for these disappointing results is the quality of the endometrial factor that is affected during pharmacological treatments (HRT and COH), and this can be proved by the results obtained when sharing oocytes between IVF donors and oocyte donation recipients. Also, when implantation starts, an even higher amount of early embryonic wastage occurs after ART compared with natural cycles.[5]

For these reasons, the implantation process constitutes the limiting factor to increase pregnancy rates in ART and the fundamental question is: could implantation be improved in ART up to physiological levels, therefore increasing the chances of pregnancy of our patients? The answer is definitively yes.

In this chapter, we analyse the basic aspects of human implantation and what we have learned from ART. Based on this knowledge we consider current and future strategies to improve embryonic implantation in patients undergoing ART.

## BASIC ASPECTS OF HUMAN IMPLANTATION

Implantation is a progressive process in which the embryo has to appose and attach itself to the maternal endometrium, and invade it. The most intriguing aspect of implantation is that it involves two outstanding players: the maternal endometrium and the embryo. Communication between them, and the reciprocal effect on each other, constitute an exciting and as yet unsolved paradigm in reproductive medicine.

This process consists in the fixation of the blastocyst to the maternal endometrium and requires a receptive endometrium, a functional normal embryo at the blastocyst stage, and a dialogue or cross-communication between these two organisms which are immunologically and genetically different. Embryonic implantation consists of three distinct, related and consecutive phases: apposition, adhesion and invasion. During apposition the human blastocyst 'finds its implantation place', is guided towards a specific area in the maternal uterus, generally in the posterior wall, with its embryonic pole directed towards the superficial endometrial epithelium. On the adhesion phase that occurs between day 6 and 7 after ovulation, the direct contact between endometrial epithelium and the blastocyst trophoectoderm is produced. Finally, during invasion the embryonic trophoblast penetrates and displaces the endometrial epithelium, destroys the basal membrane and is introduced into the stroma, invading up to the uterine vessels.

The time period in which this initial dialogue takes place is termed 'window of implantation' (days 20–24 after ovulation), corresponding to the period of maximum uterine receptivity with a hatched blastocyst present. Nowadays, in addition to the histological criteria, we have biochemical and morphological markers of endometrial receptivity that allow us a better understanding and detection of this endometrial state.

The most reliable biochemical markers are the presence of a specific pattern of endometrial adhesion molecules. Specifically, integrins are membrane glycoproteins composed of two subunits ($\alpha$ and $\beta$) forming homologous groups.

Their primary function is to mediate cell-to-cell and cell-to-extracellular matrix (ECM) binding by specialized cell attachment sites, such as the tripeptide sequence Arg–Gly–Asp (RGD) which is a target sequence for integrin binding.[6] During this period $\beta_3$, $\alpha_4$ and $\alpha_1$ integrins are considered potential markers of uterine receptivity.[7–10] The $\alpha_1$ subunit is present only during the luteal phase (days 15–28).[8–10] The $\alpha_4$ integrin is expressed during days 14–24[8–10] whereas the $\beta_3$ subunit appears only on day 20 of the menstrual cycle and continues in the midluteal phase.[8,10] Therefore co-expression of $\beta_3$, $\alpha_4$ and $\alpha_1$ integrins occurs on the glandular epithelium during the implantation window, and as a consequence alterations in this endometrial integrin pattern have been associated with infertility of unknown aetiology.[7] Also, the embryonic ability to modulate human endometrial receptivity has been described. Human blastocyst selectively upregulates $\beta_3$ integrin in human endometrial epithelial cells compared with arrested embryos. It is worth noting that the embryonic upregulation of endometrial $\beta_3$ integrin is mediated, at least in part, by the embryonic interleukin 1 (IL-1) system[11] (Figure 1).

The most important morphological marker is the presence, at the endometrial epithelial surface, of apical protrusion with sacular aspect-denominated pinopodes. In humans, as in rodents, there are morphological changes in the plasma membrane of uterine epithelial cells in the peri-implantation period which are essential for endometrial receptivity. At the apical surface, long, thin, regular microvilli are gradually converted into irregular, flattened projections and pinopodes that last about 24–48 hours. This process is known as 'plasma membrane transformation'[12] (Figure 2). The function of pinopodes seems to be the absorption of molecules and fluids from the lumen, facilitating the proximity between embryo and endometrium, favouring apposition.

The crucial role of steroid hormones in order to prepare and drive the endometrium for successful embryonic implantation is beyond any doubt. However, it is clear that steroid hormones are not the final effectors, but rather they

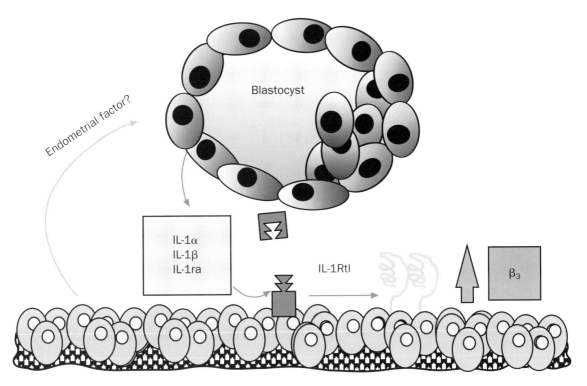

**Figure 1** In response to an unknown endometrial factor (*), the human embryo secretes the complete IL-1 system (IL-1$\alpha$, IL-1$\beta$/IL-1ra) as demonstrated by the selective release in the presence of endothelial-epithelial cells (EEC).[55] The human blastocyst upregulates the endometrial epithelial $\beta_3$ subunit and this activation is triggered by the binding and activation of embryonic IL-1$\alpha$ + IL-1$\beta$ to the endometrial epithelial IL-1R tl. The endometrial $\beta_3$ upregulation is functionally relevant because it increases the ability of the mouse blastocyst to adhere to the EEC monolayer.[11]

may initiate a 'downstream' cascade of molecular events through local paracrine/autocrine molecules such as chemokines, cytokines, growth factors, adhesion molecules and invasive proteases, which account for the intimate molecular mechanisms of apposition, adhesion and invasion (Figure 3).

In humans, the apposition phase is controlled by the embryo's developmental lineage, the uterine microenvironment and at least partly by the presence of chemokines such as IL-8[13], MCP-1 (monocyte chemotactic protein-1)[14] and RANTES (regulated on activated normal T cells expressed and secreted)[15] produced by the uterine epithelium.[16] Alterations in this phase will determine the existence of an ectopic

or eutopic pregnancy and, even in the intrauterine pregnancy, the localization of the placenta will be determined in this process. For the adhesion phase, a general hypothesis has been postulated wherein cytokines, such as leukaemia inhibitory factor (LIF), the IL-1 system,[17] heparan-binding endothelial growth factor (HB-EGF), and possibly others, as well as their specific receptors properly distributed throughout the endometrium and embryo, and adequately controlled at the endocrine (hormonal) and paracrine/autocrine (cytokine and growth factor) levels, may start the mutual recognition of implanting blastocyst and endometrium by activating endometrial adhesion molecules that will provide the physical

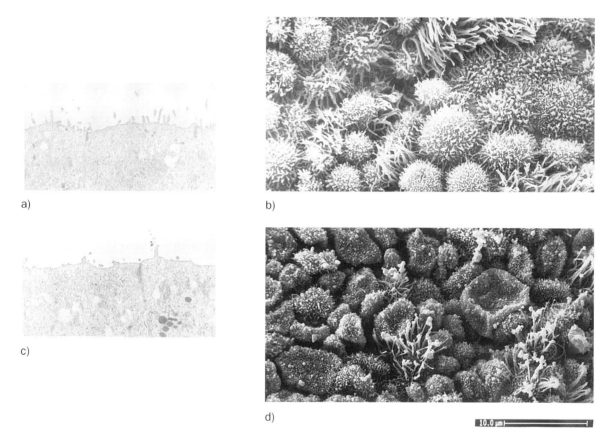

**Figure 2** Transmission electron microscopy (TEM) and scanning electron microscopy (SEM) of the plasma membrane transformation. Non-receptive endometrium with numerous and longer microvilli covering the cell surface (a) by TEM and (b) by SEM. Receptive endometrium with a flattened surface profile with irregular flattened projections and a few low microvilli and pynopods (c) by TEM and (d) by SEM.

contact between embryo and uterus.[17] The pathology of this phase is involved in the infertility of unknown aetiology, implantation failure after repeated embryo transfer (in IVF or oocyte donation) and early pregnancy loss (EPL) before menstruation occurs.[5] Invasion is a self-controlled proteolytic process; 8 days after ovulation the blastocyst is embedded in the stroma and the site of entry is covered by fibrin over which the epithelial cells grow. In humans, the basement membrane is the first barrier that must be breached, and trophoblast further invades the stromal compartment, and then penetrates the maternal blood vessels. This action is mediated by several proteases that degrade the ECM such as serine proteases, metalloproteases and collagenases.[18] Urokinase-type (uPA) and tissue-type (tPA) plasminogen activates are serine proteases that catalyse the conversion of plasminogen to plasmin, with a broad proteolytic action capable of direct action on the degradation of the ECM. The matrix metalloproteases (MMPs) are a family of zinc-dependent endopeptidases with proteolytic

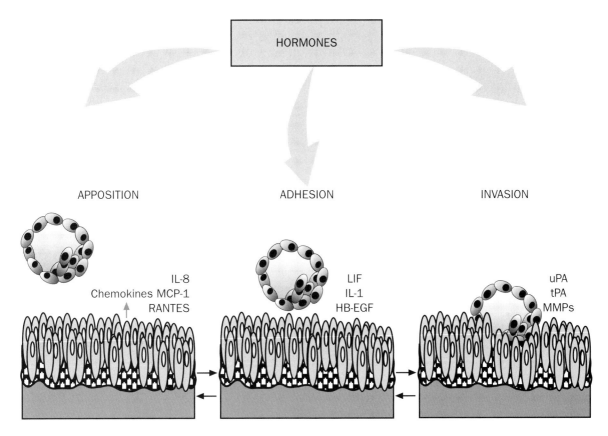

**Figure 3** Schematic diagram of the chemokine–cytokine–adhesion molecule-invasive protease hypothesis. Apposition: chemokines may direct the embryo towards a specific part of the uterus or ectopic localizations. Adhesion: cytokines controlled at the endocrine (hormonal) and paracrine/autocrine (cytokines and growth factors) levels may start the mutual recognition of implanting blastocyst and endometrium. Adhesion molecules provide the physical contact between embryo and uterus. Invasion: invasive proteases have a close connection with adhesion molecules and they are regulated by hormones, growth factors and cytokines.

activities against several components of the ECM.[19] Activated enzymes digest the ECMs and, according to their substrate specificity, this family is composed of three groups: collagenases, gelatinases and stromelysins. Collagenases include MMP-1 and MMP-8; these enzymes digest collagen types I, II, III, VII and X. Gelatinases digest collagen type IV and denatured collagen. Stromelysins degrade fibronectin, laminin, collagens IV, V and VII as well as proteoglycans. Tight regulation of this process is required to prevent pathological

invasion by excess, as occurs in placenta accreta or by defect as in pre-eclampsia.[20]

## CURRENT STRATEGIES TO IMPROVE IMPLANTATION IN PATIENTS UNDERGOING ART

Learning from the basics of this process, we believe that implantation in patients undergoing ART cycles must and can be improved. For this purpose we consider separately possible strategies directed to improve implantation in IVF and oocyte donation. A frequent pitfall found in the literature is the consideration that implantation is the result of good embryonic quality. Although this is completely true, it is not the only truth because maternal endometrium is at least of equal relevance. In IVF, the main problem is an altered endometrial factor, because of abnormally high ovarian steroid levels as a consequence of gonadotrophin treatment. In ovum donation, the endometrial factor could also be improved by individualizing the implantation window in each patient. In both techniques the embryonic factor could be clearly improved by transferring embryos at the blastocyst stage, which have been co-cultured in conditions that improved their ability to implant. In this section we analyse our experience with these strategies to optimize human implantation in patients undergoing ART.

## Improving endometrial receptivity in IVF patients

Uterine receptivity deteriorates during COH used for IVF. This is not surprising considering that the aim of ovulation-induction drugs is to recruit more oocytes, and as a consequence supraphysiological levels of steroid hormones are produced. High oestradiol levels, which are known to be interceptive,[21] and altered oestradiol/progesterone ratios, are also associated with the impairment of endometrial receptivity.[22] These clinical observations are reinforced by the morphological changes detected in the secretory endometrium from COH patients by histology[23] and scanning electron microscopy (SEM),[24] and also by the biochemical patterns found in the endometrial fluid in COH patients compared with HRT patients.[25]

Based on the above-mentioned considerations, we designed a series of studies aimed at developing clinical strategies to improve endometrial receptivity while using COH to produce multiple embryos in IVF. We chose, as a model, high-responder patients in whom ovarian response is abnormally high and, as a consequence, endometrial receptivity is even worse.

We have previously defined the concept of high response based on a regression analysis of the proportion of unfertilized oocytes and the number of oocytes retrieved per patient.[26] According to our data, we considered high response as the retrieval of 15 or more follicles after ovarian stimulation.[27] We have demonstrated that high serum oestradiol levels (> 3000 pg/ml) on the day of human chorionic gonadotrophin (hCG) administration in these patients, regardless of the number of oocytes retrieved and serum progesterone levels, are detrimental to uterine receptivity without affecting embryo quality.[28] In fact, pregnancy and implantation rates in recipients of embryos derived from high responders are similar to those in normal responders.[28] Furthermore, we documented an increase in serum oestradiol and progesterone levels during the preimplantation period in high responders compared with normal responder patients. The oestradiol:progesterone ratio was significantly different between normal and high responders during the preimplantation period. Pregnancy and implantation rates decreased as serum oestradiol levels increased on days 4–6 after oocyte retrieval (preimplantation period), suggesting that this abnormal endocrine milieu could be responsible for an impaired implantation.[29]

Based on this evidence we proposed one possible strategy. The concept is to reduce the ovarian response in these patients (and therefore the oestradiol levels) by eliciting recruitment and maturation of a relatively small number of follicles, mimicking the dynamics of the follicle-stimulating hormone (FSH) in natural cycles.[30] The step-down principle developed by Fauser et al[31] allows us to stimulate follicles to full maturation using a decremental dose regimen while reducing the number of functionally active mature follicles. Moreover, luteinizing hormone (LH) was not administered. The objective of this strategy was to produce a small 'FSH window'. Initially, we have to reach the FSH threshold, then gonadotrophin doses should be reduced to

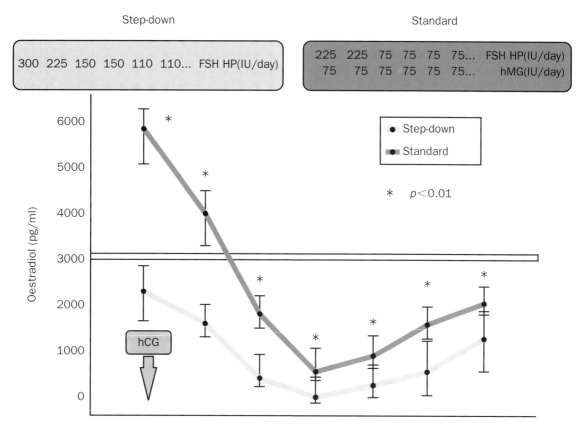

**Figure 4** Dose regimen and circulating levels of oestradiol during the preimplantation period (from days 0 to 6) in patients undergoing step-down regimen versus the previously failed cycle.

obtain FSH levels that dip below the FSH threshold (Figure 4).

In patients who have failed at least one IVF attempt with three to four good quality embryos transferred and oestradiol levels over 3000 pg/ml at the day of hCG, the comparison between the step-down regimen and standard protocol in the following cycle (Figure 4) revealed that oestradiol levels at the day of hCG were significantly lower in the step-down regimen compared with the standard ($1919 \pm 477$ vs $5271 \pm 613$ pg/ml); $p = 0.001$), as well as throughout the preimplantation period. As expected, the number of oocytes collected were also lower in the step-down regimen compared with the standard protocol ($18.1 \pm 2.1$ vs $23.1 \pm 1.6$; $p = 0.001$). Never-

theless, similar fertilization rates were obtained (74.2% vs 76.1%) and the number of good quality embryos transferred was also similar ($3.3 \pm 0.2$ vs $3.4 \pm 0.2$). However, implantation and pregnancy rates were significantly improved in patients undergoing the step-down regimen compared with those stimulated with the standard protocol (29.3% and 64.2% vs 8.5% and 24.2%, respectively; $p = 0.02$ and $p = 0.0002$, respectively). These clinical results again indicate that, in high responders to COH, endometrial receptivity can be improved by lowering abnormally high oestradiol levels mimicking physiological conditions.[32] The major problem within the step-down protocol is to determine the individual FSH threshold in clinical practice. For this reason, five cycles

(17.2%) were cancelled because the FSH threshold was not reached and follicle development was arrested, as demonstrated by an abrupt drop in oestradiol levels.

The possible mechanism(s) responsible for our clinical observation remain(s) unknown. But the implication of an altered regulation of steroid receptors in human endometrium can be expected because, in COH cycles, a significant reduction in the nuclear receptors for progesterone and oestradiol in both the glands and the stroma has been demonstrated.[33]

These clinical data confirm that high oestradiol levels are detrimental to embryonic implantation and indicate that, in high responders to COH, endometrial receptivity can be improved by lowering abnormally high oestradiol levels.[32]

## Improving endometrial receptivity in ovum donation patients

Ovum donation is a programme in which patients receive oocytes donated by young women. As a consequence ovum recipients are not stimulated with gonadotrophins, and the endometrial factor is better than in IVF patients. Nevertheless, implantation could be improved by optimizing the timing of embryo transfer, taking into consideration the individualized period of pinopode apparition, development and regression detected by SEM. The objective is to achieve a better individual synchronization between embryo and endometrium at the moment of embryo transfer. To this end, we have designed a controlled and prospective study in order to evaluate the clinical value of this endometrial marker in patients of our oocyte donation programme. Patients with ovarian function were desensitized with leuprolide acetate 0.2 ml/day in the secretory phase of the previous cycle. Hormone replacement started on day 1 of the cycle with administration of oestradiol valerate (EV, Progynova, Schering Spain, Madrid): 2 mg/day on days 1–8; 4 mg/day from days 9 to 11; and 6 mg/day from day 12 onwards. Natural micronized progesterone 800 mg/day was administered

vaginally from day 15 onwards and leuprolide acetate was discontinued. During this mock cycle, two endometrial biopsies were taken on days 6 and 8 of the progesterone phase, and analysed by histology and SEM. The most receptive day of the cycle corresponds to the pinopodes that are completely developed. A transfer HRT cycle followed where synchronization with the donor was arranged so that the predicted most receptive day coincides with embryonic age day 6.

A total of 19 cycles was studied, in six of which day-2 embryos were transferred at the proposed day of embryo transfer according to SEM: the results are explained in Table 1.[34] Although mainly a result of the scarce number of patients studied, this approach may be useful to tune up endometrial receptivity in patients undergoing oocyte donation.

## Improving embryo quality in IVF and ovum donation

The current trend is to transfer embryos at the blastocyst stage because the implantation rate is higher.[35,36] The main problem is to obtain an adequate number of embryos that achieve the blastocyst stage with appropriate quality. The concept that human preimplantation development and implantation ability may be improved by co-culturing embryos in the presence of another cell type (cells helping cells) has led to the concept of co-culture system. Multiple cell types have been used for this purpose, from human reproductive tissues,[37–41] human non-reproductive cells,[42–45] to non-human cell lines,[36,46–50] and even cells from ovarian carcinoma.[51] As a consequence, the reported embryonic effects of using this technology are cell, tissue and species non-specific. The suggested beneficial effects of co-cultures are the secretion of embryotrophic factors such as nutrients and substrates, growth factors and the removal of potentially harmful substances such as heavy metals, ammonium and free radical formation detoxifying the culture medium. All that matters is to increase the metabolic chances of the

| Patient | Age (years) | Ovarian function | Histological dating P6/P8 | Pinopodes P6 or P8 | Proposed day of embryo transfer | Actual day of embryo transfer | No. of embryos | No. of sacs |
|---------|-------------|------------------|---------------------------|--------------------|-------------------------------|------------------------------|----------------|-------------|
| A | 27 | No | 14/irregular | Moderate | P3 | P3 | 4 | 2 |
| B | 47 | No | 15–16/18–19 | Abundant | P4 | P4 | 4 | 1 |
| C | 30 | Yes | 15–16/19 | Moderate | P3 | P3 | 4 | 2 |
| D | 31 | Yes | 16/18–19 | ND | ND | P3 | 4 | 1 |
| E | 38 | Yes | 15–16/ND | Abundant | P4 | P3 | 4 | 0 |
| F | 33 | Yes | 17–18/19–20 | Moderate | P3 | P3 | 4 | 4 |

**Table 1** Data for the six completed cycles

ND = not determined.
P6/P8, day 6 or 8 of progesterone phase.

human embryo to achieve the blastocyst stage and implant.

Unfortunately, there is no general agreement on the efficacy of any of the co-culture systems employed,[52] not even the utility of the co-culture system itself compared with a chemically defined medium.[47,53,54] Even using the most extensive system – the Vero cell co-culture – results are discrepant.[47] Also, when co-culture systems are employed, in addition to the goal of high yield production of viable blastocysts, there are other important issues that must also be considered as endpoints, such as medical, ethical and practical feasibility. Recently, our group has demonstrated that not only is a co-culture system with autologous human endometrial epithelial cells (EEC) beneficial to the human blastocyst because of the induction of secretion of embryonic paracrine molecules,[55] but also the embryo co-cultured under these conditions improves uterine receptivity by increasing EEC adhesion molecules such as $\beta_3$.[11]

We have performed a total of 279 co-culture cycles corresponding to 91 ovum donation and 188 IVF cycles in patients with implantation failure, who underwent at least three previ-

ously failed ovum donation or IVF attempts with three to four good quality embryos transferred.[56] The protocol for ovarian stimulation, oocyte recovery and manipulation as well as luteal support has been reported elsewhere.[57] For embryo co-culture, EECs were isolated from human secretory endometrium and cultured in DMEM (Dulbecco's modified Eagle's medium)–MCDB with 10% FBS (fetal bovine serum) until confluence. Forty-eight hours after insemination, two- to four-cell embryos were co-cultured on the prepared monolayer of human EEC in 1 ml Hatch 50 (Scandinavian IVF) for 5 days (from day 2 until day 7 of embryonic development). The medium was changed every 24 h. On days 5, 6 or 7 embryos were checked for blastocyst formation and then transferred back to the mother using a Frydman catheter (Figure 5). In ovum donation, the mean age of the patients was $39.3 \pm 0.7$ years and the number of previously failed attempts was $3.2 \pm 0.3$. A mean of $6.8 \pm 0.3$ embryos started co-culture resulting in 59.1% of blastocyst formation. Ten cycles (12.1%) were cancelled. We transferred a mean of $2.1 \pm 0.1$ blastocysts per cycle and clinical pregnancy rate was 50.8%

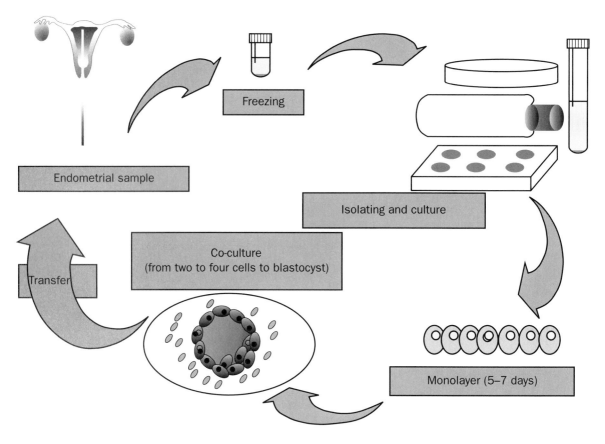

**Figure 5** Diagram of the steps involved in embryonic EEC co-culture.

with an implantation rate per blastocyst of 28.2%. Eight multiple pregnancies were obtained (24.2%) and, with six sets of twins and two of triplets, seven miscarriages (21.2%) and no ectopic pregnancies (14.3%) have occurred so far. In IVF, the mean age of the patients was $33.4 \pm 0.2$ years and the number of previously failed attempts was $3.8 \pm 0.2$. A mean of $8.2 \pm 0.3$ embryos started co-culture, resulting in 44.8% blastocyst formation. Eighteen cycles (9.6%) were cancelled. We transferred a mean of $2.1 \pm 0.1$ blastocysts per cycle and clinical pregnancy rate was 15% with an implantation rate per blastocyst of 12.2%. Six multiple pregnancies were obtained (24.0%) and, with three sets of twins and three of triplets, three miscarriages (12%) and two ectopic pregnancies (8%) have occurred so far.[56]

The fact that implantation rates of blastocysts obtained by co-culture were different when transferred to patients treated with gonadotrophins reinforces the concept that the endometrial factor is crucial in determining the success of embryo implantation.

Therefore, for implantation failure we view the ideal co-culture system as an autologous EEC system which in addition to improving embryonic preimplantation development and implantation as a crucial endpoint, could also be feasible, medically and ethically. The indications for blastocyst transfer using this co-culture system are: repeated failures of implantation (three or more transfers with three good quality embryos), avoidance of multiple gestations and for preimplantation diagnosis (PGD). However, embryonic quality can be improved but not fabricated and therefore, in ageing patients or patients with bad quality embryos, this technique is not indicated.

## Selecting chromosomally normal embryos in recurrent aborter patients

Recurrent miscarriage is defined as three or more non-consecutive clinical pregnancy losses before 20 weeks of gestation. This enigmatic pathological condition is induced by maternal and embryonic causes. For this reason recurrent miscarriage patients undergo a standard work-up consisting of: (1) endocrine tests, serum LH, serum FSH, prolactin, triiodothyronine, thyroxine, thyroid-stimulating hormone, progesterone and glucose levels; (2) morphological examination: transvaginal ultrasonography, hysterosalpingography, hysteroscopy; (3) parental genetic karyotyping and measurement of human leukocyte antigens; and (4) immunological tests: lupus anticoagulants and anticardiolipin antibodies. The most common finding is that, after the standard work-up, in up to 60% of patients the cause remains unknown. In these patients, our hypothesis is that non-inheritable abnormalities which arise from random errors produced any where from fertilization to embryonic development signify an important aetiology in recurrent abortion.

We have conducted a prospective study to determine the real incidence of aneuploidy for autosomes 13, 16, 18, 21, 22 and for gonosomes in preimplantation human embryos obtained from patients with recurrent pregnancy loss after ovarian stimulation in an IVF/ET programme. Our results indicate that aneuploidy for the chromosomes analysed is abnormally high in embryos obtained after IVF from recurrent abortion patients (58%), compared with that from non-recurrent abortion patients

undergoing IVF (5.5%). Furthermore, monosomies are four times more frequent than trisomies (23:7) in preimplantation embryos from recurrent abortion patients. In addition, pregnancy rates are similar to those in regular IVF patients (30%) and pregnancies can be carried to the first trimester.[58] Based on the present study, PGD of embryos obtained from patients with recurrent miscarriage could prove advantageous in diagnosing abnormal embryos and selecting normal embryos for transfer.[58]

## FUTURE STRATEGIES TO IMPROVE IMPLANTATION IN PATIENTS UNDERGOING ART

We are convinced that, at the endometrial site, the future direction will be to obtain a receptive endometrium similar to a natural cycle while performing COH to obtain oocytes. Currently, we are working on several research projects targeting the improvement of endometrial receptivity within gonadotrophin stimulation: first, to analyse molecular mechanisms regulating the phosphatase enzyme(s) involved in plasma membrane transformation, therefore facilitating their manipulation (activation or inhibition) in stimulated cycles; second, to investigate the effect of a selective aromatase inhibitor administered after oocyte retrieval, the aim of which is to decrease oestradiol levels during the peri-implantation period.

From the embryonic point of view, in addition to obtaining blastocysts using the most physiological and reliable system, the next step is to select embryos for transfer. Selection could consist of using biochemical markers obtained from the embryo-conditioned media or chromosomal selection of the blastocysts by blastomere biopsy and fluorescence in situ hybridization analysis.

## REFERENCES

1. Miller JF, Williamson E, Glue J, et al. Fetal losses after implantation. *Lancet* 1980;**ii**:554–6.
2. Hertig AT, Rock J, Adams EC, Menkin MC. Thirty-four fertilized human ova, good, bad and indifferent, recovered from 210 women of known fertility: a study of biologic wastage in early human pregnancy. *Pediatrics* 1959; **23**:202–11.
3. Wilcox AJ, Weinberg CR, O'Connor JF, et al. Incidence of early losses of pregnancy. *N Engl J Med* 1988;**319**:189–94.
4. Society for Assisted Reproductive Technology and The American Society for Reproductive Medicine. Assisted reproductive technology in the United States and Canada: 1994 results generated from the American Society for Reproductive Medicine/Society for Assisted Reproductive Technology Registry. *Fertil Steril* 1996;**66**:697–705.
5. Simón C, Landeras J, Zuzuarregui J, et al. Early embryonic losses after oocyte donation. LIII Annual Meeting of the ASRM. *Fertil Steril* 1997;**145**(suppl):114.
6. Ruoslahti E, Pierschbacher MD. New perspectives in cell adhesion: RGD and integrins. *Science* 1987;**238**:491–7.
7. Lessey BA, Castelbaum AJ. Integrins in the endometrium. *Reprod Med Rev* 1995;**4**:43–58.
8. Lessey BA, Damjanovich L, Coutifaris C, et al. Integrins adhesion molecules in the human endometrium. Correlation with the normal and abnormal menstrual cycle. *J Clin Invest* 1992; **90**:188–95.
9. Tabibzadeh S. Patterns of expression of integrin molecules in human endometrium throughout the menstrual cycle. *Hum Reprod* 1992;**7**:876–82.
10. Lessey BA, Castelbaum AJ, Buck CA, et al. Further characterization of endometrial integrins during the menstrual cycle and in pregnancy. *Fertil Steril* 1994;**62**:497–506.
11. Simón C, Gimeno MJ, Mercader A, et al. Embryonic regulation of integrins β3, α4 and α1 in human endometrial epithelial cells in vitro. *J Clin Endocrinol Metab* 1997;**82**:2607–16.
12. Murphy CR. The cytoskeleton of uterine epithelial cells: A new player in uterine receptivity and the plasma membrane transformation. *Hum Reprod Update* 1995;**1**:567–80.
13. Arici A, Head JR, MacDonald PC, Casey ML. Regulation of interleukin-8 gene expression in human endometrial cells in culture. *Mol Cell Endocrinol* 1993;**94**:195–204.
14. Wood G, Hausmann E, Cloudluri R. Relative role of CSF-1, MCP-1/JE and RANTES in macrophage recruitment during successful pregnancy. *Mol Reprod Develop* 1997;**46**:62–70.
15. Horung D, Tseng JF, Ryan IP, et al. Transcriptional regulation Rantes of gene expression in human endometrial cells. XIII Annual Meeting of the ESHRE. *Hum Reprod* Abstract book, 1997;**O-009**:55–6.
16. Simón C, Caballero-Campos P, García-Velasco J, et al. Implications of chemokines in the reproductive function. *J Reprod Immunol* 1998; in press.
17. Simón C, Gimeno MJ, Mercader A, et al. Cytokines-adhesion molecules-invasive proteinases. The missing paracrine/autocrine link in embryonic implantation? *Mol Hum Reprod* 1996;**2**:405–24.
18. Alexander CM, Werb Z. Extracellular matrix degradation. In: *Cell Biology of Extracellular Matrix* (Hay ED, ed.). New York: Plenum Press, 1991: 255–302.
19. Matrisian LM. Metalloproteinases and their inhibitors in matrix remodeling. *Trends Genet* 1990;**6**:121–5.
20. Zhou Y, Damsky CH, Chiu K, et al. Preeclampsia is associated with abnormal expression of adhesion molecules by invasive cytotrophoblasts. *J Clin Invest* 1993;**91**:950–60.
21. McLean-Morris J, Van Wagenen G. Interception: The use of the preovulatory estrogens to prevent implantation. *Am J Obstet Gynecol* 1973; **115**:101–6.
22. Gidley-Baird AA, O'Neil C, Sinosich MJ, et al. Failure of implantation in human in vitro fertilization and embryo transfer patients: The effects of altered progesterone/estrogen ratios in human and mice. *Fertil Steril* 1986;**45**:69–75.
23. García JE, Acosta AA, Hsiu JG, Jones HW. Advanced endometrial maturation after ovulation induction with human menopausal gonadotropin/human chorionic gonadotropin for in vitro fertilization. *Fertil Steril* 1984;**41**:31–7.
24. Bladford AJ, Najmabadi S, Paulson RJ. Ultrastructural characteristics of the luteal phase endometrium in donors undergoing controlled ovarian hyperstimulation. *Fertil Steril* 1997; **67**:625–30.
25. Simón C, Mercader A, Frances A, et al. Hormonal regulation of serum and endometrial

IL-1a, IL-1b and IL-1ra: IL-1 endometrial microenvironment of the human embryo at the apposition phase under physiological and supra-physiological steroid level conditions. *J Reprod Immunol* 1996;**31:**165–84.

26. Tarín JJ, Sampaio MC, Catalayud C, et al. Relativity of the concept 'high responder to gonadotrophins'. *Hum Reprod* 1992;**7:**19–22.

27. Pellicer A, Ruiz A, Castellví RM, et al. Is the retrieval of high number of oocytes desirable in patients treated with gonadtrophin-releasing hormone analogues (GnRHa) and gonado-trophins? *Hum Reprod* 1989;**4:**536–40.

28. Simon C, Cano F, Valbuena D, et al. Clinical evidence for a detrimental effect on uterine receptivity of high serum oestradiol concentrations in high and normal responder patients. *Hum Reprod* 1995;**10:**2432–7.

29. Pellicer A, Valbuena D, Cano F, et al. Lower implantation rates in high responders: Evidence for an altered endocrine milieu during the preimplantation period. *Fertil Steril* 1996; **65:**1190–5.

30. Hillier SG. Regulation of follicle estrogen biosynthesis: a survey of current concepts. *J Endocrinol* 1981;**89**(suppl):3–18.

31. Fauser BCJM, Donderwinkel P, Schoot DC. The step-down principle in gonadotrophin treatment and the role of GnRH analogues. *Baillière's Clin Obstet Gynaecol* 1993;**7:**309–30.

32. Simón C, García Velasco J, Valbuena D, et al. Increased uterine receptivity by decreasing estradiol levels during the preimplantation period in high responder patients by using an FSH step-down regimen. *Fertil Steril* 1998; in press.

33. Hadi FH, Chantler E, Anderson E, et al. Ovulation induction and endometrial steroid receptors. *Hum Reprod* 1994;**9:**2405–10.

34. Nikas G, García Velasco J, Pellicer A, Simon C. Assessment of uterine receptivity and timing of embryo transfer using the detection of pinopodes. Abstract presented for the XIII Annual Meeting of the European Society of Human Reproduction and Embryology. *Hum Reprod* Abstract book, 1997;**O-069:**32.

35. Scholtes MCW, Zeilmaker GH. A prospective, randomized study of embryo transfer results after 3 or 5 days of embryo culture in 'in vitro' fertilization. *Fertil Steril* 1996;**65:**1245–8.

36. Menezo Y, Hasout A, Dumant M, et al. Co-culture of embryos on Vero cells and transfer of blastocysts in human. *Hum Reprod* 1992;**7:**101–6.

37. Yeung WSB, Ho PC, Lan EYL, Chan STH. Improved development of human embryos in vitro by a human oviductal cell co-culture system. *Hum Reprod* 1992;**7:**1144–9.

38. Bongso A, Ng SC, Fong CY, et al. Improved pregnancy rate after transfer of embryos grown in human fallopian tubal cell co-culture. *Fertil Steril* 1992;**58:**569–74.

39. Bongso A, Fong CY, Ng SC, et al. Human embryonic behavior in a sequential human oviduct–endometrial coculture system. *Fertil Steril* 1994;**61:**976–8.

40. Plachot M, Alvarez S, Merviel P, et al. Role of endometrial cells in 'in vitro' embryo development. *Assist Reprod Rev* 1994;**4:**85–95.

41. Jayot S, Parneix Y, Verdaguer S, et al. Coculture of embryos on homologous endometrial cells in patients with repeated failures of implantation. *Fertil Steril* 1995;**63:**109–14.

42. Saito H, Hirayama T, Koine K, et al. Cumulus mass maintains embryo quality. *Fertil Steril* 1994; **62:**555–8.

43. Quinn P, Margalit R. Beneficial effects of coculture with cumulus cells on blastocyst formation in a prospective trial with the supernumerary human embryo. *J Assist Reprod Genet* 1996;**13:**9–14.

44. Plachot M, Antoime JM, Alvarez S, et al. Granulosa cells improve human embryo development in vitro. *Hum Reprod* 1993;**8:**2133–40.

45. Freeman MR, Witworth CM, Hill GA. Granulosa cell co-cultures enhances human embryo development and pregnancy rate following in vitro fertilization. *Hum Reprod* 1995;**10:**408–14.

46. Neimer KE, Hoffman DI, Maxson WS, et al. Embryonic morphology and rate of implantation of human embryos following co-culture on bovine oviductal epithelial cells. *Hum Reprod* 1993;**8:**97–101.

47. Van Blerkom J. Development of human embryos to the hatched blastocyst stage in the presence or absence of a monolayer of Vero cells. *Hum Reprod* 1993;**8:**1525–39.

48. Schillaci R, Ciriminna R, Cefali E. Vero cell effect on in vitro human blastocyst development: preliminary results. *Hum Reprod* 1994;**9:**1131–5.

49. Sakkas D, Jaquenoud N, Leppens G, Campana A. Comparison of results after in vitro fertilized human embryos are cultured in routine medium and coculture on Vero cells: a randomized study. *Fertil Steril* 1994;**61:**521–5.

50. Guerin JF, Nicollet B. Interest of co-cultures for embryos obtained by in-vitro fertilization: a French collaborative study. *Hum Reprod* 1997;**12:**1043–6.

51. Ben-Chetrit A, Jurisicova A, Casper RF. Coculture with ovarian cancer cell enhances human blastocyst formation in vitro. *Fertil Steril* 1996;**65:**664–6.

52. Tucker MJ, Morton PC, Wright G. Enhancement of outcome from intracytoplasmic sperm injection: Does co-culture or assisted hatching improve implantation rates. *Hum Reprod* 1996;**11:**2434–7.

53. Bavister BD. Co-culture for embryo development is it really necessary? *Hum Reprod* 1992;**7:**1339–41.

54. Schramm RD, Bavister BD. Development of in vitro fertilized primate embryos into blastocyst in a chemically defined, protein-free culture medium. *Hum Reprod* 1996;**11:**1690–7.

55. De los Santos MJ, Mercader A, Frances A, et al. Immunoreactive human embryonic interleukin-1 system and endometrial factors regulating their secretion during embryonic development. *Biol Reprod* 1996;**54:**563–74.

56. Simón C, Mercader A, García Velasco J. Co-culture of human embryos with autologous human endometrial epithelial cells in patients with repeated implantation failures. *J Clin Endocrinol Metab* 1998; submitted.

57. Gil-Salom M, Mínguez Y, Rubio C, et al. Efficacy of intracytoplasmic sperm injection using testicular spermatozoa. *Hum Reprod* 1995;**10:**3166–70.

58. Simón C, Rubio C, Vidal F, et al. Increased chromosome abnormalities in human preimplantation embryos after in vitro fertilization in patients with recurrent miscarriages. *J Reprod Fertil Develop* 1998; in press.

# 37

# Clinical assessment of uterine receptivity

Seang Lin Tan, Marinko M Biljan

**Histological and hormonal assessment of uterine receptivity** • **Ultrasonography** • **Doppler ultrasonography studies of uterine arteries** • **Conclusion**

As a result of improvements in ovarian stimulation regimens,[1] oocyte collection techniques[2–4] and advances in laboratory management, over the past 15 years, in vitro fertilization (IVF) has become an increasingly successful treatment for infertility caused by organic pelvic disease, male factor infertility or ovarian dysfunction, or of unexplained etiology. Its results compare favorably with those of spontaneous conception in the natural menstrual cycle in fertile women.[5] Nevertheless, a high proportion of IVF treatment cycles are unsuccessful, and although most patients have at least two to three good quality embryos for transfer, only 30–40% achieve clinical pregnancy. This relatively poor result is primarily because of the low embryo implantation rate which, even in the best centers, has remained at about 15–17%. The transfer of more than one embryo increases the pregnancy rate, but results in an increased incidence of multiple gestation. Uterine receptivity is a crucial element in achieving implantation and appropriate endometrial maturation is necessary. To achieve optimal endometrial growth and differentiation, the proliferative phase must be followed by timely secretory changes during the luteal phase with stromal decidualization.

This sequence of events is probably regulated by locally produced growth factors and is altered by the hormonal environment. The interaction of different elements and the importance of factors, such as the various endometrial proteins, uterine and ovarian perfusion, are still not fully understood. The influence of age on uterine receptivity in humans is also not clear.

In animal studies it has been shown that the decline in fecundity is at least partly caused by age-related morphological and physiological changes of the uterus.[6,7] To investigate the effect of aging on the uterus, Sauer et al[8] studied 122 functionally agonadal women, aged 25–60, during a hormone replacement cycle leading to oocyte donation. Ultrasonography and endometrial biopsy, which were performed on day 21 of the cycle in this group of patients, showed no age-related difference in ultrasonographic appearance, endometrial histology, or the presence of estrogen or progesterone receptors. In a separate study, Guanes et al[9] investigated the age-related difference in uterine response to early pregnancy. They followed 21 patients who achieved a singleton pregnancy longitudinally after oocyte donation and found no difference in either hormone levels or uterine artery resistance when patients of different age groups were compared. These data suggest that the increase in miscarriage rate seen in older patients is not the result of decreased uterine perfusion. The best model for assessing the effect of age on uterine receptivity is to share oocytes from the same donor between recipients of different ages. This study model was used in two prospective[10,11] and two retrospective[12,13] studies. In a prospective study, Navot et al[10] found no difference in either the pregnancy rate or the miscarriage rate between younger and older patients. In a similar study, however, Cano et al[11] observed significantly higher pregnancy loss rates in a group of older patients. In a retrospective study, Borini et al[12] found reduced pregnancy rates in patients over the age of 40.

In another retrospective study, Abdalla et al[13] compared pairs of patients separated by at least 5 years of age receiving oocytes from the same donors. Cycles where there were comparable fertilization rates and embryo quality and in which a similar number of embryos were transferred were included in the analysis. Their findings suggested no difference in implantation, pregnancy, miscarriage or live-birth rates between younger and older patients.

Finally, in a recent review, Meldrum[14] reported a marked decrease in the live-birth rate in women aged over 40 years. However, when the progesterone dosage for luteal support was increased from 50–100 mg/day, recipients aged over 40 years had a marked increase in pregnancy rate when compared with younger patients. From the above, it appears that, unlike the quality of oocytes, which clearly declines with age, endometrial receptivity remains relatively constant, perhaps compromised only marginally by a delay in steroid synthesis. In practice, oocyte donation using oocytes from young donors, and possibly using hormone preparations with an increased dosage of progesterone, results in high pregnancy rates even in older patients.

An additional factor that plays an important role in implantation is embryo quality. Differentiation between these two factors is not always obvious in an individual patient. The role of uterine receptivity is likely to be more important in cases where excellent embryos are replaced, such as in young patients or in oocyte donation patients where the donor is young. Unfortunately, there are no universally accepted measures related to uterine receptivity. Recently a number of investigators have tried to correlate different histological, hormone and ultrasonic measures with uterine receptivity. Here we will make a critical assessment of some of these approaches.

## HISTOLOGICAL AND HORMONAL ASSESSMENT OF UTERINE RECEPTIVITY

The traditional method of assessing endometrial receptivity involves histological dating of the endometrium,[15] or quantification of the expression of endometrial proteins in response to circulating sex steroids. In addition, several groups have recently reported the potential value of assessing the endometrial epithelial surface by scanning electron microscopy (SEM). By using this technique they described apical protrusions, called pinopods, which were noted to develop and regress over a short period during the midluteal phase spanning days 4–7 after administration of human chorionic gonadotrophin (hCG).[16] Initial pinopod development begins in the region of the glandular orifices, with substantially fewer occurring outside this region. It is postulated that the appearance of pinopods marks the duration of the endometrial implantation window.

In a recent study investigating 40 patients undergoing oocyte donation, Reddy and colleagues[17] carried out endometrial biopsies in the pre-treatment assessment cycle. They reported an 83% pregnancy rate in patients who developed pinopods, and no pregnancies in patients who had no pinopods upon endometrial biopsy. This technique of predicting implantation may prove promising if confirmed by other studies. Unfortunately all the tests described above require endometrial biopsy. The potential disadvantage of removing a strip of endometrium to assess uterine receptivity in the same cycle in which embryo transfer is performed is evident. The biopsy may cause trauma and bleeding at the implantation site with a potential reduction in the chance of pregnancy. To avoid this problem, some centers advocate the performance of a mock replacement cycle, with a timed endometrial biopsy in frozen or egg donation cycles.[18] This, however, requires an additional preparatory cycle, which increases costs and is inconvenient to the patient.

Serum levels of reproductive hormones appear to be of relatively little value in predicting endometrial maturation, although there is a correlation between endometrial thickness and serum estrogen levels in both natural[19] and stimulated cycles.[20] Estrogen levels alone express the activity of granulosa cells and not the maturity of the endometrium. The latter probably depends upon estrogen receptor development, which is genetically coded for each individual and, therefore, similar levels of estrogen can initiate different levels of endometrial maturity in different individuals. This discrepancy has been shown in both natural[19] and assisted conception[21] cycles.

It is clear from this that histological and hormone assessment are not reliable predictors of endometrial status. Pinopod assessment, although promising, is expensive and experimental. It is therefore important to find alternative, non-invasive methods of assessing uterine receptivity. Turnbull et al[22] have demonstrated the potential value of magnetic resonance imaging (MRI) in distinguishing conceptional and non-conceptional cycles. However, as a result of its high cost, MRI is unlikely to be incorporated into routine infertility practice. In the last few years, ultrasonography has been proposed as an alternative tool in the assessment of endometrial receptivity. Here we review existing data concerning its value in predicting endometrial maturation, and the likelihood of conception.

## ULTRASONOGRAPHY

Two ultrasonographic techniques have been proposed for the assessment of endometrial receptivity, the assessment of endometrial appearance, and the assessment of endometrial vascularization by Doppler ultrasonography. To be of practical value, the results of any diagnostic test should be available, at the latest, on the day of hCG administration, allowing time for hormone manipulation, delay of embryo transfer, or preparation for embryo cryopreservation.

## Endometrial appearance

Two anatomical measures have been suggested for the evaluation of the endometrium by ultrasonography: endometrial thickness and endometrial pattern.

### Endometrial thickness

Endometrial thickness is defined as the maximal distance between the echogenic interfaces of the myometrium and the endometrium measured in the plane through the central longitudinal axis of the uterus (Figure 1). It is an easily measurable ultrasonic characteristic, and it represents a bioassay of the estrogenic activity. Endometrial thickness is unrelated to endometrial

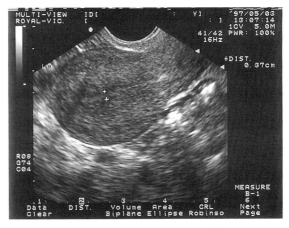

**Figure 1** Measurement of thin endometrium.

pattern.[23] In natural cycles, on the day of ovulation, the endometrium has been reported to be significantly thicker in conceptual cycles.[24] Dynamic changes in endometrial thickness in assisted conception cycles were first described by Rabinowicz et al.[21] In conception cycles, a rapid increase in endometrial thickness was noted from 11 days after embryo transfer (ET); reaching a significantly greater thickness than in non-conceptual cycles 17 days after ET. Using transvaginal ultrasonography, Gonen et al,[23] in a retrospective analysis, suggested that endometrial thickness, on the day before oocyte recovery, was significantly greater in the pregnant than in the non-pregnant woman, and postulated that it may predict the likelihood of implantation. However, Glissant et al,[24] Fleicher et al,[25] and Welker et al[26] found that measurement of endometrial thickness had no predictive value for pregnancy. Moreover, Li et al[27] reported no correlation between endometrial thickness, measured by abdominal ultrasonography, and histological dating of the endometrium.

In their study of endometrial thickness, Dickey et al[28] found an increased rate of early miscarriage in a group of patients with very thin (<6 mm) or thick endometrium (>13 mm). Krampel and Feichtinger,[29] however, found no correlation between endometrial thickness and the likelihood of miscarriage. Imoedemhe et al[30] compared the endometrial thickness in three groups of patients who were prescribed three different ovulation-induction regimens. They found that the endometrial thickness in all three groups of patients was similar and comparable to that observed in a group of spontaneously ovulating, fertile patients, despite significantly higher serum estradiol concentrations in all the hyperstimulated cycles. Their findings suggest that there is a maximum endometrial response, inducible by estrogen, which is virtually achieved in the normal menstrual cycle.

Recently, Freidler et al[31] reviewed 2665 assisted conception cycles from 25 reports. Eight reports found that the difference in the mean endometrial thickness of conception and non-conception cycles was statistically significant, whereas 17 reports found no significant difference. They concluded that the results from various trials are conflicting and that there are insufficient data to describe a linear correlation between endometrial thickness and the probability of conception. The main advantage of measuring endometrial thickness lies in its high negative predictive value in cases where there is minimal endometrial thickness. Gonen et al[32] reported an absence of pregnancies in donor insemination cycles where the endometrium did not reach at least 6 mm in cross-section.

Similarly, in a group of oocyte recipients, no pregnancies were reported in women who had an endometrial thickness of less than 5 mm in diameter, whereas several pregnancies occurred in patients with an endometrium thinner than 7.5 mm.[33] Finally, in IVF cycles, Kalifa et al[34] reported a minimal endometrial thickness of 7 mm to be compatible with pregnancy.

In summary, although a few studies suggest that there is a linear correlation between endometrial thickness and the prevalence of conception, in the context of assisted conception most reports do not support this. However, a very thin endometrium (<7 mm) (Figure 1) seems to be accepted as a reliable sign of suboptimal implantation potential.

### Endometrial pattern

Endometrial pattern is defined as the relative echogenicity of the endometrium and the adjacent myometrium, as demonstrated on a longitudinal ultrasonic scan. In principle, the central echogenic line represents the uterine cavity; the outer lines represent the basal layer of the endometrium, or the interface between the endometrium and myometrium. The relatively hypoechogenic regions between two outer lines and the central line may represent the functional layer of endometrium.[35] Classification of the types of endometrium have been simplified over time. The first classification proposed four patterns describing a gradual change from a fully echogenic endometrium (grade A) to a distinct echogenic black region surrounding the midline.[36] Nowadays, intermediate patterns are often discarded and the endometrium is simply described as multilayered, the so-called triple line appearance (Figure 2),

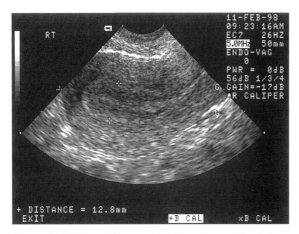

**Figure 2** Thick multilayered endometrium with triple line appearance.

or non-multilayered (Figure 3).[37] In a prospective study, Serafini et al[38] found the multilayered pattern to be more predictive of implantation than any other measure. Sher et al[37] correlated a non-multilayered echo pattern with advanced age and uterine abnormalities. In the literature, of 13 studies that examined the value of endometrial pattern in predicting pregnancy, only four failed to confirm its predictive value. It is, however, important to emphasize that a poor endometrial pattern does not exclude pregnancy. Many authors have demonstrated that pregnancies can occur in patients with a non-multilayered pattern of endometrium, albeit at a lower frequency.[28,38] The endometrial pattern does not appear to be influenced by the type of ovarian stimulation and it is of prognostic value in both fresh IVF and frozen ET cycles.

## DOPPLER ULTRASONOGRAPHY STUDIES OF UTERINE ARTERIES

### Uterine blood flow

Generally, blood flow studies have been confined to arteries. Doppler ultrasonography studies of the venous circulation provide no information about flow impedance and it is assumed that changes in venous circulation are a poor predictor of functional changes in organ perfusion.

Initial Doppler ultrasonography studies in assisted conception cycles were performed using the transabdominal approach. However, this approach requires the presence of a distended bladder which increases the distance between the Doppler probe and the vessels under investigation, so that low-pulse repetition frequencies, which are relatively inaccurate, have to be used. Another disadvantage of the abdominal approach is that the distended bladder may alter blood flow in the smaller arteries. Finally, patients can rarely tolerate an uncomfortably full bladder long enough for the Doppler ultrasonography study to be completed.[39] In contrast, vaginal ultrasonography obviates the need for a full bladder and the ultrasonic probe can be placed close to the vessel under investigation, so that the optimal pulse-repetition frequency can be chosen. Our group has investigated the accuracy of transvaginal and transabdominal Doppler assessment of uterine arteries in the subfertile population, and we have found the transvaginal assessment to be easier to perform and significantly more reproducible.[39]

With regard to the size of blood vessels, it is unlikely that blood flow in large vessels such as the external or internal iliac artery would have

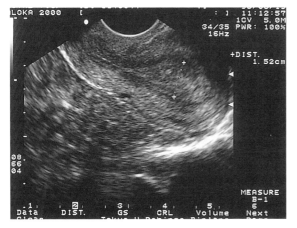

**Figure 3** Non-multilayered endometrium.

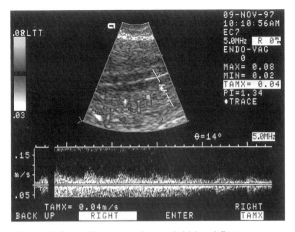

**Figure 4** Pulsatile subendometrial blood flow.

a significant effect on physiological changes during the implantation period and there have therefore been no attempts to investigate these vessels. So far the most commonly studied blood vessel in relation to implantation has been the uterine artery. However, with the development of power-Doppler ultrasonography, attention has been drawn to the importance of smaller uterine blood vessels, such as the subendometrial and arcuate arteries (Figure 4).[40] The graphic display of the temporal changes in Doppler frequency, which shifts across the full cross-section of the vessel throughout each cardiac cycle, is called the flow velocity waveform (FVW). The maximum outline, that is, the shape, of the FVW indicates the degree of resistance to flow in the artery under investigation. Absence of Doppler frequency shifts during the diastolic phase of the cycle is typically found in large arteries, for example, the external iliac artery, supplying high-resistance vascular beds. In contrast, high end-diastolic velocities are usually present in smaller arteries supplying organs such as the uterus and ovaries. The FVW is most easily quantified by calculating an index of resistance of impedance to blood flow. The indices most commonly used clinically are the resistance index (RI) and the pulsatility index (PI). Both indices are based on the ratio between the peak systolic and end-diastolic velocities, and they are both independent of the angle of insonation. This is important because FVW analysis can, therefore, be used for blood flow studies even in small arteries that are not clearly visualized, and which have an undefined angle of insonation. Of the various indices, we favor use of the PI because it has been demonstrated to correlate most closely with changes in blood flow volume[41] and can be used even when there is absence of diastolic velocities or reverse flow in the diastolic phase.

## Clinical application

Taylor et al[42] were the first to point out the possibility of investigating normal ovarian and uterine blood flow by means of Doppler ultrasonography. Its use for investigating implantation potential was suggested by Goswamy and Steptoe.[43] Using the transabdominal route, these authors examined, in the late luteal phase, 153 patients who had a history of three previous unsuccessful IVF attempts in spite of the transfer of good quality embryos. They reported a 55% incidence of poor perfusion, defined as an absence of end-diastolic flow, in this group of patients and postulated that suboptimal flow could possibly be an independent cause of infertility.

Steer et al[44] were the first to use transvaginal color Doppler ultrasonography to study the uterine arteries in infertility. Daily measurements of the PI of both uterine arteries were made in 23 normally cycling women. They noted that the lowest uterine artery PI was found 9 days after the luteinizing hormone (LH) peak, which is consistent with maximum uterine perfusion at the time of peak luteal function, and expected implantation. Steer et al[45] also showed that the uterine artery impedance was different in the midluteal phase in subfertile women compared with normal women. We used transvaginal color Doppler ultrasonography to study the uterine arterial

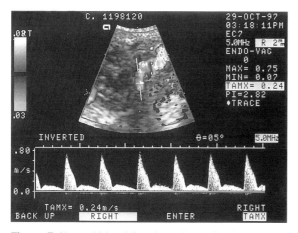

**Figure 5** Normal blood flow impedance in the uterine artery.

blood flow in 82 women undergoing IVF treatment on the day of embryo transfer.[46] The PI was calculated and the patients were grouped according to whether the PI was low (1–1.99), medium (2–2.99) (Figure 5) or high (3.0+) (Figure 6). There were no pregnancies in the high PI group and the PI was significantly lower in women who became pregnant, compared with those who did not. Moreover, we found a significant correlation between uterine blood flow indices and biochemical markers of uterine receptivity, including protein of molecular weight 24 kDa, uterine estradiol receptor, and endometrial histology dating.[47]

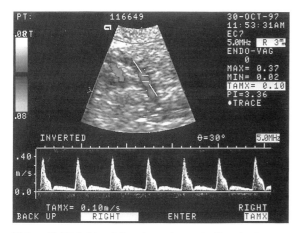

**Figure 6** High blood flow impedance in the uterine artery.

Similar findings have since been reported by others. Coulam et al[48] found that significantly more non-conception than conception cycles ($p < 0.001$) had a high uterine artery PI (> 3.3.). It was interesting that Tekay et al[49] were not able to confirm data reported by other groups. In their study, which included only 30 non-selected patients, the authors found no difference in uterine perfusion between pregnant and non-pregnant patients. This difference could be attributed to an inconsistency in patient preparation and timing of Doppler investigations. In an interesting study, Dickey et al[50] examined the influence of patient position on Doppler readings. The patients were first examined in the recumbent and subsequently in the upright position; after standing for 9–14 min, the uterine artery blood flow decreased by an average of 34% and RI increased by 70%. In addition, the number of cycles with absent end-diastolic flow increased. We have recently shown that the time of day at which Doppler measurements are made has a major impact on the results.[51,52] We found that blood flow in the uterine arteries follows a circadian rhythm, with the PI values being lowest during the early morning hours and increasing towards the evenings.[51,52] To obtain consistent and comparable data it is, therefore, important to allow patients to remain in a recumbent position and to perform investigations on all patients at about the same time of day.

Although blood flow impedance on the day of embryo transfer may be able to predict pregnancy, it would be more useful to detect flow abnormalities earlier in the cycle. To investigate this we recently measured uterine artery PI in 135 women undergoing IVF on the day of hCG injection.[53] We found significantly diminished implantation rates in women with a uterine artery PI of over 3.0. With regard to subendometrial blood flow, we found that the absence of pulsatile subendometrial blood flow on the day of hCG administration was an excellent prognostic value for the absence of pregnancy.[54] The ability to predict implantation before the administration of hCG allows the clinician the option to delay giving it until the uterine artery PI and subendometrial blood flow improve. An alternative approach would be to try to improve uterine perfusion by the administration of glyceryl trinitrate (GTN).

In a preliminary study Cacciatore et al[55] reported, in a group of patients with increased uterine artery PI, a 20% increase in uterine blood flow after the administration of GTN throughout the normal menstrual cycle. It has been suggested that the administration of GTN may increase pregnancy rates in women with poor uterine perfusion. However, no randomized studies have been carried out to address this issue. In a study investigating intrauterine circulation, Achiron et al[40] investigated subendometrial flow in 18 patients with premature ovarian failure (POF) and 12 healthy controls. They observed a decreased vascular impedence in the late follicular phase, with a gradual increase during an early and late luteal phase in both groups of patients. In the patients with POF, they observed a significantly higher vascular resistance in the early follicular phase. This difference disappeared after administration of hormone replacement therapy. These authors concluded that increased subendometrial blood flow resistance could be a sign of diminished implantation potential, and hormone replacement therapy enables normalization of subendometrial blood flow and creates a vascular status compatible with pregnancy.

## CONCLUSION

A better understanding of implantation is crucial for further improvement of success rates in assisted conception. Recent advances in ultrasonographic assessment of endometrium and blood flow, as well as histological evaluation of the endometrium, are helpful in identifying women who have suboptimal chances of implantation. The advent of three-dimensional ultrasonography in infertility research may also prove helpful in clinical studies of uterine receptivity.[56,57] Additional research is needed to investigate methods of improving endometrial receptivity and implantation rates in assisted conception treatment.

## REFERENCES

1. Tan SL, Maconochie N, Doyle P, et al. Cumulative conception and live-birth rates after in vitro fertilization with and without the use of long, short, and ultrashort regimens of the gonadotropin-releasing hormone agonist buserelin. *Am J Obstet Gynecol* 1994;**171**:513–20.
2. El Hussein E, Balen AH, Tan SL. A prospective study comparing the outcome of oocytes retrieved in the aspirate with those retrieved in the flush during transvaginal ultrasound directed oocyte recovery for in-vitro fertilization. *Br J Obstet Gynaecol* 1992;**99**:841–4.
3. Tan SL, Waterstone J, Wren M, Parsons J. A prospective randomized study comparing aspiration only with aspiration and flushing for transvaginal ultrasound-directed oocyte recovery. *Fertil Steril* 1992;**58**:356–60.
4. Biljan MM, Dean N, Bissonnette F, Hemmings R, Tan SL. Prospective randomized trial on effect of two flushing media on oocyte collection and fertilization rates following in vitro fertilization. *Fertil Steril* 1997;**68**:1132–4.
5. Tan SL, Royston P, Campbell S, et al. Cumulative conception and livebirth rates after in-vitro fertilisation. *Lancet* 1992;**339**:1390–4.
6. Harman SM, Talbert GB. Effect of maternal age on synchronization of ovulation and mating and on tubal transport of ova in mice. *J Gerontol* 1974;**29**:493–8.
7. Adams CE. Effects of maternal age on ovulation, fertilization and embryonic development. In: *Aging Gametes* (Blandau RJ, ed.). Basel: Karger, 1975;231–48.
8. Sauer MV, Miles RA, Dahmoush L, Paulson RJ, Press M, Moyer D. Evaluating the effect of age on endometrial responsiveness to hormone replacement therapy: a histologic ultrasonographic, and tissue receptor analysis. *J Assist Reprod* 1993;**10**:47–52.
9. Guanes PP, Remohi J, Gallardo E, Valbuena D,

Simon C, Pellicer A. Age does not affect uterine resistance to vascular flow in patients undergoing oocyte donation. *Fertil Steril* 1996;**66:**265–70.

10. Navot D, Drews MR, Bergh PA, et al. Age-related decline in female fertility is not due to diminished capacity of the uterus to sustain embryo implantation. *Fertil Steril* 1994;**61:**97–101.

11. Cano F, Simon C, Remohi J, Pellicer A. Effect of aging on the female reproductive system: evidence for a role of uterine senescence in the decline in female fecundity. *Fertil Steril* 1995;**64:**584–9.

12. Borini A, Bianchi L, Violini F, Maccolini A, Cattoli M, Flamigni C. Oocyte donation program: pregnancy and implantation rates in women of different ages sharing oocytes from single donor. *Fertil Steril* 1996;**65:**94–7.

13. Abdalla HI, Wren ME, Thomas A, Korea L. Age of the uterus does not affect pregnancy or implantation rates; a study of egg donation in women of different ages sharing oocytes from the same donor. *Hum Reprod* 1997;**12:**827–9.

14. Meldrum DR. Female reproductive aging-ovarian and uterine factors. *Fertil Steril* 1993;**59:**1–5.

15. Noyes RW, Hertig AT, Rock J. Dating the endometrial biopsy. *Fertil Steril* 1997;**1:**23.

16. Kolb BA, Najmabadi S, Paulson RJ. Ultrastructural characteristics of the luteal phase endometrium in patients undergoing controlled ovarian hyperstimulation. *Fertil Steril* 1997;**67:**625–30.

17. Reddy N, Ryder TA, Mobberley MA, Nikas G, Wiston RML. Positive correlation of pregnancy with the presence of endometrial pinopods in oocyte recipients: a preliminary study. *Hum Reprod* 1997;**12:**32(abstract).

18. Sauer MV, Paulson RJ, Moyer DL. Assessing the importance of endometrial biopsy prior to oocyte donation. *J Assist Reprod Genet* 1997;**14:**125–7.

19. Hackeloer BJ. Ultrasound scanning of the ovarian cycle. *J in vitro Fertil Embryo Transf* 1984;**1:**217–20.

20. Fleischer AC, Herbert CM, Hill GA, Kepple DM, Worrell JA. Transvaginal sonography of the endometrium during induced cycles. *J Ultrasound Med* 1991;**10:**93–5.

21. Rabinowitz R, Laufer N, Lewin A, et al. The value of ultrasonographic endometrial measurement in the prediction of pregnancy following in vitro fertilization. *Fertil Steril* 1986;**45:**824–8.

22. Turnbull LW, Rice CF, Horseman A, Robinson J, Killick SR. Magnetic resonance imaging and transvaginal ultrasound of the uterus prior to embryo transfer. *Hum Reprod* 1994;**9:**2438–43.

23. Gonen Y, Casper RF, Jacobson W, Blankier J. Endometrial thickness and growth during ovarian stimulation: a possible predictor of implantation in in vitro fertilization. *Fertil Steril* 1989;**52:**446–50.

24. Glissant A, de Mouzon J, Frydman R. Ultrasound study of the endometrium during in vitro fertilization cycles. *Fertil Steril* 1985;**44:**786–90.

25. Fleischer AC, Herbert CM, Sacks GA, Wentz AC, Entman SS, James AE Jr. Sonography of the endometrium during conception and nonconception cycles of in vitro fertilization and embryo transfer. *Fertil Steril* 1986;**46:**442–7.

26. Welker BG, Gembruch U, Diedrich K, al-Hasani S, Krebs D. Transvaginal sonography of the endometrium during ovum pickup in stimulated cycles for in vitro fertilization. *J Ultrasound Med* 1989;**8:**549–53.

27. Li TC, Nuttall L, Klentzeris L, Cooke ID. How well does ultrasonographic measurement of endometrial thickness predict the results of histological dating? *Hum Reprod* 1992;**7:**1–5.

28. Dickey RP, Olar TT, Curole DN, Taylor SN, Rye PH. Endometrial pattern and thickness associated with pregnancy outcome after assisted reproduction technologies. *Hum Reprod* 1992;**7:**418–21.

29. Krampl E, Feichtinger W. Endometrial thickness and echo patterns [letter; comment]. *Hum Reprod* 1993;**8:**1339.

30. Imoedemhe DA, Shaw RW, Kirkland A, Chan R. Ultrasound measurement of endometrial thickness on different ovarian stimulation regimens during in-vitro fertilization. *Hum Reprod* 1987;**2:**545–7.

31. Freidler S, Schenker JG, Herman A, Lewin A. The role of ultrasonography in the evaluation of endometrial receptivity following assisted reproductive treatments: a critical review. *Hum Reprod Update* 1996;**2:**323–35.

32. Gonen Y, Calderon M, Direnfeld M, Abramovici H. The impact of sonographic assessment of the endometrium and meticulous hormonal monitoring during natural cycle in patients with failed donor artificial insemination. *Ultrasound Obstet Gynecol* 1991;**1:**122–6.

33. Abdalla HI, Brooks AA, Johnson MR, Kirkland A, Thomas A, Studd JW. Endometrial thickness: a predictor of implantation in ovum recipients? *Hum Reprod* 1994;**9:**363–5.

34. Khalifa E, Brzyski RG, Oehninger S, Acosta AA, Muasher, SJ. Sonographic appearance of the endometrium: the predictive value for the outcome of in-vitro fertilization in stimulated cycles. *Hum Reprod* 1992;**7**:677–80.

35. Forrest TS, Elyaderani MK, Muilenburg MI, Bewtra C, Kable WT, Sullivan P. Cyclic endometrial changes: US assessment with histologic correlation. *Radiology* 1988;**167**:233–7.

36. Smith B, Porter R, Ahuja K, Craft I. Ultrasonic assessment of endometrial changes in stimulated cycles in an in vitro fertilization and embryo transfer program. *J in vitro Fertil Embryo Transf* 1984;**1**:233–8.

37. Sher G, Herbert C, Maassarani G, Jacobs MH. Assessment of the late proliferative phase endometrium by ultrasonography in patients undergoing in-vitro fertilization and embryo transfer (IVF/ET). *Hum Reprod* 1991;**6**:232–7.

38. Serafini P, Batzofin J, Nelson J, Olive D. Sonographic uterine predictors of pregnancy in women undergoing ovulation induction for assisted reproductive treatments. *Fertil Steril* 1994;**62**:815–22.

39. Steer CV, Williams J, Zaidi J, Campbell S, Tan SL. Intra-observer, interobserver, interultrasound transducer and intercycle variation in colour Doppler assessment of uterine artery impedance. *Hum Reprod* 1995;**10**:479–81.

40. Achiron R, Levran D, Sivan E, Lipitz S, Dor J, Mashiach S. Endometrial blood flow response hormone replacement therapy in women with premature ovarian failure: a transvaginal Doppler study. *Fertil Steril* 1995;**63**:550–4.

41. Tan SL, Zaidi J, Campbell S, Doyle P, Collins W. Blood flow changes in the ovarian and uterine arteries during the normal menstrual cycle. *Am J Obstet Gynecol* 1996;**175**:625–31.

42. Taylor KJ, Burns PN, Wells PN, Conway DI, Hull MG. Ultrasound Doppler flow studies of the ovarian and uterine arteries. *Br J Obstet Gynaecol* 1985;**92**:240–6.

43. Goswamy RK, Steptoe PC. Doppler ultrasound studies of the uterine artery in spontaneous ovarian cycles. *Hum Reprod* 1988;**3**:721–6.

44. Steer CV, Campbell S, Pampiglione JS, et al. Transvaginal colour flow imaging of the uterine arteries during the ovarian and menstrual cycles. *Hum Reprod* 1990;**5**:391–5.

45. Steer CV, Tan SL, Mason BA, Campbell S. Midluteal-phase vaginal color Doppler assessment of uterine artery impedance in a subfertile population. *Fertil Steril* 1994;**61**:53–8.

46. Steer CV, Campbell S, Tan SL, et al. The use of transvaginal color flow imaging after in vitro fertilization to identify optimum uterine conditions before embryo transfer. *Fertil Steril* 1992;**57**:372–6.

47. Steer CV, Tan SL, Dillon D, Mason BA, Campbell S. Vaginal color Doppler assessment of uterine artery impedance correlates with immunohistochemical markers of endometrial receptivity required for the implantation of an embryo. *Fertil Steril* 1995;**63**:101–8.

48. Coulam CB, Bustillo M, Soenksen DM, Britten S. Ultrasonographic predictors of implantation after assisted reproduction. *Fertil Steril* 1994;**62**:1004–10.

49. Tekay A, Martikainen H, Jouppila P. Blood flow changes in uterine and ovarian vasculature, and predictive value of transvaginal pulsed colour Doppler ultrasonography in an in-vitro fertilization programme. *Hum Reprod* 1995;**10**:688–93.

50. Dickey RP, Hower JF, Matulich EM, Brown GT. Effect of standing on non-pregnant uterine flow. *Ultrasound Obstet Gynecol* 1994;**4**:480–7.

51. Zaidi J, Jurkovic D, Campbell S, Okokon E, Tan SL. Circadian variation in uterine artery blood flow indices during the follicular phase of the menstrual cycle. *Ultrasound Obstet Gynecol* 1995;**5**:406–10.

52. Zaidi J, Jurkovic D, Campbell S, Pittrof R, McGregor A, Tan SL. Description of circadian rhythm in uterine artery blood flow during the peri-ovulatory period. *Hum Reprod* 1995;**10**:1642–6.

53. Zaidi J, Pittrof R, Shaker A, Kyei-Mensah A, Campbell S, Tan SL. Assessment of uterine artery blood flow on the day of human chorionic gonadotropin administration by transvaginal color Doppler ultrasound in an in vitro fertilization program. *Fertil Steril* 1996;**65**:377–81.

54. Zaidi J, Campbell S, Pittrof R, Tan SL. Endometrial thickness, morphology, vascular penetration and velocimetry in predicting implantation in an in vitro fertilization program. *Ultrasound Obstet Gynecol* 1995;**6**:191–8.

55. Cacciatore B, Tiitinen A, Ylikorkala O. Is it possible to improve uterine blood flow in infertile women? *Ultrasound Obstet Gynecol* 1996;**8**:204 (abstract).

56. Kyei-Mensah A, Maconochie N, Zaidi J, Pittrof R, Campbell S, Tan SL. Transvaginal three-dimensional ultrasound: reproducibility of ovarian and endometrial volume measurements. *Fertil Steril* 1996;**66**:718–22.

57. Kyei-Mensah A, Zaidi J, Pittrof R, Shaker A, Campbell S, Tan SL. Transvaginal three-dimensional ultrasound: accuracy of follicular volume measurements. *Fertil Steril* 1996;**65:** 371–6.

# Index

Abbreviations used in subheadings are: ET = Embryo transfer; FSH = Follicle-stimulating hormone; GnRH = Gonadotrophin releasing hormone; hCG = Human chorionic gonadotrophin; hMG = Human menopausal gonadotrophin; ICSI = Intracytoplasmic sperm injection; IUI = Intrauterine insemination; IVF = In vitro fertilization; IVM = In vitro maturation; LH = Luteinizing hormone; OHSS = Ovarian hyperstimulation syndrome; PCOS = Polycystic ovary syndrome; r-hFSH = Recombinant human FSH; r-hLH = Recombinant human LH; u-hFSH = Urine-derived human FSH; ZP = Zona pellucida